The Massachusetts Eye and Ear Infirmary Illustrated Manual of Ophthalmology

The Massachusetts Eye and Ear Infirmary Illustrated Manual of Ophthalmology

PETER K. KAISER, MD
Director, Clinical Research Center
Cole Eye Institute, The Cleveland Clinic Foundation
Cleveland, Ohio

NEIL J. FRIEDMAN, MD
Private Practice
Palo Alto, California;
Clinical Instructor, Department of Ophthalmology
Stanford University School of Medicine
Stanford, California

Associate author
Roberto Pineda II, MD
Assistant Professor of Ophthalmology
Harvard Medical School
Cornea and Refractive Surgery Service
Massachusetts Eye and Ear Infirmary
Boston, Massachusetts

SECOND EDITION

SAUNDERS
An Imprint of Elsevier

SAUNDERS
An Imprint of Elsevier

The Curtis Center
Independence Square West
Philadelphia, Pennsylvania 19106

THE MASSACHUSETTS EYE AND EAR INFIRMARY
ILLUSTRATED MANUAL OF OPHTHALMOLOGY

ISBN 0-7216-0140-5

NOTICE

Ophthalmology is an ever-changing field. Standard safety precautions must be followed, but as new research and clinical experience broaden our knowledge, changes in treatment and drug therapy may become necessary or appropriate. Readers are advised to check the most current product information provided by the manufacturer of each drug to be administered to verify the recommended dose, the method and duration of administration, and contraindications. It is the responsibility of the licensed prescriber, relying on experience and knowledge of the patient, to determine dosages and the best treatment for each individual patient. Neither the publisher nor the author assumes any liability for any injury and/or damage to persons or property arising from this publication.

Previous edition copyrighted 1998

International Standard Book Number 0-7216-0140-5

Acquisitions Editor: Natasha Andjelkovic
Developmental Editor: Heather Krehling
Publishing Services Manager: Patricia Tannian
Project Manager: John Casey
Book Design Manager: Gail Morey Hudson
Book and Cover Design: Jonel Sofian

Printed in China

Last digit is the print number: 9   8   7   6   5   4   3   2   1

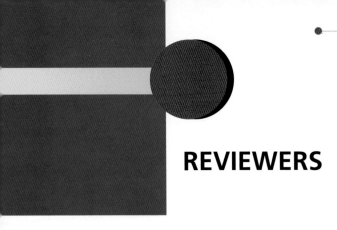

REVIEWERS

The contribution of the following colleagues, who have reviewed parts of this text, is greatly appreciated:

Michael Lee, MD, Careen Lowder, MD, Darius Moshfeghi, MD, Victor Perez, MD, Julian D. Perry, MD, Scott Smith, MD, Elias Traboulsi, MD, Michelle Young, MD, and Kang Zhang, MD
Cole Eye Institute
Cleveland Clinic Foundation
Cleveland, Ohio

Aaron Fay, MD, Mark Hatton, MD, and Shahzad Mian, MD
Massachusetts Eye and Ear Infirmary
Harvard Medical School
Boston, Massachusetts

Maria Braun, MD, Chris Engelman, MD, Anne Fung, MD, and Danny Lin, MD
Department of Ophthalmology
Stanford University School of Medicine
Stanford, California

Peter K. Kaiser, MD
Neil J. Friedman, MD
Roberto Pineda II, MD

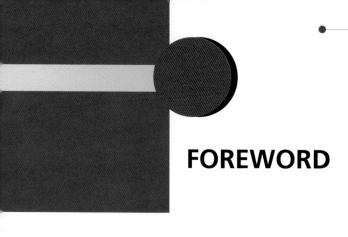

FOREWORD

"Omit needless words."
William Strunk, Jr.
The Elements of Style

This small, handsome manual provides a wealth of information for a broad spectrum of ophthalmic professionals. The task of writing a concise book for medical students, residents in ophthalmology, optometrists, ophthalmic technicians, and ophthalmologists requires special talents. Selecting the essential information and the appropriate illustrations is a process of elimination that requires a deep knowledge of the subject in order to separate the important from the trivial. The presentation of different disorders from definition and etiology to symptoms, signs, evaluation, and management involves critical judgment and very good writing. This becomes even more challenging when the goal is to present this information in an organized fashion so that it can be quickly reviewed in one to three pages. These achievements are obvious to the readers of the second edition of *The Massachusetts Eye and Ear Infirmary Illustrated Manual of Ophthalmology*. Drs. Kaiser, Friedman, and Pineda have succeeded admirably in their goal. The text is concise, well written, and easy to read. The book is beautifully illustrated with excellent photographs, most of them in color. The objective of the book is laudable, and the execution successful. This manual is a worthy addition to the library of anyone who has an interest in ophthalmology.

I feel proud that all the authors were associated with Harvard Medical School and that two of them were residents at The Massachusetts Eye and Ear Infirmary. The second edition of this book is a proof of its success, and I am sure that more will follow. It deserves to be a classic.

Evangelos S. Gragoudas, MD

Professor of Ophthalmology and Acting Chairman
Department of Ophthalmology
Harvard Medical School;
Director of Retina Service
The Massachusetts Eye and Ear Infirmary
Boston, Massachusetts

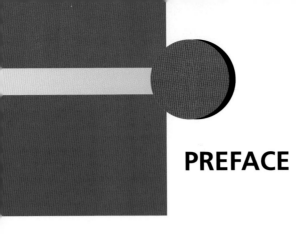

PREFACE

In the first edition of this book, our goal was to produce a concise manual that covered a broad variety of ophthalmic disorders and present it in a user-friendly diagnostic atlas. We were pleasantly surprised by the wide acceptance of the first edition, as well as by the positive comments it garnered.

In the 5 years since its publication, many areas of ophthalmology have undergone significant changes. We believe it is time for a second edition that expands on our original goal: to provide the practicing ophthalmologist, optometrist, fellow, resident, and medical student with an easy-to-read, comprehensive ophthalmology manual.

We have made a number of specific improvements to build on the strengths of the first edition. New diagnoses have been added throughout the book. We have added a plethora of new illustrations and improved the overall quality of current illustrations by increasing the number in color and adding arrows and lead lines to most figures to highlight specific details. To further enhance the illustrations, the descriptions in most figure legends have been expanded. All chapters have been updated with the latest diagnostic and therapeutic modalities, and many sections have been completely rewritten. Moreover, current residents, fellows, and staff physicians have added their particular expertise to improve various chapters throughout this edition. In the first edition, treatment options were intentionally left broad to guide readers in the management of the various disorders and not to serve as a therapeutic "bible." In this edition, we have expanded the treatment details for all diagnoses and have added more precise treatment parameters.

In this edition, we wanted to retain the ease of use of the first edition and have added features to make it even easier to navigate, including color-coding chapters and improving the index. Finally, additions to the appendix, including a history and examination primer, a new drug guide with drugs listed by classes and uses, and a suggested readings list have been incorporated into this edition.

We would like to thank the residents and fellows from the Cole Eye Institute, Stanford University Department of Ophthalmology, and the Massachusetts Eye and Ear Infirmary who have contributed greatly to the completion of this project. In addition, we thank the unnamed contributors from academic institutions around the world who have provided ideas to improve this edition. And, of course, a special thanks goes to our families, without whose support this project could never have been completed. We hope that readers will find this edition even more useful than the first.

Peter K. Kaiser, MD
Neil J. Friedman, MD
Roberto Pineda II, MD

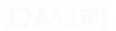

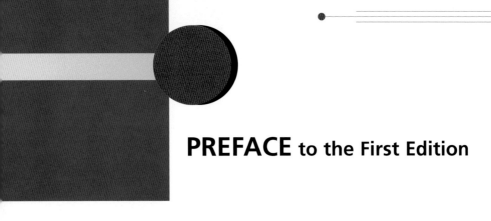

PREFACE to the First Edition

One of the special aspects of ophthalmology is its visual nature. Because most ocular pathology is directly visible, accurate diagnosis depends on careful examination of all ocular structures. Therefore, it is important for the examiner to be familiar with the symptoms and signs as well as the appearance of every disorder.

The purpose of this book is twofold: to present concise, useful information on a broad range of ophthalmic disorders, and to direct this information to a wide audience. Thus, we have created a user-friendly diagnostic atlas that also integrates essential therapeutic information. It is geared toward anyone who administers eye care regardless of training, including medical students, residents, primary care and emergency medicine physicians, ophthalmic technicians, optometrists, and ophthalmologists.

We have organized the book into sections corresponding to each ocular structure and the different aspects of a routine eye examination. For most disease processes, we provide the classic symptoms and signs and figures illustrating typical presentations. This allows the pertinent diagnostic information on any given disorder to be quickly and easily accessed without any previous ophthalmic training or knowledge of the entity. Moreover, once a disorder is identified, the epidemiology, work-up, treatment, and prognosis are available to guide its management.

To maintain this easy-to-use format and prevent the text from becoming too unwieldy, only a limited amount of information is presented for each diagnosis. Therefore, we have used an outline format to include all essential data for making a diagnosis and properly managing most common ophthalmic disorders. The summaries should not be considered definitive or exhaustive, which is beyond the scope of this book. Rather, this manual should be used as a diagnostic guide to aid the examiner in making the correct diagnosis as well as to help him or her learn about the disorder and formulate a treatment plan.

One additional word of caution regarding using this text solely as a therapeutic "bible," which is not our intent; rather, the treatment sections include typical strategies and favored options that we have been exposed to during our training. They are meant to be guidelines, not rigid orders. As in any speciality, management choices exist and often change with time; therefore, a certain degree of clinical judgement is necessary, and in difficult or uncertain cases other sources should be consulted. In addition, every effort was made to ensure that the drug selections and dosages were in accordance with current therapeutic guidelines; however, these recommendations are continually evolving. Therefore, we advise referring to the individual package inserts or the *Physicians' Desk Reference* for more specific information and warnings. We have also provided a list of some of the standard textbooks that contain more detailed coverage related to etiology, diagnosis, and management of these disorders.

We wish that a similar book existed during our training, and we hope that you will find it a useful addition to your library, white coat, or black bag.

Neil J. Friedman, MD
Roberto Pineda II, MD
Peter K. Kaiser, MD

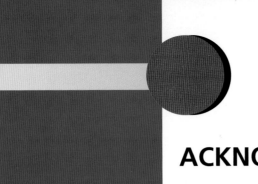

ACKNOWLEDGMENTS

As this work becomes more mature, the number of people who we must thank continually grows. We gratefully acknowledge the faculty, staff, fellows, residents, colleagues, and peers at our various training programs including the Bascom Palmer Eye Institute, the Cole Eye Institute, the Cullen Eye Institute, the Massachusetts Eye and Ear Infirmary, the New York Eye and Ear Infirmary, and Stanford University for their guidance, instruction, and support of this project at all stages of its development. We owe a special debt of gratitude to a number of individuals who helped review chapters and made invaluable comments and suggestions.

In addition, we would like to especially acknowledge the expert assistance of Tami Fecko, Nicole Drozda, Deborah Ross, Shawn Perry, Louise Carr-Holden, Ditte Hesse, Kit Johnson, Bob Masini, Audrey Melacan, and Jim Shigley, as well as the dedicated members of their photography departments for all the wonderful pictures without which this book would not be possible. We would also like to thank the many physicians who contributed photographs to complete the vast collection of ophthalmic disorders found in this manual.

Finally, we are indebted to our families, including Maureen, Peter (PJ), Stephanie, Peter, Anafu, Christine, Alan, Diane, Lisa, Roberto, Anne, Gabriela, Nicole, and Susannah, for their love, support, and encouragement during the course of this project.

Peter K. Kaiser, MD
Neil J. Friedman, MD
Roberto Pineda II, MD

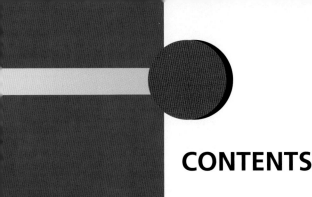

CONTENTS

Figure Courtesy Lines

The following illustrations are courtesy of the Cole Eye Institute:
1-2,1-3,1-5, 1-20, 1-23, 1-24, 1-25, 1-26, 3-2, 3-9, 3-12, 3-16, 3-19, 3-20, 3-32, 3-38, 3-40, 3-41, 3-47, 3-55, 4-6, 4-16, 4-20, 4-24, 4-26, 4-34, 4-38, 4-43, 4-48, 4-49, 4-60, 4-61, 5-1, 5-2, 5-15, 5-19, 5-29, 5-30, 5-33, 5-34, 5-42, 5-48, 5-51, 5-55, 5-73, 5-76, 5-77, 5-78, 5-79, 6-10, 6-11, 7-22, 7-35, 8-4, 8-8, 8-9, 8-10, 8-11, 8-21, 8-24, 9-2, 9-5, 10-2, 10-11, 10-13, 10-14, 10-15, 10-16, 10-17, 10-19, 10-21, 10-22, 10-24, 10-25, 10-29, 10-30, 10-31, 10-32, 10-36, 10-38, 10-40, 10-41, 10-42, 10-44, 10-47, 10-48, 10-49, 10-50, 10-55, 10-59, 10-60, 10-61, 10-62, 10-63, 10-64, 10-65, 10-66, 10-68, 10-70, 10-71, 10-74, 10-75, 10-76, 10-77, 10-78, 10-79, 10-83, 10-87, 10-91, 10-92, 10-95, 10-96, 10-97, 10-98, 10-99, 10-100, 10-102, 10-103, 10-104, 10-108, 10-114, 10-116, 10-117, 10-118, 10-120, 10-121, 10-122, 10-123, 10-124, 10-131, 10-132, 10-133, 10-139, 10-140, 10-141, 10-142, 10-143, 10-144, 10-147, 10-148, 10-149, 10-150, 10-151, 10-152, 10-153, 10-157, 10-161, 10-163, 10-164, 10-165, 10-166, 10-167, 10-168, 10-169, 10-174, 10-175, 10-176, 10-178, 10-179, 10-180, 10-184, 10-189, 10-197, 10-200, 10-201, 10-204, 10-212, 10-213, 10-214, 10-218, 11-2, 11-4, 11-10, 11-1, 11-12, 11-16, 11-18, 11-19, 11-20, 11-25, 12-3, 12-4, 12-7, 12-8, 12-10, 12-11, and 12-15

The following illustrations are courtesy of the Massachusetts Eye and Ear Infirmary:
1-1, 1-4, 1-6, 1-7, 1-8, 1-9, 1-10, 1-11, 1-12, 1-13, 1-14, 1-21, 1-27, 2-1, 2-2, 2-3, 2-6, 2-9, 2-10, 2-11, 2-14, 2-15, 2-16, 3-3, 3-6, 3-10, 3-11, 3-14, 3-17, 3-18, 3-21, 3-22, 3-24, 3-36, 3-37, 3-39, 3-48, 3-53, 3-54, 3-56, 4-2, 4-3, 4-4, 4-7, 4-8, 4-9, 4-11, 4-12, 4-13, 4-14, 4-15, 4-17, 4-19, 4-21, 4-22, 4-25, 4-27, 4-28, 4-30, 4-31, 4-32, 4-33, 4-37, 4-42, 4-44, 4-45, 4-50, 4-51, 4-53, 4-54, 4-55, 4-57, 5-3, 5-4, 5-10, 5-11, 5-12, 5-13, 5-14, 5-16, 5-17, 5-18, 5-21, 5-22, 5-23, 5-27, 5-28, 5-32, 5-35, 5-36, 5-40, 5-43, 5-46, 5-47, 5-50, 5-52, 5-59, 5-60, 5-61, 5-63, 5-66, 5-68, 5-70, 5-71, 5-72, 5-74, 6-1, 6-2, 6-3, 6-5, 6-12, 7-1, 7-2, 7-3, 7-6, 7-8, 7-11, 7-15, 7-18, 7-20, 7-21, 7-24, 7-27, 7-28, 7-29, 7-30, 7-31, 7-32, 7-33, 7-34, 7-36, 8-1, 8-3, 8-5, 8-7, 8-12, 8-13, 8-15, 8-16, 8-17, 8-18, 8-22, 8-23, 8-26, 8-35, 8-39, 8-40, 9-1, 9-3, 10-4, 10-20, 10-23, 10-37, 10-53, 10-56, 10-57, 10-58, 10-80, 10-84, 10-86, 10-88, 10-89, 10-90, 10-93, 10-101, 10-107, 10-115, 10-126, 10-127, 10-128, 10-129, 10-130, 10-134, 10-135, 10-138, 10-146, 10-156, 10-159, 10-173, 10-177, 10-186, 10-188, 10-190, 10-191, 10-193, 10-198, 10-202, 11-3, 11-5, 11-6, 11-8, 11-21, 11-23, 11-24, and 12-6.

The following illustrations are courtesy of the New York Eye and Ear Infirmary:
3-5, 3-13, 3-29, 3-34, 3-50, 4-10, 4-18, 4-29, 4-39, 4-40, 4-41, 4-47, 4-52, 4-56, 5-9, 5-37, 5-39, 5-41, 5-44, 5-45, 5-49, 5-75, 7-5, 7-7, 7-9, 7-17, 8-14, 8-25, 8-28, 8-31, 8-33, 8-38, 9-4, 9-7, 10-3, 10-7, 10-8, 10-9, 10-12, 10-18, 10-27, 10-43, 10-51, 10-67, 10-82, 10-113, 10-136, 10-137, 10-145, 10-156, 10-162, 10-172, 10-181, 10-182, 10-183, and 11-9.

The following illustrations are courtesy of the Bascom Palmer Eye Institute:
3-8, 4-1, 4-36, 4-46, 4-58, 5-5, 5-8, 5-20, 5-26, 5-31, 5-38, 5-53, 5-54, 5-58, 5-62, 5-64, 5-67, 6-7, 6-8, 6-9, 7-4, 7-10, 7-13, 7-14, 8-6, 8-19, 8-32, 8-34, 8-36, 9-6, 10-1, 10-5, 10-6, 10-10, 10-26, 10-28, 10-33, 10-34, 10-35, 10-39, 10-45, 10-46, 10-52, 10-54, 10-69, 10-72, 10-73, 10-81, 10-85, 10-94, 10-105, 10-106, 10-109, 10-110, 10-111, 10-112, 10-119, 10-125, 10-154, 10-155, 10-158, 10-160, 10-170, 10-171, 10-185, 10-187, 10-192, 10-194, 10-195, 10-196, 10-199, 10-203, 10-205, 10-206, 10-207, 10-208, 10-209, 10-210, 10-211, 10-215, 10-216, 10-217, 11-13, 11-15, and 11-17.

The following illustrations are courtesy of Warren Chang, MD: 2-7 and 2-8.

The following illustrations are courtesy of Cullen Eye Institute: 5-65 and 11-14.

The following illustrations are courtesy of Ronald L. Gross, MD: 5-57, 6-4, 6-6, 7-16, 7-19, 7-25, and 11-22.

The following illustrations are courtesy of M. Bowes Hamill, MD: 3-1, 4-5, 4-21, 4-23, 4-35, 4-59, 5-6, 5-7, 5-18, 5-69, 7-23, and 7-26.

The following illustrations are courtesy of Douglas D. Koch, MD: 5-24, 5-25, 5-56, 8-2, 8-20, 8-27, 8-28, 8-29, 8-30, 8-37, 12-5, 12-9, and 12-18.

The following illustrations are courtesy of Andrew G. Lee, MD: 2-12, 2-13, 2-17, 7-12, 11-1, and 11-7.

The following illustrations are courtesy of Peter S. Levin, MD: 1-17, 1-22, 3-7, 3-25, 3-33, 3-43, 3-49, 3-51, and 3-52.

The following illustration is courtesy of Thomas Loarie: 12-17.

The following illustrations are courtesy of Edward E. Manche, MD: 12-12, 12-13, 12-14, and 12-16.

The following illustrations are courtesy of James R. Patrinely, MD: 1-15, 1-18, 1-19, 3-4, 3-15, 3-23, 3-26, 3-27, 3-28, 3-30, 3-31, 3-35, 3-42, 3-44, 3-45, and 3-46.

The following illustrations are courtesy of Paul G. Steinkuller, MD: 1-16, 2-4, 2-5, and 12-1.

The following illustration is courtesy of Anneke Worst: 12-2.

The Massachusetts Eye and Ear Infirmary Illustrated Manual of Ophthalmology

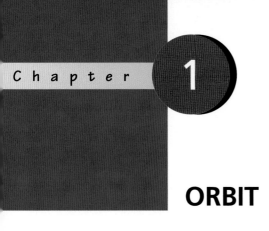

ORBIT

Trauma

Definition

Blunt or lacerating injury. Sequelae reflect mechanism and magnitude of injury.

Blunt Trauma

Orbital Contusion

Periocular bruising caused by blunt trauma; often with injury to the globe, paranasal sinuses, and bony socket; traumatic optic neuropathy or orbital hemorrhage may be present. Patients report pain and decreased vision. Signs include lid edema and ecchymosis, and ptosis. Isolated contusion is a preseptal (eyelid) injury and typically resolves without sequelae. Traumatic ptosis secondary to levator muscle contusion may take up to 3 months to resolve; however, most surgeons observe for 6 months prior to surgical repair.

- In the absence of orbital signs (afferent pupillary defect, visual field defect, limited extraocular motility, and proptosis) imaging studies are not required. Ominous mechanism of injury (e.g., motor vehicle accident [MVA], massive trauma, or loss of consciousness) is an indication for orbital computed tomography (CT), even in the absence of orbital signs.
- When the globe is intact and vision unaffected, use ice compresses every hour for 20 minutes during the first 48 hours to decrease swelling.
- Concomitant injuries should be treated accordingly.

Orbital Hemorrhage or Orbital Compartment Syndrome

Diffuse accumulation of blood throughout the intraorbital tissues due to surgery or trauma (retrobulbar hemorrhage). May cause proptosis, distortion of the globe, and optic nerve stretching and compression (orbital compartment syndrome). No discrete hematoma is formed; therefore, surgical evacuation is not possible. Patients report pain and decreased vision. Signs include bullous, subconjunctival hemorrhage, tense orbit, proptosis, resistance to retropulsion of globe, limitation of ocular movements, lid ecchymosis, and increased intraocular pressure. Immediate recognition and treatment is critical in determining outcome.

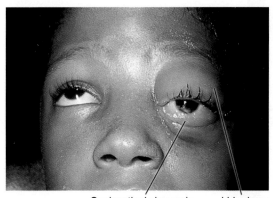

Figure 1-1 • Retrobulbar hemorrhage of the left eye demonstrating proptosis, lid swelling, chemosis, and restricted extraocular motility on upgaze.

Conjunctival chemosis   Lid edema

Ophthalmic Emergency

- If orbital compartment syndrome is suspected, lateral canthotomy and cantholysis should be performed emergently.
- Lateral canthotomy is performed by compressing the lateral canthus with a hemostat. Stevens scissors are then used to make a full-thickness incision from the lateral commissure (lateral angle of the eyelids) posterolaterally to the lateral orbital rim. The inferior crus of the lateral canthal tendon is then transected by elevating the lateral lower lid margin away from the face, placing the scissors between the cut edges of lower lid conjunctiva and lower lid skin, palpating the tendon with the tips of the scissors, and transecting it. If the inferior eyelid is not extremely mobile, the inferior crus has not been transected adequately and the procedure should be repeated. If the intraocular pressure remains elevated and the orbit remains tense, the superior crus of the lateral canthal tendon may be cut. However, this is an extremely rare occurrence and suggests an inadequate inferior cantholysis.
- Emergent inferior orbital floor fracture, while advocated by some, is fraught with complications and is not advised for surgeons with little experience in orbital surgery; however, it should be considered in emergent situations with risk of blindness.
- Canthoplasty can be scheduled electively approximately 1 week after the hemorrhage.
- Orbital CT scan (without contrast, direct coronal and axial views, 3-mm slices) once visual status has been determined and emergent treatment (if necessary) administered (i.e., after canthotomy and cantholysis). Magnetic resonance imaging (MRI) is *contraindicated* in acute trauma and is not the study of choice for orbital imaging.
- If vision is stable and intraocular pressure is elevated (>25 mm Hg), topical hypotensive agents may be administered (bromindione 0.15% [Alphagan P] 1 gtt tid, timolol 0.5% 1 gtt bid, and/or dorzolamide 2% [Trusopt] 1 gtt tid).

Orbital Fractures

Fracture of the orbital walls may occur in isolation (e.g., blow-out fracture) or with displaced or nondisplaced orbital rim fractures. There may be concomitant ocular, optic nerve, maxillary, mandibular, or intracranial injuries.

Orbital floor or blow-out fracture   Most common orbital fracture. Usually involves maxillary bone and posterior medial floor (weakest point), but may extend laterally to the infraorbital canal. Orbital contents may prolapse or become entrapped in maxillary sinus. Signs and symptoms include diplopia on upgaze (anterior fracture) or downgaze (posterior fracture), enophthalmos, globe ptosis, and infraorbital nerve hypesthesia. Orbital and lid emphysema tend to develop 24-48 hours later when patient blows his nose.

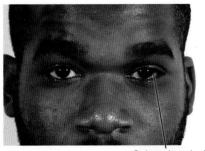

Subconjunctival
hemorrhage

Orbital floor fracture
with entrapment

Figure 1-2 • Orbital floor blow-out fracture with enophthalmos and globe dystopia and ptosis of the left eye.

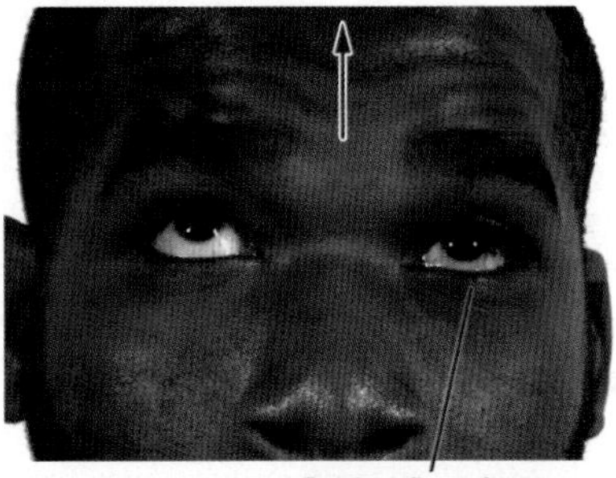

Figure 1-3 • Same patient as Figure 1-2 demonstrating entrapment of the left inferior rectus and inability to look up.

- Orbital CT need not be obtained in the absence of orbital signs.
- Surgery, when indicated, typically is delayed 1 week to allow for reduction of swelling.

Pediatric floor fractures differ significantly from adult fractures because the bones are pliable rather than brittle. A "trap door" phenomenon is created where the inferior rectus muscle or perimuscular tissue can be entrapped in the fracture site. In this case, enophthalmos is unlikely, but supraduction is limited dramatically, halting abruptly on upgaze as if it is "tethered." Nausea is common, and the eye is typically quiet.

- Urgent surgery is indicated (<24 hours) in pediatric cases with entrapment.

Medial wall or nasoethmoidal fracture   Involves lamina papyracea, lacrimal, and maxillary bones. Occasionally associated with depressed nasal fracture, traumatic telecanthus (in severe cases), and orbital floor fracture. Complications include nasolacrimal duct injury, severe epistaxis due to anterior ethmoidal artery damage, and orbit and lid emphysema. Medial rectus entrapment is rare, but enophthalmos due to medial rectus herniation is not uncommon. Patients should anticipate persistent tearing due to nasolacrimal duct obstruction.

- May require dacryocystorhinostomy after 6 months.

Orbital roof   Uncommon fracture usually secondary to blunt or projectile injuries. May involve frontal sinus, cribriform plate, and brain. May have cerebrospinal fluid (CSF) rhinorrhea or pneumocephalus.

* Neurosurgery and otolaryngology consultations are advised, especially in the presence of CSF rhinorrhea or pneumocephalus.

Orbital apex   May be associated with other facial fractures and involve optic canal and superior orbital fissure. Direct traumatic optic neuropathy likely. Complications include carotid-cavernous fistula and fragments impinging on optic nerve. Difficult to manage owing to proximity of multiple cranial nerves and vessels.

* Treatment of traumatic optic neuropathy is controversial but may include surgery or high-dose systemic steroids or both (see Chapter 11).

Zygomatic or tripod fracture   Involves three or more fracture sites, including the inferior orbital rim (maxilla), zygomaticofrontal suture (superotemporal orbital rim), and zygomatic arch. The fracture invariably extends through the orbit floor. The defect may not be appreciated at the time of the injury but becomes evident following anterior distraction of the impacted zygoma. Patients report pain, tenderness, binocular diplopia, and trismus (pain on opening mouth or chewing). Signs include orbital rim discontinuity or palpable "step off," malar flattening, enophthalmos, infraorbital nerve hypesthesia, orbital, conjunctival, or lid emphysema, limitation of ocular movements, epistaxis, rhinorrhea, ecchymosis, and ptosis. Enophthalmos may not be appreciated on exophthalmometry due to retrodisplaced lateral orbital rim.

Maxillary fractures have been further classified by Le Fort:

Le Fort I   low transverse maxillary bone; no orbital involvement.

Le Fort II   nasal, lacrimal, and maxillary bones (medial orbital wall); may involve nasolacrimal duct.

Le Fort III   orbital floor, lateral and medial wall (craniofacial dysjunction); may involve optic canal.

* Orbital CT (without contrast, direct axial and coronal views, 3-mm slices) is indicated in the presence of orbital signs (afferent papillary defect, diplopia, limited extraocular motility, proptosis, and enophthalmos) or ominous mechanism of injury (e.g., MVA, massive facial trauma). MRI is *contraindicated* in acute trauma and does not highlight fractures as well as CT.
* Otolaryngology consultation is indicated in the presence of CSF rhinorrhea or displaced nasal fracture. Nondisplaced nasal fracture can be referred to otolaryngology for outpatient treatment.
* Oral surgery consultation is indicated in the presence of mandibular fracture.
* Orbital surgery consultation is indicated in the presence of isolated orbital and trimalar fractures.
* Obvious impingement by a bone fragment on the optic nerve may require immediate surgical intervention by an oculoplastic surgeon or neurosurgeon. High-dose systemic steroids may be given for traumatic optic neuropathy (see Chapter 11).
* Instruct patient to avoid blowing nose. "Suck-and-spit" technique should be used to clear nasal secretions.
* Nasal decongestant (oxymetazoline hydrochloride [Afrin nasal spray] bid for 10 days; *Note:* may cause urinary retention in men with prostatic hypertrophy).

- Ice compresses for first 48 hours.
- Systemic oral antibiotics (amoxicillin-clavulanate [Augmentin] 250-500 mg po tid for 10 days) are advocated by some but may be avoided in minor cases.
- Orbital surgery consultation should be considered especially in the setting of diplopia, large floor fractures that are prone to enophthalmos, trismus, facial asymmetry, inferior rectus entrapment, and enophthalmos. Consider surgical repair after 1 week except in cases of entrapment causing oculocardiac reflex where emergent repair is advocated.
- Nondisplaced zygomatic fractures may become displaced after initial evaluation due to masseter and temporalis contraction. Orbital or otolaryngology consultation is indicated for evaluation of open reduction and internal fixation.

Penetrating Trauma

May result from either projectile (e.g., pellet gun) or stab (e.g., knife, tree branch) injury. Foreign body should be suspected even in the absence of significant external wounds.

Optic Nerve Avulsion

Typically results from stab-type injury, although optic nerve can be severed by bullets or other projectiles. Entry at the lateral commissure, where globe exposure is greatest, is most common. Globe may be entirely subluxed. Symptoms include no light perception vision and strong afferent pupillary defect in an otherwise quiet eye. Orbital CT demonstrates transection of optic nerve. Retrobulbar avulsion may produce intraocular hemorrhage. Extraocular muscle dysfunction is usually evident, but does not necessarily indicate direct injury to the muscles.

Intraorbital Foreign Body

Retained orbital foreign body (FB) with or without associated ocular and optic nerve involvement. Inert FB (e.g., glass, lead, BB, plastics) may be well tolerated, and should be evaluated by orbital surgeon in a controlled setting. Organic matter carries significant risk of infection and should be removed surgically. Long-standing iron FB can produce iron toxicity (siderosis) including retinopathy.

Patients may be asymptomatic or may report pain or decreased vision. Critical signs include eyelid or conjunctival laceration. Other signs may include ecchymosis, lid edema and erythema, conjunctival hemorrhage or chemosis, proptosis, and limitation of ocular movements.

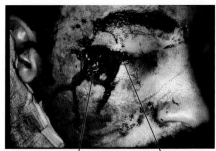

Avulsion of globe   Optic nerve

Figure 1-4 • Traumatic avulsion of the globe. The entire globe is extruded from the orbit but still attached to the optic nerve.

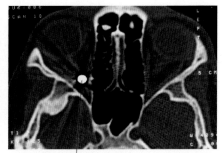

Intraorbital foreign body

Figure 1-5 • Orbital CT demonstrating intraorbital foreign body.

A positive relative afferent pupillary defect (RAPD) may be present. Prognosis is generally good if the globe and optic nerve are not affected.

- Precise history (may be necessary to isolate a minor child from the parents while obtaining history) is critical in determining the nature of any potential FB.
- Orbital CT (without contrast, direct coronal and axial views, 1.5-mm to 3-mm slices depending on suspected FB) to determine character and position of foreign body. MRI is *contraindicated*.
- **Lab tests:** Culture entry wound for bacteria and fungus.
- If there is no ocular or optic nerve injury, small inert and posterior foreign bodies usually are not removed but observed.
- Patients are placed on systemic oral antibiotics (amoxicillin-clavulanate [Augmentin] 500 mg po tid for 10 days) and are followed up the next day.
- Tetanus booster (tetanus toxoid 0.5mL IM) if necessary for prophylaxis (>10 years since last tetanus shot or if status is unknown).

Indications for surgical removal include fistula formation, infection, optic nerve compression, intolerable foreign body, large foreign body, or easily removable foreign body (usually anterior to the equator of the globe). Should be performed by an orbital plastic surgeon. Organic material is removed more urgently.

■ Carotid-Cavernous Fistula

Spontaneous high-flow fistula formation between the cavernous sinus and internal carotid artery (carotid-cavernous fistula). Occurs in patients with atherosclerosis and hypertension or secondary to closed head trauma (basal skull fracture). Patients often hear a "swishing" noise (venous souffle). Signs may include orbital bruit, pulsating proptosis, chemosis, epibulbar injection and vascular tortuosity (conjunctival corkscrew vessels), congested retinal vessels, and increased intraocular pressure.

Alternatively, small meningeal arterial branches may cause low-flow fistula formation with the dural walls of the cavernous sinus (dural sinus fistula). Slower onset compared with the carotid-cavernous variant with only mild proptosis and orbital congestion. Up to 70% of dural sinus fistulas may resolve spontaneously.

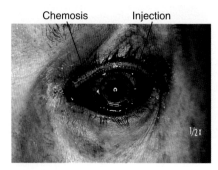

Figure 1-6 • Carotid-cavernous fistula with conjunctival injection and chemosis.

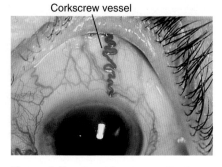

Figure 1-7 • Carotid-cavernous fistula with dilated, corkscrew, episcleral, and conjunctival vessels.

Differential Diagnosis

Orbital varices that expand in a dependent position or during Valsalva maneuvers and may produce hemorrhage with minimal trauma.

* Orbital CT or MRI: enlargement of superior ophthalmic vein.
* Arteriography usually is required to identify the fistula.
* Consider periodic compression of ipsilateral internal carotid artery in neck (use contralateral hand).

Consider treatment with selective embolization or ligation for severely symptomatic patients (uncontrolled increase in intraocular pressure, severe proptosis, retinal ischemia, optic neuropathy, severe bruit, involvement of the cortical veins). Treatment for all cases of carotid-cavernous fistula has been advocated but is controversial.

■ Infections

Preseptal Cellulitis

Definition

Infection and inflammation located anterior to the orbital septum and limited to the superficial periorbital tissues and eyelids. The globe and orbit are not involved.

Etiology

Usually follows periorbital trauma or dermal infection. Suspect *Staphylococcus aureus* in traumatic cases. *Haemophilus influenzae* in children less than 5 years old is uncommon now that they receive *H. influenzae* vaccination.

Symptoms

Eyelid swelling, redness, ptosis, and pain; low-grade fever.

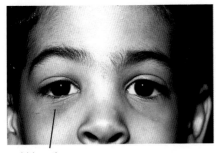

Lid erythema

Figure 1-8 • Mild preseptal cellulitis with right eyelid erythema in a young child.

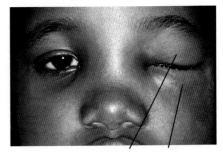

Lid edema   Erythema

Figure 1-9 • Moderate preseptal cellulitis with left eyelid edema and erythema.

Signs

Eyelid erythema, edema, ptosis, and warmth (may be quite dramatic); visual acuity is normal when lid is elevated; full ocular motility without pain; no proptosis; the conjunctiva and sclera appear uninflamed; an inconspicuous lid wound may be visible.

Differential Diagnosis

Orbital cellulitis, idiopathic orbital inflammation, eyelid abscess, dacryoadenitis, dacryocystitis, conjunctivitis, trauma, rhabdomyosarcoma (children).

Evaluation

- Complete ophthalmic history with attention to trauma, sinus disease, recent dental work or infections, history of diabetes or immunosuppression.
- Complete eye examination with attention to acuity, color vision, pupils, motility, exophthalmometry, lids, conjunctiva, and sclera.
- Check vital signs, head and neck lymph nodes, meningeal signs (nuchal rigidity), and sensorium.
- Orbital and sinus CT scan in the absence of trauma or in the presence of orbital signs: paranasal sinus opacification.
- **Lab tests**: Complete blood count (CBC) with differential, blood cultures; wound culture if appropriate.

Management

MILD PRESEPTAL CELLULITIS

- Systemic oral antibiotics:
  Amoxicillin-clavulanate [Augmentin] 250-500 mg po tid *or*
  Cefaclor [Ceclor] 250-500 mg po tid *or*
  Trimethoprim-sulfamethoxazole [Bactrim] 1 double-strength tablet po bid, in penicillin-allergic patients.
- Warm compresses tid.
- Topical antibiotics (bacitracin or erythromycin ointment qid) for concurrent conjunctivitis.
- Consider surgical drainage of abscess (avoid orbital septum and levator aponeurosis).

MODERATE TO SEVERE PRESEPTAL CELLULITIS

- Systemic intravenous antibiotics:
  Cefuroxime 1 g IV q8h *or*
  Ampicillin-sulbactam [Unasyn] 1.5-3.0 g IV q6h.
- Systemic intravenous treatment also indicated for septic patients, outpatient noncompliant patients, children less than 5 years old, and patients who fail oral antibiotic treatment after 48 hours.
- Daily follow-up in all cases until improvement noted.

Prognosis

Usually good when treated early.

Orbital Cellulitis

Definition

Infection and inflammation within the orbital cavity producing orbital signs and symptoms. May also involve the eyelids.

Etiology

Most commonly secondary to ethmoid sinusitis. May also result from frontal, maxillary, or sphenoid infection. Other causes include dacryocystitis, dental caries, intracranial infections, trauma, and orbital surgery. *Streptococcus* and *Staphylococcus* species are most common isolates. *Haemophilus influenzae* is uncommon in children under 5 years old now that they receive *H. influenzae* vaccination. Fungi in the group *Phycomycetes* (*Absidia*, *Mucor*, or *Rhizopus*) are the most common causes of fungal orbital infection causing necrosis, vascular thrombosis, and orbital invasion. Fungal infections usually seen in patients with diabetes mellitus, metabolic acidosis, malignancy, or immunosuppression; and can be fatal due to spread along ophthalmic artery to cranium.

Symptoms

Decreased vision, pain, red eye, headache, diplopia, "bulging" eye, lid swelling, and fever.

Signs

Decreased visual acuity, fever, lid edema, erythema, and tenderness; limitation of or painful ocular movements, proptosis, positive relative afferent pupillary defect, conjunctival injection and chemosis; there may be optic disc swelling; fungal infection usually manifests with proptosis and orbital apex syndrome (see Chapter 2). Cranial nerve (CN) V signs suggest orbital apex/cavernous sinus involvement.

Lid edema/erythema

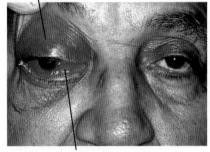
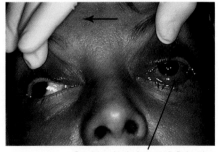

Conjunctival chemosis/injection

Conjunctival chemosis/injection

Figure 1-10 • Orbital cellulitis with right-sided proptosis, lid edema and erythema, conjunctival injection and chemosis, and right exotropia (note decentered right corneal light reflex at the limbus).

Figure 1-11 • Mucormycosis of the left orbit with eyelid edema, conjunctival injection, chemosis, and gaze restriction.

Differential Diagnosis

Thyroid ophthalmopathy (adults), idiopathic orbital inflammation, subperiosteal abscess, orbital tumors, lacrimal gland tumors, orbital vasculitis, trauma, carotid-cavernous fistula, cavernous sinus thrombosis, cranial nerve palsy.

Evaluation

- Complete ophthalmic history with attention to trauma, sinus disease, recent dental work or infections, history of diabetes or immunosuppression.
- Complete eye examination with attention to acuity, color vision, pupils, motility, exophthalmometry, conjunctiva, cornea (including corneal sensitivity), CN V sensation, and ophthalmoscopy.
- Check vital signs, head and neck lymph nodes, meningeal signs (nuchal rigidity), and sensorium.
- CT scan of orbits and paranasal sinuses (with contrast, direct coronal and axial views, 3-mm slices): look for sinus opacification or abscess.
- **Lab tests**: CBC with differential, blood cultures (results usually negative in phycomycosis); wound culture, if present.

Management

- Systemic intravenous antibiotics (1-week course):
    Nafcillin 1-2 g IV q4h and ceftriaxone 1-2 g IV q12-24h *or*
    Ampicillin-sulbactam (Unasyn) 1.5-3.0 g IV q6h.
- Topical antibiotics (bacitracin or erythromycin ointment qid) for conjunctivitis or corneal exposure.
- Daily follow-up required to monitor visual acuity, color vision (red desaturation), ocular movements, proptosis, intraocular pressure, cornea, and optic nerve.
- Systemic oral antibiotics (10-day course) after improvement on intravenous therapy:
    Amoxicillin-clavulanate (Augmentin) 250-500 mg po tid *or*
    Cefaclor (Ceclor) 250-500 mg po tid *or*
    Trimethoprim-sulfamethoxazole (Bactrim) 1 double-strength tablet po bid
    in penicillin-allergic patients.
- Subperiosteal abscess requires urgent referral to orbital surgeon for systemic oral antibiotics (see above) and close observation, or surgical drainage.
- Otolaryngology consultation is indicated to obtain tissue diagnosis for opacified sinuses and if phycomycosis suspected.
- Diabetic or immunocompromised patients are at high risk for phycomycosis (mucormycosis). Given the very high mortality rate, emergent debridement and biopsy, systemic intravenous antifungal medications (amphotericin B 0.25-1.0 mg/kg IV divided equally q6h), and management of underlying medical disorders.

Prognosis

Depends on organism and extent of inflammation. May develop orbital apex syndrome, cavernous sinus thrombosis, or meningitis, which produce permanent neurologic deficits. Mucormycosis is potentially fatal.

Inflammation

Thyroid-Related Ophthalmopathy

Definition

An immune-mediated disorder linked to the thyroid gland that causes a spectrum of ocular abnormalities. Also called *dysthyroid orbitopathy* or *ophthalmopathy*, and *Graves' ophthalmopathy* (inappropriate).

Epidemiology

Most common cause of unilateral or bilateral proptosis in adults; female predilection (8:1); 80% of patients have abnormal thyroid function test results; hyperthyroidism (particularly Graves' disease) is most common, although patients may be hypothyroid or euthyroid (25%); associated with myasthenia gravis.

Symptoms

Note: Signs and symptoms reflect four clinical components of this disease process as follows: eyelid disorders, eye surface disorders, ocular motility disorders, and optic neuropathy.

Usually asymptomatic. May have red eye, foreign body sensation, tearing, decreased vision, dyschromatopsia, diplopia, prominent ("bulging") eyes, or retracted eyelids.

Signs

Eyelid retraction, edema, lagophthalmos, lid lag (von Graefe's sign), reduced blinking, superficial keratopathy, conjunctival injection, exophthalmos, limitation of extraocular movements (supraduction most common), resistance to retropulsion of globe, decreased visual acuity and color vision, positive RAPD, and visual field defect. A minority of cases may have acute congestion of the socket and periocular tissues.

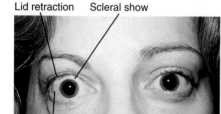

Lid retraction   Scleral show

Proptosis

Figure 1-12 • Thyroid ophthalmopathy with proptosis, lid retraction, and superior and inferior scleral show of the right eye.

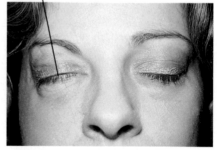

Lagophthalmos

Figure 1-13 • Same patient as shown in Figure 1-12, demonstrating lagophthalmos on the right side with eyelid closure (note the small incomplete closure of the right eyelids).

Differential Diagnosis

Idiopathic orbital inflammation, orbital and lacrimal gland tumors, orbital vasculitis, trauma, cellulitis, arteriovenous fistula, cavernous sinus thrombosis, gaze palsy, aberrant regeneration of CN III, physiologic exophthalmos.

Evaluation

- Complete medical history, with attention to history of thyroid disease, autoimmune disease, or cancer; history of hyperthyroid symptoms such as heat intolerance, weight loss, palpitations, sweating, irritability.
- Complete eye examination, with attention to cranial nerves, acuity, color vision, pupils, motility, forced ductions, eyelid position, Hertel exophthalmometry, cornea, tonometry, and ophthalmoscopy.
- Obtain automated visual field test for baseline study in early cases and to rule out optic neuropathy in advanced cases.
- **Lab tests:** Thyroid function tests (thyroid stimulating hormone [TSH], thyroxine [total and free T4], and triiodothyronine [T3]).
- **Orbital CT scan** (with contrast, direct coronal and axial views, 3-mm slices): extraocular muscle enlargement with sparing of the tendons; inferior rectus is most commonly involved, followed by medial, superior, and lateral. Isolated lateral rectus involvement suggests another diagnosis.
- Endocrinology consultation.

Management

- Irreversible interventions are deferred until a 6-month stable interval is recorded, except in cases of optic neuropathy or extreme proptosis causing severe exposure keratopathy with corneal ulceration.
- Surgical reconstruction after a 6-month quiescent interval proceeds in stepwise fashion, moving posteriorly to anteriorly: orbital bony decompression, strabismus surgery, then eyelid reconstruction as indicated.
- Underlying thyroid disease should be managed by endocrinologist, but may not alter the acute orbital process.

EXPOSURE

- Topical lubrication with artificial tears (see Appendix) up to q1h while awake and ointment (Refresh P.M.) at bedtime.
- Consider lid taping or humidifying goggles at bedtime.
- Punctal occlusion for more severe dry eye symptoms.
- Permanent lateral tarsorrhaphy or canthorrhaphy useful in cases of lateral chemosis or widened lateral palpebral fissure.

EYELID RETRACTION

- Surgical eyelid recession (lengthening) after a 6-month stable interval.

Management—cont'd

DIPLOPIA

- Systemic steroids (prednisone 80-100 mg po qd for 1-2 weeks, then taper over 1 month) for acute diplopia and congestive orbitopathy; not as effective for restrictive myopathy, lid retraction, or proptosis.
- Fresnel (temporary) prisms to glasses.
- Strabismus surgery (rectus muscle recessions) considered after a 6-month stable interval and after orbital surgery completed.

OPTIC NEUROPATHY

- Immediate treatment with systemic steroids (prednisone 100 mg po qd for 2-14 days); some reports recommend external beam irradiation (15-30 Gy).
- Orbital decompression for compressive optic neuropathy via either Caldwell-Luc (greater access to posterior orbit) or transcutaneous/transconjunctival approach; should be performed by orbital surgeon.

Prognosis

Generally good. May require multiple surgeries if extensive orbital involvement exists.

Idiopathic Orbital Inflammation or Orbital Pseudotumor

Definition

Acute or chronic idiopathic inflammatory disorder of the orbital tissues sometimes collectively termed *orbital pseudotumor*. Any of the orbital tissues may be involved: lacrimal gland (dacryoadenitis), extraocular muscles (myositis), sclera (scleritis), optic nerve sheath (optic perineuritis), orbital fat; Tolosa-Hunt syndrome is a form of idiopathic orbital inflammation involving the orbital apex and/or anterior cavernous sinus that produces painful external ophthalmoplegia.

Epidemiology

Occurs in all age groups; usually unilateral, although bilateral disease is more common in children; adults require evaluation for systemic vasculitis (e.g., Wegener's granulomatosis, polyarteritis nodosa) or lymphoproliferative disorders.

Symptoms

Acute onset of orbital pain, decreased vision, binocular diplopia, red eye, headaches, and constitutional symptoms. (Constitutional symptoms including fever, nausea, and vomiting are present in 50% of children with idiopathic orbital inflammation.)

Signs

Marked tenderness of involved region, lid edema and erythema, lacrimal gland enlargement, limitation of and pain on extraocular movements (myositis), proptosis, decreased orbital retropulsion, induced hyperopia, conjunctival chemosis, reduced corneal sensation (due to CN VI involvement), increased intraocular pressure; papillitis or iritis may occur in children.

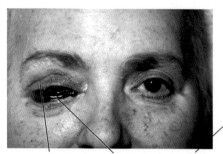   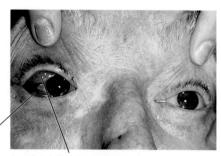

Lid erythema   Conjunctival chemosis   Lacrimal gland enlargement

Figure 1-14 • Idiopathic orbital inflammation of the right orbit with lid edema, ptosis, and chemosis.

Figure 1-15 • Idiopathic orbital inflammation of the right orbit with lacrimal gland involvement. Note the swollen, prolapsed, lacrimal gland superiorly.

Differential Diagnosis

Thyroid-related ophthalmopathy, orbital cellulitis, orbital tumors, lacrimal gland tumors, orbital vasculitis, trauma, cavernous sinus thrombosis, cranial nerve palsy, herpes zoster ophthalmicus.

Evaluation

- Complete ophthalmic history, with attention to previous episodes and history of cancer or other systemic disease.
- Complete eye examination, with attention to eyelid and orbital palpation, pupils, motility, exophthalmometry, lids, cornea, tonometry, and ophthalmoscopy.
- **Lab tests** for bilateral or unusual cases (vasculitis suspected): CBC with differential, erythrocyte sedimentation rate (ESR), antinuclear antibodies (ANA), blood urea nitrogen (BUN), creatinine, fasting blood glucose, antineutrophil cytoplasmic antibodies (ANCA), and urinalysis.
- **Orbital CT scan:** thickened, enhancing sclera (ring sign), extraocular muscle enlargement with involvement of the tendons, or lacrimal gland involvement, diffuse inflammation with streaking of orbital fat.
- Consider orbital biopsy for steroid-unresponsive or unusual cases.

Management

- Systemic steroids (prednisone 80-100 mg po qd for 1 week, then taper slowly over 6 weeks); check purified protein derivative (PPD) reaction, blood glucose, and chest radiographs before starting systemic steroids.
- Add H_2-blocker (ranitidine HCl [Zantac] 150 mg po bid) or proton pump inhibitor when giving systemic steroids.
- Topical steroid (prednisolone acetate 1% up to q2h initially, then taper over 3-4 weeks) if iritis present.
- Patients should respond dramatically to systemic corticosteroids within 24-48 hours. Failure to do so strongly suggests another diagnosis.
- Orbital decompression rarely is indicated and considered only in the presence of compressive optic neuropathy.

Prognosis

Generally good for acute disease, although recurrences are common. The sclerosing form of this disorder has a more insidious onset and is often less responsive to treatment.

Congenital Anomalies

Usually seen with developmental syndromes, rarely in isolation.

Congenital Anophthalmia

Absence of globe with normal-appearing eyelids; extraocular muscles are present and insert abnormally into orbital soft tissue Extremely rare condition that produces a hypoplastic orbit that becomes accentuated with contralateral hemifacial maturation. Usually bilateral and sporadic. Characteristic "purse stringing" of the orbital rim. Orbital CT, ultrasonography, and examination under anesthesia are required to make the diagnosis.

Microphthalmos (small, malformed eye) and nanophthalmos (small eye with normal structures) are more common than true anophthalmos; present similar orbital challenges. True anophthalmia and severe microphthalmia can be differentiated only on histologic examination.

* Treatment is aimed at progressive orbital expansion for facial symmetry and includes serial orbital implants requiring multiple orbitotomies over the first several years of life, expandable orbital implants, and serial conjunctival conformers. Avoid enucleation in cases of microphthalmos.
* Reconstructive surgery can be undertaken after the first decade of life.

Infantile Enucleation

More common condition that mimics congenital anophthalmia. Age of orbital maturation is not known, but elective enucleation should be deferred in early childhood. Enucleation before the age of 9 years may produce significant orbital asymmetry (radiographically estimated deficiency up to 15%), while enucleation after 9 years leads to no appreciable asymmetry.

Craniofacial Disorders

Midfacial clefting syndromes can involve the medial superior or medial inferior orbit (sometimes with meningoencephalocele) and can produce hypertelorism (increased bony expanse between the medial walls of the orbit). Hypertelorism is also seen in craniostenoses such as Crouzon's syndrome (craniofacial dysostosis) and Apert's syndrome (arachno-encephalodactyly) in which there is premature closure of cranial sutures. Exorbitism and lateral canthal dystopia are also seen in these syndromes.

* Craniofacial surgery by experienced orbital plastic surgeon.

Pediatric Orbital Tumors

Benign Pediatric Orbital Tumors

Orbital dermoid or dermoid cyst   Common, benign, palpable, smooth, painless choristoma composed of connective tissue and containing dermal adnexal structures including sebaceous glands and hair follicles. Most common pediatric orbital tumor. Usually manifests in childhood (90% in first decade of life) and may enlarge slowly. Most common location is superotemporal at the zygomaticofrontal suture, leading to downward globe displacement. Symptoms include ptosis, proptosis, and diplopia. There may be components external or internal to the orbit, or both ("dumbbell" dermoid).

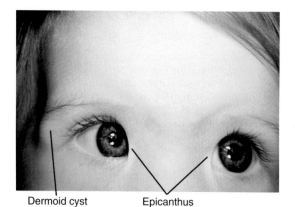

Figure 1-16 • Dermoid cyst of the right orbit appearing as a mass at the lateral orbital rim. Also note the epicanthus causing pseudostrabismus.

Dermoid cyst   Epicanthus

- **Orbital CT scan** (with contrast, direct coronal and axial views, 3-mm slices): well circumscribed, cystic mass with bony molding.
- Complete surgical excision should be performed by an oculoplastic surgeon in cases of amblyopia and intractable diplopia; preserve capsule and avoid rupturing cyst to prevent acute inflammatory process.

Lymphangioma

No-flow malformations misnamed *lymphangioma*. Benign, nonpigmented choristoma characterized by lymphatic fluid–filled spaces lined by flattened endothelial cells; vascular channels do not contain red blood cells; patients do not produce true lymphatic vessels. May appear blue through the skin. Commonly associated with head and neck components. Becomes apparent during the first decade of life with an infiltrative growth pattern or with abrupt onset due to hemorrhage within the tumor ("chocolate cyst"). May enlarge during upper respiratory tract infections (reactive lymphoid hyperplasia). Strabismus and amblyopia are common complications. Slow, relentless progression is common; may regress spontaneously.

- CT scan of orbit, paranasal sinuses, and pharynx with contrast: nonencapsulated, irregular mass with cystic spaces; infiltrative growth pattern.
- Complete surgical excision is impossible. Limited excision indicated for ocular damage or severe cosmetic deformities; should be performed by an oculoplastic surgeon. Children should undergo pediatric otolaryngologic examination to rule out airway compromise.

Orbital needle aspiration of hemorrhage ("chocolate cysts") or surgical exploration for acute orbital hemorrhage with compressive optic neuropathy; tumor recurrence common.

Juvenile Xanthogranuloma

Nevoxanthoendothelioma, composed of histiocytes and Touton giant cells, that rarely involves the orbit. Appears between birth and 1 year of age. Associated with yellow-orange cutaneous lesions, and may cause destruction of bone. Spontaneous resolution often occurs.

- No treatment recommended because of frequent spontaneous regression.
- Consider local steroid injection (controversial).
- Surgical excision rarely indicated.

Malignant Pediatric Orbital Tumors

Rhabdomyosarcoma

Most common primary pediatric orbital malignancy and most common pediatric soft tissue malignancy; mean age 7-8 years; 90% of cases occur in patients under 15 years old; male predilection (5:3). Presents with rapid onset, progressive, unilateral proptosis, eyelid edema, and discoloration. Epistaxis, sinusitis, and headaches indicate sinus involvement. History of trauma may be misleading. Predilection for superonasal orbit. CT scan commonly demonstrates bony orbital destruction. Arises from primitive mesenchyme, not extraocular muscles. Urgent biopsy necessary for diagnosis. Four histologic forms:

Embryonal   Most common (70%); cross striations seen in 50% of cells.

Alveolar   Most malignant, worst prognosis, inferior orbit, second most common (20-30%); few cross-striations seen.

Botryoid   Grapelike, originates within paranasal sinuses or conjunctiva; rare.

Pleomorphic   Rarest (<10%), most differentiated, seen in older patients, best prognosis; 90-95% 5-year survival rate if limited to orbit; cross-striations in most cells.

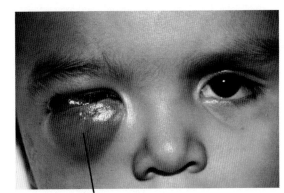

Figure 1-17 • Rhabdomyo-sarcoma of the right orbit with marked lower eyelid edema, discoloration, and chemosis.

Eyelid edema/discoloration

- Emergent diagnostic biopsy with immunohistochemical staining in all cases. Should be coordinated with pediatric oncologist.
- Pediatric oncology consultation for systemic evaluation including abdominal and thoracic CT, bone marrow biopsy, and lumbar puncture.

- Current modes of treatment involve combinations of surgery, systemic chemotherapy, and radiotherapy.

Neuroblastoma

Most common pediatric orbital metastatic tumor (second most common orbital tumor behind rhabdomyosarcoma). Occurs in children during first decade of life. Usually arises from a primary tumor in the abdomen (adrenals in 50%), mediastinum, or neck from undifferentiated embryonic cells of neural crest origin. Patients typically have sudden proptosis with eyelid ecchymosis ("raccoon eyes") that may be bilateral. Associated with lateral orbital wall destruction and displacement of the globe. Prognosis is poor.

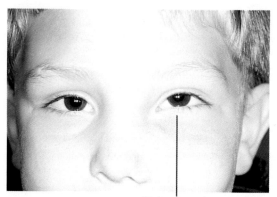

Figure 1-18 • Neuroblastoma of the left orbit with resulting globe dystopia.

Globe dystopia

- Orbital CT: poorly defined mass with bony erosion (usually lateral wall).
- Pediatric oncology consultation for systemic evaluation.
- Treatment is with local radiotherapy and systemic chemotherapy.

Leukemia

Advanced leukemia, particularly the acute lymphocytic type, may appear with proptosis; granulocytic sarcoma (chloroma), an uncommon subtype of myelogenous leukemia, may also produce orbital proptosis, often prior to hematogenous or bone marrow signs; both forms usually occur during first decade.

- Pediatric oncology consultation.
- Treatment is with systemic chemotherapy.

Adult Orbital Tumors

Benign Adult Orbital Tumors

Cavernous Hemangioma

This misnamed tumor is a vascular hamartoma and the most common adult orbital tumor. Probably present from birth, but typically appears during the fourth to sixth decades. One of the four periocular tumors that are more common in females (meningioma, sebaceous carcinoma, and choroidal osteoma). Patients usually have painless, decreased visual acuity or diplopia. Signs include slowly progressive proptosis and compressive optic neuropathy. May have induced hyperopia, strabismus, increased intraocular pressure, and chorioretinal folds due to posterior pressure on the globe. May enlarge during pregnancy.

* **Orbital CT scan** (in cases of suspected tumor, CT scans are ordered with contrast): well-circumscribed intraconal or extraconal lesion; no bony erosion; adjacent structures may be displaced, but are not invaded or destroyed.
* **Orbital MRI:** tumor appears hypointense on T1-weighted images and hyperintense on T2-weighted images with heterogenous internal signal density.
* **A-scan ultrasonography:** high internal reflectivity.
* Complete surgical excision (usually requires lateral orbitotomy with bone removal) indicated for severe corneal exposure, compressive optic neuropathy, intractable diplopia, or exophthalmos; should be performed by an orbital plastic surgeon.

Mucocele

Cystic sinus mass due to obstructed excretory ducts, lined by pseudostratified ciliated columnar epithelium and filled with mucoid material. May invade the orbit wall through bony erosion. Patients usually have a history of chronic sinusitis (frontal and ethmoidal sinuses). Associated with cystic fibrosis; usually seen in the superonasal orbit; must be differentiated from encephalocele and meningocele.

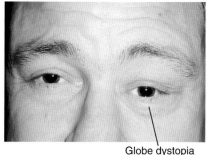
Globe dystopia

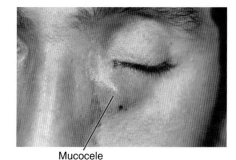
Mucocele

Figure 1-19 • Mucocele of the orbit with left globe dystopia.

Figure 1-20 • Mucocele of the left eye.

* Head and orbital CT scan: orbital lesion and orbital wall defect with sinus opacification.
* Complete surgical excision should be performed by an orbital or otolaryngology plastic surgeon. May require obliteration of frontal sinus; add preoperative and postoperative systemic antibiotics (ampicillin-sulbactam [Unasyn] 1.5-3.0 g IV q6h).

Neurilemoma or Schwannoma

Rare, benign tumor (1% of all orbital tumors) that occurs in young to middle-aged individuals. Patients have gradual, painless proptosis and globe displacement. May be associated with neurofibromatosis type 1. One of two truly encapsulated orbital tumors. Histologic examination demonstrates two patterns of Schwann cell proliferation enveloped by perineurium: Antoni A (solid, nuclear palisading, Verocay bodies) and Antoni B (loose, myxoid areas).

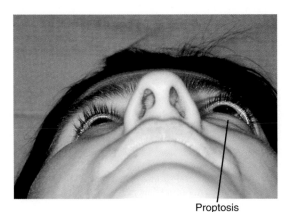

Figure 1-21 • Neurilemoma (Schwannoma) producing proptosis of the left eye.

Proptosis

- **Orbital CT scan:** well-circumscribed lesion; virtually indistinguishable from "cavernous hemangioma"; may have cystic areas.
- **A-scan ultrasonography:** low internal reflectivity.
- Complete surgical excision should be performed by an orbital plastic surgeon; recurrence and malignant transformation are rare.

Meningioma

Symptoms relate to specific location, but proptosis, globe displacement, diplopia, and optic neuropathy are common manifestations. Median age at diagnosis is 38 years with female predilection (3:1). See Chapter 11 for complete discussion.

Primary orbital meningioma   Typically arises from the optic nerve (see Chapter 11).

Sphenoid meningioma   Usually arises intracranially with expansion into the orbit.

- Surgical treatment is deferred, because complete excision usually involves injury or transection of the optic nerve.

Histiocytic Tumors

Initially designated *Histiocytosis X,* the Langerhans' cell histiocytoses comprise a spectrum of related granulomatous diseases seen most frequently in children ages 1-4 years. Immuno-histochemical staining and electron microscopy reveals atypical (Langerhans') histiocytes with characteristic Birbeck's (cytoplasmic) granules.

Hand-Schüller-Christian disease   Chronic, recurrent form. Classic triad of proptosis, lytic skull lesions, and diabetes insipidus.

- Systemic glucocorticoids and chemotherapy.

Letterer-Siwe disease   Acute, systemic form. Occurs during infancy with hepatosplen-omegaly, thrombocytopenia, and fever, and with very poor prognosis for survival.

- Systemic glucocorticoids and chemotherapy.

Eosinophilic granuloma, localized Form   Most likely to involve the orbit. Bony lesion with soft tissue involvement that typically produces proptosis and more often is located in the superior orbit as a result of frontal bone disease.

• Local incision and curettage, intralesional steroid injection, or radiotherapy.

Fibrous Histiocytoma

Most common mesenchymal orbital tumor, but extremely rare. Firm, well-defined lesion that is usually located in the superonasal quadrant. Occurs in middle-aged adults. Less than 10% have metastatic potential. Histologically, cells have a cartwheel or storiform pattern.

• Complete surgical excision should be performed by an orbital plastic surgeon; recurrence is often more aggressive, with possible malignant transformation.

Fibro-Osseous Tumors

Fibrous dysplasia   Nonmalignant, painless, bony proliferation often involving single (monostotic) or multiple (polyostotic) facial and orbital bones, seen in Albright's syndrome. Most appear during first decade of life, with rapid growth during puberty and little growth during adulthood. Most patients will have pathologic long bone fractures.

• Orbital radiographs: diffuse bony sclerosis with ground glass appearance, radiolucent lesions, thickened occiput.

Osteoma   Rare, slow-growing, benign bony tumor frequently involving frontal and ethmoid sinuses. Causes globe displacement away from tumor.

• **Orbital CT scan:** well-circumscribed lesion with calcifications.
• Osteoma usually can be excised completely if visual function threatened or intracranial extension; surgical intervention in other lesions is usually palliative and clinical cure almost impossible.
• Should be evaluated by orbital plastic surgeon; otolaryngology consultation may be required.

Cholesterol granuloma   Idiopathic hemorrhagic lesion of orbital frontal bone, usually occurring in males. Causes proptosis, blurred vision, diplopia, and a palpable mass. Surgical excision is curative.

• **Orbital CT scan:** Well-defined superotemporal mass with bony erosion.

Aneurysmal Bone Cyst   Idiopathic, osteolytic, expansile mass typically found in long bones of the extremities or less commonly in the superior orbit. Occurs during adolescence. Intralesional hemorrhage produces proptosis, diplopia, and cranial nerve palsies.

• **Orbital CT scan:** Well-defined soft tissue mass with bony lysis.

Malignant Adult Orbital Tumors

Lymphoid Tumors

Lymphoid infiltrates account for 10% of orbital tumors. The noninflammatory orbital lymphoid infiltrates are classified as reactive lymphoid hyperplasia and malignant lymphoma.

Often clinically indistinguishable, the diagnosis is made by microscopic morphology and immunophenotyping. Most common in patients 50-70 years old; extremely rare in children; more common in women than in men (3:2). Patients have painless proptosis, diplopia, decreased visual acuity (induced hyperopia), or a combination of these symptoms. Lesions may be intraconal, extraconal, or both. Fifty percent of patients with orbital lymphoma eventually develop systemic involvement; risk of systemic disease is lower in cases of mucosa-associated lymphoid tissue (MALT) lymphomas. Radiation adequately controls local disease in nearly 100% of cases. Systemic disease treated with radiation to the orbit and systemic chemotherapy. Good prognosis with 90% 5-year survival.

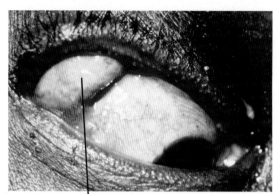

Figure 1-22 • Lacrimal gland enlargement due to reactive lymphoid hyperplasia.

Lacrimal gland enlargement

- **Orbital CT scan:** unencapsulated solid tumor that molds to surrounding structures; bony changes are usually absent.
- Tissue biopsy and immunohistochemical studies on fresh (not preserved) specimens required for diagnosis.
- Reactive infiltrates demonstrate follicular hyperplasia without a clonal population of cells.
- Lymphoma is diagnosed in the presence of monoclonality, or sufficient cytologic and architectural atypia; nearly always extranodal B-cell non-Hodgkin's lymphomas; greater than 50% are MALT-type lymphomas.
- Multiclonal infiltrates not fulfilling the criteria to be diagnosed as lymphoma may progress to malignant lymphoma.

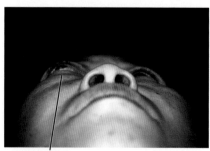

Proptosis

Figure 1-23 • Right proptosis from orbital tumor.

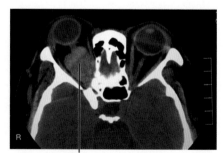

Orbital tumor

Figure 1-24 • Orbital CT of same patient as Figure 1-23 demonstrating the orbital tumor.

- Systemic evaluation by internist or oncologist in the presence of biopsy-proven orbital lymphoma: includes thoracic, abdominal, and pelvic CT scan, CBC with differential, serum protein electrophoresis, erythrocyte sedimentation rate, bone marrow biopsy, and possibly bone scan.
- Low-dose, fractionated radiotherapy for localized orbital lesions (15-20 Gy for benign lesions; 20-30 Gy for malignancy) and chemotherapy with or without adjunctive ocular radiotherapy for systemic disease.

Fibro-Osseous Tumors

Chondrosarcoma   Usually occurs after age 20 with slight female predilection; often bilateral with temporal globe displacement. Intracranial extension is often fatal.

- **Orbital CT scan:** irregular lesion with bony erosion.

Osteosarcoma   Common primary bony malignancy; usually occurs before age 20.

- **Orbital CT scan:** lytic lesion with calcifications.

Metastatic Tumors

Metastases account for 10% of all orbital tumors but are the most common orbital malignancy. Most common primary sources are breast, lung (bronchogenic), prostate, and gastrointestinal tract. Symptoms include rapid-onset, painful proptosis, limitation of extraocular movements, and diplopia. Visual acuity may be normal. CT demonstrates bony erosion and destruction of adjacent structures. Scirrhous breast cancer characteristically causes enophthalmos from orbital fibrosis.

- Local radiotherapy for palliation should be performed by a radiation oncologist experienced in orbital processes.
- Carcinoid may be treated with wide orbital excision.
- Hematology and oncology consultation.

▇ Acquired Anophthalmia

Common condition resulting from enucleation or evisceration of the globe; more common in men than women; initial complaints include copious mucopurulent discharge, pain greater in one direction of eye movement, or serosanguinous tears; pain is qualitatively different from preenucleation pain; signs may include inflamed conjunctiva, dehiscence or erosion of conjunctiva with exposure of implant, blepharitis, or cellulitis.

- Eyelids should be observed for cellulitis, ptosis, or retraction.
- Superior tarsal conjunctiva must be examined for giant papillae (see Chapter 4).
- In the absence of conjunctival defect or lesion, treat with broad-spectrum antibiotic drops (gentamicin or polymyxin B sulfate [Polytrim] 1 gtt qid).
- If conjunctival defect is observed, refer to orbital surgeon for evaluation. Treatment may include removal of avascular portion of porous implant, secondary implant, dermis fat graft placement, or other techniques.

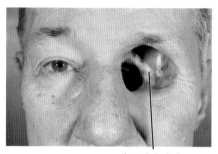

Anophthalmia

Figure 1-25 • Acquired anophthalmia of the left eye secondary to evisceration for orbital tumor.

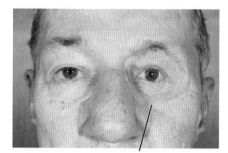

Prosthesis

Figure 1-26 • Same patient as Figure 1-25 with prosthesis in place.

- Exposed implant is at risk for orbital cellulitis and should be treated with systemic oral antibiotics, surgically, or both (see above).
  Cephalexin 250-500 mg po qid or
  Amoxicillin-clavulanate [Augmentin] 250-500 mg po tid.
- Orbital prosthesis should be replaced with orbital conformer during period of infection. If conjunctival defect is present, the prosthesis must be reconstructed by ocularist postoperatively while conformer is used for 1 month.
- Socket should not be left without prosthesis or conformer for longer than 24 hours (controversial) due to conjunctival cicatrization, forniceal foreshortening, and socket contracture.

Atrophia Bulbi and Phthisis Bulbi

Progressive functional ocular decompensation, after either accidental or surgical trauma, the end stage of which is called *phthisis bulbi*. Three stages exist.

Atrophia Bulbi Without Shrinkage

Globe shape and size are normal, but with cataract, retinal detachment, synechiae, or cyclitic membranes.

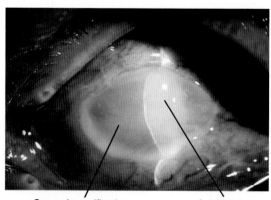

Figure 1-27 • Phthisis bulbi demonstrating shrunken globe. The cornea is opaque, edematous, and thickened, and the anterior chamber is shallow.

Corneal opacification   Calcification

Atrophia Bulbi With Shrinkage

Soft and smaller globe with decreased intraocular pressure; collapse of the anterior chamber; edematous cornea with vascularization, fibrosis, and opacification.

Atrophia Bulbi With Disorganization or Phthisis Bulbi

Globe approximately two thirds normal size with thickened sclera, intraocular disorganization, and calcification of cornea, lens, and retina; spontaneous hemorrhages or inflammation can occur, and bone may be present in the uveal tract. These eyes usually have no vision, and they carry an increased risk of intraocular malignancies.

* B-scan ultrasonography should be performed annually to rule out intraocular malignancies.
* Blind, painful eyes are first treated with topical steroid (prednisolone acetate 1% qid) and a cycloplegic agent (atropine 1% tid). Consider retrobulbar alcohol or chlorpromazine (Thorazine) injection for severe ocular pain.
* Cosmetic shell can be created by an ocularist and is worn over the phthisical eye to improve appearance and support the eyelid.
* Enucleation typically relieves pain permanently and can improve cosmesis in many cases.
* Modern enucleation techniques involve porous orbital implants with extraocular muscles attached, allowing for natural-appearing movement of the prosthesis.

2

Chapter

OCULAR MOTILITY AND CRANIAL NERVES

▓ Strabismus

Definition

Ocular misalignment that may be idiopathic or acquired; horizontal or vertical; comitant (same angle of deviation in all positions of gaze) or incomitant (angle of deviation varies in different positions of gaze [paralytic or restrictive causes]); latent, manifest, or intermittent.

Phoria   Latent deviation.

Tropia   Manifest deviation.

Esotropia   Inward deviation.

Exotropia   Outward deviation.

Hypertropia   Upward deviation.

Hypotropia   Downward deviation (vertical deviations usually are designated by the hypertropic eye, but if the process clearly is causing one eye to turn downward, this eye is designated *hypotropic*).

Etiology

See below for full description of the various types of strabismus (horizontal, vertical, miscellaneous forms). See also cranial nerve palsy, chronic progressive external ophthalmoplegia (CPEO), and myasthenia gravis.

Hypertropia

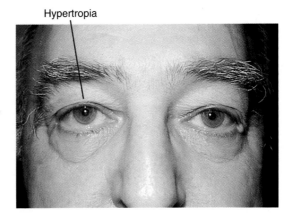

Figure 2-1 • Hypertropia of the right eye.

Symptoms

Asymptomatic; may have eye turn, head turn, head tilt, decreased vision, diplopia (in older children and adults), headaches, asthenopia, and eye fatigue.

Signs

Normal or decreased visual acuity (amblyopia), strabismus, limitation of ocular movements, reduced stereopsis; may have other ocular pathology (i.e., cataract, aphakia, retinal detachment, optic atrophy, macular scar, phthisis) causing a secondary sensory strabismus (usually esotropia in children <5 years old, exotropia in older children and adults).

Differential Diagnosis

See above; pseudostrabismus (epicanthal fold), negative angle kappa (pseudoesotropia), positive angle kappa (pseudoexotropia), dragged macula (e.g., retinopathy of prematurity, toxocariasis).

Evaluation

- Complete ophthalmic history and eye examination with attention to visual acuity, refraction, cycloplegic refraction, pupils, motility (versions, ductions, cover and alternate cover test), measure deviation (Hirschberg, Krimsky, or prism cover tests), measure torsional component (double Maddox rod test), Parks-Bielschowsky three-step test (identifies isolated cyclovertical muscle palsy [see Fourth Cranial Nerve Palsy section]); stereopsis (Titmus stereoacuity test, Randot stereotest), suppression/anomalous retinal correspondence (Worth 4-dot, 4PD base-out prism, Maddox rod, red glass, Bagolini's striated lens, or after-image tests), fusion (amblyoscope, Hess screen tests), forced ductions, and ophthalmoscopy.
- Orbital computed tomography (CT) or magnetic resonance imaging (MRI) in cases of muscle restriction.
- **Lab tests:** Thyroid function tests (triiodothyronine [T3], thyroxine [T4], thyrotropin [TSH]) in cases of muscle restriction, and antiacetylcholine (anti-ACh) receptor antibody titers if myasthenia gravis is suspected. Electrocardiogram in patients with CPEO, and to rule out heart block in Kearns-Sayre syndrome.

- Consider edrophonium chloride (Tensilon) test to rule out myasthenia gravis.
- Neurology consultation and brain MRI if cranial nerves are involved.
- Medical consultation for dysthyroid and myasthenia patients.

Management

- Correct any refractive component.
- In children, patching or occlusion therapy for amblyopia (see Chapter 12); initially patch dominant or fixating eye; part-time patching can be used at any age. If full-time patching is used (during all waking hours, then taper as amblyopia improves), do not occlude one eye for more than 1 week per year of age. Atropine penalization, one drop in the better seeing eye every day or every other day, is a good substitute to patching in children who are not compliant with occlusion.
- Timing of reexamination is based on patient's age (1 week per each year of age; e.g., 2 weeks for 2 year old, 4 weeks for 4 year old).
- Consider muscle surgery based on the indications outlined earlier.

Prognosis

Usually good; depends on cause.

▊ Horizontal Strabismus

Esotropia

Eye turns inward; most common ocular deviation (>50%).

Infantile Esotropia

Appears by age 6 months with a large, constant angle of deviation (80% >35 prism diopters [PD]); often cross-fixate; normal refractive error; positive family history is common; may be

Esotropia

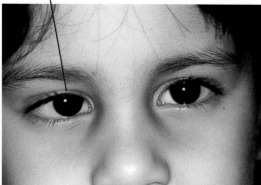

Figure 2-2 • Esotropia (inward turn) of the right eye. The corneal light reflex in the deviated eye is at the temporal edge of the pupil rather than the center.

associated with inferior oblique overaction, dissociated vertical deviation (DVD), latent nystagmus, and persistent smooth pursuit asymmetry.

- Treat amblyopia with occlusive therapy of fixating or dominant eye (see later) before performing surgery.
- Correct any hyperopia greater than 2.00 diopters (D).
- Muscle surgery should be performed early (6 months to 2 years): bilateral medial rectus recession or unilateral recession of medial rectus and resection of lateral rectus; additional surgery for inferior oblique overaction, DVD, and overcorrection and undercorrection is necessary in a large percentage of cases.

Accommodative Esotropia

Develops between age 6 months and 6 years, usually around age 2?, with variable angle of deviation (eyes usually straight as infant); initially intermittent when child is tired or sick; three types.

Refractive   Usually hyperopic (average +4.75D), normal accommodative convergence-to-accommodation (AC/A) ratio (3:1PD to 5:1PD per diopter of accommodation), esotropia at distance (ET) similar to that at near (ET'); (ET = ET').

Nonrefractive   High AC/A ratio; esotropia at near greater than at distance (ET' > ET).

- **Methods of calculating AC/A ratio**
  - *Heterophoria method:* AC/A = IPD + [(N − D) / Diopter]
    IPD, interpupillary distance (cm); N, near deviation; D, distance deviation; Diopter, accommodative demand at fixation distance.
  - *Lens gradient method:* AC/A = (WL − NL) / D.
    WL, deviation with lens in front of eye; NL, deviation with no lens in front of eye; D, dioptric power of lens used.

Mixed   Not completely correctable with single vision or bifocal glasses.

- Give full cycloplegic refraction if child is under 6 years old, and as much as tolerated if over 6 years old; if esotropia corrects to within 8PD, then no further treatment necessary.
- With high AC/A ratio and residual ET', prescribe executive-style, flat-top bifocal segment that bisects the pupil +2.50D to +3.00D) or try miotic agents, especially in infants too young for glasses (echothiophate iodide 0.125% qd; be careful not to use with succinylcholine for general anesthesia); a combination of both can be used in refractory cases.
- Muscle surgery as above should be performed if residual esotropia greater than 10PD.

Acquired Nonaccommodative Esotropia and Other Forms of Esotropia

Due to stress, sensory deprivation, divergence insufficiency (ET ≥ ET'), spasm of near reflex, consecutive (after exotropia surgery), or cranial nerve (CN) VI palsy.

- Muscle surgery can be considered either in symptomatic cases or if angle of deviation is large.
- If no evident cause, MRI indicated to rule out Arnold-Chiari malformation.

Table 2-1   Surgical Numbers for Horizontal Strabismus Surgery—Esotropia

Prism Resection Diopters	Bilateral MR Recession (mm)	Bilateral LR Resection (mm)	Recession & Resection (R & R)	
			MR Recess (mm)	LR Resect (mm)
15	3	3.5	3	3.5
20	3.5	4.5	3.5	4.5
25	4	5.5	4	5.5
30	4.5	6	4.5	6
35	5	6.5	5	6.5
40	5.5	7	5.5	7
50	6	8	6	7.5
60	6.5		6.5	8
70	7			

MR, Medial rectus; *LR,* lateral rectus.

Cyclical Esotropia

Very rare form of nonaccommodative ET (1:3000); occurs between 2 and 6 years of age; child is usually orthophoric (eyes straight) but develops esotropia for 24-hour to 48-hour periods; can progress to constant esotropia.

• Correct any hyperopia greater than +3.00D.
• Muscle surgery as above can be performed when deviation stabilizes.

Exotropia

Eye turns outward; may be intermittent (usually at age 2 years, amblyopia rare) or constant (rarely congenital, consecutive [after esotropia surgery], due to decompensated intermittent exotropia [XT] or from sensory deprivation [in children >5 years of age]); amblyopia rare due to formation of anomalous retinal correspondence.

Exotropia

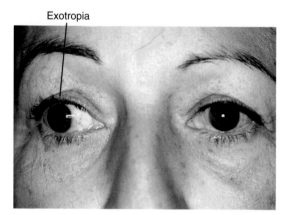

Figure 2-3 • Exotropia (outward turn) of the right eye. The corneal light reflex in the deviated eye is at the nasal edge of the iris rather than the center of the pupil.

Basic Exotropia

Exotropia at distance (XT) equal to that at near (XT′); normal AC/A ratio, normal fusional convergence.

Convergence Insufficiency

Inability to maintain convergence as object is brought in from distance to near (increased near point of convergence); exotropia at near greater than at distance (XT′ > XT); reduced fusional convergence amplitudes; rare before 10 years of age; slight female predilection; symptoms often begin during teen years with asthenopia, difficulty reading, blurred near vision, diplopia, and fatigue; may be associated with accommodative insufficiency, ciliary body dysfunction, and head trauma.

- Orthoptic exercises: near-point pencil push-ups (bring pencil in slowly from distance until breakpoint reached, then repeat 10-15 times) or prism convergence exercises (increase amount of base-out prism until breakpoint reached, then repeat starting with low prism power, 10-15 times).
- Base-out prism lenses.
- Muscle surgery: bilateral medial rectus resection is occasionally necessary.

Pseudodivergence Excess

XT > XT′ except after prolonged patching (patch test) when near deviation increases (full latent deviation); near deviation also increases with +3.00D lens; may have high AC/A ratio.

True Divergence Excess

XT > XT′ even after patch test, may have high AC/A ratio.

- Correct any refractive error and give additional minus, especially with high AC/A ratio.
- Consider base-in prism lenses.
- Muscle surgery if the patient manifests exotropia over 50% of the time and is older than 4 years old: bilateral lateral rectus recession; consecutive esotropia (postoperative diplopia) can be managed with prisms or miotics unless it lasts more than 8 weeks, then reoperate.

Table 2-2 Surgical Numbers for Horizontal Strabismus Surgery—Exotropia

Prism Resection Diopters	Bilateral LR Recession (mm)	Bilateral MR Resection (mm)	Recession & Resection (R & R)	
			LR Recess (mm)	MR Resect (mm)
15	4	3	4	3
20	5	4	5	4
25	6	5	6	5
30	7	5.5	7	5.5
35	7.5	6	7.5	6
40	8	6.5	8	6.5
50	9		9	7

MR, Medial rectus; *LR*, lateral rectus.

A-, V-, and X-Patterns

Amount of horizontal deviation varies from upgaze to downgaze.

A-pattern

Amount of horizontal deviation changes between upgaze (larger esotropia in upgaze) and downgaze (larger exotropia in downgaze); more common with exotropia; clinically significant if difference is 10PD or greater; associated with superior oblique muscle overaction; patients may have chin-up position.

- Muscle surgery if deviation is clinically significant: weakening of oblique muscles if overaction exists or transposition of horizontal muscles (medial recti moved up, lateral recti moved down) if no oblique overaction.
- Absolutely no superior oblique tenotomies if patient is bifixator with 40 seconds of arc of stereo acuity.

V-pattern

Amount of horizontal deviation changes between upgaze (larger exotropia in upgaze) and downgaze (larger esotropia in downgaze); more common with esotropia; clinically significant if difference is 15PD or greater; associated with inferior oblique muscle overaction, increased lateral rectus muscle innervation, underaction of superior rectus muscle, Apert's syndrome, and Crouzon's syndrome; patients may have chin-down position.

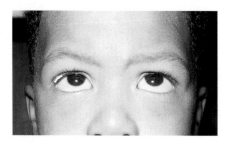 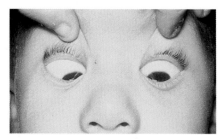

Figure 2-4 • V-pattern esotropia demonstrating reduced esotropia in upgaze.

Figure 2-5 • Same patient as shown in Figure 2-4, demonstrating increased esotropia in downgaze.

- Muscle surgery if deviation is clinically significant: weakening of oblique muscles if overaction exists or transposition of horizontal muscles (medial recti moved down, lateral recti moved up) if no oblique overaction.

X-pattern

Larger exotropia in upgaze and downgaze than in primary position; due to secondary contracture of the oblique muscles or the lateral recti, causing a tethering effect in upgaze and downgaze.

- Muscle surgery if deviation is clinically significant: staged surgery if due to oblique muscles or lateral rectus recessions if due to tether effect.

Vertical Strabismus

Brown's Syndrome

Congenital or acquired anomaly of the superior oblique tendon sheath, causing an inability to elevate the affected eye especially in adduction; elevation in abduction is normal or slightly decreased; usually hypotropia with chin-up position; positive forced duction testing that is worse on retropulsion and when moving eye up and in (differentiates from inferior rectus restriction, which is worse with proptosing eye); V-pattern (differentiates from superior oblique overaction, which is A-pattern), no superior oblique overaction, down-shoot in adduction, and widened palpebral fissures on adduction in severe cases; 10% bilateral, female predilection (3:2), and affects right eye more often than left eye; acquired forms are associated with rheumatoid arthritis, juvenile rheumatoid arthritis, sinusitis, sinus surgery, muscle surgery, retinal detachment surgery, scleroderma, hypogammaglobulinemia, postpartum, and trauma.

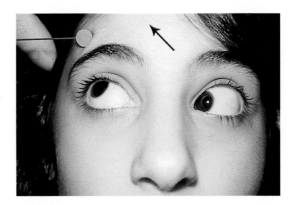

Figure 2-6 • Brown's syndrome, demonstrating inability to elevate left eye in adduction.

- No treatment usually required, especially for acquired forms, which often improve spontaneously.
- Consider injection of steroids near trochlea or oral steroids if inflammatory etiology exists.
- Muscle surgery for abnormal head position or large hypotropia in primary position: superior oblique muscle tenotomy or tenectomy or silicon band expander, with or without ipsilateral inferior oblique muscle recession.

Dissociated Strabismus Complex: Dissociated Vertical Deviation or Dissociated Horizontal Deviation

Updrift, horizontal, oblique, or torsional movement of fixating eye under cover; Bielschowsky phenomenon (downdrift of occluded eye as increasing neutral density filters are placed over fixating eye); usually bilateral, asymmetric, and asymptomatic; does not obey Hering's law (equal innervation to yoke muscles); associated with congenital esotropia (75%) more than exotropia and with exotropia more than hypertropia; also seen with latent nystagmus and after esotropia surgery.

- No treatment required usually.
- Muscle surgery if deviation is large and constant or very frequent; recess superior rectus muscle.

Table 2-3   Surgical Numbers for Vertical Strabismus Surgery

Dissociated Vertical Deviation

Magnitude	Recess SR
Mild	5 mm
Moderate	7 mm
Severe	10 mm

Inferior Oblique Overaction

Magnitude	Recess IO
Mild	10 mm
Moderate	15 mm
Severe	Myectomy

SR, Superior rectus; *IO,* inferior oblique.

Monocular Elevation Deficiency

Sporadic, unilateral defect causing total inability to elevate one eye (may have good Bell's reflex); hypotropia in primary position and increases on upgaze, ipsilateral ptosis common, may have chin-up head position to fuse; may be supranuclear, congenital, or acquired (due to cerebrovascular disease, tumor, or infection); three types:

- *Type 1:* Inferior rectus muscle restriction—unilateral fibrosis syndrome.
- *Type 2:* Elevator weakness (superior rectus, inferior oblique)—true double elevator palsy.
- *Type 3:* Combination (inferior rectus restriction and weak elevators).

Ptosis/hypotropia

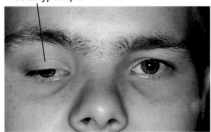

Figure 2-7 • Monocular elevation deficiency (double elevator palsy) demonstrating ptosis and hypotropia of the right eye.

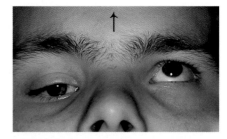

Figure 2-8 • Same patient as shown in Figure 2-7, demonstrating inability to elevate right eye.

- Muscle surgery for chin-up head position, large hypotropia in primary position, or poor fusion: inferior rectus recession for inferior rectus muscle restriction; Knapp procedure (elevation and transposition of medial and lateral recti to the side of superior rectus) for superior rectus muscle weakness.
- May require surgery to correct residual ptosis.

Skew Deviation

Comitant or incomitant acquired vertical misalignment of the eyes due to supranuclear dysfunction from brain stem or cerebellar process; hypotropic eye is ipsilateral to lesion.

Miscellaneous Strabismus

Duane's Retraction Syndrome

Congenital anomalous innervation of lateral rectus muscle by CN III due to agenesis of CN VI; 20% bilateral, female predilection (3:2), affects left eye more often than right eye (3:1); three types (type 1 more common than type 3, and type 3 more common than type 2):
- *Type 1:* Limited abduction; esotropia in primary position.
- *Type 2:* Limited adduction; exotropia in primary position.
- *Type 3:* Limited abduction and adduction.

Narrowing of palpebral fissure on adduction and widening on abduction in all three types; upshoots and downshoots (leash phenomenon) common; may have head turn to fuse; amblyopia rare; associated with deafness and less commonly with other ocular or systemic conditions.

Upshoot/limited adduction/
narrowing of palpebral fissure

Limited abduction/widened PF

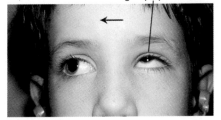 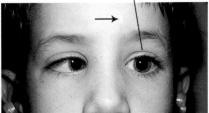

Figure 2-9 • Duane's retraction syndrome type 3, demonstrating limited adduction, upshoot (leash phenomenon) and narrowing of the palpebral fissure of the left eye.

Figure 2-10 • Same patient as shown in Figure 2-9, demonstrating limited abduction and widening of the palpebral fissure of the left eye.

- No treatment required usually.
- Correct any refractive error.
- Treat amblyopia.
- Muscle surgery if there is significant ocular misalignment in primary position, abnormal head position, or significant upshoot or downshoot: medial rectus muscle recession in type 1 or lateral rectus muscle recession in type 2; never perform lateral rectus muscle resection. Recess medial and lateral rectus muscles in type 3 with severe retraction, upshoot, and downshoot.

Möbius' Syndrome

Congenital bilateral aplasia of CN VI and VII nuclei (CN V, IX, and XII may also be affected); inability to abduct either eye past midline; associated with esotropia, epiphora, exposure keratitis, and masklike facies; patient may have limb deformities or absence of pectoralis muscle (Poland anomaly).

- Muscle surgery (bilateral medial rectus recessions) for esotropia.

Restrictive Strabismus

Various disorders that cause tethering of one or more extraocular muscles; restriction of eye movement in the direction of action of the affected muscle (these processes cause incomitant strabismus). Commonly seen in thyroid ophthalmopathy (see Chapter 1), orbital floor fracture (see Chapter 1), and congenital fibrosis syndrome.

Limited elevation/enophthalmos

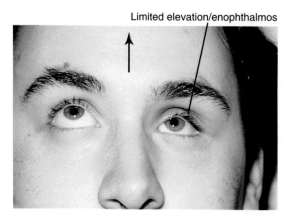

Figure 2-11 • Restrictive strabismus due to an orbital fracture of the left eye with inferior rectus entrapment, demonstrating limited elevation of the left eye; also note enophthalmos (sunken appearance of left eye).

Five types of congenital fibrosis syndrome

(1) Generalized fibrosis (autosomal dominant [AD] more common than autosomal recessive [AR], and AR more common than idiopathic): all muscles in both eyes affected, inferior rectus usually affected the worst.
(2) Congenital fibrosis of inferior rectus: only inferior rectus affected.
(3) Strabismus fixus (sporadic): horizontal muscles affected in both eyes; medial rectus more often than lateral rectus.
(4) Vertical retraction syndrome: vertical muscles affected in both eyes; superior rectus more often than inferior rectus.
(5) Congenital unilateral fibrosis (sporadic): all muscles affected in one eye; also associated with enophthalmos and ptosis.

■ Nystagmus

Definition

Involuntary, rhythmic oscillation of eyes; may be horizontal, vertical, rotary, or a combination; fast or slow; symmetric or asymmetric; pendular (equal speed in both directions) or jerk (direction designated by the fast phase component).

Etiology

Congenital Nystagmus

Nystagmus is different depending on gaze; may have null point (nystagmus slows or stops in certain eye positions); one dominant locus.

Afferent or sensory deprivation nystagmus   Pendular nystagmus due to sensory deprivation; associated with ocular albinism, aniridia, achromatopsia, congenital stationary night blindness, congenital optic nerve anomaly, Leber's congenital amaurosis, and congenital cataracts.

Efferent or motor nystagmus   Due to ocular motor disturbance; present at or shortly after birth, may be hereditary; mapped to chromosome 6p; usually horizontal; may have null point and head turn (to move eyes to the null point); decreases with convergence and stops during sleep; horizontal in all positions of gaze, no oscillopsia; may have head oscillations, a latent component, and inversion with horizontal optokinetic (OKN) testing (60%); associated with strabismus (33%).

Latent   Bilateral jerk nystagmus when one eye is covered (jerk component away from covered eye) that resolves when eye is uncovered; may be associated with congenital esotropia and DVD; only present under monocular viewing conditions; therefore, binocular visual acuity is better than when each eye is tested separately; normal OKN response; nulls with adduction.

Spasmus nutans   Triad of nystagmus (monocular or asymmetric, fine, very rapid, horizontal, and variable), head nodding, and torticollis (head turning); develops between 4 and 12 months of age, disappears by 5 years of age; otherwise neurologically intact; similar eye movements can be seen with chiasmal gliomas and parasellar tumors; therefore, check pupils for relative afferent pupillary defect and optic nerve carefully and perform neuroimaging; spasmus nutans is a diagnosis of exclusion; monitor for amblyopia.

Acquired Nystagmus

Various types of nystagmus are localizing.

Convergence-retraction   Co-contraction of extraocular muscles causes jerk convergence-retraction of eyes, especially on convergence or upgaze; seen in dorsal midbrain syndrome; also associated with aqueductal stenosis, pinealoma, trauma, brain stem arteriovenous malformation, multiple sclerosis, or basilar artery cerebrovascular accident.

Dissociated   Nystagmus is different in the two eyes; due to posterior fossa disease or internuclear ophthalmoplegia (INO).

Downbeat   Jerk nystagmus with rapid downbeat and slow upbeat; seen most easily in lateral and downgaze; null point is usually in upgaze; associated with cervicomedullary junctional lesions including Arnold-Chiari malformation, syringomyelia, multiple sclerosis, cerebrovascular accidents, and drug intoxication (lithium); may respond to clonazepam treatment.

Drug-induced   Associated with use of anticonvulsants (phenytoin, carbamazepine), barbiturates, tranquilizers, and phenothiazines; often gaze-evoked; may be absent in downgaze.

Nonspecific gaze-evoked   Jerk nystagmus in direction of gaze, no nystagmus in primary position; can be physiologic (fatigable with prolonged eccentric gaze, symmetric) or pathologic (prolonged, asymmetric); often due to medications (anticonvulsants, sedatives) or brain stem or posterior fossa lesions.

Opsoclonus (saccadomania)   Rapid, unpredictable, multidirectional saccades; absent during sleep; associated with neuroblastoma or after postviral encephalopathies in children; seen with visceral carcinomas in adults; if restricted to horizontal meridian is called *flutter*.

Periodic alternating   Very rare, horizontal jerk nystagmus present in primary gaze with spontaneous direction changes every 60 to 90 seconds, with periods as long as 10 to 15 seconds of no nystagmus; cycling persists despite fixating on targets; may be congenital or due to vestibulocerebellar disease; also associated with cervicomedullary junction lesions; usually responds to treatment with baclofen.

See-saw   One eye rises and incyclotorts while other eye falls and excyclotorts, then the process alternates; may have INO; usually due to suprasellar or diencephalon lesions; also after cerebrovascular accidents or trauma; or congenital.

Upbeat   Nystagmus occurs in primary position; usually due to anterior vermis and lower brain stem lesion; also associated with Wernicke's syndrome or drug intoxication.

Vestibular   Usually horizontal with rotary component (fast component toward normal side, slow component toward abnormal side); may have associated vertigo, tinnitus, and deafness; due to lesion of end organ, peripheral nerve (fixation inhibits nystagmus), or central (fixation does not inhibit nystagmus).

Voluntary   Usually hysterical or malingering; unable to sustain nystagmus longer than 30 seconds; usually in horizontal plane with rapid back-to-back saccades; lid fluttering may be present.

Physiologic Nystagmus

Occurs normally in a variety of situations including end gaze, OKN, caloric, and rotational.

Symptoms

Asymptomatic, may have decreased vision, oscillopsia (in acquired nystagmus), and other neurologic deficits (reduced hearing, tinnitus, vertigo).

Signs

Variable decreased visual acuity, ocular oscillations; may have better near than distance visual acuity, astigmatism, head turn, other ocular or systemic pathology (e.g., aniridia, bilateral media opacities, macular scars, optic atrophy, foveal hypoplasia, albinism).

Differential Diagnosis

See above; multiple sclerosis.

Evaluation

• Complete ophthalmic history, with attention to drug or toxin ingestion, and eye examination, with attention to monocular and binocular visual acuity, retinoscopy, pupils, motility, and ophthalmoscopy.
• Neurology or neuro-ophthalmology consultation.
• Head CT scan or MRI to rule out intracranial process.

Management

- No effective treatment in most forms.
- Consider base-out prism lenses for congenital nystagmus (dampens nystagmus by stimulating convergence).
- Consider baclofen (5-80 mg po tid) for periodic alternating nystagmus.
- Consider muscle surgery with Kestenbaum's procedure for congenital nystagmus if patient has head turn to keep eyes in null point.
- Discontinue inciting agent if condition is due to drug or toxin ingestion.

Prognosis

Usually benign; depends on etiology.

Third Cranial Nerve Palsy

Definition

Paresis of CN III (oculomotor) caused by a variety of processes anywhere along its course from the midbrain to the orbit; can be complete or partial (superior division innervates superior rectus and levator; inferior division innervates medial rectus, inferior rectus, inferior oblique, and parasympathetic fibers to iris sphincter and ciliary muscle); can be isolated with or without pupil involvement.

Etiology

Depends on age: congenital due to birth trauma or neurologic syndrome; in children due to infection, postviral illness, trauma, or tumors (pontine glioma); in adults, most commonly due to ischemia or microvascular problems (20-45% hypertension or diabetes mellitus); also associated with aneurysm (15-20%), trauma (10-15%), and tumors (10-15%); 10-30% are of undetermined cause; rarely associated with ophthalmoplegic migraine. Aberrant regeneration may occur after intracavernous aneurysm, trauma, and tumors, but never after ischemic or microvascular causes; pupil sparing usually microvascular or ischemic (80% are pupil sparing); 95% of compressive lesions involve the pupil; important to localize level of pathology.

Nuclear

Very rare, usually due to microvascular infarctions; signs include bilateral ptosis and contralateral superior rectus involvement.

Fascicular

Usually due to vascular or metastatic lesions; associated with several syndromes including Benedikt's syndrome (CN III palsy with contralateral hemitremor, hemiballismus, and loss of sensation), Nothnagel's syndrome (CN III palsy and ipsilateral cerebellar ataxia and dysmetria), Claude's syndrome (combination of Benedikt's and Nothnagel's syndromes), and Weber's syndrome (CN III palsy and contralateral hemiparesis).

Subarachnoid Space

Usually involves pupil and is due to aneurysms (notably posterior communicating artery aneurysm), trauma, or uncal herniation; rarely microvascular disease and infections.

Intracavernous Space

Usually due to cavernous sinus fistula, aneurysms, tumors, Tolosa-Hunt syndrome, infections (e.g., herpes zoster), or pituitary apoplexy; usually associated with CN IV, V, and VI findings and sympathetic abnormalities (see Multiple Cranial Nerve Palsies section); pupil usually spared (90%).

Orbital Space

Usually due to trauma and infections; often associated with CN II, IV, V, and VI findings (see Multiple Cranial Nerve Palsies section); CN III splits before superior orbital fissure, so partial (superior or inferior division) palsies may occur (however, divisional CN III palsies have been reported from fascicular and subarachnoid lesions).

Symptoms

Binocular diplopia (disappears with one eye closed), eye turn; may have pain, headache, or ipsilateral droopy eyelid.

Signs

Ptosis, ophthalmoplegia except lateral gaze, negative forced ductions, exotropia and hypotropia in primary gaze (eye is down and out); may have mid-dilated nonreactive pupil ("blown" pupil, efferent defect); in cases of aberrant regeneration: lid-gaze dyskinesis (inferior rectus or medial rectus fibers to levator causing upper lid retraction on downgaze [pseudo–von Graefe's sign] or on adduction), pupil-gaze dyskinesis (inferior rectus or medial rectus fibers to iris sphincter causing pupil constriction on downgaze or on adduction); depending on syndrome causing the paresis may have other neurologic deficits or cranial nerve palsies.

Ptosis   Dilated pupil

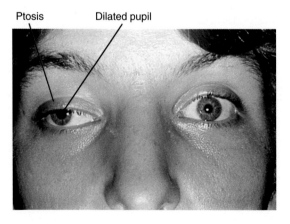

Figure 2-12 • Third cranial nerve palsy with right ptosis, pupillary dilation, exotropia, and hypotropia. This is the typical appearance of the "down and out" eye with a droopy lid and large pupil.

Differential Diagnosis

Myasthenia gravis, thyroid ophthalmopathy, migraine, CPEO.

Evaluation

- Complete ophthalmic history, neurologic examination with attention to cranial nerve examination, and eye examination with attention to pupils, lids, proptosis, motility, and forced ductions.
- MRI or magnetic resonance angiography (MRA), or both, if pupil involved in any patient, if associated with other neurologic abnormalities, if pupil spared in young patients (<45 years old), if signs of aberrant regeneration are present, or if no improvement of isolated pupil-sparing microvascular cases after 3 months is evident.
- **Lab tests:** Fasting blood glucose, complete blood count (CBC), erythrocyte sedimentation rate (ESR), Venereal Disease Research Laboratory (VDRL), fluorescent treponemal antibody absorption (FTA-ABS), antinuclear antibody (ANA).
- Check blood pressure.
- Consider cerebral angiography to rule out aneurysm (neurosurgical emergency) if pupil involved and MRI-MRA results inconclusive.
- Consider lumbar puncture if subarachnoid hemorrhage suspected.
- Consider edrophonium chloride (Tensilon) test to rule out myasthenia gravis.
- Neuro-ophthalmology or interventional neuroradiology consultation (especially if pupil involved).

Management

- Treatment depends on cause.
- Follow isolated pupil-sparing lesions closely for pupil involvement during first week.
- Occlusion with Transpore clear surgical tape or clear nail polish across one spectacle lens to help alleviate diplopia in adults.
- Aneurysms, tumors, and trauma may require neurosurgery.
- Treat underlying medical condition.

Prognosis

Depends on etiology; usually poor except microvascular palsies, which tend to resolve within 2 to 3 months (6 months maximum).

▇ Fourth Cranial Nerve Palsy

Definition

Paresis of CN IV (trochlear) caused by a variety of processes anywhere along its course from the midbrain to the orbit.

Etiology

Most commonly trauma (30-40%; especially closed head trauma with contrecoup forces) and microvascular disease (20%; e.g., hypertension or diabetes mellitus); also can be congenital (with longstanding head tilt), idiopathic (30%) or, rarely, due to a tumor, hemorrhage, or aneurysm; bilateral seen after severe head trauma (damage at anterior medullary velum); important to localize level of pathology.

Nuclear

Rare, due to trauma, vascular lesion (e.g., hemorrhage, infarction), or demyelinating disease; signs include contralateral superior oblique palsy.

Fascicular

Rare, same associations as nuclear; may get contralateral Horner's syndrome; trauma (especially near anterior medullary velum) usually causes bilateral CN IV palsies.

Subarachnoid Space

Usually due to closed head trauma; rarely tumor or infection.

Intracavernous Space

Due to trauma, tumors, and inflammation; usually associated with CN III, V, and VI findings and sympathetic abnormalities (see Multiple Cranial Nerve Palsies section).

Symptoms

Binocular vertical or diagonal diplopia; may have a torsional component, blurred vision, head tilt toward contralateral side.

Signs

Superior oblique palsy with positive Parks-Bielschowsky three-step test (see below), ipsilateral hypertropia (greatest on contralateral gaze and ipsilateral head tilt), excyclotorsion (if >10 degrees, likely bilateral), large vertical fusional amplitude in congenital cases (10PD to 15PD); chin-down position; negative forced ductions; bilateral cases have V-pattern esotropia, left hypertropia on right gaze, and right hypertropia on left gaze; other neurologic deficits if CN IV paresis is not isolated.

Differential Diagnosis

Myasthenia gravis, thyroid ophthalmopathy, orbital disease, CN III palsy, Brown's syndrome, skew deviation, superior oblique myokymia.

Evaluation

• Complete ophthalmic history, neurologic examination with attention to cranial nerve examination, and eye examination with attention to motility, head posture (check old photographs for longstanding head tilt in congenital cases), vertical fusion, double Maddox rod test (measure torsional component), and forced ductions.

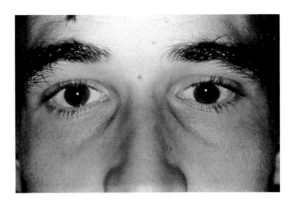

Figure 2-13 • Fourth cranial nerve palsy with right hypertropia.

- Perform Parks-Bielschowsky three-step test to determine paretic muscle.

    Step 1: Identify hypertropic eye in primary gaze (e.g., if right hypertropia then problem is with right inferior rectus/superior oblique or left superior rectus/inferior oblique).

    Step 2: Identify horizontal direction of gaze that makes the hypertropia worse (e.g., if left gaze then problem is with right superior oblique/inferior oblique or left superior rectus/inferior rectus).

    Step 3: Bielschowsky head-tilt test: identify direction of head tilt that makes the hypertropia worse (e.g., if right head tilt, then problem is with right superior oblique/superior rectus or left inferior oblique/inferior rectus).

    - After three steps, the paretic muscle will be identified (e.g., right hypertropia in primary position, worse on left gaze, and right head tilt indicates right superior oblique).

- **Lab tests:** Fasting blood glucose, CBC, ESR, VDRL, FTA-ABS, ANA.
- Check blood pressure.
- Head and orbital CT scan or MRI-MRA, or both, if history of head trauma, history of cancer, signs of meningitis, young age, associated with other neurologic abnormalities, or no improvement of isolated presumed microvascular cases after 3 to 4 months; isolated and microvascular cases do not initially require neuroimaging.
- Consider lumbar puncture.

Management

- Treatment depends on cause.
- Occlusion with Transpore clear surgical tape, clear nail polish across one spectacle lens, or prism glasses to help alleviate diplopia in adults.
- Consider muscle surgery in longstanding, stable CN IV palsy: Knapp classification for management of superior oblique palsy offers guidance, consider Harado Ito procedure (lateral transposition of superior oblique tendon) to correct torsional component.
- Aneurysms, tumors, and trauma may require neurosurgery.
- Treat underlying medical condition.

* Consider edrophonium chloride (Tensilon) test to rule out myasthenia gravis.
* Neuro-ophthalmology consultation.

Prognosis

Depends on etiology; microvascular palsies tend to resolve within 3 months.

▓ Sixth Cranial Nerve Palsy

Definition

Paresis of CN VI caused by a variety of processes anywhere along its course from the pons to the orbit.

Etiology

Depends on age: in children (0-15 years old), most commonly tumors (e.g., pontine glioma) or postviral; in young adults (15-40 years old), usually miscellaneous or undetermined (8-30%); in adults (>40 years old) usually due to trauma and microvascular disease (e.g., hypertension, diabetes mellitus [most common isolated cranial nerve palsy in diabetes: CN VI>III>IV]); also associated with multiple sclerosis, cerebrovascular accidents, increased intracranial pressure, and rarely tumors (e.g., nasopharyngeal carcinoma); important to localize level of pathology.

Nuclear

Due to pontine infarcts, pontine gliomas, cerebellar tumors, microvascular disease, and Wernicke-Korsakoff syndrome; causes an ipsilateral, horizontal gaze palsy (cannot look to side of lesion).

Fascicular

Usually due to tumors, microvascular disease, or demyelinating disease; can cause Foville's syndrome (dorsal pons lesions with horizontal gaze palsy, ipsilateral CN V, VI, VII, VIII palsies, and ipsilateral Horner's syndrome) and Millard-Gubler syndrome (ventral pons lesion with ipsilateral CN VI and VII palsies and contralateral hemiparesis).

Subarachnoid Space

Usually due to elevated intracranial pressure (30% of patients with idiopathic intracranial hypertension have CN VI palsy); also basilar tumors (e.g., acoustic neuroma, chordomas), basilar artery aneurysm, hemorrhage, inflammations, or meningeal infections.

Petrous Space

Due to trauma (e.g., basal skull fracture) and infections; can cause Gradenigo's syndrome (infection of petrous bone secondary to otitis media causing ipsilateral CN VI and VII paresis, ipsilateral Horner's syndrome, ipsilateral trigeminal pain, and ipsilateral deafness; seen in children) or pseudo–Gradenigo's syndrome (nasopharyngeal carcinoma may cause severe otitis media with findings similar to those of Gradenigo's syndrome).

Intracavernous Space

Usually due to trauma, vascular lesion, inflammation, or tumors; associated with CN III, IV, and V findings and sympathetic abnormalities (see Multiple Cranial Nerve Palsies section); isolated palsy is rare.

Symptoms

Horizontal binocular diplopia (worse at distance than near, and in direction of gaze of paretic muscle); may have eye turn.

Signs

Lateral rectus muscle palsy with esotropia and inability to abduct eye fully or slow abducting saccades; negative forced ductions; other neurologic deficits if CN VI paresis is not isolated.

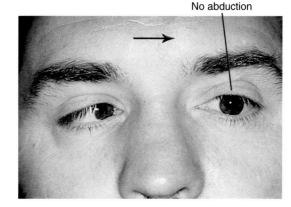

No abduction

Figure 2-14 • Sixth cranial nerve palsy demonstrating the inability to abduct the left eye on left gaze.

Differential Diagnosis

Thyroid ophthalmopathy, myasthenia gravis, orbital inflammatory pseudotumor, Duane's retraction syndrome type I, Möbius' syndrome (CN VI and VII palsy), orbital fracture with medial rectus entrapment, spasm of near reflex.

Evaluation

- Complete ophthalmic history, neurologic examination with attention to cranial nerve examination, and eye examination with attention to motility, forced ductions, and ophthalmoscopy.
- Head and orbital CT scan or MRI-MRA, or both, if in child, history of pain, history of head trauma, history of cancer, signs of meningitis, associated with other neurologic abnormalities, or no improvement of isolated, presumed microvascular cases after 3-6 months; isolated and microvascular cases in adults over 40 years old do not initially require neuroimaging.
- **Lab tests:** Fasting blood glucose, CBC, ESR, VDRL, FTA-ABS, ANA.
- Check blood pressure.
- Consider lumbar puncture if elevated intracranial pressure suspected.

- Consider edrophonium chloride (Tensilon) test to rule out myasthenia gravis.
- Neuro-ophthalmology consultation.

Management

- Treatment depends on cause.
- Occlusion with Transpore clear surgical tape or clear nail polish across one spectacle lens to help alleviate diplopia in adults.
- Consider muscle surgery in longstanding, *stable* cases.
- Aneurysms, tumors, and trauma may require neurosurgery.
- Treat underlying medical condition.

Prognosis

Depends on cause; microvascular palsies tend to resolve within 3 months.

Multiple Cranial Nerve Palsies

Definition

Multiple cranial nerve abnormalities appearing simultaneously; lesions can be located in the brain stem, subarachnoid space, cavernous sinus, or orbital space.

Etiology

Important to localize level of pathology.

Brain Stem

Due to midbrain or pons vascular lesions and tumors involving cranial nerve nuclei that are in close proximity.

Subarachnoid Space

Usually due to infections or midline tumors.

Cavernous Sinus Syndrome

Multiple cranial nerve pareses (CN III, IV, VI, V1, V2) and sympathetic involvement due to parasellar lesions, which affect these motor nerves in various combinations in the sinus or superior orbital fissure; may have Horner's syndrome due to oculosympathetic paresis; caused by aneurysms (e.g., intracavernous carotid artery), arteriovenous fistulas (e.g., carotid-cavernous fistula, dural sinus fistula), tumors (e.g., leukemia, lymphoma, meningioma, pituitary adenoma, chordoma), inflammations (e.g., Wegener's granulomatosis, sarcoidosis, Tolosa-Hunt syndrome), and infections (e.g., cavernous sinus thrombosis, herpes zoster, tuberculosis, syphilis, mucormycosis); lesions of the cavernous sinus do not necessarily affect all the cranial nerves in it.

Orbital Apex Syndrome

Multiple motor cranial nerve palsies (except no CN V2 involvement) and optic nerve (CN II) dysfunction; etiologies similar to those mentioned above.

Symptoms

Pain, diplopia, droopy eyelid, variable decreased vision.

Signs

Normal or decreased visual acuity (orbital apex syndrome), ptosis, strabismus, limitation of ocular motility, decreased facial sensation in CN V1-V2 distribution, positive relative afferent pupillary defect, miosis (Horner's syndrome), and trigeminal (facial) pain; pupil usually spared; may have proptosis, conjunctival injection, chemosis, increased intraocular pressure, bruit, and retinopathy in cases of high-flow arteriovenous fistulas; fever, lid edema, and signs of facial infection in cases of cavernous sinus thrombosis.

Differential Diagnosis

Thyroid ophthalmopathy, myasthenia gravis, giant cell arteritis, Miller-Fisher variant of Guillain-Barré syndrome, CPEO, orbital disease (see Chapter 1).

Evaluation

- Complete ophthalmic history, neurologic examination with attention to cranial nerve examination, and eye examination with attention to facial sensation, ocular auscultation, pupils, motility, Hertel exophthalmometry, tonometry, and ophthalmoscopy.
- **Lab tests:** Fasting blood glucose, CBC with differential, ESR, VDRL, FTA-ABS, ANA; consider blood cultures if infectious etiology suspected.
- Head, orbital, and sinus CT scan or MRI-MRA or both.
- Consider lumbar puncture.
- Consider cerebral angiography to rule out aneurysm or arteriovenous fistula.
- Consider edrophonium chloride (Tensilon) test to rule out myasthenia gravis.
- Neuro-ophthalmology, otolaryngology, or medical consultations as needed.

Management

- Treatment depends on cause.
- Aneurysms, tumors, and trauma may require neurosurgery.
- Systemic steroids (prednisone 60-100 mg po qd) for Tolosa-Hunt syndrome; check purified protein derivative, blood glucose, and chest radiographs before starting systemic steroids.
- Add H_2-blocker (ranitidine [Zantac] 150 mg po bid) or proton pump inhibitor when administering systemic steroids.
- Systemic antibiotic agents (vancomycin 1 g IV q12h and ceftazidime 1 g IV q8h for staphylococcus and streptococcus) for cavernous sinus thrombosis; penicillin G (2.4 million U IV q4h for 10-14 days, then 2.4 million U IM q week for 3 weeks) for syphilis.
- Systemic antifungal medications (amphotericin B 0.25-1.0 mg/kg IV over 6h) for mucormycosis.
- Treat underlying medical condition.

Prognosis

Usually poor.

Chronic Progressive External Ophthalmoplegia

Definition

Slowly progressive, bilateral, external ophthalmoplegia affecting all directions of gaze.

Etiology

Isolated or hereditary myopathy; several rare syndromes.

Kearns-Sayre Syndrome (Mitochondrial DNA)

Triad of CPEO, pigmentary retinopathy (see Chapter 10), and cardiac conduction defects (arrhythmias, heart block, cardiomyopathy); also associated with mental retardation, short stature, deafness, vestibular problems, and elevated cerebrospinal fluid protein.

MELAS (Mitochondrial Encephalopathy, Lactic Acidosis, and Stroke)

MERRF (Myoclonus Epilepsy with Ragged Red Fibers)

Myotonic Dystrophy (AD)

CPEO, bilateral ptosis, lid lag, orbicularis oculi weakness, miotic pupils, "Christmas tree" (polychromic) cataracts, and pigmentary retinopathy with associated muscular dystrophy (worse in morning), cardiomyopathy, frontal baldness, temporalis muscle wasting, testicular atrophy, and mental retardation; mapped to chromosome 19q.

Oculopharyngeal Muscular Dystrophy (AD)

CPEO with dysphagia; usually French-Canadian lineage; mapped to chromosome 14q.

Symptoms

Variable decreased vision, droopy eyelids, foreign body sensation, tearing. Usually no diplopia.

Signs

Normal or decreased visual acuity, limitation of eye movements (even with doll's head maneuvers and caloric stimulation), absent Bell's phenomenon, large-angle strabismus (usually exotropia), no restrictions on forced ductions, ptosis, orbicularis oculi weakness, superficial punctate keratitis (especially inferiorly), retinal pigment epithelial changes or pigmentary retinopathy (see Chapter 10); pupils usually spared.

Ptosis

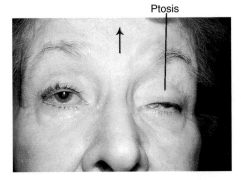

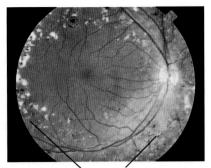

Pigmentary changes

Figure 2-15 • Chronic progressive external ophthalmoplegia, demonstrating ptosis and limited elevation in both eyes. The patient is attempting to look upward (note raised brows), yet the eyes remain in primary position (note the corneal light reflex centered over the pupil of the right eye) and the lids remain ptotic (markedly on the left side).

Figure 2-16 • Retinal pigmentary changes in a patient with Kearns-Sayre syndrome. Areas of retinal pigment epithelial hyperpigmentation, as well as atrophy, are apparent around the optic nerve and vascular arcades.

Differential Diagnosis

Downgaze palsy (lesion of rostral interstitial nucleus of the medial longitudinal fasciculus [riMLF]), upgaze palsy, progressive supranuclear palsy, dorsal midbrain syndrome, oculogyric crisis, myasthenia gravis.

Evaluation

- Complete ophthalmic history, neurologic examination with attention to cranial nerve examination, and eye examination with attention to motility, doll's head maneuvers, caloric stimulation, Bell's phenomenon, lids, pupils, and ophthalmoscopy.
- Consider muscle biopsy (deltoid) to check for "ragged red" abnormal muscle fibers or electromyography for definitive diagnosis.
- Consider edrophonium chloride (Tensilon) test to rule out myasthenia gravis.
- Consider lumbar puncture (Kearns-Sayre syndrome).
- Medical consultation for complete cardiac evaluation including electrocardiogram (Kearns-Sayre syndrome, myotonic dystrophy) and swallowing studies (oculopharyngeal dystrophy).
- Mitochondrial DNA analysis for deletions (Kearns-Sayre syndrome).

Management

- No treatment effective.
- Topical lubrication with nonpreserved artificial tears (see Appendix) up to q1h and ointment (Refresh P.M.) at bedtime if signs of exposure keratopathy exist.
- Kearns-Sayre syndrome requires a cardiology consultation; may require pacemaker.
- Ptosis surgery can be considered but risk corneal exposure.

Prognosis

Depends on syndrome; usually poor.

■ Horizontal Gaze Palsy

Definition

Internuclear Ophthalmoplegia (INO)

Lesion of medial longitudinal fasciculus (MLF) in brain stem causing gaze defects in both eyes by blocking connection between contralateral CN VI nucleus and the ipsilateral CN III nucleus; ipsilateral deficiency of adduction and contralateral abducting nystagmus (named after side of MLF lesion); convergence can be absent (mesencephalic lesion; anterior lesion) or intact (lesion posterior in the MLF); may be unilateral or bilateral (appears exotropic; WEBINO, "wall-eyed" bilateral INO).

One-and-a-Half Syndrome

So-called *INO plus* with lesion of paramedian pontine reticular formation (PPRF, the horizontal gaze center) or CN VI nucleus, *and* the ipsilateral MLF causing conjugate gaze palsy to ipsilateral side (one) and INO or inability to adduct on gaze to contralateral side (half).

Etiology

Depends on age: less than 50 years old usually multiple sclerosis (unilateral or bilateral INO) or tumor (pontine glioma for one-and-a-half syndrome); bilateral in children, often due to brain stem glioma; over 50 years old usually vascular disease (cerebrovascular accident affecting brain stem, arteriovenous malformation, aneurysm, basilar artery occlusion), multiple sclerosis, or tumor (pontine metastasis).

Symptoms

Binocular horizontal diplopia worse in contralateral gaze.

Signs

Limitation of eye movements (cannot adduct on side of lesion in INO; can abduct only on side contralateral to lesion in one-and-a-half syndrome); nystagmus in abducting contralateral eye (INO); may have upbeat nystagmus or skew deviation.

Differential Diagnosis

Medial rectus palsy, myasthenia gravis.

Evaluation

• Complete ophthalmic history, neurologic examination with attention to cranial nerve examination, and eye examination with attention to motility, doll's head maneuvers, and caloric stimulation.
• MRI with attention to brain stem and midbrain.

- Consider edrophonium chloride (Tensilon) test to rule out myasthenia gravis.
- Consider neurology or neurosurgery consultation.

Management

- Treatment depends on cause.
- Aneurysms, tumors, and trauma may require neurosurgery.
- Treat underlying neurologic or medical condition.

Prognosis

Usually poor.

■ Vertical Gaze Palsy

Definition

Progressive Supranuclear Palsy (Steele-Richardson-Olszewski Syndrome)

Degenerative neurologic disorder with parkinsonian features that causes progressive, bilateral, external ophthalmoplegia affecting all directions of gaze; usually starts with vertical gaze (downgaze first).

Dorsal Midbrain (Parinaud's Syndrome)

Supranuclear palsy of vertical gaze (upgaze first) due to lesions of the dorsal midbrain.

Etiology

Most commonly due to pineal tumor (in young men), also seen with cerebrovascular accidents, hydrocephalus, arteriovenous malformation, trauma, multiple sclerosis, or syphilis.

Symptoms

Blurred vision, binocular diplopia (at near with dorsal midbrain syndrome); may have trouble reading, foreign body sensation, tearing, or dementia (progressive supranuclear palsy [PSP]).

Signs

Progressive Supranuclear Palsy

Progressive limitation of voluntary eye movements (but doll's head maneuvers give full range of motion); may have nuchal rigidity and seborrhea, progressive dementia, dysarthria, hypometric saccades.

Dorsal Midbrain Syndrome

Supranuclear paresis of upgaze (therefore vestibular, doll's head maneuvers, and Bell's phenomenon intact), light-near dissociation, may see papilledema, convergence-retraction nystagmus (on attempted upgaze or downward OKN drum), lid retraction (Collier's sign), spasm of convergence and accommodation (causing induced myopia), skew deviation, superficial punctate keratitis (especially inferiorly).

Differential Diagnosis

Downgaze palsy (lesion of riMLF), upgaze palsy, CPEO, oculogyric crisis (bilateral tonic supraduction of eyes and neck hyperextension; occurs in phenothiazine overdose and Parkinson's disease), myasthenia gravis.

Evaluation

- Complete ophthalmic history, neurologic examination with attention to cranial nerve examination, and eye examination with attention to motility, lids, accommodation, pupils, cornea, and ophthalmoscopy.
- Head and orbital CT scan or MRI-MRA, or both, with attention to brain stem and midbrain.
- Consider edrophonium chloride (Tensilon) test to rule out myasthenia gravis.
- Consider neurology or neurosurgery consultation.

Management

- Treatment depends on cause.
- Topical lubrication with nonpreserved artificial tears (see Appendix) up to q1h and ointment (Refresh P.M.) at bedtime if signs of exposure keratopathy exist.
- Aneurysms, tumors, and trauma may require neurosurgery.
- Treat underlying neurologic or medical condition.

Prognosis

Poor; usually death within 5 years in PSP.

▌ Myasthenia Gravis

Definition

Systemic disease of the neuromuscular junction causing muscle weakness; hallmark is variability and fatigability.

Etiology

Autoantibodies to acetylcholine receptors in voluntary striated muscles seen in 70-90% of patients with generalized myasthenia but is as low as 50% in ocular myasthenia; does not affect pupils or ciliary muscle.

Epidemiology

Female predilection; positive family history in 5%; 90% have eye involvement (levator, orbicularis oculi, and extraocular muscles), 75% as initial manifestation, 20% ocular only; increased incidence of thyroid disease, thymoma (15%), and autoimmune diseases including scleroderma, systemic lupus erythematosus, rheumatoid arthritis, Hashimoto's thyroiditis, multiple sclerosis, and thyroid ophthalmopathy.

Symptoms

Asymptomatic; may have diplopia (especially when tired), droopy eyelids, dysarthria, dysphagia.

Signs

Variable, asymmetric ptosis (worse with fatigue, sustained upgaze, and at end of day), variable limitation of extraocular movements (mimics any motility disturbance), strabismus, gaze-evoked nystagmus, orbicularis oculi weakness; Cogan's lid twitch (upper eyelid twitch when patient looks up to primary position after looking down for 10-15 seconds); very rarely may have an INO.

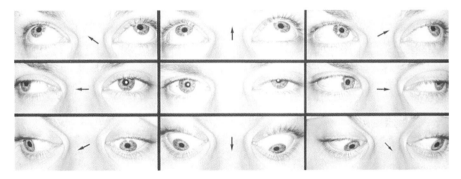

Figure 2-17 • Myasthenia gravis with left ptosis and adduction deficit. The left ptosis is most evident in primary gaze and gaze to the left; the left adduction deficit is apparent in all right gaze positions.

Differential Diagnosis

Gaze palsy, multiple sclerosis, CN III, IV, or VI palsy, INO, thyroid ophthalmopathy, CPEO, inflammatory orbital pseudotumor, levator dehiscence.

Evaluation

- Complete ophthalmic history, neurologic examination with attention to cranial nerve examination, and eye examination with attention to motility, lids, pupils, and cornea.
- **Lab tests:** Anti-ACh receptor antibodies, thyroid function tests (T3, T4, TSH), rheumatoid factor, ANA.

- **Edrophonium chloride (Tensilon) test:** Test dose of edrophonium chloride 2 mg IV with 1 mL saline flush, then observe for improvement in diplopia and lid signs over next minute; if no improvement, increase edrophonium chloride dose to 4 mg IV with 1 mL saline flush and observe for improvement in diplopia and lid signs; repeat two times; if no improvement in diplopia and lid signs after 3 to 4 minutes, the test result is negative; a negative test result does not rule out myasthenia gravis. *Note:* test should be performed with cardiac monitoring because of cardiovascular effects of edrophonium chloride; if bradycardia, angina, or bronchospasm develop, inject atropine (0.4 mg IV) immediately; consider pretreatment with atropine 0.4 mg IV.
- Consider single-fiber electromyography of peripheral or orbicularis muscles for definitive diagnosis.
- Chest CT scan to rule out thymoma.
- Neurology or medical consultation or both.

Management

- No treatment required if symptoms are mild.
- Oral anticholinesterase agent (pyridostigmine 60-120 mg po qid) for moderate symptoms.
- Consider systemic steroids (prednisone 20-100 mg po qd); check purified protein derivative, blood glucose, and chest radiographs before starting systemic steroids.
- Add H_2-blocker (ranitidine [Zantac] 150 mg po bid) or proton pump inhibitor when taking systemic steroids.
- Occlusion with Transpore clear surgical tape or clear nail polish across one spectacle lens to help alleviate diplopia in adults.
- Surgery for thymoma if present.
- Treat underlying medical condition.

Prognosis

Variable, chronic, progressive; good if ocular only.

C h a p t e r 3

LIDS, LASHES, AND LACRIMAL GLANDS

■ Eyelid Trauma

Eyelid trauma must be evaluated thoroughly, because seemingly trivial trauma may threaten the viability of the globe. Embedded foreign bodies, incomplete eyelid closure, or lacrimal system damage all can have lasting effects beyond any obvious cosmetic consequences. Trauma is typically blunt resulting from fist, motor vehicle, or athletic injury with open or closed soft tissue injury. Ominous mechanism of injury, orbital signs, or massive periocular injury may warrant orbital evaluation including computed tomography (CT) scan.

Contusion

Bruising of eyelid with edema and ecchymosis, usually secondary to blunt injury. Hematoma is not discrete but is embedded within the layers of septum and orbicularis and, therefore, cannot be evacuated surgically, so the goal of treatment is to reduce further bleeding. Ocular involvement is common; traumatic ptosis may occur (mechanical from edema and hematoma, or direct levator injury) and can take up to 6 months to resolve. Usually excellent prognosis if no ocular or bony injuries.

- Cold compresses for 10-15 minutes qid for 24-48 hours.
- Rule out and treat open globe (see Chapter 4) or other associated ocular trauma.

Preseptal hematoma (absent orbital signs) is not an indication for canthotomy. Orbital compartment syndrome does not result from preseptal edema.

Abrasion

Superficial abrasions or mild dermal epithelial abrasions usually heal by secondary intention; rarely require skin grafting.

* Antibiotic ointment lubrication (erythromycin or bacitracin ointment) helps prevent scab and scar formation.

Avulsion

Tearing or shearing injury to the eyelid resulting in partial or complete severance of eyelid tissue. Surgical repair of eyelid defect depends upon the degree of tissue loss and damage; entirely avulsed remnant should be sought and surgically replaced.

Upper Lid Defects

* Small (<25%): direct closure.
* Moderate (25-50%): Tenzel semicircular flap advancement or lateral segment lid advancement.
* Large (>50%): lower eyelid bridge flap reconstruction (Cutler-Beard procedure) or full-thickness lower eyelid flap advancement.

Lower Lid Defects

* Small (<25%): direct closure.
* Moderate (25-50%): Tenzel semicircular flap advancement or full thickness composite graft from contralateral lid.
* Large (>50%): upper eyelid tarsoconjunctival pedicle flap reconstruction (Hughes' procedure), Mustarde's rotational cheek flap, or anterior lamella reconstruction with retroauricular free skin graft or skin flap advancement.

Lid-sharing procedures should be avoided in young children due to the risk of deprivation amblyopia.

Laceration

Cut in the eyelid involving skin and deeper structures (muscle and fat), usually due to penetrating trauma. Lid lacerations are divided into: (1) no lid margin involvement, (2) lid margin involvement, and (3) canthal angle involvement (tendon and lacrimal gland system). Early, clean wounds usually are repaired successfully but can be complicated by lid notching, entropion, ectropion, or cicatrix; dirty wounds are also at risk for infection.

* Tetanus booster (tetanus toxoid 0.5 mL IM) if necessary for tetanus prophylaxis (>10 years since last tetanus shot or if status is unknown); consider rabies with animal bites.
* Fat prolapse into wound suggests orbital septum violation.

Canalicular Laceration

Laceration involving the canaliculus (tear duct) at the nasal lid margin between the punctum and the medial canthus of either eyelid; often identified on inspection as a pouting gray structure, or with probing and irrigation of the lacrimal system; good prognosis if repaired early with stent; notoriously misdiagnosed even by senior eye staff. Probing of lacrimal canaliculus required for diagnosis.

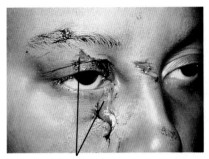

Lid lacerations

Figure 3-1 • Upper and lower eyelid margin lacerations.

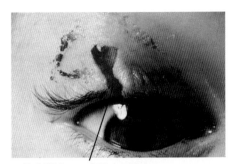

Full thickness lid laceration

Figure 3-2 • Full-thickness upper eyelid laceration.

- Surgical repair with stent (silicone intubation) placement in the nasolacrimal duct system.

- **Surgical repair of eyelid laceration not involving lid margin:** The area around the wound is infiltrated with 2% lidocaine with epinephrine 1:100,000. The area is prepped and draped using povidone-iodine [Betadine] solution. The wound is inspected carefully for the presence of foreign bodies. Deep portions of the wound are probed to the base of the wound to identify septal penetration. (Wounds involving levator muscle or levator aponeurosis require layered closure, usually with an extended incision along the major lid crease, and external repair.) Copiously irrigate with saline or bacitracin solution. All tissue should be preserved if possible; only severely necrotic tissue must be excised. Horizontal or arcuate wounds oriented along orbicularis typically are closed in a single layer that includes skin only; gaping wounds or wounds which are oriented transverse to orbicularis are closed in two layers. 6-0 polyglactin interrupted, buried sutures are used to close orbicularis; skin is closed with 6-0 nylon interrupted sutures. Wound is dressed with antibiotic ointment, and sutures are removed in 7-10 days.

- **Surgical repair of eyelid laceration involving lid margin, sparing canaliculus:** The area around the wound is infiltrated with 2% lidocaine with epinephrine 1:100,000. The area is prepped and draped using povidone-iodine [Betadine] solution. The wound is inspected carefully for the presence of foreign bodies. Canalicular involvement is assessed via lacrimal intubation. All tissue should be preserved, if possible; only severely necrotic tissue must be excised. The lid margin is reapproximated using two or three interrupted 6-0 nylon sutures. The initial suture is passed through the mucocutaneous junction, with one additional suture at the posterior lid margin and one through the lash line. It is important for each bite to be placed symmetrically with regard to its opposite counterpart. However, the three different sutures do not all have to be of equal distance from the wound margin. It is important to make the depth of each pass at equal to or greater than the width of each pass in order to avoid notching of the lid margin. These sutures are left long and may be placed untied on Steri-Strips temporarily. The tarsus is closed using interrupted lamellar 6-0 polyglactin sutures. Attention must be paid to the distance from the lid margin each suture is placed. In the upper lid it is important to avoid full-thickness bites onto the conjunctival surface, although this is safely tolerated in the lower eyelid. The lid margin sutures are now tied, and the ends are left long. Orbicularis is closed using interrupted, buried 6-0 polyglactin sutures. Skin is closed using interrupted 6-0 nylon sutures. The long ends of the lid margin sutures are incorporated into a skin suture to keep them away from the cornea. The wound is dressed with antibiotic ointment, and sutures are removed in 7-10 days.

• **Surgical repair of eyelid laceration involving lid margin and canaliculus:** The area is prepped and draped using povidone-iodine [Betadine] solution and inspected carefully with minimal manipulation. Small (0.3-mm) forceps and cotton-tipped applicators are helpful in locating the nasal end of the transected canaliculus. The area around the wound is infiltrated with 2% lidocaine with epinephrine 1:100,000. The punctum of the involved canaliculus is dilated and intubated with a Silastic stent (Crawford tube). The Crawford probe is passed entirely through the temporal portion of the canaliculus. It is then inserted into the nasal end, advanced to a hard stop against the lamina papyracea, and rotated into a superior-inferior orientation. The nasolacrimal duct is then intubated. The second arm of the tube is advanced through the opposite canaliculus, and the tubes are secured at the external naris. The canalicular tear is closed using two interrupted 7-0 polyglactin sutures which are passed through the canalicular walls, 180 degrees apart. Pericanalicular sutures are added as needed. The lid margin is repaired as described above. Tubes are removed after 3 months.

• For dirty wounds, systemic antibiotics (dicloxacillin 250-500 mg po qid for 7-10 days; consider penicillin V 500 mg po qid for animal or human bites).

■ Eyelid Infections

Blepharitis and Meibomitis

Definition

Inflammation of the eyelid margins (blepharitis) and inspissation of the oil-producing sebaceous glands of the lids (meibomitis); often occur together; extremely common in adult population and often coexist with dry eyes.

Etiology

Chronic *Staphylococcus* or *Demodex* infection, seborrhea, and eczema; angular blepharitis is associated with *Moraxella* infection.

Symptoms

Itching, red eye, burning, tearing, mild pain, foreign body sensation; often worse on awakening and late in the day.

Signs

Thickened and erythematous eyelid margins with telangiectatic blood vessels, crusting along eyelashes ("scurf" and "collarettes" in blepharitis); swollen, pitted, or blocked meibomian glands (meibomitis); may have "toothpaste sign" (gentle pressure on lids expresses columns of thick, white sebaceous material).

Flakes/collarettes Telangiectatic vessels

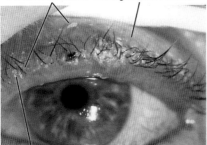

Thickened lid margin

Figure 3-3 • Blepharitis with thickened eyelid margins, flakes, and collarettes.

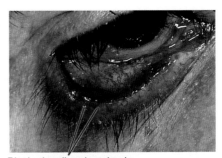

Blocked meibomian glands

Figure 3-4 • Meibomitis demonstrating inspissated right lower eyelid meibomian glands with obstructed, pouting meibomian gland orifices.

Differential Diagnosis

Acne rosacea, dry eye syndrome, herpes simplex virus, corneal foreign body, allergic or infectious conjunctivitis, chalazion or hordeolum (stye), sebaceous cell carcinoma, squamous or basal cell carcinoma, discoid lupus, medicamentosa, ocular cicatricial pemphigoid.

Evaluation

- Complete history with attention to history of skin cancer, sexually transmitted diseases, cold sores, allergies, eye medications, and chronic recurrent disease; unilateral, chronic, or refractory symptoms suggest malignancy.
- Complete eye examination with attention to lids, lashes, conjunctiva, and cornea.
- Biopsy if lesions are suspicious for malignancy (ulcerated, yellow, chronic, scarred, or unilateral lid lesions, often with concomitant corneal pathology).
- **Lab tests:** Chlamydia cultures (if there is associated chronic follicular conjunctivitis or suspicion of sexually transmitted disease).

Management

- Warm compresses for 10 minutes in both eyes qd to qid.
- Daily lid scrubs: Commercial preparations are available. Alternatively, a warm solution of baby shampoo and water (50:50 mixture) may be applied rigorously to the lids and lashes using cotton, a face cloth, or cotton-tipped applicator.
- Topical antibiotic ointment (bacitracin or erythromycin) at bedtime for 1-2 weeks.
- Consider short course (1-2 weeks) of topical antibiotic-steroid ointment (Tobradex) bid.
- Consider doxycycline 50-100 mg po qd for recalcitrant cases.
- Treat associated pathology such as rosacea or dry eye.

Prognosis

Good; recurrence common; maintenance treatment often required indefinitely.

Herpes Simplex Virus

Primary infection due to herpes simplex virus; often mild and unrecognized; patients may note pain, itching, and redness; appear as small crops of seropurulent vesicles on the eyelid that eventually rupture and crust over; marginal ulcerative blepharitis, follicular conjunctivitis, punctate or dendritic keratitis, and preauricular lymphadenopathy may also occur.

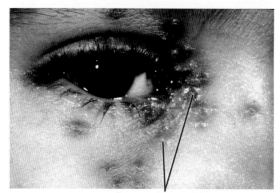

Figure 3-5 • Primary herpes simplex virus with eyelid vesicles.

Seropurulent vesicles

- Cool compresses bid to qid to affected skin area.
- Topical antiviral agents (trifluridine 0.1% 9 times/day or vidarabine 3% 5 times/day for 14 days) for patients with blepharoconjunctivitis or corneal involvement.
- Systemic antiviral (acyclovir [Zovirax] 400 mg po 5 times/day for 10 days or famciclovir [Famvir] 500 mg po tid for 7 days) when patient has constitutional symptoms.

Herpes Zoster Virus

Maculopapular skin eruption, followed by vesicular ulceration and crusting due to reactivation of latent varicella zoster virus in the first division of cranial nerve V; usually involves upper lid and does not cross the midline; patients may have fever, lymphadenopathy, headache, malaise, nausea, tingling, paresthesias, and burning over cranial nerve V1 dermatome; scarring may result with entropion, ectropion, lash loss (madarosis), canalicular and punctal stenosis, and lid retraction with exposure keratitis.

- Cool saline or aluminum sulfate-calcium acetate (Domeboro) compresses bid to tid.
- Topical antibiotic ointment (erythromycin or bacitracin bid to tid) to affected skin.
- Systemic antiviral (acyclovir [Zovirax] 800 mg po 5 times/day for 7-10 days, or famciclovir [Famvir] 500 mg po or valacyclovir 1 g po tid for 7 days); if immunocompromised, acyclovir 10-12 mg/kg/day, IV divided, q8h for 10-14 days.
- Treat postherpetic neuralgia with capsaicin ([Zostrix] 0.025% tid to qid) cream to affected skin or amitriptyline (25 mg po tid); other options include Neurontin, Lidoderm patches, and pain medications.

Vesicles with crusting

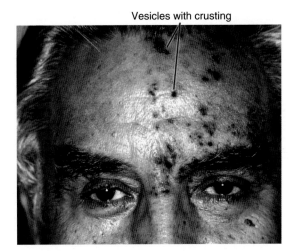

Figure 3-6 • Herpes zoster virus demonstrating unilateral VI dermatomal distribution (trigeminal ophthalmic branch).

Molluscum Contagiosum

DNA poxvirus infection, typically seen in children and spread by direct contact; usually asymptomatic; appears as shiny dome-shaped waxy papules with central umbilication on the lid or lid margin; papules may appear anywhere on the body; may be associated with chronic follicular conjunctivitis, superficial pannus, and superficial punctate keratitis; although disease is self-limited, resolution may take years; disseminated disease seen in patients with acquired immunodeficiency syndrome (AIDS).

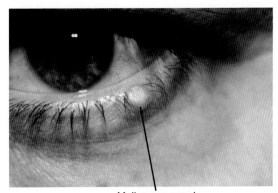

Figure 3-7 • Molluscum contagiosum demonstrating characteristic shiny, domed papule with central umbilication of the lower eyelid.

Molluscum papule

- Treatment is by curettage, cryotherapy, or cautery of one or more lesions with the intention of stimulating the immune system to eliminate satellite lesions. Suggested protocol includes excisional biopsy of one lesion with curettage of at least one additional lesion.

Demodicosis

Parasitic hair follicle infection with *Demodex folliculorum* or *D. brevis*; associated with blepharitis; very common infestation but usually asymptomatic; examination of epilated hair follicles reveals sleeves of thin, semitransparent crusting at the base of the lashes; may incite hordeolum formation.

- Lid scrubs may be effective: commercial preparations are available; alternatively, a warm solution of baby shampoo and water (50:50 mixture) may be applied rigorously to the lids and lashes using cotton, a face cloth, or cotton-tipped applicator.

Phthiriasis or Pediculosis

Infestation of eyelashes with lice *(Phthirus pubis);* usually sexually transmitted or from very close contact with an infected individual; patients note itching and burning; signs include small, pearly, white nits (eggs) attached to lashes, adult lice, preauricular lymphadenopathy, blood-tinged lids and lashes, blepharoconjunctivitis, conjunctival follicles, and conjunctival injection.

Phthirus pubis lice

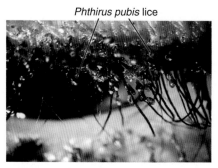

Phthirus pubis lice

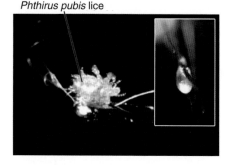

Figure 3-8 • Infestation of eyelashes with *Phthirus pubis.* Note the chronic skin changes at the base of the lashes.

Figure 3-9 • Close-up of eyelash with *Phthirus pubis.*

- Mechanical removal of lice and nits with fine forceps.
- Topical ointment (erythromycin, Lacri-Lube [white petrolatum, mineral oil, lanolin], or petroleum jelly tid for 14 days) to suffocate lice.
- Physostigmine 0.25% ointment × 1, repeat in 1 week, or fluorescein 20% 1-2 drops to lid margins plus delousing creams and shampoo (not for ocular use): permethrin cream rinse 1% (Nix), lindane 1%, γ-benzene hexachloride (Kwell), or pyrethrins liquid with piperonyl butoxide (RID, A-200 Pyrinate liquid) (Warning: Kwell and RID not recommended for pregnant women and children.)
- Discard or thoroughly wash in hot cycle all bedding, linens, and clothing.
- Treat sexual partner.

Leprosy

Chronic infectious disease caused by *Mycobacterium leprae,* a pleomorphic, acid-fast bacillus. Of the four variants, tuberculoid and lepromatous leprosy can have eyelid involvement, including loss of eyelashes and eyebrows, trichiasis, paralytic ectropion, lagophthalmos with exposure keratitis, and reduced blink rate; may develop corneal ulceration and perforation.

- Systemic multidrug treatment with dapsone (100 mg po qd) and rifampin (600 mg po qd); consider adding clofazimine (100 mg po qd).
- Reduce corneal exposure with temporary or permanent reversible tarsorrhaphy.

Eyelid Inflammations

Chalazion or Hordeolum (Stye)

Definition

Hordeolum Acute bacterial infection of sebaceous eyelid glands; most commonly meibomian glands (internal hordeolum) or the glands of Zeis or Moll (external hordeolum); associated with *Staphylococcus aureus*.

Chalazion Obstruction and inflammation of meibomian gland with leakage of sebum into surrounding tissue and resultant lipogranuloma formation; often evolving from an internal hordeolum; associated with widespread meibomitis or rosacea.

Symptoms

Painful, hot, swollen, red eyelid lump; chronic chalazia become nontender.

Signs

Erythematous subcutaneous nodule, sometimes tender with visible pointing or drainage; usually solitary, but can be multiple or bilateral; occasionally, severe swelling prevents visualization or palpation of a discrete nodule; may have signs of blepharitis and meibomitis.

Chalazion

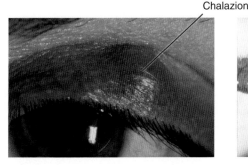 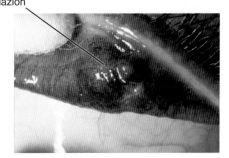

Figure 3-10 • Chalazion of the upper eyelid.

Figure 3-11 • Everted eyelid of the same patient in Figure 3-10, demonstrating the chalazion.

Differential Diagnosis

Preseptal cellulitis, sebaceous cell carcinoma, pyogenic granuloma.

Evaluation

• Complete ophthalmic history and eye examination with attention to previous episodes, fever, rosacea, meibomian gland evaluation, eyelid eversion, lashes, motility, and cornea.

Management

• Warm compresses with gentle massage for 10 minutes qid.
• Topical antibiotic ointment (erythromycin or bacitracin bid to tid) in the inferior fornix if lesion is draining.
• Consider incision and curettage after 1 month if no improvement.
• Consider intralesional steroid injection (triamcinolone acetate 40 mg/mL; inject 0.5 mL with 30-gauge needle) for chalazia near lacrimal system or if only partially responsive to incision and curettage.
• Recurrent lesion must be evaluated by biopsy to rule out malignancy.
• Treat underlying meibomitis and rosacea.
• Multiple and recurrent chalazia may respond to doxycycline 100 mg po bid or erythromycin 250 mg po qid. Tetracycline is avoided in children and women in childbearing years.

Prognosis

Good; may take weeks to months to resolve fully; recurrence is common (20%); conservative treatment is recommended; surgical drainage can lead to scarring and further episodes; steroid injection may produce hypopigmentation or local fat atrophy.

Contact Dermatitis

Definition

Acute dermatitis resulting from chemical or mechanical irritants, or from immunologic hypersensitivity to an allergic stimulus.

Symptoms

Swelling, redness, itching, tearing, foreign body sensation, and ocular and eyelid discomfort.

Signs

Erythematous, flaking, or crusting rash accompanied by edema; may have vesicular or weeping lesions; lichenified plaques suggest chronic exposure to irritant.

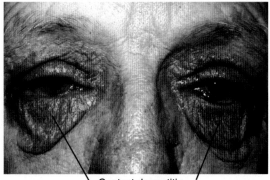

Figure 3-12 • Contact dermatitis, demonstrating bilateral erythematous, flaking rash.

Contact dermatitis

Differential Diagnosis

Herpes simplex, herpes zoster, preseptal cellulitis; chemical, ultraviolet, or thermal burns.

Evaluation

- Complete history with attention to exposure to irritants such as soaps, fragrances, cosmetics, hairspray, nail polish, jewelry, medications, poison ivy; and chemical, ultraviolet, or thermal exposure.
- Complete eye examination with attention to scalp, hair, hands, fingers, lids, and conjunctiva.

Management

- A stepwise approach is required given the wide range of severity that can be seen in eyelid dermatitis. Periocular steroids should not be used for more than 2 weeks without ophthalmic supervision.
- Identify and remove inciting agent(s); may require allergic patch testing to determine causative allergens.
- Cool compresses.
- Topical antibiotic ointment (erythromycin or bacitracin bid) to crusted or weeping lesions.
- Consider mild steroid cream (<1% hydrocortisone cream bid to tid for 7-10 days) on eyelids; avoid lid margins and ocular exposure (for this reason, it is safer to use an ophthalmic preparation, e.g., fluorometholone [FML] ointment).
- Alternatively, ophthalmic steroid solution (sulfacetamide-prednisolone [Blephamide]) may be massaged onto affected eyelids bid.
- Tacrolimus 0.1% (Protopic), a nonsteroidal ointment, is very effective in the treatment of eyelid dermatitis and can be considered a first-line medication in advance of topical steroids.
- Oral antihistamine (diphenhydramine 25-50 mg po tid to qid) for severe or widespread lesions or excessive itching.
- Consider short-term oral steroids (prednisone 40-80 mg po qd tapered over 10-14 days) for severe cases; check purified protein derivative (PPD), blood glucose, and chest radiographs before starting systemic steroids.
- Add H_2-blocker (Zantac 150 mg po bid) or proton pump inhibitor when taking systemic steroids.

Prognosis

Usually good; resolution occurs 1-2 weeks after removal of inciting agent; rebound can occur if steroids tapered too rapidly.

Blepharochalasis

Idiopathic, recurrent episodes of painless edema of the upper eyelids with or without redness and itching. Over time, repeated episodes may result in atrophy and laxity of the upper eyelid tissues. Typically occurs in young females, first episode usually occurs before the age of 20. Inflammation may be treated acutely with topical steroid (sulfacetamide-prednisolone [Blephamide] ointment); there is no treatment to prevent or shorten the episodes. Blepharoplasty may be helpful in addressing the long-term results of multiple inflammatory episodes.

Madarosis

Definition

Loss of eyelashes or eyebrows or both.

Etiology

Local   Chronic blepharitis, eyelid neoplasm (sebaceous cell carcinoma), burn, trauma, trichotillomania.

Systemic   Hypothyroidism, psoriasis, seborrheic dermatitis, chemotherapeutic agents, connective tissue disease (e.g., systemic lupus erythematosus), chronic malnutrition, alopecia syndromes.

Evaluation

• Complete ophthalmic history and eye examination with attention to eyelids and lashes. High suspicion for neoplasm, especially with focal areas of madarosis. Evaluation for underlying hormonal or nutritional deficits.

Management

• Treat underlying etiology.

Vitiligo and Poliosis

Total absence of melanin in hair follicles of the eyelashes or eyebrow (poliosis) and in skin (vitiligo), leading to focal patches of white hair or skin; associated with severe dermatitis, Vogt-Koyanagi-Harada syndrome, tuberous sclerosis, localized irradiation, sympathetic ophthalmia, and Waardenburg's syndrome (autosomal dominant, white forelock, congenital poliosis, nasal root abnormalities, synophrys, congenital deafness, iris heterochromia, and hypertelorism).

Poliosis

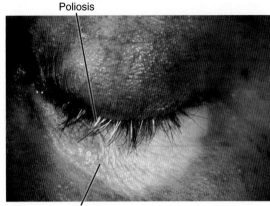

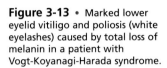

Figure 3-13 • Marked lower eyelid vitiligo and poliosis (white eyelashes) caused by total loss of melanin in a patient with Vogt-Koyanagi-Harada syndrome.

Vitiligo

• Treat underlying medical condition.

Acne Rosacea

Definition

Chronic inflammatory disorder of the midline facial skin and eyelids.

Etiology

Etiology is unknown; there is a genetic predilection and it is more common in certain ethnic backgrounds (e.g., Northern European ancestry). Rosacea may result from degenerative changes in perivascular collagen resulting in blood vessel dilation and leakage of inflammatory substances into the skin. It has also been suggested that the pathophysiology may include an inflammatory response to *D. folliculorum*.

Symptoms

Facial flushing (often resulting from a trigger such as ingestion of alcohol or spicy food), tearing, dry eye, foreign body sensation.

Signs

Acne, facial and eyelid telangiectasia, flushing most predominantly involving the nose and malar skin, persistent facial erythema, rhinophyma, blepharitis, chalazia, conjunctivitis, keratitis, peripheral corneal neovascularization, shortened tear break-up time.

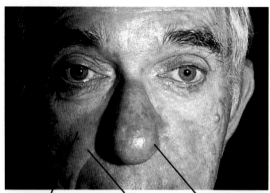

Figure 3-14 • Acne rosacea demonstrating rhinophyma (bulbous nose) and midline facial erythema in the malar and brow regions.

Erythema   Telangiectasia   Papules

Evaluation

- Complete ophthalmic history and eye examination with attention to facial skin, eyelids, conjunctiva, and cornea.

Management

DERMATOLOGIC MANIFESTATIONS

- Doxycycline 100 mg po bid for 3 weeks, followed by 100 mg po qd for 3-4 months. Tetracycline is also effective but requires more frequent dosing and is associated with more frequent gastrointestinal side effects. Neither doxycycline nor tetracycline is offered to women in their childbearing years nor to children with deciduous dentition.
- Topical metronidazole (MetroGel) 0.75% bid for 2-4 weeks.
- Avoidance of triggers of flushing (alcohol, spicy foods, extreme temperatures, prolonged sunlight exposure, caffeine).
- Advanced rhinophyma can be treated with carbon dioxide laser, incisional surgery, or electrocauterization.

OPHTHALMIC MANIFESTATIONS

- Doxycycline (see above).
- Lid hygiene: twice-daily application of warm compresses to the eyelids followed by cleansing of the lid margins with commercial lid scrub pads, or face cloth or cotton-tipped applicator soaked in dilute baby shampoo solution.

Eyelid Malpositions

Ptosis

Definition

Drooping of the upper eyelid(s).

Etiology

Aponeurotic (Involutional)

Disinsertion, central dehiscence, or attenuation of the levator aponeurosis causing poor levator function. Most common form of ptosis, often associated with advanced age, eye surgery or trauma, pregnancy, chronic eyelid swelling, and blepharochalasis; good levator function.

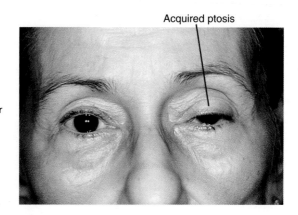

Acquired ptosis

Figure 3-15 • Significant acquired ptosis of the left eye. Most commonly caused by levator aponeurosis attenuation or dehiscence.

Mechanical

Poor upper eyelid elevation due to mass effect of tumors, or to tethering of the eyelid by scarring (cicatricial ptosis); good levator function.

Myogenic

Inherent weakness of levator palpebrae superioris due to disorders of neuromuscular junction including chronic progressive external ophthalmoplegia, myotonic dystrophy, and oculopharyngeal dystrophy; extremely poor levator function.

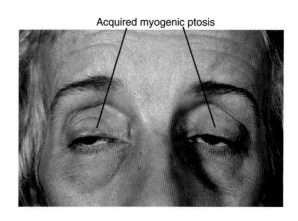

Acquired myogenic ptosis

Figure 3-16 • Bilateral acquired myogenic ptosis due to myasthenia gravis.

Neurogenic

Defects in innervation to cranial nerve III (oculomotor palsy) or sympathetic input to Müller's muscle (Horner's syndrome) or generalized dysfunction of neuromuscular junction such as myasthenia gravis; levator function varies according to etiology.

Congenital

Poor levator function from birth; usually unilateral, nonhereditary, and myogenic with fibrosis and fat infiltration of levator muscle; rarely results from aponeurosis dehiscence (possibly birth trauma), in which case good levator function would be expected. Congenital Horner's syndrome (ptosis, miosis, anhidrosis, iris hypopigmentation) with poor Müller's muscle function from decreased sympathetic tone, or congenital neurogenic with Marcus Gunn jaw-winking syndrome from aberrant connections between cranial nerve V (innervating the pterygoid muscles) and the levator muscle.

Congenital ptosis

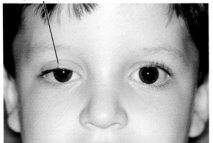

Poor levator function

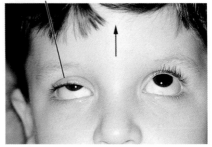

Figure 3-17 • Congenital ptosis of the right eye in a child.

Figure 3-18 • Same patient as shown in Figure 3-17, demonstrating poor levator function with upgaze of the right eye. Note reduced levator excursion.

Symptoms

Superior visual field defect, brow ache, loss of depth perception; deprivation amblyopia in congenital cases.

Signs

Drooping of upper eyelid(s) with impaired elevation on upgaze, recruitment of brow muscles with brow furrows, higher lid crease and apparently smaller eye on ptotic side, abnormally high contralateral eyelid (Hering's law); in downgaze, affected lid may be higher than contra-lateral lid in congenital ptosis (lid lag) and lower in acquired cases; may have decreased visual acuity when visual axis obscured or head tilt with chin-up position when bilateral; other associated abnormalities in congenital ptosis include lagophthalmos, decreased superior rectus function, high astigmatism, anisometropia, strabismus, amblyopia, epicanthus, and blepharophimosis.

Differential Diagnosis

Dermatochalasis (excess skin of upper eyelids, pseudoptosis), lid swelling, enophthalmos (e.g., orbital floor fracture), hypotropia, contralateral eyelid retraction causing asymmetry (e.g., thyroid ophthalmopathy), small eye (e.g., phthisis bulbi, microphthalmia, anophthalmia).

Evaluation

- Complete ophthalmic history with attention to age of onset, previous surgeries or trauma, degree of functional impairment and time of day when worst, associated symptoms such as generalized fatigue, breathing problems, diplopia.
- Complete eye examination with attention to amblyopia in children, visual acuity, pupils, motility, Bell's phenomenon, corneal sensation, and cornea.
- Eyelid measurements: margin reflex distance, palpebral fissure height, upper lid crease height (high in aponeurotic), and levator function (normal in aponeurotic, decreased in congenital).
- Consider neurologic evaluation with edrophonium chloride (Tensilon) test to rule out myasthenia gravis.
- Consider phenylephrine 2.5% to stimulate Müller's muscle and rule out Horner's syndrome; may also use topical cocaine 4-10% or hydroxyamphetamine 1% or both.
- Check visual field test with and without lids being held open by tape or finger (ptosis visual fields) to document visual impairment prior to surgery.

Management

- Ptosis is treated with surgery.
  Good levator function: levator aponeurosis advancement, levator resection, Fasanella-Servat tarsoconjunctival resection.
  Poor levator function: frontalis suspension with silicone rods, fascia lata, or frontalis flap. Maximal levator resection may be useful in some cases.
  Superior tarsal (Müller's muscle) resection in Horner's syndrome or mild ptosis with good levator function.
- Ptosis is a difficult surgical challenge that often is confused with the simpler technique of blepharoplasty. Ptosis surgery should be performed by an experienced eyelid surgeon.
- Avoid surgery or undercorrect when poor Bell's reflex or decreased corneal sensation exists.
- Treat underlying medical problems.

Prognosis

Prognosis for acquired mechanical and aponeurotic ptosis is excellent; congenital is fair to excellent; myogenic and neurogenic are variable.

Dermatochalasis

Laxity of the upper eyelid tissues resulting in redundancy of skin and subcutaneous tissue. Frequently associated with herniation of orbital fat through an attenuated orbital septum. May be associated with upper lid ptosis or pseudoptosis (mechanical effect of dermatochalasis). Profound dermatochalasis may result in superior visual field defect. Management is surgical with careful attention given preoperatively to coexisting conditions (e.g., ptosis). Lower lid dermatochalasis, on very rare occasion, may limit vision in downgaze due to extreme orbital fat herniation.

Pseudoptosis   Dermatochalasis

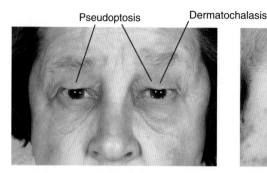 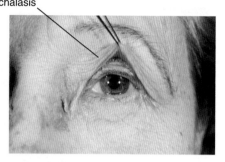

Figure 3-19 • A patient with pseudoptosis from dermatochalasis.

Figure 3-20 • Dermatochalasis with redundant upper eyelid skin and subcutaneous tissue and herniated orbital fat.

Ectropion

Definition

Eversion of the eyelid margin.

Etiology

Cicatricial

Due to burns (thermal or chemical), trauma (surgical or mechanical), or chronic inflammation with anterior lamellar contraction.

Congenital

Due to vertical shortening of anterior lamella (skin and orbicularis oculi), rarely isolated, may be associated with blepharophimosis syndrome.

Inflammatory

Due to chronic eyelid skin inflammation (atopic dermatitis, herpes zoster infections, rosacea).

Involutional

Due to horizontal lid laxity and tissue relaxation, followed by lid elongation, sagging, and conjunctival hypertrophy; usually involves lower eyelid; most frequent cause of ectropion in adults.

Mechanical

Due to lid edema, bulky lid tumors, orbital fat herniation, or lid-riding spectacles.

Paralytic

Usually follows cranial nerve VII palsy; often temporary.

Symptoms

Tearing, chronic eyelid or ocular irritation, or asymptomatic.

Signs

Eversion of eyelid margin, conjunctival keratinization, injection and hypertrophy, superficial punctate keratitis, dermatitis (from chronic tearing and rubbing).

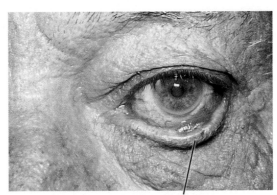

Figure 3-21 • Involutional ectropion of the left lower eyelid.

Ectropion

Evaluation

- Complete ophthalmic history with attention to history of burns, trauma, surgery, or facial droop (cranial nerve VII [Bell's] palsy).
- Complete eye examination with attention to orbicularis function, lateral canthal tendon laxity, lids, herniated fat and scarring, conjunctiva, and cornea.

Management

- Treat ectropion-related corneal and conjunctival exposure with topical lubrication with preservative-free artificial tears (see Appendix) up to q1h and ointment (Refresh P.M.) at bedtime.

CICATRICIAL

- Four-step procedure: (1) cicatrix release and relaxation, (2) horizontal lid tightening with lateral tarsal strip, (3) anterior lamella lengthening with full-thickness skin graft or cheek lift, and (4) posterior lamellar spacer (with ear cartilage or other).

CONGENITAL

- Mild ectropion often requires no treatment. Moderate or severe ectropion treated like cicatricial ectropion with horizontal lid tightening and full-thickness skin graft to vertically lengthen anterior lamella.

Management—cont'd

INFLAMMATORY

- Treat underlying dermatologic condition. Temporizing measures include taping temporal side of eyelid, using moisture chambers, and topical lubrication with preservative-free artificial tears (see Appendix) up to q1h.

INVOLUTIONAL

- Three procedures may be used individually or in combination: (1) medial spindle procedure for punctal ectropion, (2) horizontal lid shortening using lateral tarsal strip procedure, lateral lid wedge resection, or canthal tendon plication, and (3) lower lid retractor reinsertion.

MECHANICAL

- Treat mechanical force causing ectropion (tumor or fat removal, eyeglass adjustment, etc.).

PARALYTIC

- Often resolves spontaneously within 6 months if due to Bell's palsy. Temporizing measures include taping temporal side of eyelid, suture tarsorrhaphy, using moisture chambers, and topical lubrication with preservative-free artificial tears (see Appendix) up to q1h; rarely, if chronic, consider canthoplasty, lateral tarsorrhaphy, brow suspension, and horizontal lid tightening with or without middle lamellar buttress such as ear cartilage.

Prognosis

Usually good with surgical treatment; cicatricial or inflammatory ectropion is prone to recurrence; paralytic ectropion may resolve spontaneously within 6 months after Bell's palsy.

Entropion

Definition

Inversion of the eyelid margin; may affect either eyelid, although the lower lid is affected more frequently.

Etiology

Cicatricial

Due to posterior lamella (tarsus and conjunctiva) shortening with lid inversion and rubbing of lashes and lid margin on globe; associated with Stevens-Johnson syndrome, ocular cicatricial pemphigoid, trachoma, herpes zoster, ocular surgery, and ocular trauma. More common in upper eyelid.

Congenital

Due to structural tarsal plate defects, shortened posterior lamellae, or eyelid retractor dysgenesis; usually affects upper eyelid.

Involutional

Most common cause of entropion in older patients, usually affects lower lid; predisposing factors include horizontal lid laxity, overriding preseptal orbicularis, disinserted or atrophied lid retractors, and involutional enophthalmos.

Spastic

Due to ocular inflammation or irritation; often seen following ocular surgery in patients with early underlying involutional changes.

Symptoms

Tearing, foreign body sensation, red eye.

Signs

Inturned eyelid margin, keratinized eyelid margins (cicatricial), horizontal lid laxity, overriding preseptal orbicularis, enophthalmos, symblepharon (cicatricial), conjunctival injection, superficial punctate keratitis.

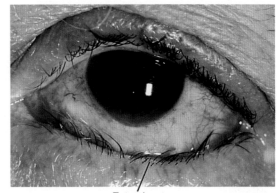

Figure 3-22 • Involutional entropion of the left lower eyelid.

Entropion

Differential Diagnosis

Trichiasis, distichiasis, blepharospasm.

Evaluation

- Complete ophthalmic history with attention to history of eye surgery, trauma, eye infections, burns.
- Complete eye examination with attention to lid tone (snapback test), lower lid margin (sagging), medial and lateral canthal tendons, inferior fornix (unusually deep), digital eversion test at the inferior border of tarsus to distinguish involutional from cicatricial entropion (involutional rotates, cicatricial does not).

Management

- If corneal involvement exists, topical antibiotic ointment (erythromycin or bacitracin bid to qid).

CICATRICIAL

- Excision of scar and consider anterior lamellar resection or recession for minimal involvement; tarsal fracture procedure for lower lid involvement; tarsal graft from preserved sclera, ear cartilage, or hard palate if the tarsus is badly damaged; may also require conjunctival and mucous membrane grafts in severe cases.

CONGENITAL

- Rarely improves and often requires surgical treatment to correct underlying anatomic defect.

INVOLUTIONAL

- Three procedures may be used individually or in combination: (1) temporizing measure with lid taping below lower lid, Quickert suture, or thermal cautery, (2) horizontal lid tightening with lateral tarsal strip procedure, and (3) lid retractor repair with full-thickness transverse blepharoplasty and eyelid margin rotation (Wies' procedure) or retractor reinsertion.

SPASTIC

- Break entropion–irritation cycle by taping inturned lid to evert margin, thermal cautery, or suture techniques to temporarily evert lid; often requires more definitive procedure as involutional changes progress (see below).

Prognosis

Good prognosis except for autoimmune or inflammatory related cicatricial entropion.

▉ Blepharospasm

Definition

Bilateral, uncontrolled, episodic contraction of orbicularis oculi.

Essential Blepharospasm

Thought to be caused by disorder of the basal ganglia; usually with gradual onset during the fifth to seventh decade; likely genetic disorder given high incidence of movement disorders among first-degree relatives.

Meige's Syndrome

Essential blepharospasm with facial grimacing; may have cog-wheeling in the neck and extremities.

Symptoms

Uncontrollable blinking, squeezing, or twitching of eyelids or facial muscles.

Signs

Spasms of orbicularis oculi or facial muscles; may prevent examiner from prying open lids during episodes; may be absent during sleep.

Differential Diagnosis

Reflex blepharospasm (caused by eyelid irritation, dry eye, entropion, trichiasis, contact lens overuse, or meningeal irritation), hemifacial spasm, facial myokymia, Tourette's syndrome, tic douloureux (trigeminal neuralgia), Parkinson's disease, Huntington's disease, basal ganglia infarct.

Evaluation

- Complete ophthalmic history with attention to causes of ocular irritation, stress and caffeine use, and history of neurologic disorders.
- Complete eye examination with attention to cranial nerves, motility, and lids.
- Head magnetic resonance imaging (MRI) with attention to the posterior fossa.

Management

- Injection of botulinum type A toxin (BTX, Botox) into the orbicularis muscle to weaken contractions; repeat injections are often required every 12 weeks as the therapeutic effect declines; transient ptosis and diplopia are uncommon side effects.
- Medical therapy with haloperidol, clonazepam, bromocriptine, or baclofen has limited success.

Prognosis

Good with appropriate therapy; in most cases, repeat injections are needed indefinitely.

■ Bell's Palsy

Definition

Acutely acquired, isolated, peripheral facial paralysis of unknown cause involving cranial nerve VII (facial nerve).

Etiology

By definition, the etiology is unknown. Neural inflammation has been identified by MRI and on autopsy. Herpes virus is thought to play a role in most cases.

Symptoms

Acute onset of unilateral facial paralysis over a period of 24 hours, often accompanied by headache and numbness; dry eye, foreign body sensation, tearing, drooling, dysarthria, and dysphagia. Long-term symptoms include ipsilateral hypertonicity, oral-ocular synkinesis, gustatory lacrimation, decreased vision, corneal irritation.

Signs

Unilateral facial paralysis including all divisions of the cranial nerve VII (facial). Chronic signs include brow ptosis, ipsilateral hypertonicity, lagophthalmos, exposure keratopathy with ulceration, and scarring.

Table 3-1   House-Brackmann Facial Nerve Grading System

Grade	Description	Characteristics
I	Normal	Normal facial function
II	Mild dysfunction	Very slight weakness seen on close inspection; good forehead function; complete and quick eyelid closure
III	Moderate dysfunction	Obvious but not disfiguring asymmetry; mild synkinesis; slight forehead movement; complete eyelid closure with effort
IV	Moderately severe dysfunction	Disfiguring asymmetry; no forehead movement; incomplete eyelid closure
V	Severe dysfunction	Barely perceptible facial movement; incomplete eyelid closure
VI	Total paralysis	No movement

Adapted from House JW, Brackmann DE: Facial nerve grading system, *Otolaryngol Head Neck Surg* 93:146, 1985.

Differential Diagnosis

Tumor of parotid gland or facial nerve, trauma (temporal bone fracture), congenital facial nerve palsy, herpes zoster cephalicus, central nervous system (CNS) disease, postsurgical.

Evaluation

* Complete history with attention to date, time, and nature of onset, duration of symptoms, evidence of improvement within first 4 months.
* Complete eye examination with attention to cranial nerves, lagophthalmos, orbicularis function, brow position, lower lid retraction, corneal sensation, corneal epithelium, epiphora.
* Delayed onset with progression over more than 1 week requires MRI of facial nerve and CT of temporal bone.
* Additional cranial nerve involvement requires further brain stem investigation.

Management

- Initially, aggressive lubrication of ocular surface with viscous artificial tears (see Appendix) up to q1h and ointment qhs. Consider taping lid closed at night, some patients prefer Tegaderm dressing instead of tape; also consider gold weight implantation or temporary lateral tarsorrhaphy.
- Follow monthly for signs of improvement. Lack of improvement after 4 months is ominous and requires further investigation (MRI and CT scan).
- Consider antiviral (acyclovir) and antiinflammatory (prednisone) treatment.
- Chronic sequelae can be treated surgically (persistent paralysis) or with botulinum toxin (aberrant regeneration).
- There is no evidence to support the use of electrical facial stimulation, nor is there strong evidence supporting the efficacy of facial physical therapy.

Prognosis

Typically excellent with most patients returning to nearly complete function (grade 2); 90% of function returns within 1 year, 99% within 2 years.

■ Floppy Eyelid Syndrome

Definition

Chronic papillary conjunctivitis with lax tarsi, spontaneous eyelid eversion, and loss of eyelid-globe contact when lying prone; often occurs in obese men with sleep apnea.

Etiology

Nocturnal lid eversion with rubbing of the tarsal conjunctiva against bedding.

Symptoms

Chronically red and irritated eyes, particularly upon awakening; mild mucous discharge.

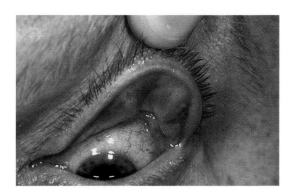

Figure 3-23 • Floppy eyelid syndrome demonstrating extreme laxity of upper eyelid. Note upper eyelid papillary conjunctivitis due to nocturnal lid eversion.

Signs

Loose, rubbery eyelids (particularly upper lids), very easily everted, palpebral conjunctival papillae, conjunctival injection, superficial punctate keratitis.

Differential Diagnosis

Giant papillary conjunctivitis, adult inclusion conjunctivitis, superior limbic keratoconjunctivitis, vernal keratoconjunctivitis, atopic keratoconjunctivitis, medicamentosa.

Evaluation

• Complete ophthalmic history and eye examination with attention to eyelid laxity, palpebral conjunctiva, and corneal surface staining with fluorescein.

Management

- Topical lubrication with preservative-free artificial tears (see Appendix) up to q1h.
- If corneal involvement exists, add topical antibiotic ointment (erythromycin or bacitracin bid to qid for 5-7 days).
- Metal eye shield when sleeping.
- Consider surgical correction using eyelid wedge resection. Sleep study with internist or otolaryngologist.

Prognosis

Excellent.

■ Trichiasis

Definition

Misdirected eyelashes.

Etiology

Entropion, cicatricial eye disease, chronic eyelid inflammation, or idiopathic.

Symptoms

Red eye, foreign body sensation, and tearing.

Signs

Eyelashes directed toward and rubbing against the eye, conjunctival injection, superficial punctate keratitis; may have corneal scarring in chronic cases.

Trichiasis

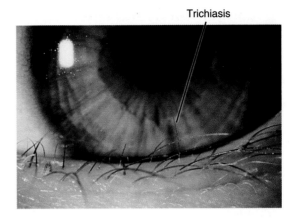

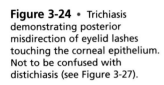

Figure 3-24 • Trichiasis demonstrating posterior misdirection of eyelid lashes touching the corneal epithelium. Not to be confused with distichiasis (see Figure 3-27).

Differential Diagnosis

Distichiasis (ectopic eyelashes).

Evaluation

- Complete ophthalmic history and eye examination with attention to lids, lashes, tarsal plate, palpebral conjunctiva, and cornea.

Management

- Topical lubrication with preservative-free artificial tears (see Appendix) up to q1h.
- If corneal involvement exists, add topical antibiotic ointment (erythromycin or bacitracin bid to qid for 5-7 days).
- Mechanical epilation using fine forceps if only a few lashes are misdirected.
- For segmental trichiasis, consider cryotherapy using a double freeze-thaw technique, lashes then mechanically removed using fine forceps; complications include lid edema, eyelid notching, and skin depigmentation.
- Electroepilation for extensive or recurrent trichiasis; use limited application because of the potential of scarring adjacent follicles and eyelid tissue.
- Consider full-thickness wedge resection with primary closure for segmental trichiasis or entropion repair (see Entropion section); should be performed by an oculoplastic surgeon.

Prognosis

Frequent recurrences with mechanical technique, usually good with permanent removal.

■ Congenital Eyelid Anomalies

Ankyloblepharon

Partial or complete eyelid fusion; severe forms may be associated with craniofacial abnormalities; prognosis usually good unless severe associated defects.

* Simple cases treated with incision of skin webs after clamping with hemostat for 10-15 seconds with reapproximation of skin and conjunctiva; severe cases may necessitate major surgical revision.

Blepharophimosis

Tight, foreshortened (vertically and horizontally) palpebral fissures with poor eyelid function and no levator fold; may be sporadic or part of congenital syndrome (autosomal dominant [AD]) with blepharophimosis, blepharoptosis, epicanthus inversus, and telecanthus; prognosis depends on extent of syndrome and need for additional surgery; mapped to chromosome 3q.

No levator fold   Telecanthus

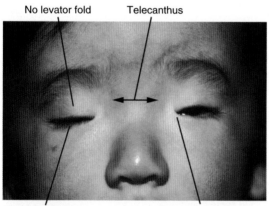

Figure 3-25 • Blepharophimosis syndrome demonstrating small palpebral fissures, lack of upper lid folds, ptosis, epicanthus inversus, and telecanthus.

Blepharophimosis   Epicanthus inversus

* Surgery usually is performed at 4-5 years of age to allow nasal bridge to develop fully.
* Congenital syndrome: consider staged oculoplastic repair with medial canthoplasty via Y-V plasty and transnasal wiring, followed by frontalis suspension for ptosis 3 to 4 months later, and finally full-thickness skin graft from periauricular or supraclavicular area.

Coloboma

Small notch to full-thickness defect of the eyelid due to incomplete union of frontonasal or maxillary mesoderm at the eyelid margin, usually superonasal and unilateral; inferolateral defects are often bilateral and associated with systemic anomalies such as mandibulofacial dysostosis (AD; Treacher Collins syndrome); corneal exposure and dryness may occur; small defects (<25%) have good prognosis; prognosis of medium and larger defects depends on location and associated abnormalities. Associated with microphthalmos, iris coloboma, and anterior polar cataract.

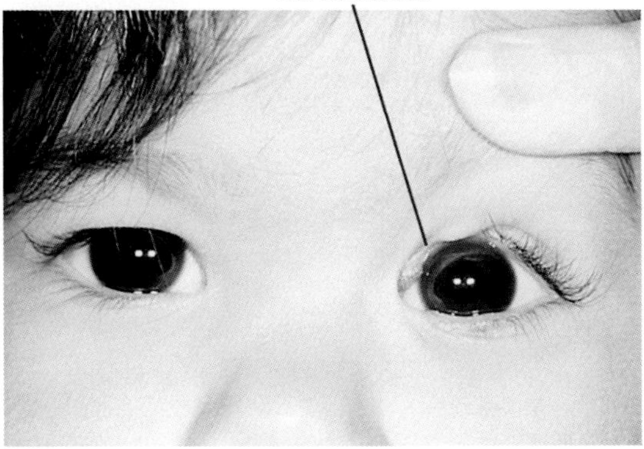

Lid coloboma

Figure 3-26 • Superonasal coloboma of left upper eyelid in a child.

- Topical lubrication with preservative-free artificial tears or ointments (see Appendix) up to q1h.
- Surgical repair (delay until preschool age): small defects (<25%) via pentagonal resection with direct layered closure, medium defects (25-50%) via Tenzel flap with or without lateral cantholysis, large defects (>50%) via myocutaneous flap or full-thickness lid rotation flap.
- Beware of lid-sharing procedures in children because occlusion amblyopia may result.

Cryptophthalmos

Congenital defects of the first, second, and third wave of neural crest migration leading to abnormal lid and anterior eye structure development, including partial or complete absence of eyebrow, palpebral fissure, eyelashes, and conjunctiva; may have hidden or buried eye with smooth skin stretching from brow to cheek; posterior structures are usually normal; prognosis often poor due to underlying structural ocular defects.

- Treatment focuses on progressive expansion of the understimulated bony orbit to prevent midfacial hypoplasia; multiple surgeries or expanding conformers often are required with eyelid reconstruction.

Distichiasis

Ectopic eyelashes growing posterior to or out of the meibomian gland orifices; may be congenital or acquired, sometimes hereditary; lashes are usually shorter, softer, and finer than normal cilia; usually well tolerated. In congenital distichiasis, the embryonic pilosebaceous units inappropriately develop into hair follicles; treat with caution, because treatment can be more damaging than disease.

- Topical lubrication with preservative-free artificial tears or ointments (see Appendix) or soft contact lens in mild cases.
- Epilation, cryotherapy, electrolysis, laser thermal ablation in more severe cases of corneal involvement.

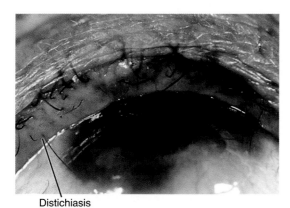

Figure 3-27 • Distichiasis with lashes originating from meibomian gland orifice.

Distichiasis

Epiblepharon

Redundant skin and orbicularis muscle leading to inward rotation of the lower eyelid margins, turning lashes against the globe; usually resolves spontaneously; more common in Asians; prognosis excellent even if surgery necessary.

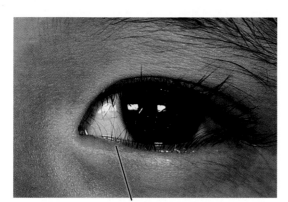

Figure 3-28 • Epiblepharon of lower eyelid demonstrating upwardly directed lashes.

Epiblepharon

- Conservative treatment in infants, because condition tends to resolve with facial maturation.
- Subciliary myocutaneous excision is extremely effective; care is taken to avoid overexcision with resultant ectropion.

Epicanthus

Crescentic vertical skin folds in the medial canthal area overlying the medial canthal tendon; usually bilateral; caused by immature facial bones or redundant skin and underlying tissue; may be most prominent superiorly (epicanthus tarsalis), inferiorly (epicanthus inversus), or equally distributed (epicanthus palpebralis); epicanthus tarsalis frequently associated with Asian eyelids, while epicanthus inversus associated with blepharophimosis syndrome; good prognosis.

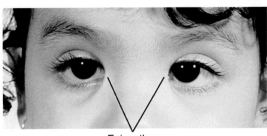

Figure 3-29 • Epicanthus demonstrating pseudostrabismus. Note vertical skin fold over medial canthal areas.

Epicanthus

- If due to facial bone immaturity, delay treatment.
- When treatment required (delay until preschool age), Z-plasty or Y-V plasty often effective; eyelid crease construction may be required.

Euryblepharon

Horizontal widening of the palpebral fissure, often temporally; usually involves the lower eyelid with an antimongoloid appearance due to inferior insertion of the lateral canthal tendon; patients have a poor blink, poor lid closure, and lagophthalmos with exposure keratitis; usually good prognosis.

- Topical lubrication with preservative-free artificial tears (see Appendix) in mild cases.
- If symptoms severe and corneal pathology exists, full-thickness eyelid resection with repositioning of lateral canthal tendon may be required. If necessary, vertical eyelid lengthening can be achieved with skin grafts.

Microblepharon

Rare, bilateral, vertical foreshortening of the eyelids, sometimes causing exposure and dry eye symptoms; may be related to cryptophthalmos; usually stable with good prognosis if no exposure keratitis exists.

- Topical lubrication with preservative-free artificial tears (see Appendix) in mild cases.
- Pedicle rotation skin flaps from cheek or brow, eyelid-sharing procedures, or full-thickness skin grafts for severe exposure with a normal globe.
- Beware of lid-sharing procedures in children because occlusion amblyopia may result.

Telecanthus

Increased distance between medial canthi caused by long medial canthal tendons (contrast with hypertelorism in which the distance between the medial walls of the orbits is increased); most frequent ocular finding in fetal alcohol syndrome; also associated with Waardenburg's syndrome and blepharophimosis syndrome; good prognosis.

Telecanthus

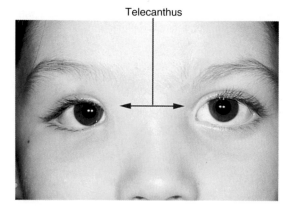

Figure 3-30 • Telecanthus. Note increased distance between medial canthi.

- Transnasal wiring to shorten distance between medial canthi and remove excess medial canthal skin.

Benign Eyelid Tumors

Pigmented Benign Eyelid Tumors

Acquired Nevus

Darkly pigmented lesion that contains modified melanocytes called nevocellular nevus cells; classified according to location in skin: junctional (epidermis), compound (epidermis and dermis), or dermal (dermis); may contain hair; malignant transformation rare, although the Halo nevus, a type of compound nevus, is associated with remote cutaneous malignant melanoma. The Spitz nevus, another type of compound nevus, may be confused histologically with malignant melanoma in children and young adults.

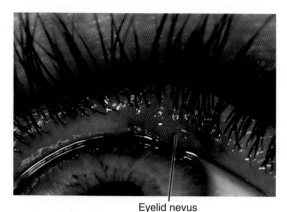

Figure 3-31 • Nevus of the upper eyelid along the lid margin.

Eyelid nevus

- No treatment usually required.
- Consider excision for cosmesis, chronic irritation, or evidence of malignant transformation.

Ephelis (Freckle)

Focal regions of cutaneous melanocytic overactivity; cells slightly larger than normal; seen in sun-exposed areas; occurs in individuals with fair complexions; no malignant potential.

• No treatment recommended.

Nevus of Ota (Oculodermal Melanocytosis)

Unilateral, blue-gray, pigmented macule; usually in the distribution of the first and second division of cranial nerve V with ipsilateral melanocytosis of the sclera and uveal tract; 10% bilateral; melanosis of the ipsilateral orbit and leptomeninges may occur; histologically, composed of dermal fusiform dendritic melanocytes. May be present at birth or during the first year of life; risk of malignant transformation is very low; however, cutaneous and ocular melanoma can occur, especially in whites.

Oculodermal melanocytosis

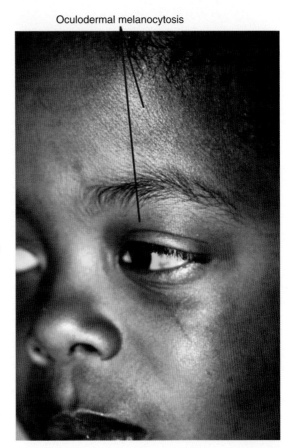

Figure 3-32 • Nevus of Ota of the left eye and orbit demonstrating unilateral, blue-gray, pigmented macule and pigmented sclera most prominent laterally.

• No treatment usually required.
• Periodic examinations to monitor for evidence of malignant transformation.

Seborrheic Keratosis

Waxy, pigmented, hyperkeratotic, plaquelike, crusty lesion often seen in the elderly; histologically, composed of intradermal proliferation of basal epithelioid cells; irritation is frequent; no malignant potential.

Seborrheic keratosis

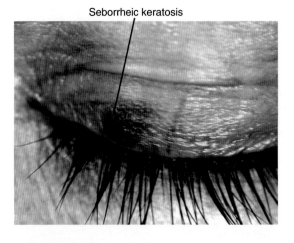

Figure 3-33 • Seborrheic keratosis at the lash line.

* Shave excision or curettage for small lesions.
* Complete surgical excision for larger lesions.

Squamous Papilloma

Most common benign eyelid growth; found in older adults; benign hyperplasia of the squamous epithelium; may be sessile or pedunculated with color similar to that of skin; grows slowly and in groups; etiology is unclear; viral papillomas are seen in groups and more common in children, while the elderly usually develop individual or widely spaced papillomas that are not thought to be viral in origin; histologically, papillomas display epithelial hyperkeratosis and acanthosis around a central vascular core.

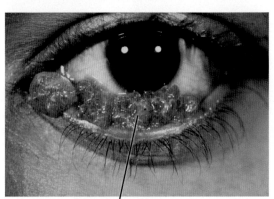

Figure 3-34 • Squamous papilloma demonstrating abundant multiple lesions of the lower eyelid.

Squamous papilloma

* Complete surgical excision.

Verruca Vulgaris (Viral Papilloma)

Viral-related growth with potential for malignant transformation; usually asymptomatic; appears as a pedunculated or sessile hyperemic mass on eyelid or tarsal conjunctiva with minimal surrounding inflammation; associated with human papillomavirus (strains 6, 11, and 16); frequently resolves spontaneously.

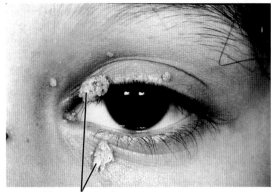

Figure 3-35 • Verruca vulgaris demonstrating multiple large and small lesions of the eyelids.

Verruca vulgaris

• Observation if small and no inflammation.

Larger or multiple lesions may be entirely excised, scraped, cauterized, or treated with cryotherapy; satellite lesions are thought to respond to initial treatment of selected lesions.

Nonpigmented Benign Eyelid Tumors

Xanthelasma

Xanthomas of the eyelids that appear as flat or slightly elevated creamy yellow plaques; usually bilateral, involving the medial upper lids; histologically composed of foamy histiocytes surrounded by localized inflammation; occurs in older patients; most patients with xanthelasma are normolipidemic; systemic diseases that demonstrate xanthomatosis include biliary cirrhosis, diabetes, pancreatitis, renal disease, and hypothyroidism; xanthelasma is the least specific of the xanthomas (nodular, tendinous, eruptive, and plaques); excellent prognosis, usually recur after excision.

Xanthelasma

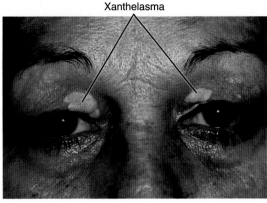

Figure 3-36 • Xanthelasma demonstrating characteristic yellow plaques on upper eyelids bilaterally.

* **Lab tests:** In extreme cases, serum cholesterol and triglycerides.
* Full-thickness excision with flaps or grafts, carbon dioxide laser treatment, or chemical cauterization with trichloroacetic acid as needed.

Moll's Gland Cyst (Hidrocystoma, Sudoriferous Cyst)

Benign cystic lesion resulting from abnormal proliferation of apocrine secretory gland (gland of Moll); also known as sudoriferous cyst or cystadenoma; smooth, translucent, and several millimeters in size; usually slow growing and painless; commonly involves the eyelid, particularly the inner canthus in a peripunctal location. No predilection for race or gender but more frequent in adults than in children. Differential diagnosis includes cystic basal cell carcinoma and milia (pilosebaceous cysts). Recurrence after complete excision is rare, but incision alone to drain the fluid contained within the hidrocystoma typically results in recurrence.

* Marsupialization or complete excision.
* Peripunctal excision may require canalicular probing to avoid or detect canalicular injury.

Epidermal Inclusion Cyst

Firm, freely mobile, subepithelial lesion (1-5 mm in diameter); cyst contains cheesy keratin material produced by cyst lining; thought to arise from occluded surface epithelium or pilosebaceous follicles; multiple epidermal inclusion cysts may be associated with Gardner's syndrome or Torre's syndrome.

* Complete surgical excision.

Inverted Follicular Keratosis

Small, solitary, benign lesion with a nodular or verrucous appearance; occurs in older adults; male predilection; may arise over months and is thought to have a viral etiology; histologically, lobular acanthosis of the epithelium with squamous and basal cell proliferation; represents a type of irritated seborrheic keratosis.

* Complete surgical excision.

Milia

Multiple, umbilicated, well-circumscribed, pinhead-sized, elevated, round, white nodules (1-3 mm in diameter); may arise spontaneously, or after trauma, radiation, herpes zoster ophthalmicus, or epidermolysis bullosa; thought to represent retention follicular cysts caused by blockage of pilosebaceous units.

* Complete surgical excision, electrolysis, or diathermy. Frequently treated with curettage using a 25-30 gauge needle.

Sebaceous (Pilar) Cyst

Yellow, elevated, smooth, subcutaneous tumor with central comedo plug caused by sebaceous or meibomian gland obstruction; occurs in the elderly; less common than epithelial inclusion cysts; may be associated with chalazia.

* Complete surgical excision with inclusion of epithelial lining.

Pilomatrixoma (Calcifying Epithelioma of Malherbe)

Small (<3 cm), solitary, firm, nodular lesion consisting of cells that demonstrate features of hair cells; slow, progressive growth; usually flesh colored but may have a red or purple hue. Occur in the head and neck, often along the brow or lid. More common in whites and slight female predilection. Differential diagnosis includes dermoid cyst, preseptal cellulitis, and cutaneous abscess. Histology reveals characteristic calcification. Recurrence after complete excision is rare.

• Biopsy or complete surgical excision.

Vascular Benign Eyelid Tumors

Eyelid Hemangioma

Most common pediatric eyelid tumor, usually appears within 1 month of life with a bluish subcutaneous mass and normal overlying dermis, or as a superficial vascular lesion (sometimes erroneously called *strawberry nevus*) representing hamartomatous growth of capillary blood vessels; rapid growth occurs in two phases with peaks at 3 and 8 months; spontaneous involution begins after 1 year and may proceed up to 10 years; slight female predilection; possible amblyopia due to occlusion of the visual axis or induced astigmatism; myopia or strabismus may occur; prognosis usually good if visual axis clear and no amblyopia.

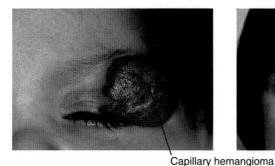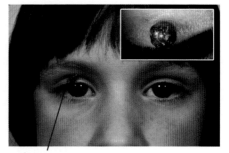

Capillary hemangioma

Figure 3-37 • Large capillary hemangioma of the left upper eyelid in an infant causing ptosis.

Figure 3-38 • Capillary hemangioma involving right upper eyelid.

• Routine follow-up visits to monitor for amblyopia and refractive error.
• Large lesions may be treated with intralesional steroid injection, systemic corticosteroids, or surgical excision. Interferon (Lupron) should be avoided due to spastic diplegia. Pulsed dye laser may be useful in treating the superficial component of some lesions.

Lymphangioma

Congenital malformation with a predilection for the head and neck. Around the eye, the orbit is more often involved. The eyelid can be involved, but is rarely involved in isolation (see Chapter 1).

Port Wine Stain (Nevus Flammeus)

Congenital venular malformation often confused with eyelid hemangioma; it is always present at birth and follows dermatomal distribution; typically lighter with a more purple hue than hemangioma; facial involvement may include any or multiple branches of the trigeminal nerve (CNV); does not blanch on palpation. Risk of glaucoma (from increased venous pressure) and the Sturge-Weber syndrome (facial port wine stain, choroidal "hemangioma," intracranial vascular anomalies) occurs primarily in patients with V1 and V2 involvement; risk of Sturge-Weber with isolated V1 involvement is extremely small.

- Early examination for choroidal involvement and glaucoma is critical.
- Pulsed dye laser treatment is recommended as early as 1 month of life.
- Cranial nerve V2 involvement is an indication for MRI of the brain.

◼ Malignant Eyelid Tumors

Basal Cell Carcinoma

Firm, pearly nodule or flatter, less well-defined lesion with central ulceration, telangiectasia, madarosis (lash loss), and inflammation; associated with ultraviolet radiation exposure and fair skin; most common (90%) malignant eyelid tumor; occurs in older adults with male predominance (2:1); usually seen on lower lid (67%) followed in frequency by upper lid (20%), medial canthus (10%), and lateral canthus (3%); locally invasive, but rarely metastatic (usually seen with canthal involvement). Two growth patterns:

Nodular   Most common; appears as small, painless, umbilicated nodule with sharp pearly borders and superficial telangiectasia that can be ulcerative ("rodent ulcer"); rarely pigmented; less invasive; nests of cells with peripheral palisading on histopathologic examination.

Morpheaform or sclerosing   Appears as flat, indurated plaque that lacks distinct margins; often ulcerated; more invasive; associated with nevoid basal cell carcinoma syndrome, linear unilateral basal cell nevus, and Bazex syndrome; excellent prognosis with appropriate treatment, but 2-10% local recurrence; metastasis in 0.02-0.1%.

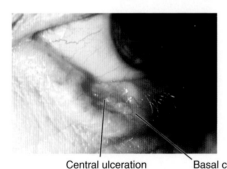 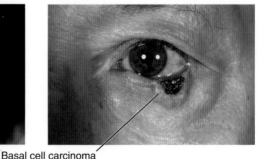

Central ulceration   Basal cell carcinoma

Figure 3-39 • Basal cell carcinoma of the lower eyelid demonstrating central ulceration with pearly, nodular border containing telangiectatic vessels.

Figure 3-40 • Basal cell carcinoma of the lower eyelid demonstrating central ulceration with scab and pearly, nodular borders.

- Protect against further sun damage.
- Complete surgical excision with margin controls (frozen sectioning); Mohs micrographic surgery sometimes useful in preserving critical eyelid tissue.
- Extremely advanced cases involving both upper and lower lids may benefit rarely from external beam irradiation.
- Canthal tumors require orbital CT to evaluate posterior (orbital) involvement. Radiation or cryotherapy should not be used in these lesions, because posterior portions of the tumor may go untreated.

Squamous Cell Carcinoma

Flat or slightly elevated, scaly, ulcerated, erythematous plaque, often arising from actinic keratosis (better prognosis), may also arise from Bowen's disease (in situ) and radiation dermatosis; constitutes less than 5% of malignant eyelid tumors (although second most common it is 40-50 times less common than basal cell carcinoma); usually seen on lower lid with lid margin involvement; risk factors include sun exposure, radiation injury, fair skin, or other irritative insults; male predominance; potentially metastatic (low) and locally invasive (faster growth than basal cell carcinoma), regional lymph node spread from eyelids occurs in 13-24% of cases; prognosis varies with tumor size, degree of differentiation, underlying etiology, and depth of tumor invasion.

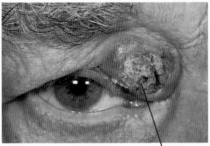 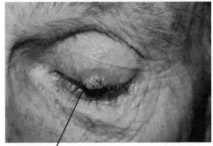

Squamous cell carcinoma

Figure 3-41 • Advanced squamous cell carcinoma of the right upper eyelid demonstrating large erythematous lesion with central scaly plaque.

Figure 3-42 • Squamous cell carcinoma of the left upper eyelid, demonstrating erythematous lesion with central scaly plaque.

- Protect against further sun damage.
- Incisional or excisional biopsy with wide surgical margins (wider than basal cell carcinoma).
- Adjunctive radiation, cryotherapy, or chemotherapy, or a combination.
- Postseptal involvement typically requires orbital exenteration.

Actinic Keratosis

Most common precancerous skin lesion; 25% develop squamous cell carcinoma; round, scaly, flat, or papillary keratotic growths with surrounding erythema; seen in sun-exposed areas; occurs in older adults with fair complexions; histologically, cellular atypia with mitotic figures and hyperkeratosis; squamous carcinoma-in-situ.

- Periocular lesions require incisional or excisional biopsy to rule out malignant lesions.
- Cryotherapy or additional surgery can be performed once diagnosis is confirmed.

Keratoacanthoma

Rapidly growing lesion usually seen in sun-exposed areas with a central ulcerated, keratin-filled crater and hyperkeratotic margins; occurs in older adults; lid or lash involvement may cause permanent damage; spontaneous resolution is common; a form of pseudoepitheliomatous hyperplasia; neither distinction is used any longer in some pathology laboratories, where these lesions are all classified as squamous carcinomas; may have viral origin; multiple keratoacanthomas seen in Ferguson-Smith syndrome.

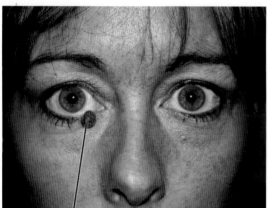

Figure 3-43 • Keratoacanthoma of the right lower lid with hyperkeratotic margins.

Keratoacanthoma

• Complete surgical excision is treatment of choice for single lesions.

Sebaceous Cell Carcinoma

Highly malignant, rare neoplasm of the sebaceous glands in the caruncle or lids; most common in fifth to seventh decades; may masquerade as chronic unilateral blepharitis (20-50% of patients) or recurrent chalazion; usually seen on upper lid; constitutes 1-15% of malignant eyelid tumors (approximately equal incidence to squamous carcinoma of the eyelid, and 40-50 times less common than basal cell carcinoma); female predilection; sometimes related to previous radiotherapy; pagetoid spread common (discontinuous areas of tumor spread through epithelium); cardinal signs include madarosis, poliosis, and thick, red lid margin inflammation; tumor is typically yellow and hard; lymphadenopathy common; poor prognosis when symptomatic for longer than 6 months (38% mortality vs. 14% for less than 6 months), size greater than 2 cm (60% mortality vs. 18% when <1 cm), upper and lower lid involvement (83% mortality), poor differentiation, and local vascular or lymphatic infiltration. Muir-Torre syndrome (multiple internal malignancies and external sebaceous tumors) is more common in sebaceous gland hyperplasia than sebaceous carcinoma.

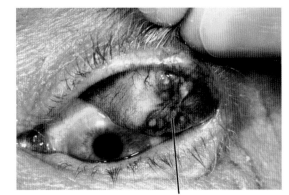

Figure 3-44 • Sebaceous cell carcinoma with chronic lid changes of the right upper eyelid.

Sebaceous cell carcinoma

- Incisional biopsy required prior to planning total resection in advanced cases, often with extensive conjunctival map biopsy (pagetoid spread). Fresh tissue should be provided for frozen section with oil-red-O stains (intracytoplasmic lipid droplets). Mohs surgery not beneficial, because skip lesions often present.
- Orbital exenteration required in advanced cases.
- Palliative radiation.

Malignant Melanoma

Tan, black, or gray nodule or plaque with irregular, notched borders; often rapidly growing with color changes. Most lethal primary skin tumor, but rare (<1% of eyelid malignancies); prognosis related to histology, depth of invasion, and tumor thickness. Acral lentiginous melanoma not seen in the eyelids; orderly growth with stage 1: localized disease without lymph node spread; stage 2: palpable regional lymph nodes (preauricular from upper lid, submandibular from lower lid); and stage 3: distant metastases; choroidal melanoma may reach lids via extrascleral extension into orbit; fair prognosis for stage 1, poor for stages 2 and 3.

Three histologic types:

Nodular melanoma   Very rare on eyelid (10% of cases), aggressive, worst prognosis.

Superficial spreading melanoma   Most common (80% of cases), onset usually 20-60 years of age; presents as flat, variegated, multicolored lesion that invades dermis, rapidly leading to raised nodule.

Lentigo malignant melanoma   Ten percent of cases, related to sun exposure, usually in the elderly; appears as flat, tan-brown lesion with irregular borders that enlarges radially with black flecks; largest when identified, often due to underdiagnosis.

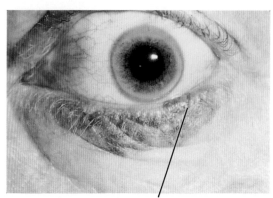

Figure 3-45 • Malignant melanoma of the lower eyelid.

Malignant melanoma

- Incisional or excisional biopsy or complete excision with or without wide margins (frozen sectioning is contraindicated); for lentigo maligna and superficial spreading this results in almost total cure; orbital exenteration and neck dissection in advanced cases.
- Dermatologic evaluation.

Merkel Cell Tumor

Rare, rapidly growing, solitary, violaceous, vascularized, occasionally ulcerated tumor of the amino precursor uptake and decarboxylation (APUD) system; usually seen in sun-exposed areas; onset in seventh decade; reported only in whites; potential for recurrence and lymphatic spread with lymph node enlargement; generally poor prognosis due to early spread after local excision alone, 39% recur locally and 46% recur regionally; after adjuvant radiation therapy or node dissection, 26% recur locally and 22% regionally; 67% tumor mortality for locoregional spread.

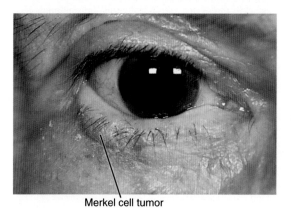

Figure 3-46 • Merkel cell tumor of the right lower eyelid.

Merkel cell tumor

- Wide local excision (immunohistochemical stains for enkephalin, calcitonin, somatostatin, corticotropin, and neuron-specific enolase).
- Lymph node resection.
- Supplemental radiation therapy.

Metastatic Tumors

Metastatic eyelid lesions are very rare; female predilection; occurs in older adults; primary sites include breast and lung (most common) carcinoma, cutaneous malignancies, gastrointestinal and genitourinary carcinomas. Three patterns: (1) single nontender nodule, (2) painless diffuse induration, (3) ulcerating lesion of eyelid skin or conjunctiva; evidence of primary tumor elsewhere, lymph node enlargement; usually poor prognosis but variable.

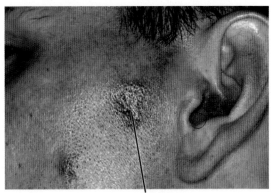

Lymphoma

Figure 3-47 • Metastatic lymphoma to left upper eyelid.

- Local excision, radiation, or observation.
- Systemic treatment for primary tumor.

Kaposi's Sarcoma of the Eyelid

Soft tissue sarcoma usually associated with acquired immunodeficiency syndrome (AIDS), may also rarely occur in Africans and older men of Mediterranean descent; very malignant in immunocompromised patients; appears as violaceous nodules on the eyelids that are nontender and progress over several months; may have associated distortion of the eyelid with entropion, edema, and misdirected lashes.

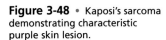

Figure 3-48 • Kaposi's sarcoma demonstrating characteristic purple skin lesion.

Kaposi's sarcoma

- Complete surgical excision.
- May require cryotherapy, radiotherapy, chemotherapy, or immunotherapy, or a combination.

Systemic Diseases

Neurofibromatosis

Definition

Neurofibromatosis (NF) is one of the classic phakomatoses and is an AD disorder of the neuroectodermal system, affecting primarily neural crest-derived tissue (Schwann cells and melanocytes), manifesting with neural, cutaneous, and ocular hamartomas. The disorder displays highly variable expressivity; two types are recognized:

NF-1 (Von Recklinghausen's disease)   Located on chromosome 17q with a prevalence of 1 in 3000; 50% of cases represent new mutations. Diagnosis requires two or more of the following criteria:

(1) Six or more café-au-lait spots 15 mm or larger in adults, 5 mm or larger in children.
(2) Two or more neurofibromas; or one plexiform neurofibroma.
(3) Axillary or inguinal freckling.
(4) Optic nerve or tract glioma.
(5) Two or more iris Lisch nodules.
(6) Characteristic osseous lesion (i.e., sphenoid dysplasia).
(7) First-degree relative with NF-1 by these criteria.

NF-2 (bilateral acoustic neurofibromatosis)   Located on chromosome 22q with a prevalence of 1 in 50,000. Diagnostic criteria include:

(1) Bilateral acoustic neuromas.
(2) First-degree relative with NF-2 and either a single acoustic neuroma or two of the following: glioma, neurilemoma, meningioma, neurofibroma, or a premature posterior subcapsular cataract.

Signs

NF-1   Café-au-lait spots, neurofibromas (fibroma molluscum), plexiform neurofibromas (bag of worms), intertriginous freckling, CNS and spinal cord gliomas, meningiomas, nerve root neurofibromas, intracranial calcifications, mild intellectual deficit, kyphoscoliosis and pseudoarthroses, gastrointestinal neurofibromas, pheochromocytoma, plus various other malignant tumors.

NF-1 ocular findings   Lisch nodules (iris melanocytic hamartomas), eyelid café-au-lait spots, neurofibromas, and plexiform neurofibroma; at times ipsilateral glaucoma, proptosis secondary to tumors or bony defects, conjunctival neurofibromas, enlarged corneal nerves, diffuse uveal thickening, choroidal hamartomas, retinal astrocytic and combined hamartomas, optic nerve glioma.

S-shaped lid deformity

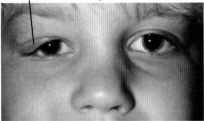

Figure 3-49 • Neurofibroma demonstrating characteristic S-shaped lid deformity of the right upper eyelid in a child with type 1 neurofibromatosis.

Eyelid neurofibroma

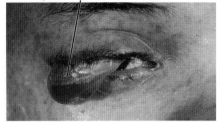

Figure 3-50 • Right eyelid neurofibroma in a patient with type 1 neurofibromatosis.

NF-2 Paucity of cutaneous lesions (few or small café-au-lait spots), bilateral acoustic neuromas, CNS and spinal cord gliomas, meningiomas, nerve root neurofibromas, intracranial calcifications, pheochromocytoma, plus various other malignant tumors.

NF-2 ocular findings Premature posterior subcapsular cataracts (40%), combined retinal hamartomas, optic nerve meningioma, and glioma; no Lisch nodules.

Evaluation

- Complete ophthalmic history and eye examination with attention to family history (examine family members), color vision, pupils, lids, corneas, tonometry, iris, lens ophthalmoscopy, visual field testing, general dermatologic evaluation (especially intertriginous regions), and neurologic screening.
- Brain and orbital MRI or CT scan.
- **Lab tests:** Complete blood count (CBC), electrolytes, and urine catecholamines (vanillylmandelic acid, metanephrine).
- Audiography for patients with NF-2.
- Intelligence testing.

Management

- Genetic counseling.
- Routine (every 6-12 months) eye examinations to monitor for glaucoma, cataracts, and ocular malignancies.
- Surgical removal of eyelid fibromas possible, but recurrence rate is high.

Prognosis

Increased morbidity if associated with CNS or other malignant neoplasm.

Sarcoidosis

Idiopathic multisystem disease, with abnormalities in cell-mediated and humoral immunity and granulomatous inflammation in many organs; commonly affects the lungs, skin, and eyes including the eyelid skin, lacrimal gland and sac, and nasolacrimal duct; may cause redness, pain, swelling of involved lids or lacrimal glands (usually bilateral), painless subcutaneous nodular masses of eyelids, ptosis, diplopia, severe cicatrizing conjunctival inflammation, conjunctival nodules, keratoconjunctivitis sicca, band keratopathy, granulomatous anterior or posterior uveitis, cataract, chorioretinitis, retinal periphlebitis or neovascularization, optic nerve disease, glaucoma, and orbital involvement; variable prognosis depending on organs involved.

- Biopsy of conjunctival, lacrimal, or eyelid nodule (with stains to rule out acid-fast bacteria).
- **Initial lab tests:** Angiotensin converting enzyme (ACE), CBC, lysozyme, serum calcium, chest radiographs, tuberculin test with anergy panel; additional tests may be ordered by pulmonologist or internist.
- Sarcoid dacryoadenitis is treated with systemic corticosteroids. Tuberculosis must be ruled out prior to initiating therapy.
- Uveitis is treated with topical corticosteroids (see Chapter 6).
- Retinal consultation as indicated.
- Treatment of systemic disease (steroids and chemotherapy) by internist.

Amyloidosis

Definition

Group of diseases (systemic or localized; primary or secondary) characterized by abnormal protein production and tissue deposition. Nonfamilial and familial forms. Familial amyloidosis (autosomal dominant [AD]) is caused by substitution errors in coding of prealbumin. Associated with multiple myeloma.

Symptoms

Asymptomatic, may notice eyelid discoloration, droopy eyelids, dryness, decreased vision, diplopia, floaters.

Signs

Systemic findings
- **Nonfamilial form:** Polyarthralgias, pulmonary infiltrates, waxy, maculopapular skin lesions, renal failure, postural hypotension, congestive heart failure, gastrointestinal bleeds.
- **Familial form:** Autonomic dysfunction, peripheral neuropathies, and cardiomyopathy.

Ocular findings   Decreased visual acuity; may have flat or nodular purpuric lesions of the eyelids, lacrimal gland, caruncle, or conjunctiva (ruptured, fragile, amyloid-infiltrated blood vessels in abnormal tissue), or may occur without hemorrhage as elevated, yellowish, waxy eyelid papules; ptosis, proptosis, ophthalmoplegia, dry eye, corneal deposits, iris stromal infiltrates, vitreous opacities, retinal vascular occlusions, cotton-wool spots, retinal neovascularization, and compressive optic neuropathy.

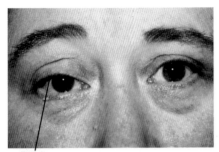

Ptosis

Figure 3-51 • Amyloidosis of the right upper eyelid causing ptosis.

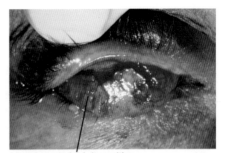

Nodular amyloid deposition

Figure 3-52 • Same patient as in Figure 3-50, demonstrating thickened everted eyelid with plaquelike appearance.

Evaluation

- Complete ophthalmic history and eye examination with attention to motility, lids, conjunctiva, cornea, iris, anterior vitreous, and ophthalmoscopy.
- **Lab tests:** Complete blood count (CBC), serum and urine protein electrophoresis, serum total protein, albumin and globulin, liver function tests, blood urea nitrogen (BUN) and creatinine, erythrocyte sedimentation rate (ESR), ANA, RF, VDRL, FTA-ABS, urinalysis, PPD, chest radiographs, electrocardiogram (ECG), bone scan.
- Diagnosis made by biopsy (birefringence and dichroism with Congo red stain, metachromasia with crystal violet, and fluorescence with thioflavine-T).
- Medical consultation.

Management

- Surgical excision/debulking, radiotherapy where feasible.
- Consider pars plana vitrectomy for vitreous opacities affecting vision.
- Underlying systemic disease should be treated by an internist.

Prognosis

Variable prognosis depending on systemic involvement; very poor when associated with multiple myeloma.

Canaliculitis

Definition

Inflammation of the canaliculus (duct between the punctum and lacrimal sac), often resulting in recurrent conjunctivitis due to viral (herpes simplex), bacterial, or fungal infections; usually insidious onset.

Etiology

Actinomyces israelii (Streptothrix), a filamentous gram-positive rod, is the most common cause; other organisms include *Candida albicans, Aspergillus, Nocardia asteroides,* and herpes simplex or zoster virus; more common in middle-aged women.

Symptoms

Medial eyelid tenderness, tearing, and redness.

Signs

Erythema and swelling of punctum and adjacent tissue ("pouting punctum"), follicular conjunctivitis around medial canthus, expression of discharge from punctum, concretions in canaliculus, grating sensation on lacrimal duct probing, dilated canaliculus on dacryocystography.

Differential Diagnosis

Conjunctivitis, dacryocystitis, nasal lacrimal duct obstruction, carunculitis.

Evaluation

- Complete ophthalmic history and eye examination with attention to history of recurrent conjunctivitis, tearing, examination of lids, punctum, lacrimal system, and conjunctiva.
- Compression medial to the punctum observing for discharge.
- **Lab tests:** Culture and Gram stain (*Actinomyces* branching filaments and sulfur granules on Gram stain).
- Probing and possible irrigation to determine patency of canalicular system.
- Consider dacryocystography to confirm a dilated canaliculus, concretions, or normal outflow function in the lower excretory system.

Management

- Warm compresses to canalicular region bid to qid.
- Marsupialization of the involved canaliculus.
- *Actinomyces israelii:* canalicular irrigation with antibiotic solution (penicillin G 100,000 U/mL) and systemic antibiotic (penicillin V 500 mg po qid for 7 days).
- *Candida albicans:* systemic antifungal agent (fluconazole 600 mg po qd for 7-10 days).
- *Aspergillus:* topical antifungal agent (amphotericin B 0.15% tid) and systemic antifungal agent (itraconazole 200 mg po bid for 7-10 days).
- *Nocardia asteroides:* topical antibiotic (sulfacetamide tid) and systemic antibiotic (trimethoprim-sulfamethoxazole [Bactrim] one double-strength tablet po qd for 7-10 days).
- Herpes simplex or zoster virus: topical antiviral agent (trifluridine 0.1% 5 times/day for 2 weeks); if stenosis present may need silicone intubation.

Prognosis

Often good; depends on infecting organism.

■ Dacryocystitis

Definition

Acute or chronic infection of the lacrimal sac, often with overlying cellulitis.

Etiology

Streptococcus pneumoniae, Staphylococcus species, and *Pseudomonas* species; *Haemophilus influenzae* in children is less common now that they receive *H. influenzae* vaccination.

Epidemiology

Conditions that cause lacrimal sac tear stasis and predispose to infection, including strictures, long and narrow nasolacrimal ducts, lacrimal sac diverticulum, trauma, dacryoliths, congenital or acquired nasolacrimal duct obstruction, and inflammatory sinus and nasal problems.

Symptoms

Pain, swelling, and redness over nasal portion of lower eyelid with tearing and crusting; may have fever.

Signs

Edema and erythema below the medial canthal tendon with lacrimal sac swelling; tenderness on palpation of the lacrimal sac, expression of discharge from the punctum; may have fistula formation or lacrimal sac cyst.

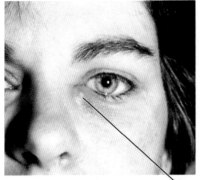 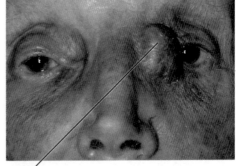

Dacryocystitis

Figure 3-53 • Dacryocystitis demonstrating erythema and swelling of lacrimal sac of the left eye.

Figure 3-54 • Dacryocystitis with massive medial canthal swelling.

Differential Diagnosis

Ethmoid sinusitis, preseptal or orbital cellulitis, lacrimal sac neoplasm, dacryocystocele (infants) and encephalocele (infants, blue mass above medial canthal tendon), facial abscess.

Evaluation

- Complete ophthalmic history with attention to history of tearing (absence of tearing calls diagnosis into question) and previous history of sinus or upper respiratory infection.
- Complete eye examination with attention to lids, lacrimal system, expression of discharge from punctum, digital massage of lacrimal sac, motility, proptosis, and conjunctiva.
- **Lab tests:** Culture and Gram stain any punctal discharge (chocolate agar in children).
- Do not probe nasolacrimal duct during acute infection.
- Orbital CT scan for limited motility, proptosis, sinus disease, or atypical cases not responding to antibiotic therapy.

Management

- Warm compresses tid.

ACUTE

- Systemic antibiotics (amoxicillin-clavulanate [Augmentin] 500 mg po tid for 10 days or amoxicillin-sulbactam [Unasyn] 15-30 mg IV q6h); if penicillin-allergic, use trimethoprim-sulfamethoxazole ([Bactrim] one double-strength tablet po bid for 10 days).
- Topical antibiotic (erythromycin ointment bid) if conjunctivitis exists.
- Percutaneous aspirate lacrimal sac contents with 18-gauge needle for culture and Gram stain.
- If pointing abscess, consider incision and drainage of lacrimal sac.
- Consider dacryocystorhinostomy once infection has resolved.

CHRONIC

- Cultures to determine antibiotic therapy (see above).
- Dacryocystorhinostomy required to relieve obstruction after infection resolved. Occasionally responds to lacrimal probing with intubation.

Prognosis

Good; usually responds to therapy, but surgery almost always required; if untreated, sequelae include mucocele formation, recurrent lacrimal sac abscess, orbital cellulitis, and infectious keratitis.

■ Nasolacrimal Duct Obstruction

Definition

Obstruction of the nasolacrimal duct; may be congenital or acquired.

Etiology

Congenital   Most frequently due to an imperforate membrane over the valve of Hasner at the nasal end of the duct; occurs clinically in 2-4% of full-term infants at 1-2 weeks of age; bilateral in one third of cases. Spontaneous opening frequently occurs 1-2 months after birth; may be complicated by acute dacryocystitis.

Acquired   Due to chronic sinus disease, involutional stenosis, dacryocystitis, or nasoorbital trauma. Involutional stenosis is the most common cause in older individuals; female predilection (2:1); may be associated with granulomatous diseases such as Wegener's granulomatosis and sarcoidosis; increased risk of dacryocystitis.

Symptoms

Tearing, discharge, crusting, recurrent conjunctivitis.

Signs

Watery eyes, eyelash crusting and debris, mucus reflux from punctum with compression over the lacrimal sac, medial lower eyelid erythema.

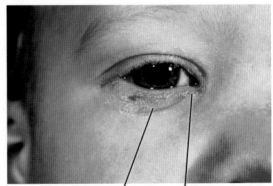

Figure 3-55 • Nasolacrimal duct obstruction with tearing, crusting of eyelids, and lower lid erythema.

Differential Diagnosis

Congenital tearing   Congenital glaucoma, trichiasis, conjunctivitis, nasal lacrimal duct anomalies (punctal atresia), dacryocystocele, corneal abrasion, corneal trauma from forceps delivery, ocular surface foreign body.

Acquired tearing   Conjunctivitis, trichiasis, entropion, ectropion, corneal abnormalities, dry eye syndrome, punctal stenosis, canalicular stenosis.

Evaluation

- Complete ophthalmic history and eye examination with attention to lid margins, lashes, puncta, conjunctiva, cornea (diameter, breaks in Descemet's membrane, staining with fluorescein), tonometry, palpate over lacrimal sac and observe for reflux of discharge from punctum.
- Dye disappearance test with fluorescein, particularly helpful in infants.
- Jones I test: fluorescein is instilled in conjunctival cul-de-sac; a cotton-tipped applicator is used to attempt fluorescein retrieval via the external naris. Positive test result indicates functional blockage.
- Jones II test: nasolacrimal irrigation with saline following positive Jones I test; fluorescein retrieval is attempted once again. Positive test result indicates anatomic blockage.
- Nasolacrimal irrigation: 23-gauge cannula mounted on 3-cc to 5-cc syringe is inserted into canaliculus, and irrigation is attempted. Retrograde flow through opposite canaliculus and punctum indicates nasolacrimal blockage. Reflux through same punctum indicates canalicular obstruction. Successful irrigation into nose and throat eliminates anatomic blockage but does not rule out functional blockage.

Management

- Treat dacryocystitis if present.

CONGENITAL

- Crigler massage bid to qid (parent places index finger over infant's canaliculi [medial corner of eyelid] and makes several slow downward strokes).
- Nasolacrimal duct probing at 13 months if no spontaneous resolution, sooner if infection or discharge occurs, probing may be repeated; consider silicone intubation of the nasolacrimal duct if initial probing does not resolve the tearing.

ACQUIRED

- Treat partial nasolacrimal duct obstruction with antibiotic-steroid preparation (neomycin-polymyxin-dexamethasone [Maxitrol] qid).
- Consider silicone intubation of the nasolacrimal duct or dacryoplasty for persistent partial obstruction.
- Complete nasolacrimal duct obstruction with patent canaliculi and functional lacrimal pump requires dacryocystorhinostomy (anastomosis between lacrimal sac and nasal cavity through a bony ostium).

Prognosis

Excellent for congenital; often good for acquired, depends on cause of obstruction.

Dacryoadenitis

Definition

Inflammation of the lacrimal gland usually of idiopathic, noninfectious origin, viral, bacterial, or rarely parasitic etiology. Chronic form is more common than acute.

Etiology

Acute Most commonly due to infection (*Staphylococcus* species, mumps, Epstein-Barr virus, herpes zoster, or *Neisseria gonorrhoeae*); palpebral lobe affected more frequently than orbital lobe; most cases associated with systemic infection; typically occurs in children and young adults.

Chronic Usually due to inflammatory disorders including idiopathic orbital inflammation, sarcoidosis, thyroid ophthalmopathy, Sjögren's syndrome, and benign lymphoepithelial lesions; also seen with syphilis and tuberculosis.

Symptoms

Acute Temporal upper eyelid redness, swelling, and pain with tearing and discharge.

Chronic Temporal upper eyelid swelling; occasional redness and discomfort.

Signs

Acute Edema, tenderness, and erythema of upper eyelid with S-shaped deformity, enlarged and erythematous lacrimal gland (palpebral lobe), preauricular lymphadenopathy, and fever; may have inferonasal globe displacement and proptosis if orbital lobe involved.

Chronic Tenderness in superotemporal area of upper eyelid, globe displacement, restricted ocular motility, and enlarged lacrimal gland.

Differential Diagnosis

Malignant lacrimal gland neoplasm, preseptal or orbital cellulitis, viral conjunctivitis, chalazion, dermoid tumor, lacrimal gland cyst (dacryops).

Evaluation

Acute
- Complete ophthalmic history and eye examination with attention to constitutional signs, palpation of parotid glands, lymph nodes, and upper lid, examination of palpebral lacrimal lobe (lift upper lid) for enlargement, globe retropulsion, and motility.
- Check Hertel exophthalmometry.
- **Lab tests:** culture and Gram stain of discharge, CBC with differential; consider blood cultures for suspected systemic involvement.
- Orbital CT scan for proptosis, motility restriction, or suspected mass.

Chronic
- Complete ophthalmic history and eye examination with attention to constitutional signs, palpation of parotid glands, lymph nodes, and upper lid; examination of palpebral lacrimal lobe (lift upper lid) for enlargement, globe retropulsion, motility, and signs of previous anterior or posterior uveitis.
- Check Hertel exophthalmometry.
- **Lab tests:** Chest radiographs, CBC with differential, ACE, VDRL test, FTA-ABS, PPD, anergy panel.
- Orbital CT scan.
- Consider lacrimal gland biopsy if diagnosis uncertain or malignancy suspected.

Management

ACUTE

- Mumps or Epstein-Barr virus: warm compresses bid to tid.
- Herpes simplex or zoster virus: systemic antiviral agents (acyclovir [Zovirax] 800 mg po 5 times/day for 10 days or famciclovir [Famvir] 500 mg po tid for 7 days); in immunocompromised patients use acyclovir 10-12 mg/kg/day IV divided into 3 doses for 7-10 days.
- *Staphylococcus* and *Streptococcus* species: Systemic antibiotic (amoxicillin-clavulanate [Augmentin] 500 mg po q8h); in severe cases ampicillin-sulbactam [Unasyn] 1.5-3 g IV q6h.
- *Neisseria gonorrhoeae:* Systemic antibiotic (ceftriaxone 1 g IV × 1); warm compresses and incision and drainage if suppurative.
- *Mycobacterium* species: surgical excision and systemic treatment with isoniazid (300 mg po qd) and rifampin (600 mg po qd) for 6-9 months, follow liver function tests for toxicity; consider adding pyrazinamide (25-35 mg/kg po qd) for first 2 months.
- *Treponema pallidum:* systemic antibiotic (penicillin G 24 million U/day IV for 10 days).

CHRONIC

- Treat underlying inflammatory disorder.
- Treat infections (rare) as above.

Prognosis

Depends on cause; most infections respond well to treatment.

■ Lacrimal Gland Tumors

Definition

Approximately 50% of all lacrimal gland masses are inflammatory; the other 50% are neoplasms. Of these, 50% are of epithelial origin while 50% are primarily lymphoproliferative. Of all epithelial tumors, 50% are pleomorphic adenomas (benign mixed tumors), and 50% are malignant. Lacrimal gland lesions appear in the superotemporal quadrant of the orbit.

Benign Mixed Cell Tumor (Pleomorphic Adenoma)

Most common epithelial tumor of the lacrimal gland, usually appearing insidiously in the fourth and fifth decade, often with inferior and medial displacement of the globe. A firm, circumscribed mass can be palpated under the superior temporal orbital rim, often with bony remodeling (not osteolytic) on radiographic images; histologically, these tumors contain a pseudocapsule, a double row of epithelial cells forming lumens, and stroma containing spindle-shaped cells with mucinous, osteoid, or cartilaginous metaplasia. Complete resection is critical in order to avoid malignant degeneration.

Malignant Mixed Cell Tumor (Pleomorphic Adenocarcinoma)

Occurs in the elderly with pain and rapid progression; contains the same epithelial and mesenchymal features of pleomorphic adenoma, but with malignant components; associated with longstanding or incompletely excised pleomorphic adenomas.

Adenoid Cystic Carcinoma (Cylindroma)

Most common malignant tumor of the lacrimal gland, rapid onset with infiltrative capacity; associated with pain due to perineural invasion; bony erosion and proptosis common; CT scan shows a poorly defined mass with adjacent bony destruction. Histologically, the tumor is composed of densely staining, packed small cells that grow in nests, tubules, or a Swiss cheese (cribriform) pattern; the basaloid pattern carries the worst prognosis.

Symptoms

Upper lid fullness, diplopia, pain.

Signs

Inferior and medial globe displacement, limitation of ocular movements, lid edema and erythema, palpable mass under the superotemporal orbital rim.

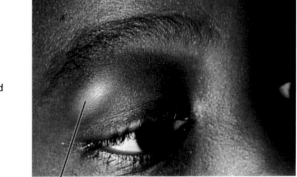

Figure 3-56 • Lacrimal gland tumor of the right orbit.

Lacrimal gland tumor

Differential Diagnosis

Dermoid, sarcoidosis, idiopathic orbital inflammation, lymphoid tumor, dacryops, benign epithelial tumor.

Evaluation

* Complete ophthalmic history with attention to duration of onset, rate of progression, pain, visual complaints, and constitutional symptoms.
* Complete eye examination with attention to lids, lacrimal gland, orbital rim, and motility.

- Orbital CT scan demonstrates well-circumscribed mass with lacrimal gland fossa enlargement (pleomorphic adenoma) or an irregular mass with or without adjacent bony erosion (adenoid cystic carcinoma).
- Fine-needle aspiration biopsy of the lacrimal gland may be useful in some cases. Incisional biopsy should be avoided.
- Consider oncology consultation.

Management

BENIGN MIXED TUMOR (PLEOMORPHIC ADENOMA)

- En bloc excision via a lateral orbitotomy; rupture of pseudocapsule may lead to recurrence and malignant transformation.

ADENOID CYSTIC CARCINOMA (CYLINDROMA)

- En bloc resection with wide margins including orbital rim at a minimum. Orbital exenteration with adjunctive chemotherapy and irradiation may be required, and must be discussed with each patient on a case-by-case basis.

PLEOMORPHIC ADENOCARCINOMA

- Same as for adenoid cystic carcinoma.

Prognosis

Benign Mixed Tumor (Pleomorphic Adenoma): excellent if tumor is excised completely.
Adenoid Cystic Carcinoma (Cylindroma): Five-year survival rate is 47%, and at 15 years is only 22%; major cause of death is intracranial extension due to perineural spread.
Pleomorphic Adenocarcinoma: similar to adenoid cystic carcinoma.

Chapter 4

CONJUNCTIVA AND SCLERA

■ Trauma

Foreign Body

Exogenous material on, under, or embedded within conjunctiva or sclera; commonly dirt, glass, metal, or cilia; patients usually note foreign body sensation and redness; good prognosis.

- Remove foreign body if present; evert lids to check for foreign body.
- Add topical broad spectrum antibiotic (polymyxin B sulfate–trimethoprim [Polytrim] or bacitracin ointment qid).

Laceration

Partial-thickness or full-thickness cut in conjunctiva with or without partial-thickness cut in the sclera; very important to rule out open globe (see below); good prognosis.

- Complete ophthalmic history and eye examination with attention to evaluating extent of laceration, tonometry, anterior chamber, and ophthalmoscopy.
- Perform Seidel test for suspected open globe (see below).
- Conjunctival and partial-thickness scleral lacerations do not require surgical repair; add topical broad spectrum antibiotic (polymyxin B sulfate–trimethoprim [Polytrim] or bacitracin ointment qid).

Slit-beam   Laceration

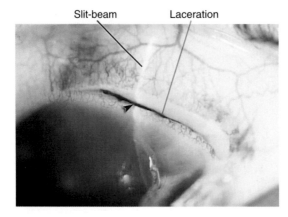

Figure 4-1 • Full-thickness corneoscleral limbal laceration with wound gape. Note discontinuity of slit beam as it crosses the wound edge *(arrowhead).*

Open Globe

Full-thickness defect in eye wall (cornea or sclera), commonly from penetrating or blunt trauma; the latter usually causes rupture at the limbus, just posterior to the rectus muscle insertions, or at previous surgical incision sites; double penetrating injuries are called *perforations;* an open globe may also be due to corneal or scleral melting. Associated signs include lid and orbital trauma, corneal abrasion or laceration, wound dehiscence, positive Seidel test, low intraocular pressure, flat or shallow anterior chamber, anterior chamber cells and flare, hyphema, peaked pupil, iris transillumination defect, sphincter tears, angle recession, iridodialysis, cyclodialysis, iridodonesis, phacodonesis, dislocated lens, cataract, vitreous and retinal hemorrhage, commotio retinae, retinal tear, retinal detachment, choroidal rupture, intraocular foreign body or gas bubbles, and extruded intraocular contents. Guarded prognosis.

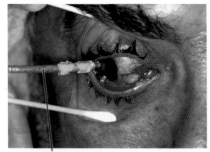

Intraorbital nail   Bulbous conjunctival hemorrhage   Uveal prolapse

Figure 4-2 • Penetrating injury with foreign body (nail) protruding from globe.

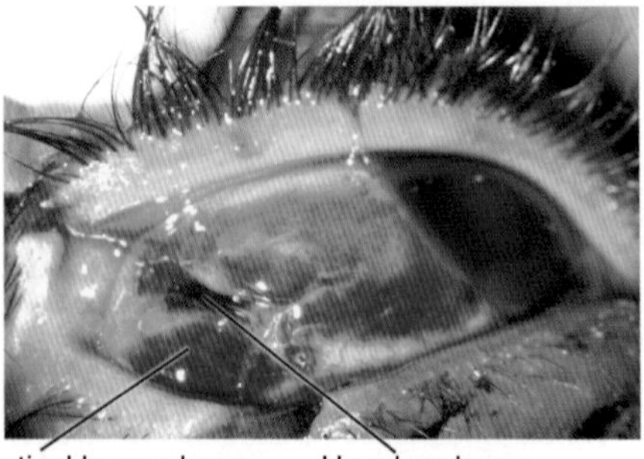

Figure 4-3 • Open globe. There is a temporal full-thickness scleral laceration with uveal prolapse. Also note the extensive subconjunctival hemorrhage and upper and lower eyelid lacerations.

Ophthalmic Emergency

- Admit for surgical exploration and repair; protect eye with metal eye shield; minimize ocular manipulations; examine globe only enough to verify the diagnosis of an open globe; remainder of examination and exploration should be performed in the operating room. Postoperatively, start antibiotics and steroids.
- Consider B-scan ultrasonography if unable to visualize the fundus.
- Consider orbital computed tomography (CT) or orbital radiographs to rule out intraocular foreign body; magnetic resonance imaging (MRI) is *contraindicated* if foreign body is metallic.
- Subconjunctival antibiotics and steroids:
  Vancomycin (25 mg).
  Ceftazidime (50-100 mg) or gentamicin (20 mg).
  Dexamethasone (12-24 mg).
- Broad spectrum fortified topical antibiotics (alternate every 30 minutes):
  Vancomycin (25-50 mg/mL q1h).
  Ceftazidime (50 mg/mL q1h).
  Topical steroid (prednisolone acetate 1% q1-2h initially) and cycloplegic agent (scopolamine 0.25% or atropine 1% tid).
- Systemic intravenous antibiotics for marked inflammation or severe cases:
  Vancomycin (1 g IV q12h).
  Ceftazidime (1 g IV q12h).
- Small corneal lacerations (<2 mm) that are self-sealing or intermittently Seidel positive may be treated with a bandage contact lens, topical broad spectrum antibiotic (gatifloxacin [Zymar] or moxifloxacin [Vigamox] q2h to q6h), cycloplegic agent (cyclopentolate 1% bid), and an aqueous suppressant (timolol maleate [Timoptic] 0.5% or brimonidine [Alphagan P] 0.15% bid); observe daily for 5-7 days; consider suturing laceration if wound has not sealed after 1 week.

Subconjunctival Hemorrhage

Diffuse or focal area of blood under conjunctiva; appears bright red, otherwise asymptomatic; may be idiopathic, associated with trauma, sneezing, coughing, straining, emesis, aspirin or anticoagulant use, or hypertension, or due to abnormal conjunctival vessel; excellent prognosis.

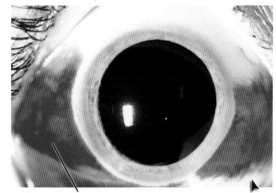

Figure 4-4 • Subconjunctival hemorrhage demonstrating bright red blood under the conjunctiva. As the hemorrhage resorbs, the edges may spread, become feathery, and turn yellowish *(arrowhead)*.

Subconjunctival hemorrhage

- Reassurance if no other ocular findings.
- Consider blood pressure measurement if recurrent.
- Medical or hematology consultation for recurrent, idiopathic, subconjunctival hemorrhages, or other evidence of systemic bleeding (ecchymoses, epistaxis, gastrointestinal bleeding, hematuria, etc.).

■ Telangiectasia

Definition

Abnormal, dilated conjunctival capillary formation.

Symptoms

Asymptomatic red spot on eye; patient may have epistaxis and gastrointestinal bleeding depending on etiology.

Signs

Telangiectasia of conjunctival vessels, subconjunctival hemorrhage.

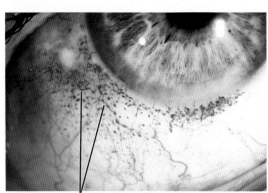

Figure 4-5 • Conjunctival telangiectasia appearing as dotlike, corkscrew, irregular vessels near the limbus.

Conjunctival telangiectasia

Differential Diagnosis

Idiopathic, Osler-Weber-Rendu syndrome, ataxia-telangiectasia, Fabry's disease, Sturge-Weber syndrome.

Evaluation

- Complete ophthalmic history and eye examination with attention to conjunctiva, cornea, lens, and ophthalmoscopy.
- Consider CT scan for multisystem disorders.
- Medical consultation to rule out systemic disease.

Management

- No treatment recommended.

Prognosis

Usually benign; may bleed; depends on etiology.

■ Microaneurysm

Definition

Focal dilation of conjunctival vessel.

Symptoms

Asymptomatic; may notice red spot on eye.

Signs

Microaneurysm; may have associated retinal findings.

Differential Diagnosis

Diabetes mellitus, hypertension, sickle cell anemia (Paton's sign), arteriosclerosis, carotid occlusion, fucosidosis, polycythemia vera.

Evaluation

- Complete ophthalmic history and eye examination with attention to conjunctiva and ophthalmoscopy.
- Check blood pressure.
- **Lab tests:** Fasting blood glucose (diabetes mellitus), sickle cell prep, hemoglobin electrophoresis (sickle cell).
- Medical consultation.

Management

- No treatment recommended.
- Treat underlying medical disease.

Prognosis

Usually benign.

Dry Eye Syndrome

Definition

Ocular irritation due to deficiency of one or more tear film components (aqueous, lipid, or mucin).

Etiology

Many conditions may produce a tear film abnormality, these can be classified by mechanism (decreased aqueous tear production or increased tear film evaporation) but are usually multifactorial.

Decreased Tear Production

Keratoconjunctivitis sicca   Characterized by hypofunction of the lacrimal gland; may be associated with Sjögren's syndrome (dry eye, dry mouth, and arthritis) manifesting with or without systemic immune dysfunction and no connective tissue disease (primary, >95% female) or with connective tissue disease, including rheumatoid arthritis and collagen vascular diseases (secondary).

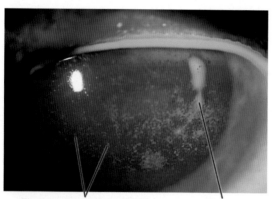

Figure 4-6 • Keratoconjunctivitis sicca demonstrating superficial punctate keratitis (SPK) and filaments stained with fluorescein dye.

Fluorescein staining of SPK   Filament

Increased Tear Evaporation

Characterized by normal lacrimal gland function, but abnormal tear film secondary to periocular disease.

Acne rosacea   Inflammatory disease causing meibomian gland dysfunction, blepharoconjunctivitis, corneal vascularization, infiltrates, and ulceration. It is associated with facial skin changes (erythema, pustules, telangiectasia, rhinophyma); may be exacerbated by certain foods (e.g., alcohol and chocolate) (see Chapter 1).

Vitamin A deficiency   Leads to conjunctival xerosis and lack of mucin that causes increased tear evaporation. It is associated with Bitot's spots (due to gas-producing bacteria *Corynebacterium xerosis*), corneal ulceration, and night blindness (nyctalopia) with progressive retinal degeneration; major cause of blindness worldwide.

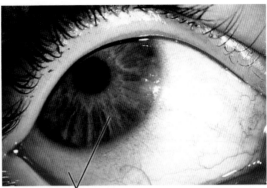

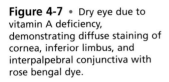

Figure 4-7 • Dry eye due to vitamin A deficiency, demonstrating diffuse staining of cornea, inferior limbus, and interpalpebral conjunctiva with rose bengal dye.

Rose bengal staining

Symptoms

Dryness, burning, foreign body sensation, tearing, red eye, discharge, blurred vision, photophobia; symptoms exacerbated by wind, smoke, and reading.

Signs

Blepharitis, conjunctival injection, decreased tear break-up time (<10 seconds), decreased tear meniscus, tear film debris, filaments, dry corneal surface, irregular and dull corneal light reflex, staining with rose bengal and fluorescein, Bitot's spot (white, foamy patch of keratinized bulbar conjunctiva [pathognomonic for vitamin A deficiency]), conjunctivochalasis (loosened bulbar conjunctiva resting on lid margin); severe cases may cause corneal ulceration, descemetocele, or perforation.

Differential Diagnosis

See above; also deficiency in aqueous (lacrimal gland tumor, lacrimal gland infiltration due to sarcoidosis and lymphoma, graft-versus-host disease, Riley-Day syndrome, radiation), lipid (blepharitis), mucin (Stevens-Johnson syndrome, ocular cicatricial pemphigoid, radiation, chemical burn, trachoma), or other (ectropion, entropion, lagophthalmos, Bell's palsy, thyroid ophthalmopathy, conjunctivitis, medicamentosa).

Evaluation

- Complete ophthalmic history and eye examination with attention to lids, conjunctiva, cornea, tear film, and rose bengal and fluorescein staining.
- **Schirmer's test:** Two tests exist, but they are usually not performed as originally described. One is done without and one is done with topical anesthesia. The inferior fornix is dried with a cotton-tipped applicator, and a strip of standardized filter paper (Whatman #41, 5-mm width) is placed over each lower lid at the junction of the lateral and middle thirds. After 5 minutes, the strips are removed and the amount of wetting is measured. Normal results are 15 mm or greater without anesthesia (basal + reflex tearing), and 10 mm or greater with topical anesthesia (basal tearing).

- **Lab tests:** Consider tear lactoferrin and lysozyme (decreased), and tear osmolarity (>310 mOsm/L).
- Electroretinogram (reduced), electro-oculogram (abnormal), and dark adaptation (prolonged) in vitamin A deficiency.
- Consider medical consultation for systemic diseases.

Management

- Topical lubrication with preservative-free artificial tears (see Appendix) up to q1h and ointment (Refresh P.M.) at bedtime.
- Consider acetylcysteine 10% (Mucomyst) qd to qid, punctal occlusion (with plugs or cautery), hydroxypropyl methylcellulose (Lacrisert), bandage contact lens, moist chamber goggles, lid taping at bedtime, and tarsorrhaphy for more severe cases.
- Consider topical cyclosporine 0.05% [Restasis] bid and autologous serum in severe cases.
- **Acne rosacea:** Doxycycline 100 mg po bid for 3 weeks, followed by 100 mg po qd for 3-4 months. Tetracycline is also effective but requires more frequent dosing and is associated with more frequent gastrointestinal side effects. Neither doxycycline nor tetracycline is offered to women in their childbearing years nor to children with deciduous dentition. Topical metronidazole (MetroGel) 0.75% bid for 2-4 weeks to facial skin.
- **Vitamin A deficiency:** Vitamin A replacement (vitamin A 15,000 IU po qd).

Prognosis

Depends on underlying condition; severe cases may be difficult to manage.

Inflammation

Definition

Chemosis

Edema of conjunctiva; may be mild with boggy appearance or massive with tense ballooning.

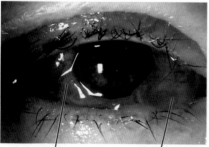

Injection   Chemosis

Figure 4-8 • Chemosis with extensive ballooning of conjunctiva and prolapse over lower lid nasally. Temporally, the edges of the elevated conjunctiva are delineated by the light reflexes from the tear film.

Follicles

Small, translucent, avascular mounds of plasma cells and lymphocytes seen in epidemic keratoconjunctivitis (EKC), herpes simplex virus, chlamydia, molluscum, or drug reactions.

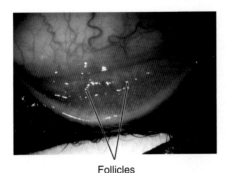

Follicles

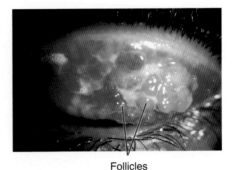

Follicles

Figure 4-9 • Follicular conjunctivitis demonstrating inferior palpebral follicles with the typical gelatinous bump appearance.

Figure 4-10 • Large, gelatinous, tarsal follicles in a patient with acute trachoma.

Granuloma

Collection of giant multinucleated cells seen in chronic inflammation from sarcoid, foreign body, or chalazion.

Hyperemia

Redness and injection of conjunctiva.

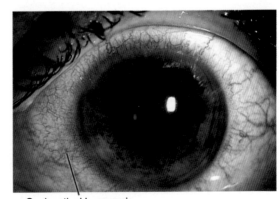

Figure 4-11 • Hyperemia. The dilated conjunctival vessels produce a diffuse redness (injection).

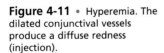

Conjunctival hyperemia

Membranes

A true membrane is a firmly adherent, fibrinous exudate that bleeds and scars when removed; seen in bacterial conjunctivitis *(Streptococcus* species, *Neisseria gonorrhoeae, Corynebacterium diphtheriae),* Stevens-Johnson syndrome, and burns; a pseudomembrane is a loosely attached, avascular, fibrinous exudate seen in EKC and mild allergic or bacterial conjunctivitis.

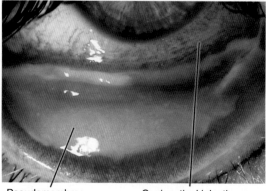

Figure 4-12 • Pseudomembrane evident as a thick yellow coating in a patient with epidemic keratoconjunctivitis.

Pseudomembrane   Conjunctival injection

Papillae

Vascular reaction consisting of fibrovascular mounds with central vascular tuft; nonspecific finding seen with any conjunctival irritation or conjunctivitis; can be large ("cobblestones" or giant papillae).

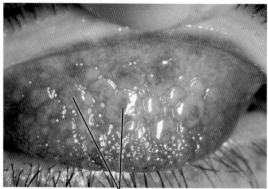

Figure 4-13 • Large papillae in a patient with vernal keratoconjunctivitis. The central vascular cores are clearly visible as dots within the papillae.

Papillae

Phlyctenule ("Blister")

Focal, nodular, vascularized infiltrate of polymorphonuclear leukocytes and lymphocytes with central necrosis due to hypersensitivity to *Staphylococcus* species, *Mycobacterium* species, *Candida* species, *Coccidioides, Chlamydia,* or nematodes; located on the bulbar conjunctiva or at the limbus; can march across cornea, causing vascularization and scarring behind the leading edge.

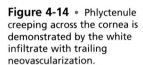

Figure 4-14 • Phlyctenule creeping across the cornea is demonstrated by the white infiltrate with trailing neovascularization.

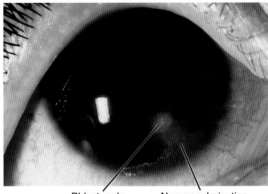

Phlyctenule   Neovascularization

Symptoms

Red eye, swelling, itching, foreign body sensation; may have discharge, photophobia, and tearing.

Signs

See above; depends on type of inflammation.

Differential Diagnosis

Any irritation of conjunctiva (allergic, infectious, autoimmune, chemical, foreign body, idiopathic).

Evaluation

- Complete ophthalmic history and eye examination with attention to preauricular lymphadenopathy, everting lids, conjunctiva, cornea, and characteristics of discharge if present.
- **Lab tests:** Cultures and smears of conjunctiva, cornea, and discharge for infectious causes.

Management

- Treatment depends on etiology; usually supportive.
- Topical vasoconstrictor, nonsteroidal antiinflammatory drug (NSAID), antihistamine, mast cell stabilizer, or mast cell stabilizer and antihistamine combination (see Table 4-1); severe cases may require topical steroid (prednisolone acetate 1% qid) or topical antibiotic (bacitracin–polymixin B sulfate [Polysporin] or erythromycin ointment qid or both).
- Membranes and pseudomembranes may require debridement.
- Discontinue offending agent if patient is allergic.

Prognosis

Depends on etiology; most are benign and self-limited (see Conjunctivitis section).

Conjunctivitis

Definition

Infectious or noninfectious inflammation of the conjunctiva classified as acute (shorter than 4-week duration) or chronic (longer than 4-week duration).

Acute Conjunctivitis

Infectious

Gonococcal

Hyperacute presentation with severe purulent discharge, chemosis, papillary reaction, preauricular lymphadenopathy, and lid swelling. *N. gonorrhoeae* can invade intact corneal epithelium and cause infectious keratitis (see Chapter 5).

Nongonococcal Bacterial

Usually caused by *Staphylococcus aureus*, *Streptococcus pneumoniae*, *Haemophilus* species, or *Moraxella catarrhalis*. Spectrum of clinical pictures ranging from mild (signs include minimal lid edema, scant purulent discharge) to moderate (significant conjunctival injection, membranes); usually no preauricular adenopathy or corneal involvement.

Mucopurulent discharge

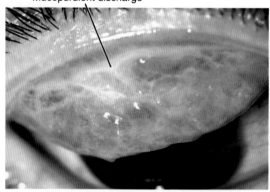

Figure 4-15 • Bacterial conjunctivitis with mucopurulent discharge adherent to the upper tarsal conjunctiva.

Adenoviral

Most common cause of viral conjunctivitis ("pink eye"); signs include lid edema, serous discharge, pseudomembranes; may have preauricular lymphadenopathy and corneal subepithelial infiltrates; transmitted by contact and contagious for 12-14 days; several different types:

- Epidemic keratoconjunctivitis: types 8 and 19.
- Pharyngoconjunctival fever: types 3 and 7.

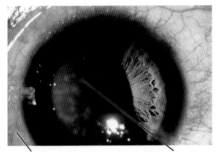

Conjunctival injection   Subepithelial infiltrates

Figure 4-16 • Adenoviral conjunctivitis due to epidemic keratoconjunctivitis with characteristic subepithelial infiltrates.

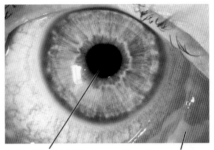

Subepithelial infiltrates   Pseudomembrane

Figure 4-17 • Adenoviral conjunctivitis due to epidemic keratoconjunctivitis demonstrating small, white, punctate subepithelial infiltrates in the central cornea and a yellow pseudomembrane in the inferior fornix.

Herpes Simplex Virus

Primary disease in children causes bilateral lid vesicles; may also have fever, preauricular lymphadenopathy, and an upper respiratory infection.

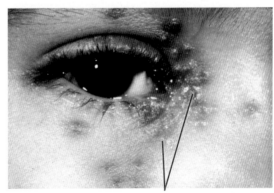

Figure 4-18 • Herpes simplex viral conjunctivitis with characteristic lid vesicles.

Seropurulent vesicles due to HSV

Pediculosis

Results from contact with pubic lice (sexually transmitted); may be unilateral or bilateral.

Allergic

Seasonal

Seen in all ages; associated with hay fever, airborne allergens.

Atopic Keratoconjunctivitis (AKC)

Occurs in adults; not seasonal; associated with atopy (rhinitis, asthma, dermatitis); similar features as vernal keratoconjunctivitis but papillae usually smaller and conjunctiva has milky edema; also thickened and erythematous lids, corneal neovascularization, cataracts (10%), and keratoconus.

Vernal Keratoconjunctivitis (VKC)

Occurs in children; seasonal (warm months); male predilection; lasts 5-10 years, then resolves; associated with family history of atopy; signs include intense itching, ropy discharge, giant papillae (cobblestones), Horner-Trantas dots (collections of eosinophils at limbus), shield ulcer, and keratitis in 50%; more than two eosinophils per high-power field is pathognomonic.

Giant papillae (cobblestones)

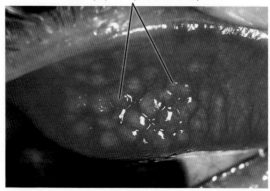

Figure 4-19 • Vernal keratoconjunctivitis demonstrating "cobblestones" (giant papillae).

Toxic

Follicular reaction due to eye drops (especially neomycin, aminoglycoside antibiotics, antiviral medications, atropine, miotic agents, brimonidine [Alphagan], apraclonidine [Iopidine], epinephrine, and preservatives including contact lens solutions).

■ Chronic Conjunctivitis

Infectious

Chlamydial

Trachoma   Leading cause of blindness worldwide; caused by serotypes A-C; signs include follicles, Herbert's pits (scarred limbal follicles), superior pannus, superficial punctate keratitis, upper tarsal scarring (Arlt's line).

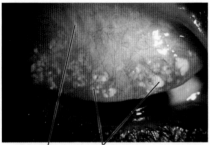

Arlt's line   Concretions

Figure 4-20 • Trachoma demonstrating linear pattern of upper tarsal scarring. Also note the abundant concretions that appear as yellow granular aggregates.

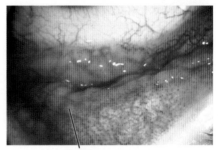

Follicles

Figure 4-21 • Chlamydial conjunctivitis with follicles in the inferior fornix.

Inclusion conjunctivitis   Caused by serotypes D-K; signs include chronic, follicular conjunctivitis, subepithelial infiltrates, and no membrane; associated with urethritis in 5%.

Lymphogranuloma venereum   Caused by serotype L; associated with Parinaud's oculoglandular syndrome (see below), conjunctival granulomas, and interstitial keratitis.

Molluscum Contagiosum

Usually appears with multiple, umbilicated, shiny nodules on the eyelid; associated with follicular conjunctivitis; with multiple lesions, consider human immunodeficiency virus (HIV).

Allergic

Giant Papillary Conjunctivitis

Occurs in contact lens wearers (>95% of giant papillary conjunctivitis cases); also secondary to prosthesis, foreign body, or exposed suture; signs include itching, ropy discharge, blurry vision, and pain with contact lens use.

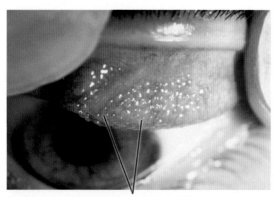

Figure 4-22 • Giant papillary conjunctivitis demonstrating large papillae in upper tarsal conjunctiva.

Giant papillary conjunctivitis

Toxic

Follicular reaction due to eye drops and contact lens solutions (see above).

Other

Superior Limbic Keratoconjunctivitis

Occurs in middle-aged females; 50% have thyroid disease; usually bilateral and asymmetric; may be secondary to contact lens use (see Chapter 5); signs include boggy edema, redundancy and injection of superior conjunctiva, superficial punctate keratitis, filaments, and no discharge; symptoms are worse than signs.

Rose bengal staining

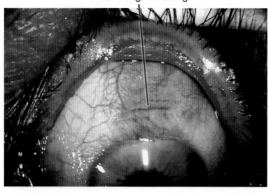

Figure 4-23 • Superior limbic keratoconjunctivitis demonstrating the typical staining of the central superior conjunctiva with rose bengal dye.

Kawasaki's Disease

Mucocutaneous lymph node syndrome of unknown etiology; seen in children under 5 years old; more common in Japanese; diagnosis based on 5 of 6 criteria: (1) fever (≥5 days), (2) bilateral conjunctivitis, (3) oral mucosal changes (erythema, fissures, "strawberry tongue"), (4) rash, (5) cervical lymphadenopathy, and (6) peripheral extremity changes (edema, erythema, desquamation); associated with polyarteritis especially of coronary arteries; may be fatal (1-2%).

Ligneous

Rare, idiopathic, bilateral, membranous conjunctivitis seen in children; develop a thick, white, woody infiltrate and plaque located on the upper tarsal conjunctiva.

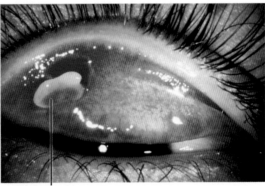

Figure 4-24 • Ligneous conjunctivitis demonstrating thick, yellow-white plaque on superior tarsal conjunctiva.

Ligneous plaque

Parinaud's Oculoglandular Syndrome

Unilateral conjunctivitis with conjunctival granulomas and preauricular/submandibular lymphadenopathy; may have fever, malaise, and rash; due to cat-scratch fever, tularemia, sporotrichosis, tuberculosis, syphilis, lymphogranuloma venereum, Epstein-Barr virus, mumps, fungi, malignancy, and sarcoidosis.

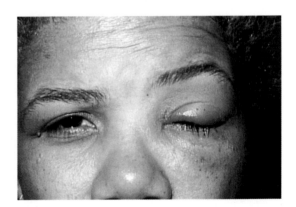

Figure 4-25 • Parinaud's oculoglandular syndrome. There is marked eyelid swelling and erythema in this patient with an affected left eye.

Ophthalmia Neonatorum

Occurs in newborns; may be toxic (silver nitrate) or infectious (bacteria [especially *N. gonorrhoeae*], herpes simplex virus, chlamydia [may have otitis and pneumonitis]).

Symptoms

Red eye, swelling, itching, burning, foreign body sensation, tearing, discharge, crusting of lashes; may have photophobia and decreased vision.

Signs

Normal or decreased visual acuity, lid edema, conjunctival injection, chemosis, papillae, follicles, membranes, petechial hemorrhages, concretions, discharge; may have preauricular lymphadenopathy, subepithelial infiltrates, punctate staining, corneal ulcers, and cataract.

Differential Diagnosis

See above; also medicamentosa (toxic reaction commonly associated with preservatives in medications, as well as antiviral medications, antibiotics, miotic agents, dipivefrin [Propine], apraclonidine [Iopidine], and atropine), dacryocystitis, nasolacrimal duct obstruction.

Evaluation

- Complete ophthalmic history and eye examination with attention to preauricular lymphadenopathy, everting lids, characteristics of discharge, conjunctiva, cornea, and anterior chamber.
- **Lab tests:** Consider cultures and smears of conjunctiva and cornea (mandatory for suspected bacterial cases).
- Consider pediatric consultation.

Management

- Treatment depends on etiology; usually supportive with medications, compresses, and debridement of membranes for symptomatic relief.

BACTERIAL

- Topical broad spectrum antibiotic (gatifloxacin [Zymar] qid or moxifloxacin [Vigamox] tid).
- May require systemic antibiotics especially in children.
- Remove discharge with irrigation and membranes with sterile cotton-tipped applicator.

VIRAL

- Topical lubrication with artificial tears (see Appendix) and topical vasoconstrictor, NSAID, antihistamine, mast cell stabilizer, or mast cell stabilizer and antihistamine combination (see Table 4-1).
- Add topical antibiotic (polymyxin B sulfate–trimethoprim [Polytrim] qid, erythromycin or bacitracin ointment qd to tid) for corneal epithelial defects.
- Add topical steroid (fluorometholone alcohol 0.1% [FML] qid) for subepithelial infiltrates in EKC.
- Add topical antiviral medication (trifluridine [Viroptic] 5 times/day) for herpes simplex.

OTHER INFECTIONS

- *N. gonorrhoeae,* chlamydia, and Parinaud's oculoglandular syndrome (e.g., cat-scratch disease, tularemia, syphilis, tuberculosis, etc.) require systemic antibiotics based on causative organism.

Management—cont'd

ALLERGIC

- Topical vasoconstrictor, NSAID, antihistamine, mast cell stabilizer, or mast cell stabilizer and antihistamine combination (Table 4-1).
- Consider mild topical steroid especially for severe allergic keratoconjunctivitis; start with fluorometholone alcohol 0.1% (FML) qid or loteprednol etabonate 0.2% (Alrex) qid, change to prednisolone 1% qid to q1h in severe cases. Solution (phosphate [Inflamase Mild, AK-Pred]) works better than suspension (acetate [Pred Mild, Econopred]).
- Consider systemic antihistamine (diphenhydramine [Benadryl] 25-50 mg po q6h prn).

GIANT PAPILLARY CONJUNCTIVITIS

- Clean, change, or discontinue use of contact lenses; change contact lens cleaning solution to preservative free (see Chapter 5).

SUPERIOR LIMBIC KERATOCONJUNCTIVITIS

- Silver nitrate solution, bandage contact lens, conjunctival cautery, or conjunctival recession and resection; steroids do not help; cromolyn sodium 4% [Crolom] qid or olopatadine hydrochloride 0.1% [Patanol] bid may be useful (see Chapter 5).

ATOPIC AND VERNAL KERATOCONJUNCTIVITIS

- Consider topical cyclosporine (1-2%) qid; also consider supratarsal steroid injection (0.25-0.50 ml dexamethasone or triamcinolone acetate [Kenalog]).

KAWASAKI'S DISEASE

- Pediatric consultation and hospital admission; systemic steroids are contraindicated.

LIGNEOUS

- May respond to topical steroids, mucolytics, or cyclosporine.

Prognosis

Usually good; subepithelial infiltrates in adenoviral conjunctivitis cause variable decreased vision for months.

◼ Conjunctival Degeneration

Definition

Secondary degenerative changes of the conjunctiva.

Table 4-1   Topical Medications Available for Management of Allergic Conjunctivitis

Mechanism	Trade Name	Pharmacologic Name	Dosage
Antihistamine	Emadine	Emadastine 0.05%	qid
	Livostin	Levocabastine 0.05%	qid
Mast cell stabilizer	Alamast	Pemirolast 0.1%	qid
	Alocril	Nedocromil 2%	bid
	Alomide	Lodoxamide 0.1%	qid
	Crolom	Cromolyn sodium 4%	qid
Mast cell stabilizer and antihistamine combination	Optivar	Azelastine 0.05%	bid
	Patanol	Olopatadine 0.1%	bid
	Zaditor	Ketotifen fumarate 0.025%	bid
Nonsteroidal antiinflammatory	Acular	Ketorolac tromethamine 0.5%	qid
Steroidal antiinflammatory	Alrex	Loteprednol etabonate 0.2%	up to qid
Vasoconstrictor	Naphcon-A	Naphazoline 0.025% and pheniramine 0.3%	up to qid
	Vasocon-A	Naphazoline 0.05% and antazoline 0.5%	up to qid

Amyloidosis

Yellow-white or salmon-colored, avascular deposits; may be due to primary (localized) or secondary (systemic) amyloidosis.

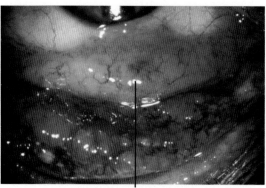

Conjunctival amyloidosis

Figure 4-26 • Yellowish avascular deposits in inferior conjunctiva from amyloidosis.

Concretions

Yellow-white inclusion cysts filled with keratin and epithelial debris in fornix or palpebral conjunctiva; associated with aging and chronic conjunctivitis; can erode overlying conjunctiva causing foreign body sensation; easily unroofed and removed with a 25-30 gauge needle if symptomatic (see Figure 4-20).

Pingueculae

Yellow-white, subepithelial deposits of abnormal collagen at the nasal or temporal limbus; due to actinic changes; elastotic degeneration seen histologically; may calcify over time.

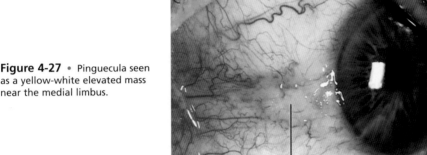

Figure 4-27 • Pinguecula seen as a yellow-white elevated mass near the medial limbus.

Pinguecula

Pterygium

Triangular fibrovascular tissue in interpalpebral space involving cornea; often preceded by pinguecula; destroys Bowman's membrane; may have iron line at leading edge (Stocker's line); induces astigmatism and may cause decreased vision.

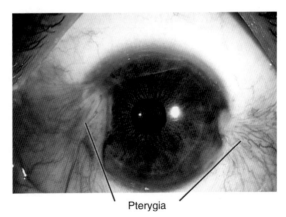

Figure 4-28 • Large nasal and smaller temporal pterygia. Note the typical triangular, wedge-shaped configuration, and also the white corneal scarring at the leading edges.

Pterygia

Symptoms

Asymptomatic; may have red eye, foreign body sensation, decreased vision; may notice bump or growth; may have contact lens intolerance.

Signs

See above.

Differential Diagnosis

Cyst, squamous cell carcinoma, conjunctival intraepithelial neoplasia, episcleritis, scleritis, phlyctenule.

Evaluation

• Complete ophthalmic history and eye examination with attention to conjunctiva and cornea.

Management

• No treatment recommended.
• Topical lubrication with artificial tears (see Appendix) up to q1h.
• Consider limited use of vasoconstrictor (naphazoline [Naphcon] qid) for inflamed pterygium, and excision of pterygium for chronic inflammation, cosmesis, contact lens intolerance, or involvement of visual axis.

Prognosis

Good; about one third of pterygia recur after simple excision, recurrences are reduced by conjunctival autograft, β-irradiation, thiotepa, or mitomycin C.

■ Ocular Cicatricial Pemphigoid

Definition

Systemic vesiculobullous disease of mucous membranes resulting in bilateral, chronic, cicatrizing conjunctivitis; other mucous membranes frequently involved, including oral (up to 90%), esophageal, tracheal, and genital; skin involved in up to 30% of cases.

Etiology

Usually idiopathic (probably autoimmune mechanism) or drug induced (may occur with epinephrine, timolol, pilocarpine, echothiophate iodide [Phospholine Iodide], or idoxuridine).

Epidemiology

Incidence of 1 in 20,000; usually occurs in females (2:1) over 60 years old; associated with HLA-DR4, DQw3.

Symptoms

Red eye, dryness, foreign body sensation, tearing, decreased vision; may have dysphagia or difficulty breathing.

Signs

Normal or decreased visual acuity, conjunctival injection and scarring, dry eye, symblepharon (fusion or attachment of eyelid to bulbar conjunctiva), ankyloblepharon (fusion or attachment of upper and lower eyelids), foreshortened fornices, trichiasis, entropion, keratitis, corneal ulcer, scarring, and vascularization, conjunctival and corneal keratinization, and oral lesions; corneal perforation and endophthalmitis can occur.

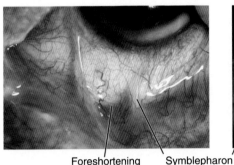

Foreshortening Symblepharon   Ankyloblepharon Neovascularization

Figure 4-29 • Ocular cicatricial pemphigoid demonstrating symblepharon and foreshortening of the inferior fornix.

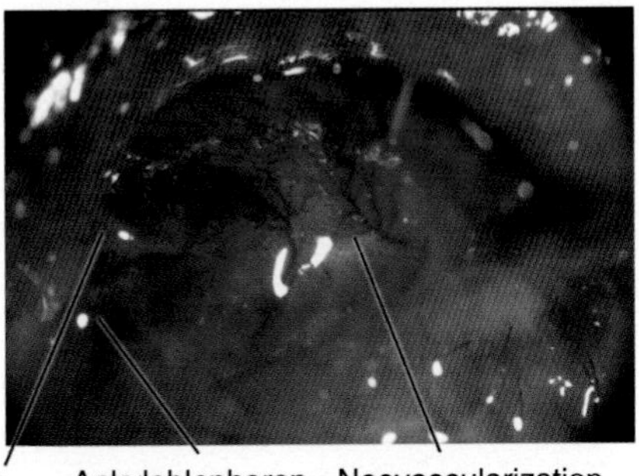

Figure 4-30 • Ocular cicatricial pemphigoid demonstrating advanced stage with corneal vascularization, symblepharon, and complete ankyloblepharon formation.

Differential Diagnosis

Stevens-Johnson syndrome, chemical burn, squamous cell carcinoma, scleroderma, infectious or allergic conjunctivitis, trachoma, sarcoidosis, ocular rosacea, radiation, linear immunoglobulin A dermatosis, practolol-induced conjunctivitis.

Evaluation

- Complete ophthalmic history and eye examination with attention to conjunctiva and cornea.
- Conjunctival biopsy (immunoglobulin and complement deposition in basement membrane).

Management

- Topical lubrication with preservative-free artificial tears (see Appendix) up to q1h and ointment (Refresh P.M.) at bedtime.
- Add topical antibiotic (polymyxin B sulfate–trimethoprim [Polytrim] qid or erythromycin ointment tid) for corneal epithelial defects.
- Consider punctal occlusion, tarsorrhaphy.
- Often requires treatment with systemic steroids or immunosuppressive agents (dapsone [contraindicated in patients with glucose 6-phosphate dehydrogenase deficiency], cyclophosphamide); should be performed by a cornea or uveitis specialist.
- Consider surgery for entropion and trichiasis, release of symblepharon, and mucous membrane grafting; keratoprosthesis used in advanced cases.

Prognosis

Poor; chronic progressive disease with remissions and exacerbations, surgery often initiates exacerbations.

Stevens-Johnson Syndrome or ■ Erythema Multiforme Major

Definition

Acute, usually self-limited (up to 6 weeks), cutaneous, bullous disease with mucosal ulceration resulting in acute membranous conjunctivitis.

Etiology

Usually drug-induced (may occur with sulfonamides, penicillin, aspirin, barbiturates, isoniazid, or phenytoin [Dilantin]) or infectious (herpes simplex virus, *Mycoplasma* species, adenovirus, *Streptococcus* species).

Symptoms

Fever, upper respiratory infection, headache, malaise, skin eruption, decreased vision, pain, red eye, swelling, and oral mucosal ulceration.

Signs

Fever, skin eruption (target lesions), mucous membrane ulceration and crusting, decreased visual acuity, conjunctival injection, discharge, membranes, dry eye, symblepharon (fusion or attachment of eyelid to bulbar conjunctiva), trichiasis, keratitis, corneal ulcer, scarring, vascularization, and keratinization.

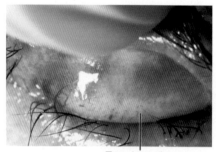

Tarsal scarring

Figure 4-31 • Stevens-Johnson syndrome demonstrating tarsal scarring.

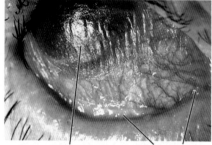

Corneal keratinization   Symblepharon

Figure 4-32 • Stevens-Johnson syndrome demonstrating keratinization of the ocular surface with a dry, wrinkled appearance. Note the resulting irregular, diffuse corneal reflex.

Differential Diagnosis

Ocular cicatricial pemphigoid, chemical burn, squamous cell carcinoma, scleroderma, infectious or allergic conjunctivitis, trachoma, sarcoidosis, ocular rosacea, radiation.

Evaluation

- Complete ophthalmic history and eye examination with attention to systemic mucous membranes, conjunctiva, and cornea.
- Medical consultation.

Management

- Supportive, topical lubrication with preservative-free artificial tears (see Appendix) up to q1h and ointment (Refresh P.M.) at bedtime.
- Add topical antibiotic (polymyxin B sulfate–trimethoprim [Polytrim] qid or erythromycin ointment tid) for corneal epithelial defects.
- Consider topical steroid (prednisolone acetate 1% up to q2h) depending on severity of inflammation.
- Consider systemic steroids (prednisone 60-100 mg po qd) in very severe cases.
- Check purified protein derivative (PPD), blood glucose, and chest radiographs before starting systemic steroids.
- Add H_2-blocker (ranitidine [Zantac] 150 mg po bid) or proton pump inhibitor when taking steroids.
- May require punctal occlusion, tarsorrhaphy for more severe cases.
- Consider surgery for trichiasis, symblepharon, or corneal scarring.

Prognosis

Fair; not progressive (in contrast to ocular cicatricial pemphigoid), recurrences are rare, but up to 30% mortality.

▊ Conjunctival Tumors

Congenital

Hamartoma

Derived from abnormal rest of cells, composed of tissues normally found at same location (e.g., telangiectasia, lymphangioma).

Choristoma

Derived from abnormal rest of cells, composed of tissues not normally found at that location.

Dermoid White-yellow, solid, round, elevated nodule, often with visible hairs on surface and lipid deposition anterior to its corneal edge; composed of dense connective tissue with pilosebaceous units and stratified squamous epithelium; usually located at inferotemporal limbus; may be part of Goldenhar's syndrome with dermoids, preauricular skin tags, and vertebral anomalies.

Dermolipoma Similar appearance to dermoid but composed of adipose tissue with keratinized surface; usually located superotemporally extending into orbit.

Epibulbar osseous choristoma Solitary, white nodule composed of compact bone that develops from episclera; freely moveable; usually located superotemporally.

Cysts

Fluid-filled cavity within the conjunctiva, defined by its lining (ductal or inclusion); often due to trauma or inflammation, can be congenital.

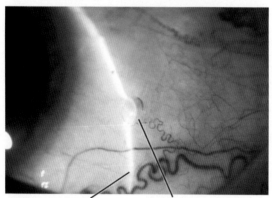

Slit-beam Conjunctival inclusion cyst

Figure 4-33 • Conjunctival inclusion cyst appears as a clear elevation over which the slit beam bends.

Epithelial

Papilloma

Red, gelatinous lesions composed of proliferative epithelium with fibrovascular cores; may be pedunculated or sessile, solitary or multiple; often associated with human papillomavirus.

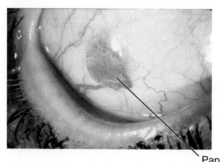

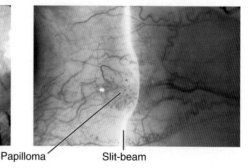

Papilloma   Slit-beam

Figure 4-34 • Papilloma demonstrating the typical elevated appearance with central vascular fronds.

Figure 4-35 • Squamous papilloma with elevated, gelatinous appearance.

Conjunctival Intraepithelial Neoplasia

White, gelatinous, conjunctival dysplasia confined to the epithelium; usually begins at limbus and is a precursor of squamous cell carcinoma.

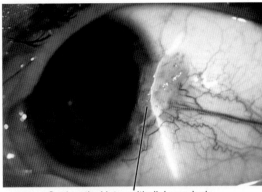

Figure 4-36 • Conjunctival intraepithelial neoplasia demonstrating pink, nodular, gelatinous, vascularized appearance at the limbus.

Conjunctival intraepithelial neoplasia

Squamous Cell Carcinoma

Interpalpebral, exophytic, gelatinous, papillary appearance with loops of vessels; may have superficial invasion and extend onto cornea; deep invasion and metastasis are rare. Suspect AIDS in patients <50 years of age.

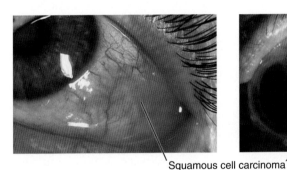 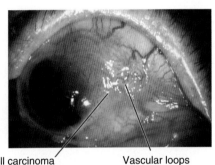

Squamous cell carcinoma   Vascular loops

Figure 4-37 • Squamous cell carcinoma appearing as a pink, diffuse, gelatinous growth.

Figure 4-38 • More advanced squamous cell carcinoma with gelatinous growth and abnormal vascular loops.

Melanocytic

Nevus

Mobile, discrete, elevated, variably pigmented lesion that contains cysts; may be junctional, subepithelial, or compound; may enlarge during puberty; rarely becomes malignant.

Ocular Melanocytosis

Unilateral, increased uveal, scleral, and episcleral pigmentation appearing as blue-gray patches; more common in whites.

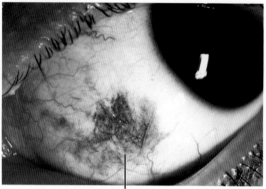

Figure 4-39 • Ocular melanocytosis demonstrating blue-gray, patchy pigmentation.

Ocular melanocytosis

Oculodermal Melanocytosis or Nevus of Ota

Increased uveal, scleral, episcleral, and periorbital skin pigmentation; more common in Asians and African Americans; uveal melanoma may rarely develop in whites (see Chapter 10).

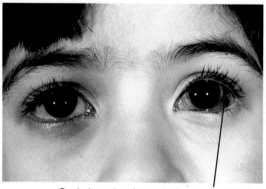

Figure 4-40 • Oculodermal melanocytosis (nevus of Ota) of the left eye. Note the prominent scleral pigmentation; the periorbital skin changes are difficult to see in this photo.

Oculodermal melanocytosis (nevus of Ota)

Primary Acquired Melanosis (PAM)

Mobile, patchy, diffuse, flat, brown lesions without cysts; indistinct margins and may grow; occurs in middle-aged adults; histologically may have atypia; malignant potential (30%).

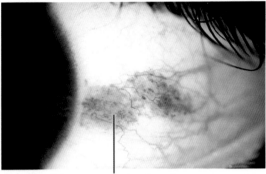

Figure 4-41 • Primary acquired melanosis demonstrating mottled, brown, patchy pigmentation.

Primary acquired melanosis

Secondary Acquired Melanosis

Hyperpigmentation due to racial variations, actinic stimulation, radiation, pregnancy, Addison's disease, or inflammation; usually perilimbal.

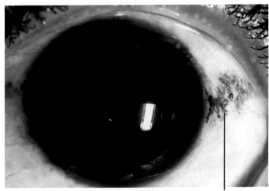

Figure 4-42 • Secondary acquired melanosis (racial pigmentation) demonstrating typical perilimbal, brown, homogeneous pigmentation.

Secondary acquired melanosis

Malignant Melanoma

Nodular, pigmented lesion containing vessels, but no cysts; may arise from primary acquired melanosis, nevi, or de novo; 20-40% mortality.

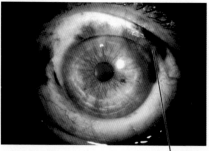

Malignant melanoma

Figure 4-43 • Malignant melanoma with nodular, pigmented, vascular lesion at the limbus.

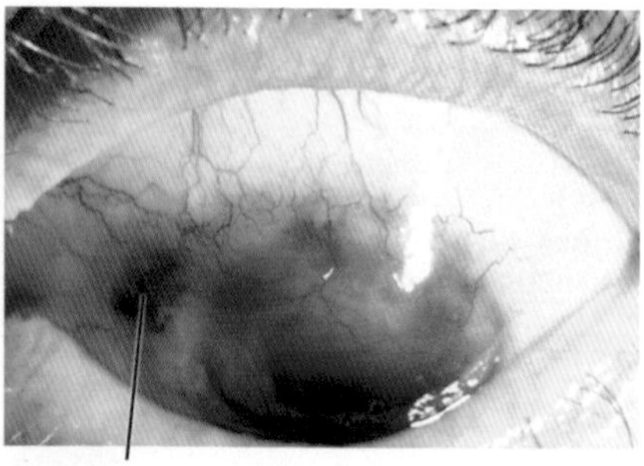

Figure 4-44 • Malignant melanoma demonstrating irregular pigmented growth at limbus and onto cornea with vascularization.

Stromal

Cavernous Hemangioma

Red patch on conjunctiva; may bleed and be associated with other ocular hemangiomas or systemic disease.

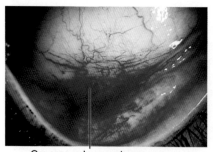

Cavernous hemangioma

Figure 4-45 • Cavernous hemangioma demonstrating red patch of dilated blood vessels in the inferior fornix.

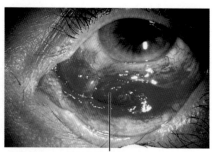

Kaposi's sarcoma

Figure 4-46 • Kaposi's sarcoma demonstrating beefy, red, large, nodular mass in the inferior fornix.

Juvenile Xanthogranuloma

Yellow-orange conjunctival nodules composed of vascularized, lipid-containing histiocytes; can also involve iris and skin; often regresses spontaneously.

Kaposi's Sarcoma

Single or multiple, flat or elevated, deep red to purple plaques (malignant granulation tissue) on palpebral conjunctiva; may involve orbit; occurs in immunocompromised individuals, especially HIV-positive patients.

Lymphangiectasis

Cluster of elevated clear cysts that represent dilated lymphatics; may have areas of hemorrhage.

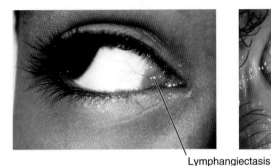
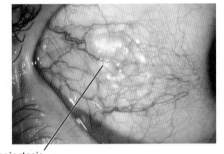

Lymphangiectasis

Figure 4-47 • Lymphangiectasis demonstrating cluster of cysts medially near the caruncle.

Figure 4-48 • Lymphangiectasis with clear cysts.

Lymphoid

Single or multiple, smooth, flat, salmon-colored patches; usually occurs in middle-aged adults; spectrum of disease from benign reactive lymphoid hyperplasia to malignant lymphoma (non-Hodgkin's); may develop systemic lymphoma (see Chapter 1).

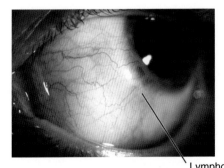
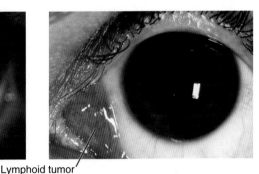

Lymphoid tumor

Figure 4-49 • Malignant lymphoma with salmon-colored lesion.

Figure 4-50 • Lymphoid tumor demonstrating typical salmon-patch appearance.

Pyogenic Granuloma

Red, fleshy, polypoid mass at the site of chronic inflammation; often follows surgical or accidental trauma; misnomer, because it is neither pyogenic nor a granuloma, but rather granulation tissue.

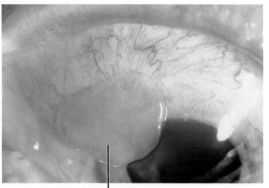

Pyogenic granuloma

Figure 4-51 • Pyogenic granuloma appearing as a large, fleshy, vascular, pedunculated growth.

Caruncle

Tumors that affect the conjunctiva may also occur in the caruncle, including (in order of frequency): papilloma, nevus, inclusion cyst, malignant melanoma, also sebaceous cell carcinoma, and oncocytoma (oxyphilic adenoma; fleshy, yellow-tan cystic mass from transformation of epithelial cells of accessory lacrimal glands; slowly progressive).

Symptoms

Asymptomatic; may notice discoloration or growth of the lesion.

Signs

Conjunctival lesion (see above), may have involvement of lids, cornea, rarely intraocular or intraorbital extension.

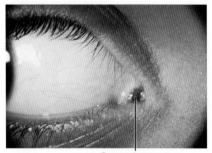

Caruncle nevus

Figure 4-52 • Nevus of the caruncle appearing as a brown pigmented spot on medial side of the caruncle.

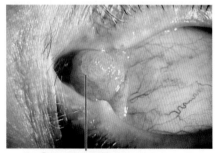

Caruncle papilloma

Figure 4-53 • Papilloma of the caruncle appearing as a large, vascular, pedunculated mass.

Differential Diagnosis

See above.

Evaluation

- Complete ophthalmic history and eye examination with attention to skin, everting lids, conjunctiva, cornea, and ophthalmoscopy.
- Consider biopsy.
- Medical consultation and systemic workup for malignant and lymphoproliferative processes.

Management

- Depends on etiology; options include observation, radiation, cryotherapy, chemotherapy (mitomycin C, interferon), excision, and enucleation; should be performed by a cornea or tumor specialist.

Prognosis

Depends on etiology; good except malignant and lymphoid tumors.

■ Episcleritis

Definition

Sectoral (70%) or diffuse (30%) inflammation of episclera.

Epidemiology

Eighty percent simple; 20% nodular; 33% bilateral.

Etiology

Idiopathic, tuberculosis, syphilis, herpes zoster, rheumatoid arthritis, other collagen vascular diseases.

Symptoms

Asymptomatic; may have mild pain and red eye.

Signs

Subconjunctival and conjunctival injection, usually sectoral; may have chemosis, episcleral nodules, anterior chamber cells and flare.

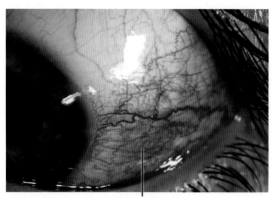

Figure 4-54 • Episcleritis demonstrating characteristic sectoral injection.

Episcleritis

Differential Diagnosis

Scleritis, iritis, phlyctenule, myositis.

Evaluation

- Complete ophthalmic history and eye examination with attention to pattern of conjunctival and scleral injection and blanching with topical phenylephrine (scleritis is painful, has violaceous hue, and does not blanch with topical vasoconstrictor [phenylephrine 2.5%]), and anterior chamber.
- Consider scleritis workup in recurrent or bilateral cases (see Scleritis section).

Management

- No treatment recommended.
- Consider limited use of vasoconstrictor (naphazoline [Naphcon] qid), mild topical steroid (fluorometholone acetate [Flarex] qid), or oral NSAID (indomethacin 50 mg po qd to bid) if severe.

Prognosis

Good; usually self-limited; may be recurrent in 67% of cases.

■ Scleritis

Definition

Inflammation of sclera, can be anterior (98%) or posterior (2%).

Epidemiology

Anterior form may be diffuse (40%), nodular (44%), or necrotizing (14%) with or without (scleromalacia perforans) inflammation; more than 50% are bilateral; associated systemic disease in 50% of cases.

Etiology

Collagen vascular disease in 30% of cases (most commonly rheumatoid arthritis, ankylosing spondylitis, systemic lupus erythematosus, polyarteritis nodosa, Wegener's granulomatosis, and relapsing polychondritis); also herpes zoster, syphilis, tuberculosis, leprosy, gout, porphyria, postsurgical, and idiopathic.

Symptoms

Pain, photophobia, swelling, red eye, decreased vision (except scleromalacia).

Signs

Normal or decreased visual acuity, subconjunctival and conjunctival injection with violaceous hue, chemosis, scleral edema, scleral nodule(s), globe tenderness to palpation; may have anterior chamber cells and flare (30%), corneal infiltrate or thinning, scleral thinning (30%); posterior type may have chorioretinal folds and focal serous retinal detachment.

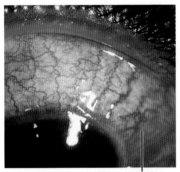

Scleritis

Figure 4-55 • Diffuse anterior scleritis demonstrating characteristic deep red, violaceous hue.

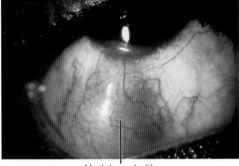

Nodular scleritis

Figure 4-56 • Nodular anterior scleritis. Note the elevated nodule within the deep, red, sectoral injection.

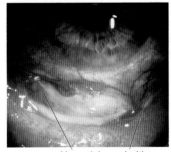

Necrotizing scleritis

Figure 4-57 • Necrotizing scleritis demonstrating thinning of sclera superiorly with increased visibility of the underlying blue uvea.

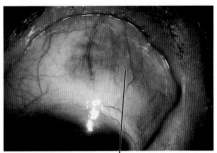

Scleromalacia perforans

Figure 4-58 • Scleromalacia perforans demonstrating characteristic blue appearance due to visible uvea underneath thin sclera.

Differential Diagnosis

Episcleritis, iritis, phlyctenule, retrobulbar mass, myositis, scleral ectasia, and staphyloma.

Evaluation

- Complete ophthalmic history and eye examination with attention to pattern of conjunctival and scleral injection and failure of area to blanch with topical vasoconstrictor (phenylephrine 2.5%), cornea, anterior chamber, and ophthalmoscopy.
- B-scan ultrasonography: thickened sclera and "T-sign" in posterior scleritis.
- **Lab tests:** Complete blood count (CBC), rheumatoid factor (RF), antinuclear antibody (ANA), antineutrophil cytoplasmic antibody (ANCA), Venereal Disease Research Laboratory (VDRL) test, fluorescent treponemal antibody absorption (FTA-ABS) test, PPD and controls, and chest radiographs.
- Medical consultation.

Management

- Depending on severity, consider using one or a combination of the following:
- Systemic NSAID (indomethacin 50 mg po bid to tid, Dolobid 500 mg po qd to bid, Celebrex 200 mg po bid).
- Systemic steroids (prednisone 60-100 mg po qd); *Note:* topical steroids and NSAIDs are ineffective.
- Check PPD, blood glucose, and chest radiographs before starting systemic steroids.
- Add H_2-blocker (ranitidine [Zantac] 150 mg po bid) or proton pump inhibitor when taking oral NSAIDs or steroids.
- Consider immunosuppressive agents (see Anterior Uveitis section in Chapter 6) in severe cases; should be administered by a uveitis specialist.
- Sub-Tenon's steroid injection is contraindicated.
- May require surgery (patch graft) for globe perforation.

Prognosis

Depends on etiology; poor for necrotizing form, which may perforate; scleromalacia perforans rarely perforates; recurrences common.

▮ Scleral Discoloration

Definition

Alkaptonuria or Ochronosis

Recessive inborn error of metabolism (accumulation of homogentisic acid) causing brown pigment deposits in eyes, ears, nose, joints, and heart; triangular patches in interpalpebral space near limbus, pigmentation of tarsus and lids.

Ectasia or Staphyloma

Congenital, focal area of scleral thinning usually near limbus; underlying uvea is visible and may bulge through defect; perforation is uncommon.

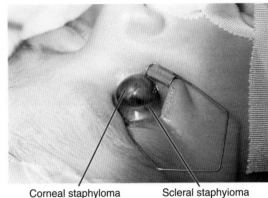

Figure 4-59 • Scleral and corneal staphylomas with bulging blue appearance.

Corneal staphyloma Scleral staphyioma

Osteogenesis Imperfecta

Congenital disorder of collagen; sclera is thin and appears blue due to underlying uvea (also seen in Ehlers-Danlos syndrome).

Scleral Icterus

Yellow sclera seen in hyperbilirubinemia.

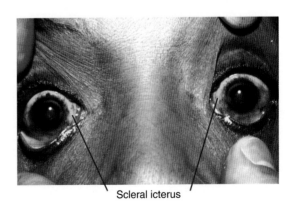

Figure 4-60 • Scleral icterus in patient with jaundice.

Scleral icterus

Senile Scleral Plaque

Blue-gray discoloration of sclera located near horizontal rectus muscle insertions due to hyalinization; seen in elderly patients.

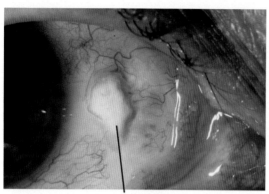

Figure 4-61 • Senile scleral plaque demonstrating discoloration of sclera near horizontal rectus muscle insertions due to hyalinization.

Scleral plaque

Symptoms

Asymptomatic; may notice scleral discoloration.

Signs

Focal or diffuse discoloration of sclera in one or both eyes.

Differential Diagnosis

See above; also foreign body, melanoma, mascara, intrascleral nerve loop, adrenochrome deposits (epinephrine), scleromalacia perforans.

Evaluation

- Complete ophthalmic history and eye examination with attention to conjunctiva, sclera, and ophthalmoscopy.
- B-scan ultrasonography and gonioscopy to rule out suspected extension of uveal melanoma.
- Medical consultation for systemic diseases.

Management

- No treatment recommended.
- Treat underlying disorder.

Prognosis

Good; discoloration itself is benign.

CORNEA

Trauma

Birth Trauma

Vertical or oblique breaks in Descemet's membrane due to forceps injury at birth; acute corneal edema and breaks or scars in Descemet's membrane that usually resolve; associated with astigmatism and amblyopia in later life.

- No treatment required.

Chemical or Thermal Burn

Corneal tissue destruction (epithelium and stroma) due to chemical (acid or base) or thermal (e.g., welding, intense sunlight, tanning lamp) injury; alkali causes most severe injury and may cause perforation; patients note pain, foreign body sensation, photophobia, tearing, and red eye; may have normal or decreased visual acuity, conjunctival injection, ciliary injection, epithelial defects that stain with fluorescein, and scleral or limbal blanching due to ischemia in severe chemical burns; prognosis variable, worst for severe alkali burns.

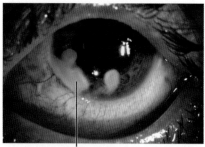

Corneal alkali burn

Figure 5-1 • Alkali burn demonstrating corneal burns and conjunctival injection on the day of the accident.

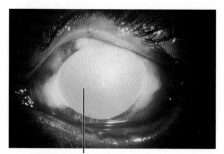

Corneal alkali burn

Figure 5-2 • Complete corneal tissue destruction 7 days after alkali burn.

Ophthalmic Emergency

- Immediate copious irrigation with sterile water, saline, or Ringer's solution.
- Measure pH before and after irrigation, continue irrigation until pH is neutralized.
- Remove any chemical particulate matter from surface of eye and evert lids to sweep fornices with sterile cotton swab.
- Topical lubrication with preservative-free artificial tears (see Appendix) up to q1h and ointment (Refresh P.M.) at bedtime, broad spectrum topical antibiotic (gatifloxacin [Zymar] or moxifloxacin [Vigamox] qid), and cycloplegic agent (cyclopentolate 1%, scopolamine 0.25%, or atropine 1% bid to qid depending on severity).
- For more severe damage, consider topical steroids (prednisolone acetate 1% up to q2h then taper; only use during first week, then if steroids are still necessary, change to medroxyprogesterone [Provera 1%]), topical citrate (10% qid), or sodium ascorbate (10% qid and 2 g po qid), collagenase inhibitor (acetylcysteine [Mucomyst] up to q4h).
- May require treatment of increased intraocular pressure (see Chapter 11).
- In severe cases, surgery may be required, including symblepharon lysis, conjunctival and mucous membrane transplantation, and tarsorrhaphy; later consider penetrating keratoplasty or keratoprosthesis.

Corneal Abrasion

Corneal epithelial defect usually due to trauma; patients note pain, foreign body sensation, photophobia, tearing, and red eye; may have normal or decreased visual acuity, conjunctival injection, and an epithelial defect that stains with fluorescein.

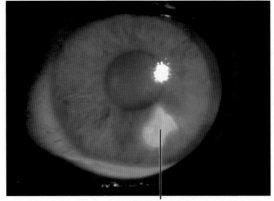

Figure 5-3 • Corneal abrasion demonstrating fluorescein staining of small inferior epithelial defect.

Corneal abrasion

- Topical antibiotic drop (polymyxin B sulfate–trimethoprim [Polytrim] or tobramycin [Tobrex] qid) or ointment (polymyxin B sulfate–bacitracin [Polysporin] qid).
- Consider topical nonsteroidal antiinflammatory drugs (NSAID) (ketorolac tromethamine [Acular] or diclofenac sodium [Voltaren] tid for 48-72 hours) for pain.
- Consider topical cycloplegic agent (cyclopentolate 1% bid) for pain and photophobia.
- Pressure patch or bandage contact lens if area larger than 10 mm² (*Note:* do not patch if patient is contact lens wearer, there is corneal infiltrate, or injury caused by plant material, because these scenarios represent high risk for infectious keratitis if patched; no patching necessary if area of abrasion is <10 mm².)

Foreign Body

Foreign material on or in cornea; usually metal, glass, or organic material; may have associated rust ring if metallic; patients note pain, foreign body sensation, photophobia, tearing, and red eye; may have normal or decreased visual acuity, conjunctival injection, ciliary injection, foreign body, rust ring, epithelial defect that stains with fluorescein, corneal edema, anterior chamber cells and flare; may be asymptomatic if deep and chronic; good prognosis unless rust ring or scarring involves visual axis.

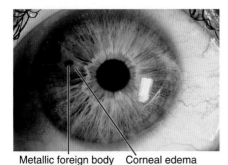

Metallic foreign body   Corneal edema

Figure 5-4 • Metallic foreign body appears as brown spot on cornea.

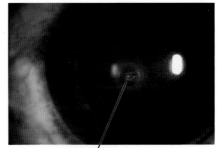

Rust ring

Figure 5-5 • Rust ring from iron foreign body in central cornea.

- Removal of foreign material with needle or foreign body removal instruments unless it is deep, nonpenetrating, unexposed, and inert material (may be observed).
- Remove rust ring with Alger brush or automated burr.
- Seidel test if deep foreign body to rule out open globe (see below).
- Topical antibiotic (polymyxin B sulfate–trimethoprim [Polytrim], moxifloxacin [Vigamox], or tobramycin [Tobrex] qid) and cycloplegic agent (cyclopentolate 1% bid).
- Pressure patch or bandage contact lens as needed (same indications as for corneal abrasion; see above).

Laceration

Partial or full-thickness cut in cornea (see Open Globe section in Chapter 4) due to trauma; patients note pain, foreign body sensation, photophobia, tearing, and red eye; may have normal or decreased visual acuity, conjunctival injection, ciliary injection, intraocular foreign body, corneal laceration, corneal edema, breaks or scars in Descemet's membrane, anterior chamber cells and flare, low intraocular pressure; good prognosis unless laceration crosses visual axis.

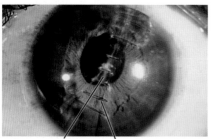

Corneal laceration   Nylon sutures

Figure 5-6 • Large corneal laceration through visual axis. Note the linear scar from the wound and around the multiple, interrupted, nylon sutures of various lengths used to repair the laceration.

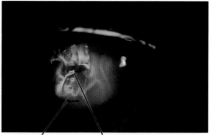

Nylon sutures   Positive Seidel test

Figure 5-7 • Corneal laceration demonstrating positive Seidel test (bright stream of fluorescein around the central suture).

- **Seidel test** (to rule out open globe): concentrated fluorescein is used to cover the suspected leakage site by placing a drop of sterile 2% fluorescein in the eye or wetting a sterile fluorescein strip and painting the area of the wound. Slit-lamp examination is then performed looking for a stream of diluted fluorescein emanating from the wound. This will appear as a fluorescent yellow area on a dark blue background with the cobalt blue light, or a light yellow-green area on a dark orange background with the white light.
- Partial thickness lacerations require topical broad spectrum antibiotic (gatifloxacin [Zymar] or moxifloxacin [Vigamox] qid) and cycloplegic agent (cyclopentolate 1% or scopolamine 0.25% tid).
- Daily follow-up until wound has healed.
- Pressure patch or bandage contact lens as needed; if wound gape exists, consider surgical repair.
- Full-thickness lacerations usually require surgical repair (see Open Globe section in Chapter 4).

- Consider orbital radiographs or computed tomography (CT) to rule out intraocular foreign body when full-thickness laceration exists; magnetic resonance imaging (MRI) contraindicated if foreign body is metallic.

Recurrent Erosion

Recurrent bouts of pain, foreign body sensation, photophobia, tearing, red eye, and spontaneous corneal epithelial defect usually upon awakening; associated with anterior basement membrane dystrophy in 50% of cases, or previous traumatic corneal abrasion (usually from fingernail, paper, plant, or brush); also seen in Meesman's, Reis-Bücklers, lattice, granular, Fuchs', and posterior polymorphous dystrophies.

- Same treatment as for corneal abrasion until reepithelialization occurs, then add hypertonic saline ointment (Adsorbonac or Muro 128 5% at bedtime for 3 months).
- Topical lubrication with preservative-free artificial tears (see Appendix) up to q1h or Muro 128 drops.
- Consider debridement, bandage contact lens, anterior stromal puncture or reinforcement, Nd:YAG laser reinforcement, or phototherapeutic keratectomy for multiple recurrences.
- Consider doxycycline 50 mg po bid for 2 months (matrix metalloproteinase-9 inhibitor) and topical steroid tid for 2-3 weeks (experimental).

■ Peripheral Ulcerative Keratitis

Definition

Marginal Keratolysis

Acute corneal ulceration or melting due to autoimmune or collagen vascular disease (systemic lupus erythematosus, rheumatoid arthritis, polyarteritis nodosa, and Wegener's granulomatosis); rapid progression, usually in one sector; corneal epithelium absent; may perforate; melting resolves after healing of overlying epithelium.

Mooren's Ulcer

Idiopathic, inflammatory, painful, progressive, peripheral thinning and ulceration that spreads circumferentially and then centrally with undermining of the leading edge; neovascularization may occur; two types:

(1) More common (75%), benign, and unilateral; seen in older patients; responds to conservative management.
(2) Progressive and bilateral; seen in younger patients; more common in black males; may perforate; may be associated with coexistent parasitemia.

Symptoms

Asymptomatic; may have pain, discharge, photophobia, red eye, and decreased vision.

Signs

Normal or decreased visual acuity, blepharitis, conjunctival injection, ciliary injection, corneal infiltrate with or without overlying epithelial defect, corneal thinning, corneal edema, anterior chamber cells and flare, hypopyon; may have associated scleritis in marginal keratolysis.

Slit-beam   Mooren's ulcer

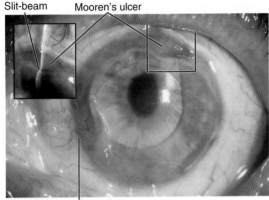

Neovascularization

Figure 5-8 • Mooren's ulcer demonstrating circumferential thinning and ulceration of almost the entire peripheral cornea. The leading edge of the ulcer can be seen as the thin, white, irregular line above the midsection of the iris from the 2 o'clock to 8 o'clock positions (counterclockwise) and then extending to the peripheral cornea. Neovascularization is most evident extending from the limbus at the 8 o'clock position. The inset demonstrates undermining of the ulcer's leading edge seen with a fine slit beam.

Differential Diagnosis

Infectious ulcer, sterile ulcer (diagnosis of exclusion), ocular rosacea, pellucid marginal degeneration, staphylococcal marginal keratitis (peripheral, white, corneal infiltrate(s) and ulceration 1-2 mm from limbus with intervening clear zone); often stains with fluorescein; due to immune response (hypersensitivity) to *Staphylococcus aureus;* associated with staphylococcal blepharitis, rosacea, phlyctenule, and vascularization; may progress to ring ulcer or become superinfected).

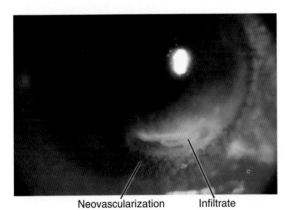

Figure 5-9 • Staphylococcal marginal keratitis demonstrating circumlimbal location of ulceration and infiltrate with intervening clear zone.

Neovascularization   Infiltrate

Evaluation

• Complete ophthalmic history and eye examination with attention to lids, keratometry, cornea, fluorescein staining, anterior chamber, and ophthalmoscopy.
• Consider corneal topography (computerized videokeratography).
• **Lab tests:** Complete blood count (CBC), erythrocyte sedimentation rate (ESR), rheumatoid factor (RF), antinuclear antibody, antineutrophil cytoplasmic antibody (ANCA); consider hepatitis C antigen (Mooren's ulcer).

- Consider cultures or smears to rule out infectious etiology.
- Medical or rheumatology consultation for systemic disorders or when treatment with immunosuppressive medications is anticipated.

Management

- Lid hygiene with warm compresses and lid scrubs for blepharitis.
- Consider oral doxycycline (50-100 mg po qd) for recurrent blepharitis.
- Consider protective eye wear to prevent perforation.
- Topical lubrication with preservative-free artificial tears (see Appendix) up to q1h and ointment (Refresh P.M.) at bedtime.
- Topical steroid (prednisolone acetate 1% or fluorometholone qid, adjust and taper as necessary).
- Add cycloplegic agent (cyclopentolate 1% bid) if anterior chamber cells and flare exists.
- Add antibiotic (polymyxin B sulfate–trimethoprim [Polytrim] or tobramycin [Tobrex] qid) if epithelial defect exists.
- Consider collagenase inhibitor (acetylcysteine [Mucomyst] qd to qid).
- Consider oral steroids (prednisone 60-100 mg po qd) for significant, progressive thinning; check purified protein derivative (PPD), blood glucose, and chest radiographs before starting systemic steroids.
- Add H_2-blocker (ranitidine [Zantac] 150 mg po bid) or proton pump inhibitor when administering systemic steroids.
- May require immunosuppressive agents, lamellar keratectomy with conjunctival resection, or penetrating keratoplasty if significant thinning exists; should be managed by a cornea specialist.

Prognosis

Depends on etiology; poor for marginal keratolysis and Mooren's ulcer.

▪ Contact Lens–Related Problems

Definition

A variety of abnormalities induced by contact lenses. Several types of lenses exist, broadly divided into rigid and soft lenses. They are used primarily to correct refractive errors (myopia, hyperopia, astigmatism, and presbyopia), but also can serve as a therapeutic bandage lens for unhealthy corneal surfaces or even for cosmetic use (to apparently change iris color or create a pseudopupil).

Rigid Lenses

Polymethylmethacrylate (PMMA) Hard lenses impermeable to oxygen; blinking allows tear film to enter space beneath lens providing nutrition to the cornea. Used for daily wear with good visual results but can lead to corneal edema and visual blur due to corneal hypoxia.

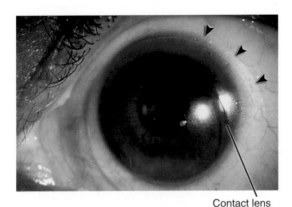

Figure 5-10 • Hard contact lens. The edge of the lens *(arrowheads)* as well as the central optical portion *(line)* are visible.

Contact lens

Gas-permeable   Rigid lenses composed of cellulose acetate butyrate, silicone acrylate, or silicone combined with polymethylmethacrylate; high oxygen permeability allows for greater comfort and improved corneal nutrition. Used for daily wear; lens of choice for patients with keratoconus and high astigmatism.

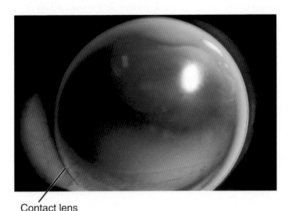

Figure 5-11 • Rigid gas-permeable contact lens demonstrating fluorescein staining pattern.

Contact lens

Soft Lenses

Daily wear   Hydrogel lenses (hydroxymethyl methacrylate); more comfortable and flexible than rigid lenses; conform to corneal surface, therefore poorly correct large degrees of astigmatism; length of time of wear depends on oxygen permeability and water content.

Extended wear   Disposable lenses discarded after extended wear from 1 week to 30 days; higher risk of infectious keratitis with overnight wear.

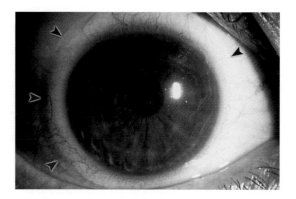

Figure 5-12 • Soft contact lens. Note the edge of the lens overlying the sclera *(arrowheads)*.

Symptoms

Foreign body sensation, decreased vision, red eye, tearing, itching, burning, pain, lens awareness, and reduced contact lens wear time.

Signs and Management

Corneal Abrasion

Corneal fluorescein staining due to epithelial defect (see Trauma: Corneal Abrasion section); contact lens–related etiologies include foreign bodies under lens, damaged lens, poor lens fit, corneal hypoxia, poor lens insertion or removal technique.

- Treat as for traumatic corneal abrasion except do not patch any size abrasion (see Trauma: Corneal Abrasion section).

Corneal Hypoxia

Acute   Conjunctival injection and epithelial defect (polymethylmethacrylate [PMMA] contact lens).

- Suspend contact lens use; topical antibiotic ointment (polymyxin B sulfate–bacitracin [Polysporin] tid for 3 days); when acute hypoxia has resolved, refit with higher Dk/L (oxygen transmissibility) contact lens.

Chronic   Punctate staining, corneal epithelial microcysts, stromal edema, and corneal neovascularization.

- Suspend contact lens use or decrease contact lens wear time; refit with higher Dk/L contact lens.

Contact Lens–Related Dendritic Keratitis

Conjunctivitis, pseudodendritic lesions.

- Suspend contact lens use until resolved.

Contact Lens Solution Hypersensitivity or Toxicity

Conjunctival injection, diffuse corneal punctate staining or erosion; seen with solutions that contain preservatives (e.g., thimerosal).

* Suspend contact lens use until resolved.
* Identify and discontinue toxic source; suspend contact lens use until corneal surface has healed; thoroughly clean, rinse, and disinfect contact lenses; educate patient on proper contact lens care or change system of care; replace soft contact lenses or polish rigid contact lens; topical antibiotic ointment (erythromycin or bacitracin tid for 3 days); do not patch.

Corneal Neovascularization

Superior corneal pannus 1-2 mm in soft contact lens wearer; larger than 2 mm is serious; may develop scarring, lipid deposits, stromal hemorrhage.

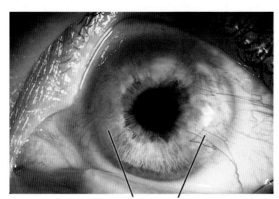

Corneal neovascularization

Figure 5-13 • Contact lens–induced corneal neovascularization and scarring.

* If neovascularization larger than 2 mm, suspend contact lens use and refit with higher Dk/L contact lens.

Corneal Warpage

Change in corneal shape (regular and irregular astigmatism) not associated with corneal edema; related to lens material (hard > rigid gas-permeable contact lens [RGP] > soft), fit, and length of time of wear. Usually asymptomatic, but some patients may notice poorer vision with glasses or contact lens intolerance; may have loss of best spectacle corrected visual acuity or change in refraction (especially axis of astigmatism); hallmark is abnormal corneal topography (computerized videokeratography).

* Suspend contact lens use; periodic evaluations with refraction and corneal topography until stabilization occurs.

Damaged Contact Lens

Pain with lens insertion and prompt relief with removal, look for chips in rigid lenses and fissures or tears in soft lenses.

• Replace defective contact lens.

Deposits on Contact Lens

Significant contact lens deposits (film or bumps), conjunctival injection, corneal erosion, excess contact lens movement, giant papillary conjunctivitis; old contact lens.

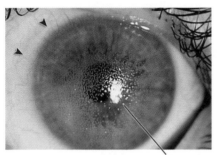
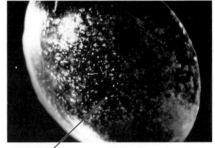

Deposits on contact lens

Figure 5-14 • Calcium phosphate deposits on soft contact lens.

Figure 5-15 • Lipid deposits on contact lens.

• Review contact lens cleaning procedures; institute regular enzyme cleaning (soft contact lens or RGP), frequent replacement schedule, or use of disposable contact lenses; polish rigid contact lens.

Giant Papillary Conjunctivitis

Due to contact lens protein deposits, conjunctival contact lens–related mechanical irritation, or soft contact lens material sensitivity reaction. Signs include large upper lid tarsal conjunctival papillae (>0.33 mm), ropy mucous discharge, contact lens coating, and possible contact lens decentration secondary to papillae; also seen with exposed sutures and ocular prosthesis (see Giant Papillary Conjunctivitis, p. 125).

• **Mild:** Replace contact lenses and reinstruct patient in thorough contact lens cleaning; decrease contact lens wear time; increase frequency of enzyme cleanings; change to frequent or disposable contact lenses, or change lens material from soft contact lens to RGP; topical lodoxamide tromethamine 0.1% (Alomide qid) or cromolyn sodium 4% (Crolom qid).
• **Severe:** Suspend contact lens use; short course of mild topical steroid (prednisolone acetate 1% or fluorometholone qid).

Infectious Keratitis

Pain, red eye, infiltrate with epithelial defect, and anterior chamber cells and flare; contact lens–related corneal infiltrates should be treated as an infection, suspect *Pseudomonas* or *Acanthamoeba;* seen more often in extended wear and soft contact lens wearers.

* See Infectious Keratitis section, p. 168.
* Suspend contact lens use.
* **Lab tests:** Cultures of cornea and contact lens solution.
* Topical broad spectrum antibiotics (fluoroquinolone [Vigamox or Zymar] or a fortified antibiotic q1h) (see Infectious Keratitis section for specific treatment); be alert for *Pseudomonas* and *Acanthamoeba;* do not patch any epithelial defects.

Sterile Corneal Infiltrates

Small (1 mm), peripheral, often multifocal, whitish, nummular, corneal lesions; corneal epithelium usually intact.

* Suspend contact lens use until condition resolves; use preservative-free solutions; must treat as corneal infection (see Infectious Keratitis section).

Poor Fit (Loose)

Upper eyelid irritation, limbal injection, excess contact lens movement with blinking, poor contact lens centration, lens edge bubbles, lens edge stand-off, variable keratometry mires with blinking, and lower portion of retinoscopy reflex darker and faster.

* Increase sagittal vault; choose steeper base curve or larger diameter contact lens.

Poor Fit (Tight)

Injection or indentation around limbus, minimal contact lens movement with blinking, blurred retinoscopic reflex, corneal edema, and distorted keratometry mires clear with blinking.

* Decrease sagittal vault; choose flatter base curve or smaller diameter contact lens.

Superior Limbic Keratoconjunctivitis

Contact lens–related causes include contact lens hypersensitivity reaction and poor contact lens fit. Upper tarsal micropapillae, superior limbal injection, fluorescein staining of superior bulbar conjunctiva, and 12 o'clock micropannus are seen (see Superior Limbic Keratoconjunctivitis in Chapter 4).

* Suspend contact lens use; replace or clean contact lenses; use preservative-free contact lens solutions (no thimerosal); for persistent cases, consider topical steroid (prednisolone acetate 1% or fluorometholone qid) or silver nitrate 0.5-1.0% solution.

Superficial Punctate Keratitis

Contact lens–related etiologies include poor lens fit, dry eye, and contact lens solution reaction; punctate fluorescein staining of corneal surface.

* Suspend contact lens use until corneal surface has healed; topical lubrication with artificial tears (see Appendix) up to q1h; refit contact lens; consider punctal plugs for dry eyes.

Evaluation

- Complete ophthalmic history with attention to contact lens wear and care habits.
- Complete eye examination with attention to contact lens fit, contact lens surface, everting upper lids, conjunctiva, keratometry, cornea, and fluorescein staining.
- Consider corneal topography (computerized videokeratography).
- Consider dry eye evaluation: tear meniscus, tear break-up time, rose bengal staining, and Schirmer's testing (see Chapter 4).
- **Lab tests:** Cultures or smears of cornea, contact lens, contact lens case, and contact lens solutions if infiltrate exists to rule out infection.

Prognosis

Usually good except for severe or central corneal infections.

■ Miscellaneous

Definitions

Dellen

Areas of corneal thinning secondary to corneal drying from an adjacent area of tissue elevation; appears as focal thinning with overlying pooling of fluorescein dye; usually seen near pterygium or filtering bleb.

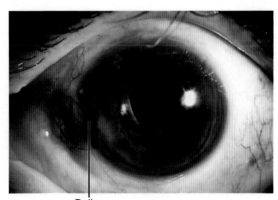

Figure 5-16 • Dellen appears as depression or thinning of cornea nasally.

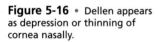

Dellen

Exposure Keratopathy

Drying of cornea with subsequent epithelial breakdown; due to neurotrophic (cranial nerve V palsy, cerebrovascular accident, aneurysm, multiple sclerosis, tumor, herpes simplex, herpes zoster), neuroparalytic (cranial nerve VII palsy), lid malposition, nocturnal lagophthalmos, or any cause of proptosis with lagophthalmos; sequelae include filamentary keratitis, corneal ulcer, and corneal vascularization.

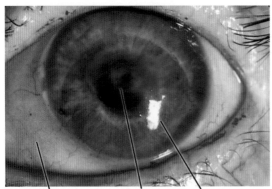

Figure 5-17 • Exposure keratopathy with interpalpebral rose bengal staining, a neurotrophic ulcer in the central cornea, and an irregular light reflex on the cornea.

Rose bengal stain   Ulcer   Irregular reflex

Filamentary Keratitis

Strands of mucus and desquamated epithelial cells adherent to corneal epithelium due to many conditions including any cause of dry eye, patching, recurrent erosion, bullous keratopathy, superior limbic keratoconjunctivitis, herpes simplex, medicamentosa, or ptosis; blinking causes pain as filaments pull on intact epithelium.

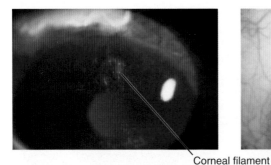

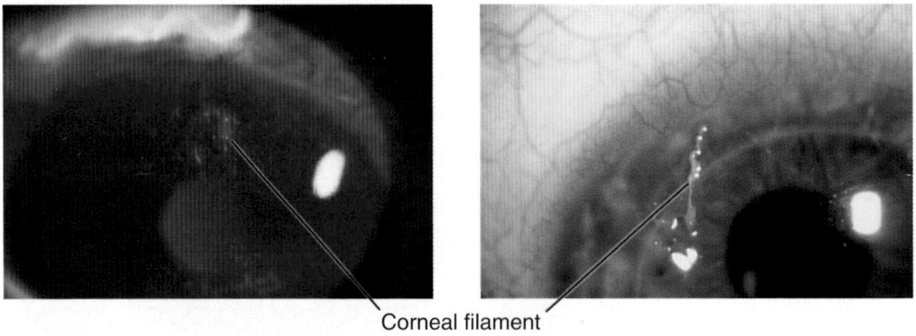

Corneal filament

Figure 5-18 • Filamentary keratitis demonstrating diffuse fluorescein staining of cornea and brighter staining of corneal filaments.

Figure 5-19 • Corneal filament appears as a thin vertical strand adherent to the superior cornea.

Keratic Precipitates

Fine, medium, or large deposits of inflammatory cells on the corneal endothelium due to a prior episode of inflammation; usually round white spots, but can be translucent or pigmented; may have mutton fat (in granulomatous uveitis) or stellate (in Fuchs' heterochromic iridocyclitis) appearance; often melt or disappear or become pigmented with time.

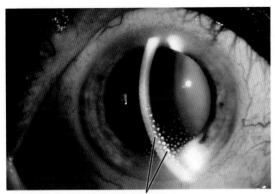

Figure 5-20 • White, mutton fat, granulomatous, keratic precipitates on the central and inferior corneal endothelium in a patient with toxoplasmosis.

Keratic precipitates

Superficial Punctate Keratitis

Nonspecific, pinpoint, epithelial defects; punctate staining with fluorescein; associated with blepharitis, any cause of dry eye, trauma, foreign body, trichiasis, ultraviolet or chemical burn, medicamentosa, contact lens–related, exposure, and conjunctivitis.

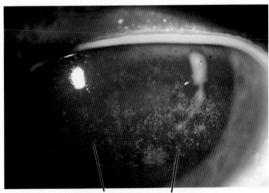

Figure 5-21 • Superficial punctate keratitis demonstrating diffuse epithelial staining of the central cornea with fluorescein.

Superficial punctate keratitis

Thygeson's Superficial Punctate Keratitis

Bilateral, recurrent, gray-white, slightly elevated lesions (similar to subepithelial infiltrates in adenoviral keratoconjunctivitis) in a white and quiet eye, minimal or no staining with fluorescein; unknown etiology; usually occurs in second to third decade.

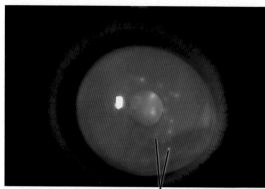

Figure 5-22 • Thygeson's superficial punctate keratitis demonstrating multiple, white, stellate, corneal opacities with cobalt blue light.

Thygeson's superficial punctate keratitis

Symptoms

Asymptomatic; may have dryness, foreign body sensation, discharge, tearing, photophobia, red eye, and decreased vision.

Signs

Normal or decreased visual acuity, lagophthalmos, conjunctival injection, decreased corneal sensation, corneal staining, superficial punctate keratitis (inferiorly or in a central band in exposure keratopathy), filaments (stain with fluorescein), subepithelial infiltrates, keratic precipitates, anterior chamber cells and flare.

Differential Diagnosis

See above.

Evaluation

- Complete ophthalmic history and eye examination with attention to lids, conjunctiva, cornea, anterior chamber, and cranial nerve testing.

Management

- Topical lubrication with preservative-free artificial tears (see Appendix) up to q1h and ointment (Refresh P.M.) at bedtime.
- Add antibiotic ointment (erythromycin, Polysporin, or bacitracin tid) for moderate superficial punctate keratitis and exposure keratitis; consider cycloplegic agent (cyclopentolate 1% or scopolamine 0.25% bid) and pressure patch (except in contact lens wearer) if severe.
- Consider punctal occlusion, lid taping at bedtime, moist chamber goggles, bandage contact lens, or tarsorrhaphy for moderate to severe dry eye symptoms and exposure keratitis.

Management—cont'd

- Clean, change, or discontinue contact lens use.
- Debridement of filaments with sterile cotton-tipped applicator, consider collagenase inhibitor (acetylcysteine [Mucomyst] qd to qid) or bandage contact lens for prolonged episodes of filamentary keratitis.
- Add mild topical steroid (fluorometholone qid for 1-2 weeks then taper slowly) for Thygeson's superficial punctate keratitis.
- Consider bandage contact lens for comfort.

Prognosis

Usually good.

Corneal Edema

Definition

Focal or diffuse hydration and swelling of corneal stroma (stromal edema due to endothelial dysfunction) or corneal epithelium (intercellular or microcystic edema due to increased intraocular pressure or epithelial hypoxia).

Symptoms

Asymptomatic; may have photophobia, foreign body sensation, tearing, pain, halos around lights, decreased vision.

Signs

Normal or decreased visual acuity, poor corneal light reflex, thickened cornea, epithelial microcysts and bullae, nonhealing epithelial defects, superficial punctate keratitis, stromal haze, Descemet's folds, guttata, anterior chamber cells and flare, decreased or increased intraocular pressure, iridocorneal touch, aphakia, pseudophakia, vitreous in anterior chamber.

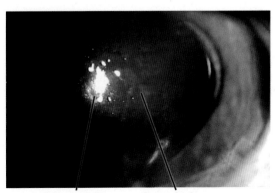

Figure 5-23 • Pseudophakic bullous keratopathy demonstrating corneal edema with central corneal folds, hazy stroma, and distorted light reflex.

Irregular reflex   Corneal edema

Differential Diagnosis

Inflammation, infection, Fuchs' dystrophy, posterior polymorphous dystrophy, congenital hereditary endothelial dystrophy, hydrops (keratoconus or pellucid marginal degeneration), acute angle-closure glaucoma, congenital glaucoma, previous ocular surgery (aphakic or pseudophakic bullous keratopathy or graft failure), contact lens overwear, hypotony, birth trauma, iridocorneal endothelial syndrome, Brown-McLean syndrome (peripheral edema in aphakic patients possibly from endothelial contact with floppy iris), anterior segment ischemia.

Evaluation

• Complete ophthalmic history and eye examination with attention to cornea, pachymetry (central thickness >0.610 mm indicates edema), tonometry, anterior chamber, gonioscopy, iris, and specular microscopy.

Management

• Symptomatic relief with hypertonic saline ointment (Adsorbonac or Muro 128 5% tid); consider topical steroid (prednisolone acetate 1% up to qid) and cycloplegic agent (scopolamine 0.25% bid to qid).
• Add broad spectrum topical antibiotic (polymyxin B sulfate–trimethoprim [Polytrim], moxifloxacin [Vigamox], or tobramycin [Tobrex] qid) for epithelial defects; consider bandage contact lens or tarsorrhaphy for persistent epithelial defects.
• Treat underlying cause (e.g., penetrating keratoplasty for aphakic or pseudophakic bullous keratopathy, Fuchs' dystrophy, and congenital hereditary endothelial dystrophy; intraocular pressure control and iridotomy for angle-closure glaucoma; observation and symptomatic relief for acute hydrops and birth trauma).

Prognosis

Depends on etiology.

▋ Graft Rejection or Failure

Definition

Graft rejection   Allograft rejection may occur early or late after corneal transplant surgery. Epithelial rejection is rare but occurs early, stromal rejection may appear with subepithelial infiltrates, and endothelial rejection usually does not occur before 2 weeks after transplantation.

Graft failure   Corneal edema and opacification due to primary donor failure (graft does not clear within 6 weeks after surgery), allograft rejection, recurrence of disease, glaucoma, or neovascularization.

Symptoms

Pain, photophobia, red eye, and decreased vision.

Signs

Decreased visual acuity, conjunctival injection, ciliary injection, corneal edema, vascularization, subepithelial infiltrates, epithelial rejection line, endothelial rejection line (Khodadoust line), keratic precipitates, anterior chamber cells and flare; may have increased intraocular pressure.

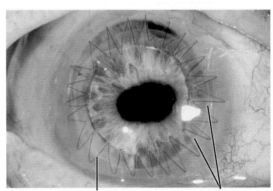

Figure 5-24 • Clear corneal graft with running suture. The edge of the graft is visible as a faint white scar between the suture bites; also note anterior chamber intraocular lens implant.

Running suture   Graft interface

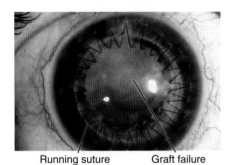

Running suture   Graft failure

Figure 5-25 • Graft failure with opaque central cornea. Once again note the running suture and the edge of the graft (*white line* under suture).

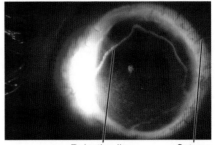

Rejection line   Sutures

Figure 5-26 • Graft failure with rejection line and keratic precipitates.

Differential Diagnosis

Endophthalmitis, herpes simplex virus (HSV) keratitis, adenoviral keratoconjunctivitis, anterior uveitis, anterior segment ischemia.

Evaluation

• Complete ophthalmic history and eye examination with attention to conjunctiva, cornea, pachymetry, suture integrity, tonometry, and anterior chamber.

Management

- Topical steroid (prednisolone acetate 1% up to q1h initially, taper slowly), cycloplegic agent (cyclopentolate 1% or scopolamine 0.25% tid); consider systemic steroids (prednisone 60-80 mg po qd initially, then taper rapidly over 5-7 days), or sub-Tenon steroid injection (triamcinolone acetonide 40 mg/mL); check PPD, blood glucose, and chest radiographs before starting systemic steroids.
- Add H_2-blocker (ranitidine [Zantac] 150 mg po bid) or proton pump inhibitor when administering systemic steroids.
- Topical cyclosporine is controversial.
- Treat recurrent HSV keratitis if this is the inciting event with systemic antivirals (acyclovir 400 mg po tid for 10-21 days, then bid for 12-18 months).
- May require treatment of increased intraocular pressure (see Chapter 11).

Prognosis

Thirty percent of patients have rejection episodes within 1 year after surgery. Often good if treated early and aggressively; poorer prognosis for a penetrating keratoplasty secondary to prior graft failure, HSV keratitis, acute corneal ulcer, chemical burn, and eyes with other ocular disease (dry eye syndrome, exposure keratopathy, ocular cicatricial pemphigoid, Stevens-Johnson syndrome, uveitis, and glaucoma); better prognosis for a penetrating keratoplasty secondary to corneal edema (aphakic or pseudophakic bullous keratopathy, Fuchs' dystrophy), keratoconus, corneal scar or opacity, and dystrophy.

■ Infectious Keratitis (Corneal Ulcer)

Definition

Destruction of corneal tissue (epithelium and stroma) due to inflammation from an infectious organism. Risks include contact lens wear, trauma, dry eyes, exposure keratopathy, bullous keratopathy, neurotrophic cornea, and lid abnormalities.

Etiology

Bacterial

Most common infectious source; usually due to *Pseudomonas aeruginosa, Staphylococcus aureus, Staphylococcus epidermidis, Streptococcus pneumoniae, Haemophilus influenzae, Moraxella catarrhalis;* beware of *Neisseria* species, *Corynebacterium diphtheriae, Haemophilus aegyptius,* and *Listeria* because they can penetrate intact epithelium; *Streptococcus viridans* causes crystalline keratopathy (central branching cracked glass appearance without epithelial defect; associated with chronic topical steroid use).

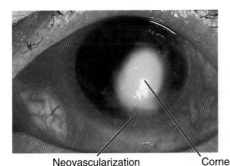
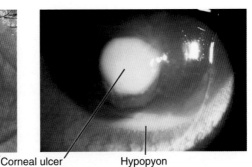

Neovascularization   Corneal ulcer   Hypopyon

Figure 5-27 • Bacterial keratitis demonstrating large, central, *Streptococcus pneumoniae* corneal ulcer. Note the dense, white, corneal infiltrate and the extreme conjunctival injection.

Figure 5-28 • Bacterial keratitis demonstrating *Pseudomonas aeruginosa* corneal ulcer with surrounding corneal edema and hypopyon.

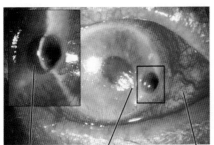

Iris plug   Corneal ulcer   Conjunctival injection   Crystalline keratopathy

Figure 5-29 • Perforated corneal ulcer. The cornea is opaque, scarred, and vascularized, and there is a paracentral perforation with iris plugging the wound. Inset shows slit beam over iris plugging perforated wound.

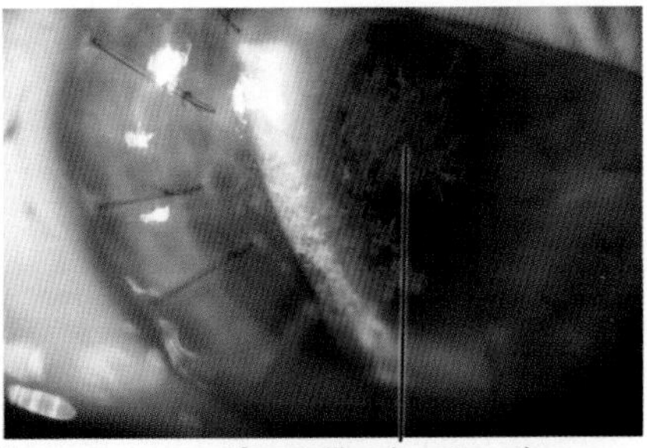

Figure 5-30 • Crystalline keratopathy due to *Streptococcus viridans*.

Fungal

Usually *Aspergillus, Candida,* or *Fusarium* species; often have satellite infiltrates, feathery edges, endothelial plaques; can penetrate Descemet's membrane; associated with trauma, especially involving vegetable matter.

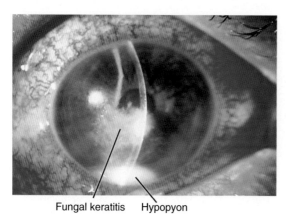

Figure 5-31 • Fungal keratitis demonstrating a central corneal infiltrate with feathery borders, severe conjunctival injection, and a small hypopyon.

Fungal keratitis   Hypopyon

Parasitic

Acanthamoeba   Resembles HSV epithelial keratitis early, perineural and ring infiltrates later; usually seen in contact lens wearers who use nonsterile water or have poor contact lens cleaning habits. Patients usually have pain out of proportion to signs.

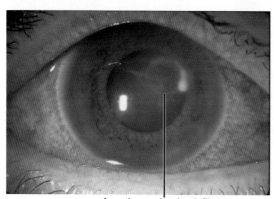

Figure 5-32 • *Acanthamoeba* keratitis demonstrating the characteristic ring infiltrate.

Acanthamoeba ring infiltrate

Microsporidia   Causes diffuse epithelial keratitis with small, white, intraepithelial infiltrates (organisms); seen in patients with acquired immunodeficiency syndrome (AIDS).

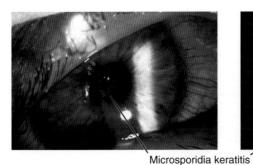

Microsporidia keratitis   Intraepithelial infiltrate

Figure 5-33 • Microsporidia keratitis demonstrating diffuse, whitish epithelial keratitis.

Figure 5-34 • Same patient as Figure 5-33 demonstrating the intraepithelial infiltrates of microsporidia keratitis.

Viral

Herpes simplex virus   Recurrent HSV is the most common cause of central infectious keratitis; associated with sun exposure, fever, stress, menses, trauma, illness, and immuno-suppression; recurrence rate = 25% during first year, 50% during second year; several types of HSV infection exist:

Epithelial Keratitis   Can appear as a superficial punctate keratitis, dendrite (ulcerated, classically with terminal bulbs), or geographic ulcer; associated with scarring and decreased corneal sensation.

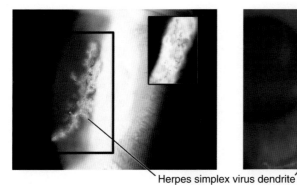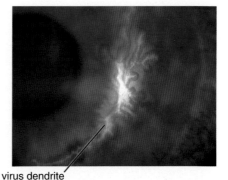

Herpes simplex virus dendrite

Figure 5-35 • Herpes simplex epithelial keratitis demonstrating dendrite with terminal bulbs; inset shows staining of dendrite with rose bengal.

Figure 5-36 • Same patient as shown in Figure 5-35 demonstrating staining of herpes simplex virus dendrite with fluorescein.

Disciform Keratitis   Self-limited (2-6 months), cell-mediated, immune reaction with focal disclike area of stromal edema, folds, fine keratic precipitates, and scarring.

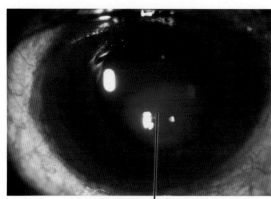

Figure 5-37 • Herpes simplex disciform keratitis demonstrating central round area of hazy edema.

Herpes simplex virus disciform keratitis

Necrotizing Interstitial Keratitis   Antigen-antibody-complement mediated; dense stromal inflammation and ulceration with severe iritis.

Endotheliitis   Corneal edema, keratic precipitates, increased intraocular pressure, anterior chamber cells and flare.

Herpes zoster virus (HZV)   Causes a pseudodendrite (coarser, heaped-up epithelial plaque without terminal bulbs) or superficial punctate keratitis with iritis and increased intraocular pressure; may develop sector iris atrophy.

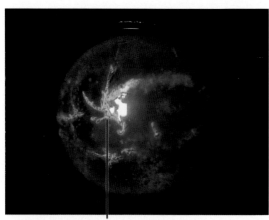

Figure 5-38 • Herpes zoster ophthalmicus demonstrating staining of coarse, pseudodendrites with fluorescein. The pseudodendrite has heaped-up epithelium without terminal bulbs.

Herpes zoster virus pseudodendrite

Symptoms

Pain, discharge, tearing, photophobia, red eye, decreased vision; may notice white spot on cornea.

Signs

Normal or decreased visual acuity, conjunctival injection, ciliary injection, white corneal infiltrate with overlying epithelial defect that stains with fluorescein, satellite lesions (fungal), corneal edema, Descemet's folds, dendrite (HSV), pseudodendrite (HZV), cutaneous herpes vesicles, perineural and ring infiltrates *(Acanthamoeba)*, corneal thinning, descemetocele, anterior chamber cells and flare, hypopyon, mucopurulent discharge, increased intraocular pressure.

Differential Diagnosis

Sterile ulcer, shield ulcer (vernal keratoconjunctivitis), staphylococcal marginal keratitis, epidemic keratoconjunctivitis subepithelial infiltrates, ocular rosacea, marginal keratolysis, Mooren's ulcer, Terrien's marginal degeneration, corneal abrasion, recurrent erosion, stromal scar, Thygeson's superficial punctate keratitis, metaherpetic or trophic ulcer (noninfectious, nonhealing epithelial defect with heaped-up gray edges due to HSV basement membrane disease with possible neurotrophic component), anesthetic abuse (nonhealing epithelial defect usually with ragged edge and "sick"-appearing surrounding epithelium with or without haze or an infiltrate), tyrosinemia (pseudodendrite).

Evaluation

- Complete ophthalmic history with attention to contact lens use and care regimen.
- Complete eye examination with attention to cornea (sensation, size and depth of ulcer, character of infiltrate, fluorescein and rose bengal staining, amount of thinning), tonometry, and anterior chamber.
- **Lab tests:** Scrape corneal ulcer with sterile spatula or blade and smear on microbiology slides; send for routine cultures (bacteria), Sabouraud's media (fungi), chocolate agar *(H. influenzae, Neisseria gonorrhoeae),* Gram stain (bacteria), Giemsa stain (fungi, *Acanthamoeba*); consider calcofluor white *(Acanthamoeba)* and acid fast *(Mycobacteria)* if these entities are suspected.
- Consider biopsy for progressive disease, culture-negative ulcer, or deep abscess (usually fungal, *Acanthamoeba,* crystalline).

Management

- Suspend contact lens use.
- May require treatment of increased intraocular pressure (see Chapter 11), especially HZV.
- Consider bandage contact lens or tarsorrhaphy to heal persistent epithelial defects; glue and contact lens to seal small perforations; and penetrating keratoplasty; never patch corneal ulcer.
- Ulcers require daily follow-up initially, and severe ones require hospital admission.
- If organism is in doubt, treat as a bacterial ulcer until culture results return.

BACTERIAL

- **Small Infiltrates (<2 mm):** broad spectrum topical antibiotic (gatifloxacin [Zymar] or moxifloxacin [Vigamox] q1h initially, then taper slowly).

Continued

Management—cont'd

- **Larger Ulcers:** broad spectrum fortified topical antibiotics (tobramycin 13.6 mg/mL and cefazolin 50 mg/mL or vancomycin 50 mg/mL [in patients allergic to penicillin and cephalosporin] alternating q1h [which means taking a drop every 30 minutes] for 24-72 hours, then taper slowly); consider subconjunctival antibiotic injections in noncompliant patients.
- Tailor antibiotic choices as culture and Gram stain results return.
- Topical cycloplegic agent (scopolamine 0.25% or atropine 1% bid to qid).
- Topical steroid (prednisolone acetate 1% dosed at lower frequency than topical antibiotics) should be avoided until improvement is noted (usually after 48-72 hours).
- Systemic antibiotics for corneal perforation or scleral involvement.

FUNGAL

- Topical antifungal agent (natamycin 50 mg/mL q1h, amphotericin B 1.0-2.5 mg/mL q1h, or miconazole 10 mg/mL q1h for 24-72 hours, then taper slowly).
- For severe infection, add systemic antifungal agent (ketoconazole 200-400 mg po qd or amphotericin B 1 mg/kg IV over 6 hours).
- Topical cycloplegic agent (scopolamine 0.25% or atropine 1% bid to qid).
- Topical steroids are *contraindicated.*

PARASITIC

- *Acanthamoeba:* topical agents (combination of propamidine isethionate [Brolene] 0.1% or hexamidine 0.1%, and miconazole 1% or clotrimazole 1%, and polyhexamethylene biguanide [Baquacil] 0.02% or chlorhexidine 0.02%, q1h for 1 week, then taper very slowly over 2-3 months), topical broad spectrum antibiotic (neomycin or paromomycin q2h), and oral antifungal agent (ketoconazole 200 mg or itraconazole 100 mg po bid).
- Topical steroids are controversial, consider for severe necrotizing keratitis (prednisolone phosphate 1% qid).
- Topical cycloplegic agent (scopolamine 0.25% or atropine 1% bid to qid).
- *Microsporidia:* topical fumagillin up to q2h initially, then taper slowly.

VIRAL

- **HSV Epithelial Keratitis:** topical antiviral (trifluridine [Viroptic] 9 times/day or vidarabine monohydrate [Vira-A] 5 times/day for 10-14 days); consider oral antiviral agent (acyclovir 400 mg po tid for 10-21 days, then prophylaxis with 400 mg bid for up to 1 year [or longer after penetrating keratoplasty]), débride dendrite.
- **HSV Disciform or Endotheliitis:** topical steroid (prednisolone phosphate 0.12-1.0% qd to qid depending on severity of inflammation, adjust and then taper slowly over months depending on response); consider cycloplegic agent (scopolamine 0.25% bid to qid); add topical antiviral (trifluridine [Viroptic] qid) if epithelium is involved or prophylactically when using steroid doses greater than prednisolone phosphate 0.12% bid (alternatively, can use acyclovir 400 mg po bid).

Management—cont'd

- **HSV Metaherpetic or Trophic Ulcer:** topical lubrication with preservative-free artificial tears (see Appendix) up to q1h and ointment (Refresh P.M.) at bedtime; broad spectrum topical antibiotic (polymyxin B sulfate–trimethoprim [Polytrim], tobramycin [Tobrex], gatifloxacin [Zymar], or moxifloxacin [Vigamox] qid), bandage contact lens; add mild topical steroid (fluorometholone qd to bid) if stromal inflammation exists.
- Long-term suppressive therapy with acyclovir (400 mg po bid) for 1 year with 6-month additional follow-up reduces the incidence of recurrent keratitis by almost 50% (Herpetic Eye Disease Study conclusion).
- **HZV:** systemic antiviral agent (acyclovir 800 mg po 5 times a day for 7-10 days, or famciclovir 500 mg po or valacyclovir 1 g po tid for 7 days), topical steroids (prednisolone acetate 1% qid to q4h, then taper slowly over months), cycloplegic agent (scopolamine 0.25% bid to qid); add topical antibiotic ointment (erythromycin or bacitracin tid) if conjunctival or corneal involvement. Consider tricyclic antidepressants, Neurontin, pain medications, capsaicin cream, or Lidoderm patches for postherpetic neuralgia.

Prognosis

Depends on organism, size, location, and response to treatment; sequelae may range from a small corneal scar without alteration of vision to corneal perforation requiring emergent grafting; poor prognosis for fungal and *Acanthamoeba* keratitis; herpes simplex and *Acanthamoeba* commonly recur in corneal graft.

Interstitial Keratitis

Definition

Diffuse or sectoral vascularization and scarring of corneal stroma due to nonnecrotizing inflammation and edema; may be acute or chronic.

Etiology

Most commonly congenital syphilis (90% of cases), tuberculosis, and herpes simplex; also herpes zoster, leprosy, onchocerciasis, mumps, lymphogranuloma venereum, sarcoidosis, and Cogan's syndrome (triad of interstitial keratitis, vertigo, and deafness).

Symptoms

Acute   Decreased vision, pain, photophobia, red eye.

Chronic   Usually asymptomatic.

Signs

Normal or decreased visual acuity.

Acute   Conjunctival injection, salmon patch (stromal vascularization), stromal edema, anterior chamber cells and flare, keratic precipitates.

Chronic   Deep corneal haze, scarring, thinning, vascularization, ghost vessels; other stigmata of congenital syphilis (optic nerve atrophy, salt-and-pepper fundus, deafness, notched teeth, saddle nose, sabre shins).

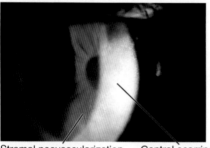

Stromal neovascularization   Central scarring

Figure 5-39 • Interstitial keratitis demonstrating diffuse stromal scarring of the central cornea and extensive corneal neovascularization.

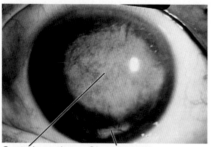

Central scarring   Ghost vessels

Figure 5-40 • Interstitial keratitis demonstrating ghost vessels that appear as clear, linear, branching lines within the dense, white, corneal scarring.

Evaluation

- Complete ophthalmic history and eye examination with attention to lids, conjunctiva, cornea, anterior chamber, and ophthalmoscopy.
- **Lab tests:** Venereal Disease Research Laboratory (VDRL), fluorescent treponemal antibody absorption test (FTA-ABS), PPD, and chest radiographs; consider angiotensin converting enzyme (ACE).
- Consider medical and otolaryngology (Cogan's syndrome) consultation.

Management

ACUTE

- Topical steroid (prednisolone acetate 1% qid to q4h, then taper) and cycloplegic agent (scopolamine 0.25% bid to qid).

CHRONIC

- Treat underlying cause (e.g., syphilis, tuberculosis).
- May require penetrating keratoplasty if vision is affected by corneal scarring.
- Early oral steroids in Cogan's syndrome may prevent permanent hearing loss.

Prognosis

Good; corneal opacity is nonprogressive.

Pannus

Definition

Superficial vascularization and scarring of peripheral cornea due to inflammation; histologically, fibrovascular tissue between epithelium and Bowman's layer; two types:

Inflammatory   Bowman's layer destruction, with inflammatory cells.

Degenerative   Bowman's layer intact, with areas of calcification.

Symptoms

Asymptomatic; may have decreased vision if visual axis is involved.

Signs

Vascularization and opacification of cornea past the normal peripheral vascular arcade; micropannus (1-2 mm), gross pannus (>2 mm).

Neovascularization   Pannus

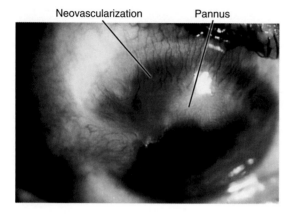

Figure 5-41 • Large pannus demonstrating scarring and vascularization of the superior cornea in a patient with a chemical burn.

Differential Diagnosis

Trachoma, contact lens–related neovascularization, vernal keratoconjunctivitis, superior limbic keratoconjunctivitis, atopic keratoconjunctivitis, staphylococcal blepharitis, ocular rosacea, herpes simplex, chemical injury, phlyctenulosis, ocular cicatricial pemphigoid, Stevens-Johnson syndrome, aniridia, or idiopathic.

Evaluation

• Complete ophthalmic history and eye examination with attention to everting lids, conjunctiva, and cornea.

Prognosis

Good; may progress.

Management

• Treat underlying cause.

▮ Degenerations

Definition

Acquired lesions secondary to aging or previous corneal insult.

Arcus Senilis

Bilateral, white ring in peripheral cornea; seen in elderly individuals due to lipid deposition at level of Bowman's and Descemet's membrane; clear zone exists between arcus and limbus; check lipid profile if patient is over 40 years old; unilateral is due to contralateral carotid occlusive disease; congenital form is called *arcus juvenilis.*

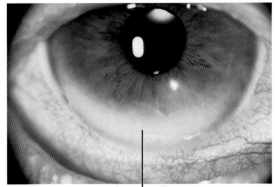

Figure 5-42 • Arcus senilis evident as a peripheral white ring in the inferior cornea.

Arcus senilis

Band Keratopathy

Interpalpebral, subepithelial, patchy calcific changes in Bowman's membrane; Swiss cheese pattern; seen in chronic ocular inflammation (edema, uveitis, glaucoma, interstitial keratitis, phthisis, dry eye syndrome), hypercalcemia, gout, mercury vapors, or hereditary.

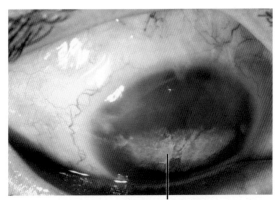

Figure 5-43 • Band keratopathy demonstrating characteristic Swiss cheese pattern of central corneal opacification.

Band keratopathy

Crocodile Shagreen

Bilateral, gray-white opacification at level of Bowman's layer (anterior) or the deep stroma (posterior); mosaic or cracked ice pattern.

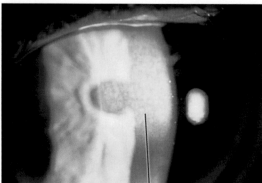

Figure 5-44 • Posterior crocodile shagreen with hazy, cracked ice appearance.

Posterior crocodile shagreen

Furrow Degeneration

Corneal thinning in the clear zone between arcus senilis and limbus (more apparent than real); perforation is rare; nonprogressive.

Lipid Keratopathy

Yellow-white, subepithelial and stromal infiltrate with feathery edges due to lipid deposition from chronic inflammation and vascularization.

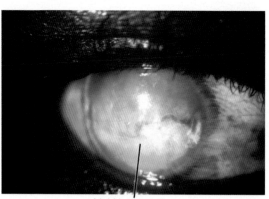

Figure 5-45 • Lipid keratopathy demonstrating dense white corneal infiltration.

Lipid keratopathy

Spheroidal Degeneration (Actinic, Labrador Keratopathy, Bietti's Nodular Dystrophy)

Bilateral, elevated, interpalpebral, yellow, stromal droplets due to sun exposure; male predilection; associated with band keratopathy.

Salzmann's Nodular Degeneration

Elevated, smooth, opaque, blue-white, subepithelial, hyaline nodules due to chronic keratitis; female predilection.

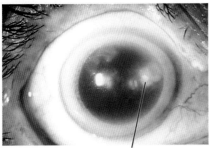

Salzmann's nodular degeneration

Figure 5-46 • Salzmann's nodular degeneration with several white, elevated, nummular opacities.

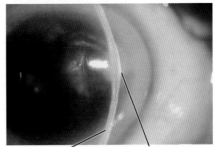

Slit-beam   Elevation of nodule

Figure 5-47 • Same patient as shown in Figure 5-46, demonstrating elevation of nodule with fine slit beam.

Terrien's Marginal Degeneration

Noninflammatory, slowly progressive, peripheral thinning of cornea with pannus; starts superiorly and spreads circumferentially; epithelium intact; slight male predilection; causes progressive against-the-rule astigmatism; rarely perforates.

Figure 5-48 • Terrien's marginal degeneration with superior thinning (note how slit beam dives downward) bounded by white scarring.

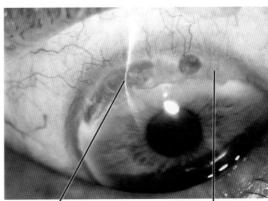

Peripheral thinning   Neovascularization

White Limbal Girdle of Vogt

Bilateral, white, needle-like opacities in interpalpebral peripheral cornea; seen in elderly patients; two types:

Type I   Calcific (lucid interval at limbus).

Type II   Elastotic (no lucid interval).

Symptoms

Asymptomatic; may have tearing, photophobia, decreased vision, and foreign body sensation.

Signs

Normal or decreased visual acuity, corneal opacity.

Differential Diagnosis

See above, corneal dystrophy, metabolic disease, corneal deposition.

Evaluation

- Complete ophthalmic history and eye examination with attention to cornea.

Management

- No treatment recommended.
- Consider 3% topical sodium ethylenediaminetetraacetic acid (EDTA) chelation, superficial keratectomy, phototherapeutic keratectomy, or penetrating keratoplasty for band keratopathy.
- Salzmann's nodules often respond to superficial keratectomy.

Prognosis

Good, most are benign incidental findings; poor for band and lipid keratopathy, because these are secondary to chronic processes.

▌Ectasias

Definition

Keratoconus

Bilateral, asymmetric, cone-shaped deformity of the cornea due to progressive paracentral corneal thinning; patients develop irregular astigmatism, corneal striae, superficial scarring from breaks in Bowman's membrane, acute painful stromal edema from breaks in Descemet's membrane (hydrops); usually sporadic, but may have positive family history (10% of cases); associated with atopy and vernal keratoconjunctivitis (eye rubbing), Down's syndrome, Marfan's syndrome, and contact lens wear (polymethylmethacrylate).

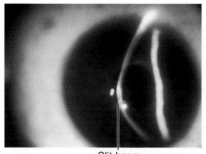

Slit-beam   Pupil   Inferior "sagging"

Figure 5-49 • Keratoconus demonstrating central "nipple" cone as seen with a fine slit beam. Note the central scarring at the apex of the cone.

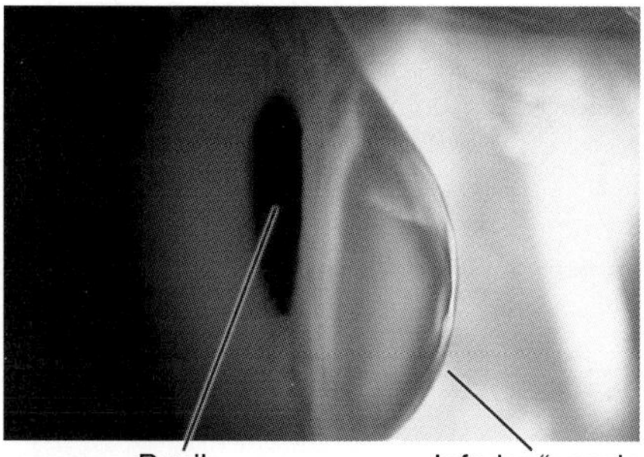

Figure 5-50 • Keratoconus demonstrating inferior "sagging" cone as viewed from the side. Note that the apex of the cone is below the center of the pupil.

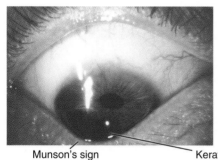

Munson's sign   Keratoconus   Hydrops

Figure 5-51 • Munson's sign in a patient with keratoconus demonstrating protrusion of lower eyelid with downgaze.

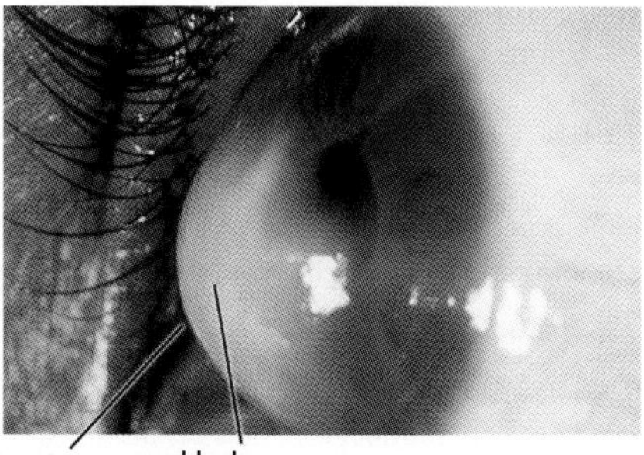

Figure 5-52 • Hydrops in a patient with keratoconus demonstrating hazy, white, central edema.

Keratoglobus

Rare, globular deformity of the cornea due to diffuse thinning that is maximal at the base of the protrusion; sporadic; associated with Ehlers-Danlos syndrome.

Pellucid Marginal Degeneration

Bilateral, inferior, peripheral corneal thinning (2 mm from limbus) with protrusion above thinned area; patients develop irregular astigmatism; no scarring, cone, or striae seen.

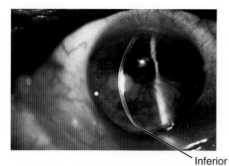 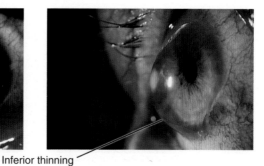

Inferior thinning

Figure 5-53 • Pellucid marginal degeneration demonstrating inferior thinning. Note how thin the slit beam is at the inferior cornea.

Figure 5-54 • Side view of same patient as shown in Figure 5-53 demonstrating protrusion of cornea inferiorly.

Symptoms

Decreased vision; may have sudden loss of vision, pain, photophobia, tearing, and red eye in hydrops.

Signs

Decreased visual acuity, abnormally shaped cornea, astigmatism, irregular keratometer mires; in keratoconus may have central thinning, scarring, Fleischer's ring (epithelial iron deposition around base of cone, best seen with blue light), Vogt's striae (deep, stromal, vertical stress lines at apex of cone), Munson's sign (protrusion of lower lid with downgaze), and Rizzuti's sign (triangle of light on iris from penlight beam focused by cone); in keratoconus and pellucid marginal degeneration may have hydrops (opaque edematous cornea, ciliary injection, and anterior chamber cells and flare).

Differential Diagnosis

See above; Terrien's marginal degeneration.

Evaluation

• Complete ophthalmic history and eye examination with attention to cornea, keratometry, retinoscopy reflex, and anterior chamber.
• Corneal topography (computerized videokeratography).

Management

• Correct refractive errors with spectacles or RGP.
• Consider penetrating keratoplasty when acuity declines or if patient is intolerant of contact lenses.

Management—cont'd

- Supportive treatment for acute hydrops with hypertonic saline ointment (Adsorbonac or Muro 128 5% qid); add topical broad spectrum antibiotic (polymyxin B sulfate–trimethoprim [Polytrim], moxifloxacin [Vigamox], or tobramycin [Tobrex] qid) for epithelial defect; consider topical steroid (prednisolone acetate 1% qid) and cycloplegic agent (cyclopentolate 1% tid) for severe pain.
- Corneal refractive surgery contraindicated in these unstable corneas.

Prognosis

Good; penetrating keratoplasty has high success rate for keratoconus and keratoglobus.

▉ Congenital Anomalies

Definition

Cornea Plana (Autosomal Dominant [AD] or Autosomal Recessive [AR])

Flat cornea (curvature often as low as 20-30 diopters); corneal curvature equal to scleral curvature is pathognomonic; associated with sclerocornea and microcornea; increased incidence of angle-closure glaucoma; mapped to chromosome 12q.

Dermoid

Choristoma composed of dense connective tissue with pilosebaceous units and stratified squamous epithelium; usually located at inferotemporal limbus, can involve entire cornea; may cause astigmatism and amblyopia; may be associated with preauricular skin tags and vertebral anomalies (Goldenhar's syndrome).

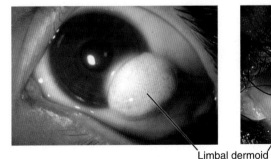
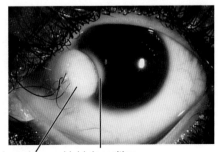

Limbal dermoid   Lipid deposition

Figure 5-55 • Limbal dermoid at inferotemporal limbus.

Figure 5-56 • Limbal dermoid with central hairs and lipid deposition along the corneal edge.

Haab's Striae

Horizontal breaks in Descemet's membrane due to increased intraocular pressure in children with congenital glaucoma.

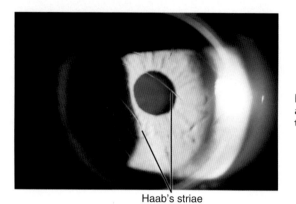

Haab's striae

Figure 5-57 • Haab's striae appear as clear parallel lines in the cornea.

Megalocornea (X-Linked)

Enlarged cornea (horizontal diameter ≥13 mm); male predilection (90%); usually isolated, nonprogressive, and bilateral; associated with weak zonules and lens subluxation.

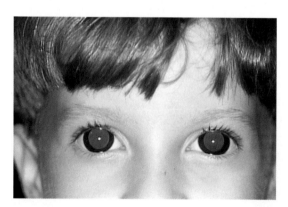

Figure 5-58 • Megalocornea demonstrating abnormally large diameter of both corneas.

Microcornea (AD and AR)

Small cornea (diameter <10 mm); increased incidence of hyperopia and angle-closure glaucoma.

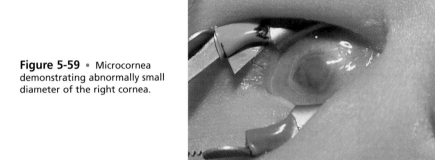

Figure 5-59 • Microcornea demonstrating abnormally small diameter of the right cornea.

Posterior Keratoconus

Focal, central indentation of posterior cornea with scarring; rare, usually unilateral, and nonprogressive; female predilection; no change in anterior corneal surface.

Sclerocornea

Scleralized peripheral or entire cornea; nonprogressive, 50% sporadic, 50% hereditary (AR more severe); 90% bilateral; 80% associated with cornea plana.

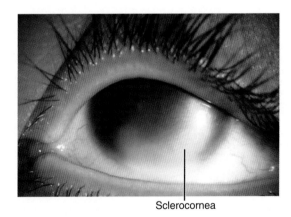

Figure 5-60 • Sclerocornea demonstrating peripheral opacification due to scleralized cornea.

Sclerocornea

Symptoms

Asymptomatic; may have decreased vision.

Signs

Normal or decreased visual acuity, abnormal corneal size or shape, corneal opacity, edema, or scarring; may have other anterior segment abnormalities (angle, iris, or lens) and increased intraocular pressure.

Differential Diagnosis

Microphthalmos, nanophthalmos, congenital glaucoma (buphthalmos), interstitial keratitis, anterior keratoconus, birth trauma.

Evaluation

• Complete ophthalmic history and eye examination with attention to refraction, cornea, keratometry, tonometry, gonioscopy, iris, lens, and ophthalmoscopy.
• May require examination under anesthesia in a child.

Management

• Correct any refractive error.
• May require patching or occlusion therapy for amblyopia (see Chapter 12), treatment of increased intraocular pressure (see Congenital Glaucoma section in Chapter 11), or even penetrating keratoplasty in severe cases.
• Consider surgical excision of dermoid.

Prognosis

Depends on etiology.

■ Dystrophies

Definition

Primary, inherited, corneal diseases without prior corneal pathology or systemic disease; usually bilateral, symmetric, and progressive with early onset.

Anterior (Epithelial and Bowman's Membrane)

Anterior Basement Membrane (ABMD) (Epithelial Basement Membrane [EBMD], Map-Dot-Fingerprint [MDF], Cogan's Microcystic) (AD)

Most common anterior corneal dystrophy; intraepithelial and subepithelial basement membrane reduplication causing abnormal epithelial adhesion and recurrent erosions; intraepithelial microcysts (dots) and subepithelial ridges and lines (maplike and fingerprint-like) are also seen; 10% with ABMD develop recurrent erosions, whereas 50% of patients with recurrent erosions have ABMD; may develop scarring and decreased vision starting after age 30 years; slight female predilection.

Gelatinous Droplike (AR)

Rare, subepithelial, central, mulberry-like, protuberant opacity; composed of amyloid; lack Bowman's membrane; decreased vision, photophobia, and tearing occur in first decade.

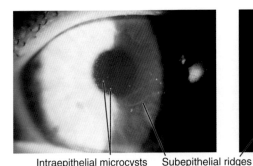

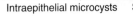
Intraepithelial microcysts   Subepithelial ridges

Figure 5-61 • Anterior basement membrane dystrophy demonstrating central dots and lines.

Figure 5-62 • Anterior basement membrane dystrophy demonstrating dots and lines as viewed with retroillumination.

Meesman's (AD)

Intraepithelial microcystic blebs concentrated in the interpalpebral zone extending to the limbus; surrounded by clear epithelium; blebs contain periodic acid–Schiff (PAS)-positive material ("peculiar substance") and appear as numerous dots with retroillumination; rare and bilateral; develop recurrent erosions, but retain good vision.

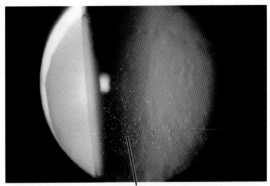

Figure 5-63 • Meesman's dystrophy demonstrating dotlike blebs as viewed with retroillumination.

Intraepithelial microcystic blebs

Reis-Bücklers (AD)

Progressive subepithelial opacification and scarring of Bowman's membrane with honeycomb appearance; recurrent erosions early, often in the first or second decade; often recurs after penetrating keratoplasty; mapped to chromosome 5q (*BIGH3* gene).

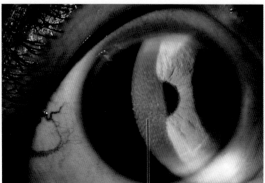

Figure 5-64 • Reis-Bücklers dystrophy demonstrating central honeycomb pattern of opacification.

Subepithelial honeycomb opacification

Stromal

Avellino (AD)

Combination of granular and lattice (see below) with discrete granular appearing opacities; intervening stroma contains lattice-like branching lines and dots (not clear like granular); composed of a combination of hyaline and amyloid that stains with Congo red and Masson's trichrome; mapped to chromosome 5q (*BIGH3* gene).

Central Cloudy (François) (AD)

Small, indistinct, cloudy gray areas in central posterior stroma with intervening clear cracks (like crocodile shagreen, but does not extend to periphery); nonprogressive; usually asymptomatic.

Central Crystalline (Schnyder's) (AD)

Central, yellow-white ring of fine, needle-like, polychromatic crystals with stromal haze; also have dense arcus and limbal girdle; composed of cholesterol and neutral fats that stain with oil-red-O; very rare and nonprogressive; associated with hyperlipidemia, genu valgum, and xanthelasma; usually asymptomatic; mapped to chromosome 1p.

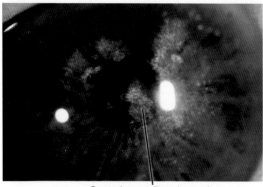

Figure 5-65 • Central crystalline dystrophy demonstrating crystalline deposits and stromal haze.

Central crystalline dystrophy

Congenital Hereditary Stromal (CHSD) (AD)

Superficial, central, feathery, diffuse opacity; alternating layers of abnormal collagen lamellae; nonprogressive; associated with amblyopia, esotropia, and nystagmus.

Fleck (François-Neetans') (AD)

Subtle, gray-white, dandruff-like specks that extend to the limbus; composed of abnormal glycosaminoglycans that stain with Alcian blue; can be unilateral and asymmetric; nonprogressive and usually asymptomatic.

Granular (AD)

Most common stromal dystrophy; central, discrete, white, breadcrumb or snowflake-like opacities; intervening stroma usually clear, but may become hazy late; corneal periphery spared; composed of hyaline that stains with Masson's trichrome; decreased vision late, erosions rare; mapped to chromosome 5q (*BIGH3* gene).

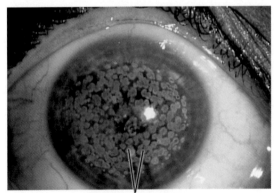

Figure 5-66 • Granular dystrophy demonstrating abundant central opacities.

Granular dystrophy

Lattice (AD)

Refractile branching lines, white dots, and central haze; intervening stroma becomes cloudy, with ground glass appearance; composed of amyloid that stains with Congo red; recurrent erosions common, decreased vision in third decade; often recurs after penetrating keratoplasty; mapped to chromosome 5q (*BIGH3* gene).

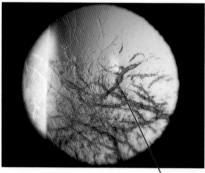

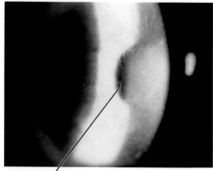

Refractile branching lines

Figure 5-67 • Lattice dystrophy demonstrating branching lines, dots, and central haze as viewed with retroillumination.

Figure 5-68 • Lattice dystrophy demonstrating branching lines.

Macular (AR)

Diffuse haze with focal, irregular, gray-white spots that have a sugar-frosted appearance; extends to limbus; composed of abnormal glycosaminoglycans that stain with Alcian blue; rare; decreased vision early, recurrent erosions occasionally; mapped to chromosome 16q.

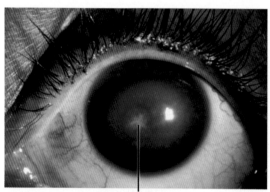

Macular dystrophy

Figure 5-69 • Macular dystrophy demonstrating diffuse central haze with focal area of white spots.

Pre-Descemet's (Deep Filiform) (AD)

Fine, gray, posterior opacities; various morphologies; composed of lipid; onset in fourth to seventh decade; four types: pre-Descemet's, polymorphic stromal, cornea farinata, and pre-Descemet's associated with ichthyosis and pseudoxanthoma elasticum; usually asymptomatic.

Posterior (Endothelial)

Congenital Hereditary Endothelial (CHED) (AR > AD)

Opacified, edematous corneas at birth due to endothelial dysfunction; rare; mapped to chromosome 20p; two types:

(1) More common, autosomal recessive, no pain or tearing, nonprogressive.

(2) Autosomal dominant, delayed onset (age 1-2 years old); painful with tearing; progressive; may require penetrating keratoplasty.

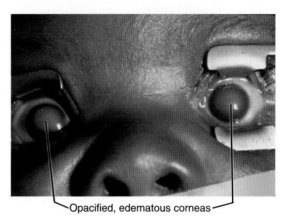

Figure 5-70 • Congenital hereditary endothelial dystrophy demonstrating bilateral corneal edema and opacification.

Opacified, edematous corneas

Fuchs' Endothelial (AD)

Cornea guttata (thickened Descemet's membrane with PAS-positive excrescences [orange peel appearance]) and endothelial dysfunction; decreased endothelial cell density, increased pleomorphism, and increased polymegathism; early stromal edema, late epithelial edema, bullae, and fibrosis; female predilection; may have decreased vision (worse in the morning), pain with ruptured bullae, and subepithelial scarring.

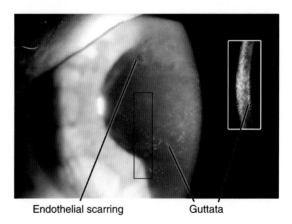

Figure 5-71 • Fuchs' endothelial dystrophy demonstrating endothelial pigment, guttata and endothelial scarring; inset demonstrates guttata and corneal edema when viewed with fine slit beam.

Endothelial scarring   Guttata

Posterior Polymorphous (PPMD) (AD)

Asymmetric patches of grouped vesicles, scalloped bands, and geographic, gray, hazy areas; epithelial-like endothelium (loss of contact inhibition with proliferation and growth over angle and iris); may develop stromal edema, iris and pupil changes similar to those in iridocorneal endothelial syndrome (see Chapter 7), broad peripheral anterior synechiae, and glaucoma; usually asymptomatic; mapped to chromosome 20q.

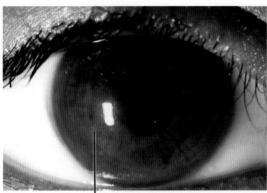

Figure 5-72 • Posterior polymorphous dystrophy demonstrating diffuse, hazy, endothelial opacities.

Posterior polymorphous dystrophy

Symptoms

Asymptomatic; may have pain, foreign body sensation, tearing, photophobia, decreased vision.

Signs

Normal or decreased visual acuity, corneal opacities.

Differential Diagnosis

See above, corneal degeneration, corneal deposition, metabolic diseases.

Evaluation

*   Complete ophthalmic history and eye examination with attention to refraction, cornea, tonometry, gonioscopy, iris, and ophthalmoscopy.
*   B-scan ultrasonography if unable to visualize the fundus.
*   Consider pachymetry and specular microscopy for Fuchs' dystrophy.
*   **Lab tests:** Lipid profile for Schnyder's central crystalline.

Management

*   No treatment recommended.
*   Topical lubrication with preservative-free artificial tears (see Appendix) up to q1h, hypertonic saline ointment (Adsorbonac or Muro 128 5% at bedtime).
*   May require treatment of recurrent erosions (see Trauma: Recurrent Erosion section).
*   May require superficial keratectomy, phototherapeutic keratectomy, lamellar keratoplasty, or penetrating keratoplasty if scarring across the visual axis exists.

Prognosis

Usually good; may recur in graft (Reis-Bücklers' > macular > granular > lattice); may develop glaucoma in posterior polymorphous.

Metabolic Diseases

Definition

Hereditary (AR) enzymatic deficiencies that result in accumulation of substances in various tissues as well as bilateral corneal opacities.

Etiology

Mucopolysaccharidoses, mucolipidoses, sphingolipidoses, gangliosidosis type 1; corneal clouding not seen in Hunter's or Sanfilippo's syndromes.

Symptoms

Decreased vision, white cornea.

Signs

Decreased visual acuity and corneal stromal opacification; may have nystagmus, cataracts, retinal pigment epithelial changes, macular cherry red spot, optic nerve atrophy, and other systemic abnormalities.

Table 5-1   Ocular Involvement of the Metabolic Diseases

Disease	Conjunctiva	Cornea	Retina	Optic nerve
Mucopolysaccharidoses (autosomal recessive)				
MPS I-H (Hurler)	-	+	+	+
MPS I-S (Scheie)	-	+	+	+
MPS II (Hunter; X-linked recessive)	-	-	+	+
MPS III (Sanfilippo)	-	-	+	+
MPS IV (Morquio)	-	+	-	+
MPS VI (Maroteaux-Lamy)	-	+	-	+
MPS VII (Sly)	-	+	-	-
Lipidoses (autosomal recessive)				
GM2 gangliosidosis type I (Tay-Sachs)	-	-	+	+
GM2 gangliosidosis type II (Sandhoff)	-	-	+	+
Fabry's disease (X-linked recessive)	+	+	+	-
Niemann-Pick disease	-	-	+	+

MPS, Mucopolysaccharidoses.

Differential Diagnosis

See above; congenital glaucoma, congenital hereditary endothelial dystrophy, birth trauma, Peter's anomaly, sclerocornea, dermoid.

Evaluation

- Complete ophthalmic history and eye examination with attention to cornea, tonometry, lens, and ophthalmoscopy.
- Pediatric consultation.

Management

• Treat underlying disease.
• May require penetrating keratoplasty.

Prognosis

Poor.

■ Corneal Deposits

Definition

Pigment or crystal deposition at various levels of the cornea.

Calcium

Yellow-white deposits in Bowman's membrane (see Degenerations: Band Keratopathy section).

Copper

Chalcosis   Green-yellow pigmentation of Descemet's membrane and iris; causes sunflower cataract; seen with intraocular foreign body composed of less than 85% copper; pure copper causes suppurative endophthalmitis.

Wilson's disease   95% have Kayser-Fleischer ring at Descemet's membrane (brown-yellow-green peripheral pigmentation that starts inferiorly, no clear interval at limbus); best identified by gonioscopy.

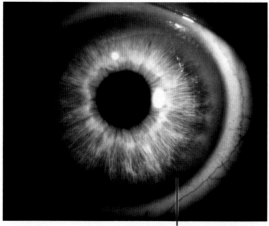

Kayser-Fleischer ring

Figure 5-73 • Copper deposition in a patient with Wilson's disease, demonstrating peripheral, brown, Kayser-Fleischer ring.

Cysteine (Cystinosis)

Stromal, polychromatic crystals.

Drugs

Epinephrine   Black, conjunctival and corneal adrenochrome deposits.

Ciprofloxacin   White, corneal precipitate over epithelial defect.

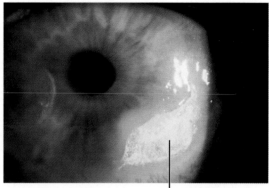

Figure 5-74 • Drug deposition demonstrating chalky, white, ciprofloxacin (Ciloxan) precipitates in the bed of a corneal ulcer.

Ciprofloxacin precipitates

Gold (chrysiasis)   Deposits in conjunctival and stromal periphery; dose related.

Mercury   Preservative in drops causes orange-brown band in Bowman's membrane.

Silver (argyrosis)   Conjunctival and deep stromal deposits.

Thorazine or stelazine   Brown, stromal deposits; also anterior subcapsular lens deposits.

Immunoglobulin (Multiple Myeloma)

Stromal deposits (also seen in Waldenström's macroglobulinemia and benign monoclonal gammopathy).

Iron

Blood staining   Stromal deposits, after hyphema.

Ferry line   Epithelial deposits, under filtering bleb.

Fleischer ring   Epithelial deposits, at base of cone in keratoconus.

Hudson-Stahli line   Epithelial deposits, across inferior one third of cornea.

Siderosis   Stromal deposits, from intraocular metallic foreign body.

Stocker line   Epithelial deposits, at head of pterygium.

Lipid or Cholesterol (Dyslipoproteinemias)

Hyperlipoproteinemia   Arcus in types 2, 3, and 4.

Fish-eye disease   Diffuse corneal clouding, denser in periphery.

Lecithin-cholesterol acyltransferase (LCAT) deficiency   Dense arcus and diffuse, fine, gray, stromal dots.

Tangier's disease   Familial high-density lipoprotein deficiency; diffuse or focal, small, deep, stromal opacities.

Melanin

Krukenberg spindle   Endothelial deposits, central vertical patch seen in pigment dispersion syndrome.

Scattered endothelial pigment   Ingested by abnormal endothelial cells (Fuchs' dystrophy).

Tyrosine (Tyrosinemia)

Epithelial and subepithelial pseudodendritic opacities; may ulcerate and lead to vascularization and scarring.

Urate (Gout)

Epithelial, subepithelial, and stromal, fine, yellow crystals; may form brown, band keratopathy with ulceration and vascularization.

Verticillata

Brown, epithelial, whorl pattern involving inferior and paracentral cornea; seen in Fabry's disease (X-linked recessive) including carriers (women); also from amiodarone, chloroquine, indomethacin, chlorpromazine, or tamoxifen deposits.

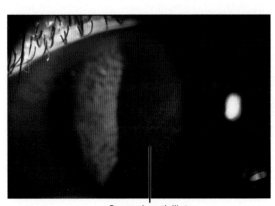

Corneal verticillata

Figure 5-75 • Corneal verticillata demonstrating golden brown deposits in a whorl pattern in the inferior central cornea of a Fabry's disease carrier.

Symptoms

Asymptomatic; may have photophobia and, rarely, decreased vision.

Signs

Normal or decreased visual acuity, corneal deposits, may have iris heterochromia (siderosis and chalcosis), cataract (Wilson's disease, intraocular metallic foreign body, tyrosinemia).

Differential Diagnosis

See above; dieffenbachia plant sap, ichthyosis (may have fine, white, deep, stromal opacities), hyperbilirubinemia.

Evaluation

- Complete ophthalmic history and eye examination with attention to conjunctiva, cornea, anterior chamber, iris, and lens.
- Electroretinogram (ERG) for intraocular metallic foreign body.
- Medical consultation for systemic diseases.

Management

- Treat underlying disease, remove offending agent.
- May require surgical removal of intraocular metallic foreign body.

Prognosis

Good except for siderosis, chalcosis, Wilson's disease, and multiple myeloma.

■ Enlarged Corneal Nerves

Definition

Prominent, enlarged corneal nerves.

Etiology

Multiple endocrine neoplasia type IIb (MEN-IIb), leprosy, Fuchs' dystrophy, amyloidosis, keratoconus, ichthyosis, Refsum's syndrome, neurofibromatosis, congenital glaucoma, trauma, posterior polymorphous dystrophy, and idiopathic.

Symptoms

Asymptomatic.

Signs

Prominent, white, branching, linear opacities in cornea.

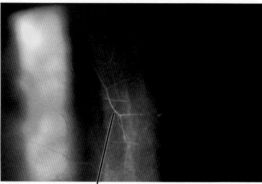

Figure 5-76 • Enlarged corneal nerves appear as prominent, white, branching lines.

Enlarged corneal nerves

Differential Diagnosis

See above; lattice dystrophy.

Evaluation

* Complete ophthalmic history and eye examination with attention to cornea, tonometry, lens, and ophthalmoscopy.
* Medical consultation for systemic diseases.

Management

* No treatment recommended.
* Treat underlying medical disorder.

Prognosis

Enlarged nerves are benign; underlying cause may have poor prognosis (MEN-IIb).

▮ Tumors

Definition

Corneal intraepithelial neoplasia (CIN) or squamous cell carcinoma involving the cornea; usually arises from conjunctiva near limbus.

Epidemiology

Usually unilateral; male predilection (95%); associated with ultraviolet radiation, human papillomavirus, and heavy smoking. Suspect AIDS in patients <50 years of age.

Symptoms

Asymptomatic; may have foreign body sensation, red eye, decreased vision, or notice growth (white spot) on cornea.

Signs

Gelatinous, thickened, white, nodular or smooth, limbal or corneal mass; may also have vascularization, conjunctival injection, and abnormal vessels.

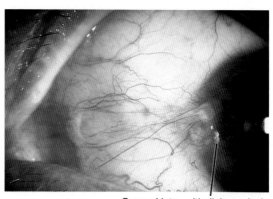

Figure 5-77 • Corneal intraepithelial neoplasia demonstrating thickened, white, gelatinous lesion at limbus with vascularization.

Corneal intraepithelial neoplasia

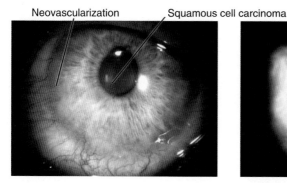

Neovascularization   Squamous cell carcinoma

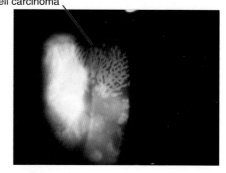

Figure 5-78 • Squamous cell carcinoma of the cornea.

Figure 5-79 • Same patient as Figure 5-78 demonstrating a close-up of the gelatinous, granular lesion.

Differential Diagnosis

Pinguecula, pterygium, pannus, dermoid, Bitot's spot, papilloma, pyogenic granuloma, pseudoepitheliomatous hyperplasia (PEH), benign hereditary intraepithelial dyskeratosis (BHID).

Evaluation

• Complete ophthalmic history and eye examination with attention to conjunctiva and cornea.

Management

• Excision with cryotherapy, radiation, or mitomycin C by a cornea or tumor specialist.

Prognosis

Good if completely excised; 50% recur; rarely invasive or metastatic.

ANTERIOR CHAMBER

Angle-Closure Glaucoma

Primary Angle-Closure Glaucoma

Definition

Glaucoma due to obstruction of trabecular meshwork by peripheral iris; classified as acute, subacute (intermittent), or chronic.

Etiology or Mechanism

Pupillary block (most common)   Lens-iris apposition interferes with aqueous flow and causes iris to bow forward and occlude the trabecular meshwork.

Plateau iris syndrome (without pupillary block)   Peripheral iris occludes angle in patients with atypical iris configuration (anteriorly positioned peripheral iris with steep insertion due to anteriorly rotated ciliary processes) (see Chapter 7).

Epidemiology

Female predilection (4:1); higher incidence in Asians and Eskimos; approximately 5% of the general population over 60 years old have occludable angles, 0.5% of these develop angle-closure; usually bilateral (develops in 50% of untreated fellow eyes within 5 years); associated with hyperopia, nanophthalmos, anterior chamber depth less than 2.5 mm, thicker lens, and lens subluxation.

Symptoms

Acute angle-closure   Pain, red eye, photophobia, decreased or blurred vision, halos around lights, headache, nausea, emesis.

Subacute angle-closure   May be asymptomatic or have symptoms of acute form but less severe; episodes evolve over the course of days or weeks and resolve spontaneously.

Chronic angle-closure   Asymptomatic; may have decreased vision or constricted visual fields in late stages.

Signs

Acute angle-closure Decreased visual acuity, increased intraocular pressure, ciliary injection, corneal edema, anterior chamber cells and flare, shallow anterior chamber, narrow angles on gonioscopy, mid-dilated, nonreactive pupil, iris bombé; may have signs of previous attacks including sector iris atrophy, anterior subcapsular lens opacities (glaukomflecken), dilated irregular pupil, and peripheral anterior synechiae (PAS).

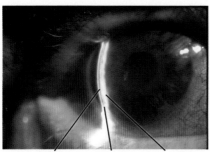

Posterior cornea   Slit-beam   Iris surface

Figure 6-1 • Primary angle-closure glaucoma with very shallow anterior chamber and iridocorneal touch (no space between slit beam view of cornea and iris).

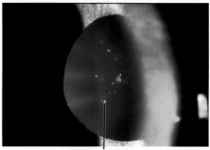

Glaukomflecken

Figure 6-2 • Dotlike anterior subcapsular lens opacities (glaukomflecken) due to lens epithelial cell ischemia and necrosis from high intraocular pressure.

Subacute and chronic angle-closure Narrow angles; may have increased intraocular pressure, PAS, glaukomflecken, visual field defects, and optic nerve cupping.

Evaluation

• Complete ophthalmic history and eye examination with attention to pupils, cornea, tonometry, anterior chamber, iris, indentation gonioscopy (Zeiss lens), lens, and ophthalmoscopy.
• Check visual fields.
• Consider provocative testing (prone test, dark room test, prone dark room test, and pharmacologic dilation; intraocular pressure increase of >8 mm Hg is considered positive).

Management

ACUTE ANGLE-CLOSURE

• Topical β-blocker (timolol [Timoptic] 0.5% q 15 minutes × 2, then bid), α-agonist (apraclonidine [Iopidine] 1% q 15 minutes × 2), and topical steroid (prednisolone acetate 1% q 15 minutes × 4, then q1h).
• Topical miotic (pilocarpine 1-2% × 1 initially, then qid if effective; usually not effective if intraocular pressure >40 mm Hg due to iris sphincter ischemia; in 20% of patients pilocarpine will exacerbate the situation due to forward displacement of the lens-iris diaphragm); can also consider topical α-antagonist (thymoxamine 0.5% q 15 minutes for 2-3h).

Management

- Systemic acetazolamide (Diamox 500 mg po STAT, then bid) and hyperosmotic (isosorbide up to 2 g/kg po of 45% solution).
- **Laser peripheral iridotomy (LPI) with or without iridoplasty:** Definitive treatment after acute attack is broken medically; may require application of topical glycerin (Ophthalgan) to clear corneal edema for adequate visualization for laser.
  - *Procedure parameters:* a contact lens is used to stabilize the eye, better focus the beam, and place laser spots peripherally; patency of the iridotomy is confirmed by visualization of the lens capsule (often a rush of aqueous fluid through the hole is seen) *not* by the appearance of a red reflex.
  - *Argon laser (depends on iris pigmentation)*
        Dark brown: 0.02-0.05 sec duration, 50 μ spot size, 600-1000 mW power; then 0.1sec and 400-600 mW through pigment epithelium.
        Medium brown: 0.1-0.2 sec duration, 50 μ spot size, 600-1000 mW power.
        Blue: 0.05 sec duration, 500 μ spot size, 200-500 mW power contraction burns; then 0.1 sec duration, 50 μ spot size, 600-1000 mW power through stroma and 400-600 mW through pigment epithelium.
  - *Nd:YAG laser:* 4-10 mJ power.
- Prophylactic laser peripheral iridotomy in fellow eye with narrow angle to prevent an acute attack in the future.
- If unable to perform laser peripheral iridotomy, consider surgical iridectomy.
- Consider goniosynechiolysis for recent peripheral anterior synechiae (<12 months).
- Plateau iris syndrome may require long-term miotic therapy and peripheral iridectomy to reduce risk of pupillary block; consider argon laser iridoplasty or gonioplasty.
  - *Procedure parameters:* 0.2-0.5 sec duration, 200-500 μ spot size, 200-400 mW power, approximately 10 spot applications per quadrant, a contact lens is used to stabilize the eye and better focus the beam, spots are placed on the iris as peripheral as possible and the power setting is adjusted until movement of the iris is observed.

SUBACUTE AND CHRONIC ANGLE-CLOSURE

- Laser peripheral iridotomy even without evidence of pupillary block.
- Treatment of increased intraocular pressure (see Primary Open Angle Glaucoma section in Chapter 11); may require trabeculectomy or glaucoma drainage implant to lower pressure adequately.

Prognosis

Good if prompt treatment is initiated for acute attack; poorer for chronic cases but depends on extent of optic nerve damage and subsequent intraocular pressure control.

Secondary Angle-Closure Glaucoma

Definition

Acute or chronic angle-closure glaucoma caused by a variety of ocular disorders.

Etiology or Mechanism

With pupillary block   Lens-induced (e.g., phacomorphic, dislocated lens, microspherophakia), seclusio pupillae, aphakic or pseudophakic pupillary block, silicone oil, nanophthalmos.

Without pupillary block

Posterior "Pushing" Mechanism   Mechanical or anterior displacement of lens-iris diaphragm.

* Anterior rotation of ciliary body due to:
  * Inflammation (scleritis, uveitis, panretinal photocoagulation).
  * Congestion (scleral buckling, nanophthalmos).
  * Choroidal effusion (hypotony; uveal effusion).
  * Suprachoroidal hemorrhage.
* Aqueous misdirection (malignant glaucoma).
* Pressure from posterior segment (tumor, expanding gas, exudative retinal detachment).
* Persistent hyperplastic primary vitreous.
* Retinopathy of prematurity.

Anterior "Pulling" Mechanism   Adherence of iris to trabecular meshwork or membranes over trabecular meshwork.

* Epithelial (downgrowth or ingrowth).
* Endothelial (iridocorneal endothelial syndrome, posterior polymorphous dystrophy).
* Neovascular (neovascular glaucoma; see Chapter 7).
* Postinflammatory peripheral anterior synechiae.
* Adhesion from trauma.

Symptoms

Acute angle-closure   Pain, red eye, photophobia, decreased or blurred vision, halos around lights, headache, nausea, emesis.

Chronic angle-closure   Asymptomatic; may have decreased vision or constricted visual fields during late stages.

Signs

Acute angle-closure   Decreased visual acuity, increased intraocular pressure, ciliary injection, corneal edema, anterior chamber cells and flare, shallow anterior chamber, narrow angles on gonioscopy, mid-dilated nonreactive pupil, iris bombé; signs of underlying etiology.

Chronic angle-closure   Narrow angles, increased intraocular pressure, peripheral anterior synechiae, signs of underlying etiology; may have visual field defects and optic nerve cupping.

Evaluation

* Complete ophthalmic history and eye examination with attention to pupils, cornea, tonometry, anterior chamber, iris, indentation gonioscopy, lens, and ophthalmoscopy.
* Check visual fields.

Management

- Treat underlying problem.
- Laser peripheral iridotomy for pupillary block.
- Topical cycloplegic agent (scopolamine 0.25% qid or atropine 1% bid) for malignant glaucoma, microspherophakia, after scleral buckle or after panretinal photocoagulation (do not use miotic agents); may require pars plana vitrectomy and lens extraction in refractory cases of malignant glaucoma or Nd:YAG laser disruption of the anterior hyaloid face in patient with pseudophakia and aphakia.
- Topical cycloplegic agent (scopolamine 0.25% qid), steroid (prednisolone acetate 1% qid), and panretinal photocoagulation for neovascular glaucoma.
- Cataract extraction may be necessary in some cases of lens-induced angle-closure glaucoma.

Prognosis

Poorer than primary angle-closure because usually due to chronic process; depends on extent of optic nerve damage and subsequent intraocular pressure control.

Hypotony

Definition

Low intraocular pressure (<10 mm Hg); functional and structural changes usually occur with pressures less than or equal to 5 mm Hg.

Symptoms

Asymptomatic; may have pain and decreased vision.

Signs

Normal or decreased visual acuity, low intraocular pressure; may have corneal folds, anterior chamber cells and flare, shallow anterior chamber, chorioretinal folds, choroidal effusion, cystoid macular edema, positive Seidel test, filtering bleb, optic disc edema, squared-off globe.

Differential Diagnosis

Trauma (blunt, penetrating, or surgical), wound leak, bleb overfiltration, ciliary body shutdown, cyclodialysis, choroidal effusion, retinal detachment, pharmacologic, systemic disorder (bilateral hypotony), uveitis, cyclitic membrane, and phthisis.

Evaluation

- Complete ophthalmic history and eye examination with attention to cornea, tonometry, anterior chamber, gonioscopy, and ophthalmoscopy.

• Check Seidel test (see Chapter 5, Trauma: Laceration section) to rule out open globe or wound leak in traumatic or postsurgical cases.

Management

- Treat underlying problem.
- Topical cycloplegic agent (cyclopentolate 1%, scopolamine 0.25%, atropine 1% bid to tid).
- Add topical antibiotic for wound leak (gatifloxacin [Zymar] or moxifloxacin [Vigamox] qid).
- May require surgical repair of wound leak, retinal detachment, ciliary body detachment, or drainage of choroidals.
- Bandage contact lens or pressure patch may work with small leaks.
- Consider Simmons' shell for bleb overfiltration.
- Use topical steroids or transseptal injection of steroid (triamcinolone acetonide 40 mg/mL) in cases of hypotony associated with uveitis.

Prognosis

Depends on etiology.

█ Hyphema

Definition

Blood in the anterior chamber. Hyphema forms a layer of blood, whereas a microhyphema cannot be visualized with the naked eye (can only see red blood cells floating in anterior chamber with slit-lamp examination).

Etiology

Usually a result of trauma (60% also have angle recession); may be spontaneous when associated with neovascularization of the iris or angle, iris lesions, or malpositioned or loose intraocular lens (IOL).

Symptoms

Decreased vision; may have pain, photophobia, red eye.

Signs

Normal or decreased visual acuity, red blood cells in the anterior chamber (layer or clot); may have subconjunctival hemorrhage, increased intraocular pressure, rubeosis, iris sphincter tears, iris lesion, unusually deep anterior chamber, angle recession, iridodonesis, iridodialysis, cyclodialysis, and other signs of ocular trauma; may have iris lesion or pseudophacodonesis of IOL implant.

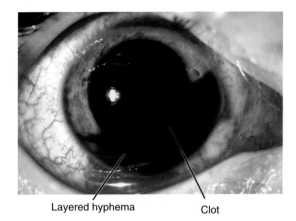

Figure 6-3 • Hyphema demonstrating layered blood inferiorly and suspended red blood cells and clot.

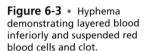

Differential Diagnosis

Trauma, uveitis-glaucoma-hyphema (UGH) syndrome, juvenile xanthogranuloma, leukemia, child abuse, postoperative, Fuchs' heterochromic iridocyclitis, rubeosis irides, malpositioned or loose IOL.

Evaluation

- Complete ophthalmic history and eye examination with attention to cornea, tonometry, anterior chamber, iris, and ophthalmoscopy; wait 2-4 weeks to perform gonioscopy and scleral depression in traumatic cases.
- **Lab tests:** Sickle cell prep and hemoglobin electrophoresis to rule out sickle cell disease.
- B-scan ultrasonography if unable to visualize the fundus to rule out open globe; consider ultrasound biomicroscopy to evaluate angle structures.

Management

- Topical steroid (prednisolone acetate 1% up to q1h initially, then taper over 3-4 weeks as hyphema and inflammation resolve).
- Topical cycloplegic agent (scopolamine 0.25% or atropine 1% bid to tid).
- Consider aminocaproic acid ([Amicar] 50-100 mg/kg q4h).
- Intraocular pressure control as needed (see Chapter 11; do not use carbonic anhydrase inhibitors in patients with sickle cell disease; do not use miotic agents).
- Counsel patient to avoid aspirin-containing products, sleep with head of bed elevated at 30-degree angle, metal eye shield over injured eye at all times, and bed rest.
- Daily examination for first 5 days (when risk of recurrent bleed is highest) then slowly space out visits.
- May require anterior chamber washout for corneal blood staining, uncontrolled elevated intraocular pressure, persistent clot, rebleed (8-ball hyphema); IOL removal or exchange for UGH syndrome and malpositioned IOLs.

Prognosis

Good in traumatic cases if intraocular pressure is controlled and there is no rebleed; may be at risk for angle recession glaucoma in the future.

Anterior Chamber Cells and Flare

Definition

Cells and increased protein (flare) in the anterior chamber due to breakdown of the blood–aqueous barrier by inflammation.

Cells   Appear as small particles floating in the aqueous; usually white blood cells; sometimes red blood cells (microhyphema) or pigment cells (from iris after dilation and in pigment dispersion syndrome). If severe, cells settle inferiorly in anterior chamber and form layer (hypopyon, hyphema, or pseudohypopyon).

Flare   Appears as hazy or cloudy aqueous; severe fibrinous exudate produces jelly-like plasmoid aqueous appearance with strands of fibrin (4^+ flare).

Etiology

Exudation from blood vessels due to anterior segment inflammation; usually uveitis, trauma, postoperative, scleritis, and keratitis.

Symptoms

Variable pain, photophobia, tearing, red eye, decreased vision; may be asymptomatic.

Signs

Normal or decreased visual acuity, ciliary injection, miosis, anterior chamber cells and flare (best seen when viewed with a short narrow slit-lamp beam directed at an angle through the pupil producing an effect similar to shining a flashlight through a dark room; cells demonstrate brownian motion and flare looks like smoke in the light beam; graded on a 1 to 4 scale [i.e., $1^+ = 0$-10 cells; $2^+ = 11$-20 cells; $3^+ = 21$-50 cells; $4^+ = >50$ cells]); may have keratic precipitates, keratitis, iris nodules, posterior synechiae, increased or decreased intraocular pressure, hypopyon, hyphema, pseudohypopyon, cataract, vitritis, or retinal or choroidal lesions.

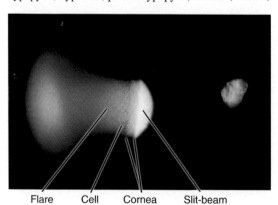

Figure 6-4 • Grade 4^+ anterior chamber cells and flare visible with fine slit beam between the cornea and iris.

Flare   Cell   Cornea   Slit-beam

Differential Diagnosis

See below.

Evaluation

- Complete ophthalmic history and eye examination with attention to cornea, tonometry, anterior chamber, gonioscopy, iris, lens, and ophthalmoscopy.
- Consider uveitis workup (see Anterior Uveitis section).

Management

- Treat underlying cause.
- Topical steroid (prednisolone acetate 1% up to q1h initially, then taper slowly) and cycloplegic agent (cyclopentolate 1%, scopolamine 0.25%, or atropine 1% bid to tid).
- May require intraocular pressure control (see Chapter 11; do not use miotic agents), sub-Tenon steroid injection (triamcinolone acetonide 40 mg/mL), systemic steroids (prednisone 60-100 mg po qd), or cytotoxic agents after ruling out infectious etiologies (see Anterior Uveitis section).

Prognosis

Depends on etiology.

■ Hypopyon

Definition

Layer of white blood cells in anterior chamber.

Etiology

Usually due to inflammation (uveitis) or infection (corneal ulcer, endophthalmitis).

Symptoms

Pain, red eye, and decreased vision.

Signs

Normal or decreased visual acuity, conjunctival injection, hypopyon, and anterior chamber cells and flare; may have corneal infiltrate, keratic precipitates, iris nodules, cataract, vitritis, vitreous hemorrhage, tumor, retinal or choroidal lesions.

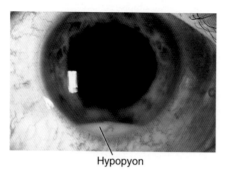

Hypopyon

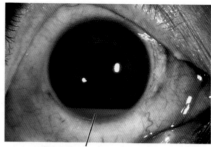

Pseudohypopyon

Figure 6-5 • Hypopyon demonstrating layered white blood cells inferiorly.

Figure 6-6 • Pseudohypopyon composed of khaki-colored ghost cells layered inferiorly.

Differential Diagnosis

Corneal ulcer, uveitis, endophthalmitis, pseudohypopyon (pigment cells, ghost cells, tumor cells, macrophages).

Evaluation

- Complete ophthalmic history and eye examination with attention to cornea, tonometry, anterior chamber, iris, lens, and ophthalmoscopy.
- B-scan ultrasonography if unable to visualize the fundus.
- **Lab tests:** Cultures or smears for infectious keratitis (see Chapter 5) or endophthalmitis (see Endophthalmitis section).
- Consider uveitis workup (see Anterior Uveitis section).

Management

- Antimicrobial medications if infectious (see Infectious Keratitis in Chapter 5 and Endophthalmitis sections below).
- Topical cycloplegic agent (cyclopentolate 1%, scopolamine 0.25%, or atropine 1% bid to tid).
- Topical steroid and cycloplegic agent if uveitic (see Anterior Uveitis section).
- Monitor treatment response by hypopyon resorption.
- Rarely requires surgery, except in cases of endophthalmitis.

Prognosis

Depends on etiology and treatment response.

Endophthalmitis

Definition

Intraocular infection; may be acute, subacute, or chronic; localized or involving anterior and posterior segments.

Etiology

Postoperative (70%)

Acute postoperative (<6 weeks after surgery) Ninety-four percent gram-positive bacteria including coagulase-negative *staphylococci* (70%), *Staphylococcus aureus* (10%), *Streptococcus* species (11%); only 6% gram-negative organisms.

Delayed postoperative (>6 weeks after surgery) *Propionibacterium acnes,* coagulase-negative *staphylococci,* and fungi (*Candida* species).

Conjunctival filtering bleb associated *Streptococcus* species (47%), coagulase-negative *staphylococci* (22%), *Haemophilus influenzae* (16%).

Posttraumatic (20%)

Bacillus (B. cereus) species (24%), *Staphylococcus* species (39%), and gram-negative organisms (7%).

Endogenous (8%)

Rare, usually fungal (*Candida* species); bacterial endogenous is usually due to *Staphylococcus aureus* and gram-negative bacteria; seen in debilitated, septicemic, or immunocompromised patients, especially after surgical procedures.

Epidemiology

Incidence of endophthalmitis following penetrating trauma is 3-7%, may be as high as 30% after injuries in rural settings; risk factors include retained intraocular foreign body, delayed surgery (>24 hours), rural setting (soil contamination), disrupted crystalline lens. Incidence of endophthalmitis following cataract surgery is less than 0.1%; risk factors include loss of vitreous, disrupted posterior capsule, poor wound closure, and prolonged surgery.

Symptoms

Pain, photophobia, discharge, red eye, decreased vision; may be asymptomatic or have chronic uveitis appearance in delayed onset and endogenous cases.

Signs

Decreased visual acuity (usually severe; only 14% of patients in the Endophthalmitis Vitrectomy Study (EVS) had better than 5/200 vision), lid edema, proptosis, conjunctival injection, chemosis, wound abscess, corneal edema, keratic precipitates, anterior chamber cells and flare, hypopyon, vitritis, poor red reflex; may have positive Seidel test result and other signs of an open globe (see Chapter 4).

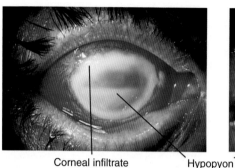
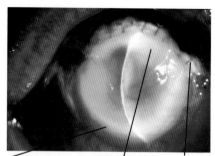

Corneal infiltrate   Hypopyon   Ring infiltrate   Sutures

Figure 6-7 • Endophthalmitis with large hypopyon (almost 50% of anterior chamber height). There is severe inflammation with 4+ conjunctival injection and a white ring corneal infiltrate at the limbus.

Figure 6-8 • *Staphylococcus* endophthalmitis with ring infiltrate. There is marked corneal edema and the corneal sutures across the surgical wound are visible at the superior limbus.

Differential Diagnosis

Uveitis, sterile inflammation (usually from prolonged intraoperative manipulations, especially involving vitreous, contaminants on IOL implant or surgical instruments, retained lens material, or rebound inflammation after sudden decrease in postoperative medications), intraocular foreign body, intraocular tumor, sympathetic ophthalmia, anterior segment ischemia (from carotid artery disease [ocular ischemic syndrome] or following muscle surgery [usually on three or more rectus muscles in same eye at the same surgery]).

Evaluation

* Complete ophthalmic history and eye examination with attention to visual acuity, surgical incision integrity, conjunctiva, cornea, tonometry, anterior chamber, vitreous cells, red reflex, and ophthalmoscopy.
* B-scan ultrasonography if unable to visualize the fundus.
* **Lab tests:** STAT evaluation of intraocular fluid cultures and smears; conjunctival and nasal swabs can also be collected for culture but have low yield.
* Medical consultation for endogenous endophthalmitis.

Management

OPHTHALMIC EMERGENCY

Acute Postoperative Endophthalmitis
* If vision is better than light perception (>LP), then anterior chamber and vitreous tap for collection of specimens for culture, and injection of intravitreal antibiotics (see below).
* If vision is LP only, then anterior chamber tap, pars plana vitrectomy, and injection of intravitreal antibiotics (EVS conclusions); should be managed by a vitreoretinal specialist.

Management—cont'd

- Intravitreal antibiotics or steroids:
    Vancomycin (1 mg/0.1 mL).
    Ceftazidime (2.25 mg/0.1 mL) or amikacin (0.4 mg/0.1 mL).
    Dexamethasone (0.4 mg/0.1 mL; controversial, because intravitreal steroids were not evaluated in the EVS).
- Subconjunctival antibiotics or steroids:
    Vancomycin (25 mg).
    Ceftazidime (100 mg) or gentamicin (20 mg).
    Dexamethasone (12-24 mg).
- Broad spectrum fortified topical antibiotics (alternate every 30 minutes):
    Vancomycin (50 mg/mL q1h).
    Ceftazidime (50 mg/mL q1h).
- Topical steroid (prednisolone acetate 1% q1-2h initially) and cycloplegic agent (atropine 1% tid or scopolamine 0.25% qid).
- Systemic intravenous antibiotics for marked inflammation, severe cases, or rapid onset (controversial, because EVS found no benefit with systemic antibiotics):
    Vancomycin (1 g IV q12h).
    Ceftazidime (1 g IV q12h).

Subacute, Delayed, Endogenous, Filtering Bleb Associated, and Posttraumatic

- EVS guidelines do not apply and treatment should be based on clinical situation.
- Intravitreal antibiotics or steroids similar to acute postoperative guidelines (see above); add amphotericin B (0.005 mg/0.1 mL) if endogenous fungal or delayed onset and presumed fungal etiology.
- Subconjunctival antibiotics or steroids similar to acute postoperative guidelines (see above).
- Broad spectrum fortified topical antibiotics similar to acute postoperative guidelines (see above); add amphotericin B 1.0-2.5 mg/mL q1h or natamycin 50 mg/mL q1h if fungal (poor penetration).
- Topical steroid (prednisolone acetate 1% q1-2h initially) and cycloplegic agent (atropine 1% tid).
- Systemic intravenous antibiotics for marked inflammation similar to acute postoperative guidelines (see above).
- Systemic antifungal agents (amphotericin B 0.25-1.0 mg/kg IV divided equally q6h) if disseminated disease exists.
- Delayed postoperative endophthalmitis may require partial or total capsulectomy, pars plana vitrectomy, or IOL removal or exchange.
- Consider repeat tap (or pars plana vitrectomy) and intravitreal injections if clinical picture is worse after 48-72 hours.
- Tailor antibiotic choices based on culture results.

Prognosis

Depends on etiology, duration, and organism; usually poor, especially for traumatic cases.

■ Anterior Uveitis (Iritis, Iridocyclitis)

Definition

Inflammation of the anterior uvea (iris [iritis] and ciliary body [cyclitis]) with exudation of blood cells and proteins into the anterior chamber secondary to breakdown of the blood–aqueous barrier and increased vascular permeability from a variety of disorders. Minimal spill-over into the retrolental space can be present. Classified by pathology (nongranulomatous [lymphocyte and plasma cell infiltrates] or granulomatous [epithelioid and giant cell infiltrates]), location (keratouveitis, sclerouveitis, anterior uveitis, intermediate uveitis, posterior uveitis, endophthalmitis, panuveitis), course (acute, chronic, recurrent), or etiology.

Etiology

Most commonly idiopathic or autoimmune, but it is critical to rule out causes such as infection, malignancy, medication, and trauma.

Infectious Anterior Uveitis

Herpes Simplex and Herpes Zoster Ophthalmicus

Patients often exhibit keratic precipitates underlying areas of dendritic keratitis; elevated intraocular pressure common; both herpes simplex and varicella zoster may cause sector iris atrophy.

Lyme Disease

Patients have classic cutaneous erythema chronicum migrans at the site of a tick bite; due to *Borrelia burgdorferi* transmitted by *Ixodes dammini* or *I. pacificus* tick; 1-3 months later can develop neurologic symptoms including encephalitis, meningitis; also conjunctivitis, keratitis, iritis, vitritis, and optic neuritis; late stages have chronic skin changes and chronic arthritis; may develop cardiac manifestations.

Syphilis

Chronic or recurrent granulomatous anterior uveitis can be an ocular manifestation of acquired syphilitic uveitis. This needs to be ruled out in every patient with persistent granulomatous iritis, because systemic antibiotics are necessary to prevent significant morbidity.

Tuberculosis

Chronic granulomatous iritis, may also have conjunctival nodules, phlyctenules, interstitial keratitis, and scleritis. It is rarely caused by direct ocular infection of *Mycobacterium tuberculosis* and most of the time is an immune response directed toward the organism. Patients with a chronic granulomatous iritis who are immunocompromised (acquired immunodeficiency syndrome) or come from endemic areas should be evaluated for tuberculosis. Other associated ocular findings in the anterior segment include: phlyctenules, interstitial keratitis, conjunctival nodules, or scleritis.

Noninfectious Anterior Uveitis

Nongranulomatous, Noninfectious Anterior Uveitis

Idiopathic (acute)   Responsible for most cases of anterior uveitis (50%).

HLA- B27 associated anterior uveitis (acute)   The iritis is acute, recurrent and may affect one eye at a time. Forty-seven percent of patients with anterior uveitis can have human lymphocyte antigen (HLA)-B27 without an associated systemic condition; often male and tend to develop uveitis at a younger age; distinct entity from the idiopathic form. Twenty-five percent have a seronegative spondyloarthropathy.

Seronegative spondyloarthropathies (acute)   This group of conditions share common features that include: radiographic sacroiliitis (with or without spondylitis), asymmetric peripheral arthritis without rheumatoid nodules, negative rheumatoid factor and antinuclear antibody (ANA), HLA-B27 association, variable mucocutaneous lesions and anterior uveitis.

Ankylosing Spondylitis   Thirty percent get anterior uveitis, recurrent in 40%, also episcleritis and scleritis. Patients develop lower back pain and stiffness after inactivity; also associated with aortitis and pulmonary apical fibrosis; arthritis less severe in women, but eye disease can still be severe; 88% have positive HLA-B27 test results; sacroiliac radiographs often show sclerosis and narrowing of joint spaces; untreated patients will progress to debilitating spinal fusion.

Reiter's Syndrome   Triad of nonspecific urethritis, polyarthritis (80%), and mucopurulent, papillary conjunctivitis with iritis; arthritis starts within 30 days of infection; also associated with keratoderma blennorrhagicum, circinate balanitis, plantar fasciitis, Achilles tendonitis, sacroiliitis, palate or tongue ulcers, nail pitting, prostatitis, and cystitis; seen in young males (90%); may be triggered by diarrhea or infectious organism *(Chlamydia, Ureaplasma, Yersinia, Shigella, Salmonella);* 85-95% have positive HLA-B27 test results.

Psoriatic Arthritis   May also get conjunctivitis and dry eyes; patients have "sausage" digits from terminal phalangeal joint arthritic involvement, subungual hyperkeratosis, erythematous rash, nail pitting, and onycholysis; associated with sacroiliitis; iritis is rarely seen when psoriasis appears without arthritis; associated with HLA-B27.

Inflammatory Bowel Disease   In contrast to the unilateral iritis associated with ankylosing spondylitis and Reiter's syndrome, the iritis associated with inflammatory bowel disease is usually bilateral and has a posterior component; may also get dry eyes, conjunctivitis, episcleritis, scleritis, orbital cellulitis, and optic neuritis; rare in Crohn's disease (2.4%), 5-10% in ulcerative colitis; associated with sacroiliitis, erythema nodosum, pyoderma gangrenosum, hepatitis, and sclerosing cholangitis; 60% of patients with sacroiliitis have positive HLA-B27 test results.

Whipple's Disease   Rare systemic disorder associated with *Tropheryma whippelii* infection, characterized by chronic diarrhea (due to malabsorption), joint inflammation, central nervous system manifestations, and anterior uveitis; associated with sacroiliitis, spondylitis, and increased prevalence of HLA-B27.

Behçet's disease (acute)   Triad of recurrent hypopyon iritis, aphthous stomatitis, and genital ulcers; also develop arthritis, thromboembolism, and central nervous system problems; iritis usually bilateral with posterior involvement, the hallmark is retinal vasculitis (see Chapter 10); more common in Asians and Middle Easterners; associated with HLA-B5 (subtypes Bw51 and B52) and HLA-B12.

Glaucomatocyclitic crisis (Posner-Schlossman syndrome, acute)   Unilateral, mild, recurrent iritis with markedly elevated intraocular pressure, corneal edema, fine keratic precipitates, and a mid-dilated pupil; no synechiae; self-limited episodes (hours to days); associated with HLA-Bw54.

Kawasaki's disease (acute)   Acute exanthematous disease seen in children (see Chapter 4).

Drug use (acute)   Certain systemic medications may cause anterior uveitis, specifically rifabutin and cidofovir.

Interstitial nephritis   Usually acute, bilateral, anterior uveitis that occurs more frequently in children, may have posterior inflammation; female predilection; patients have fever, malaise, arthralgias; urinalysis shows white blood cells without infection; may be due to allergic reaction to nonsteroidal antiinflammatory agent or antibiotic; can progress to renal failure if not treated (oral steroids).

Other autoimmune disease (acute and chronic)   Systemic lupus erythematosus, relapsing polychondritis, and Wegener's granulomatosis.

Juvenile rheumatoid arthritis (chronic)   Leading cause of uveitis in children, typically chronic, bilateral, anterior uveitis with minimal redness and pain; type I is pauciarticular (90%), rheumatoid factor (RF) negative, antinuclear antibody (ANA) positive, female predilection (4:1), no sacroiliitis, and earlier onset (by age 4 years); type II is pauciarticular, RF negative, ANA negative, HLA-B27 positive, slight male predilection, sacroiliitis common, and later onset (by age 8 years); both have chronic course with poor prognosis. Another subset is childhood spondyloarthropathy, which causes an acute, unilateral, self-limited, anterior uveitis; usually in males, older than 12 years, and HLA-B27 positive. Iritis is rare in Still's disease.

Fuchs' heterochromic iridocyclitis (chronic)   Usually unilateral (90%), low-grade iritis with small, white, stellate keratic precipitates, fine vascularization of the angle, diffuse iris atrophy, and no synechiae; predilection for blue-eyed patients; iris of affected eye may be lighter; associated with glaucoma (15%) and cataracts (70%); good prognosis; poor response to topical steroids (therefore, not indicated).

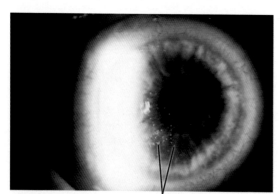

Figure 6-9 • Fuchs' heterochromic iridocyclitis with fine, white, stellate keratic precipitates.

Keratic precipitates

Postoperative or trauma (chronic)   Ocular injury including surgery produces variable anterior chamber inflammation, and the following conditions should be considered: exacerbation of preexisting uveitis, surgical trauma, retained lens fragments, UGH syndrome, endophthalmitis, and sympathetic ophthalmia.

Granulomatous NonInfectious Anterior Uveitis

Autoimmune

Sarcoidosis (see Chapter 10), Vogt-Koyanagi-Harada syndrome (see Chapter 10), sympathetic ophthalmia (see Chapter 10), Wegener's granulomatosis, multiple sclerosis, and lens-induced (phakoanaphylactic endophthalmitis; an immune-mediated [type 3] hypersensitivity reaction to lens particles after trauma or surgery causing a zonal granulomatous reaction after a latent period).

HLA associations (located on chromosome 6)

A11	Sympathetic ophthalmia.
A29	Bird-shot retinochoroidopathy.
B5	Behçet's disease (also B12).
B7	Presumed ocular histoplasmosis syndrome, serpiginous choroidopathy, ankylosing spondylitis.
B8	Sjögren's syndrome.
B12	Ocular cicatricial pemphigoid.
B27	Ankylosing spondylitis (88%), Reiter's syndrome (85-95%), inflammatory bowel disease (60%), psoriatic arthritis (also B17).
Bw54	Posner-Schlossman syndrome.
DR4	Vogt-Koyanagi-Harada syndrome, ocular cicatricial pemphigoid.

Symptoms

Pain, photophobia, tearing, red eye; may have decreased vision.

Signs

Normal or decreased visual acuity, ciliary injection, miosis, anterior chamber cells and flare; may have fine (nongranulomatous) or mutton fat (granulomatous) keratic precipitates, keratitis, iris nodules (Koeppe, Busacca), increased or decreased intraocular pressure, peripheral anterior synechiae, posterior synechiae, hypopyon (especially HLA-B27 associated and Behçet's), cataract, vitritis, retinal or choroidal lesions, cystoid macular edema.

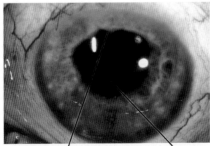

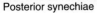
Posterior synechiae   Keratic precipitates

Figure 6-10 • Granulomatous uveitis demonstrating inflammatory iris nodules, keratic precipitates, and posterior synechiae.

Figure 6-11 • Close-up of granulomatous keratic precipitates.

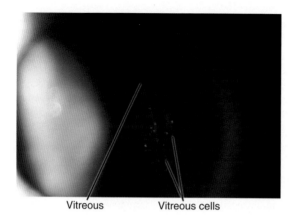

Figure 6-12 • Anterior vitreous cells visible with fine slit beam behind the lens. The cells are seen here as fine white specks among the vitreous strands.

Vitreous   Vitreous cells

Differential Diagnosis

Masquerade syndromes: retinal detachment, retinoblastoma, malignant melanoma, leukemia, large cell lymphoma (reticulum cell sarcoma), juvenile xanthogranuloma, intraocular foreign body, anterior segment ischemia, ocular ischemic syndrome, and spill-over syndromes from any posterior uveitis (most commonly toxoplasmosis).

Evaluation

- Complete ophthalmic history and eye examination with attention to corneal sensation, character of keratic precipitates, tonometry, anterior chamber, iris, vitreous cells, and ophthalmoscopy.
- Unilateral, nongranulomatous iritis is often idiopathic and treated without extensive workup.
- If uveitis is recurrent, bilateral, granulomatous, or involving the posterior segment, consider workup as clinical examination and history dictate.
- **Lab tests:** Basic testing recommended for nongranulomatous anterior uveitis with a negative history, review of systems, and medical examination: complete blood count (CBC), erythrocyte sedimentation rate (ESR), Venereal Disease Research Laboratory (VDRL) test, fluorescent treponemal antibody absorption (FTA-ABS) test or microhemagglutination for treponema pallidum (MHA-TP) (syphilis), HLA-B27.
- Other labs that should be ordered according to history or evidence of granulomatous inflammation include: ANA, RF (juvenile rheumatoid arthritis), serum lysozyme, angiotensin converting enzyme (ACE) (sarcoidosis), Lyme titer, purified protein derivative (PPD) and controls (tuberculosis), herpes simplex and herpes zoster titers, enzyme-linked immunosorbent assay (ELISA) for Lyme immunoglobulin M and immunoglobulin G, human immunodeficiency virus (HIV) antibody test, chest radiographs (sarcoidosis, tuberculosis), chest CT (sarcoidosis), sacroiliac radiographs (ankylosing spondylitis), knee radiographs (juvenile rheumatoid arthritis, Reiter's syndrome), gallium scan (sarcoidosis), urinalysis (interstitial nephritis), and urethral cultures (Reiter's syndrome).
- **Special diagnostic lab tests:** HLA typing, antineutrophil cytoplasmic antibodies (ANCA) (Wegener's granulomatosis, polyarteritis nodosa), Raji cell and C1q binding assays for circulating immune complexes (systemic lupus erythematosus, systemic vasculitides), complement proteins: C3, C4, total complement (systemic lupus erythematosus, cryoglobulinemia, glomerulonephritis), soluble interleukin-2 receptor.
- Medical or rheumatology consultation.

Management

- Topical steroid (prednisolone acetate 1% up to q1h initially, then taper very slowly over weeks to months depending on etiology and response). Patients who are steroid responsive should still be treated with prednisolone acetate 1% and the intraocular pressure treated with ocular hypotensive agents.
- Topical cycloplegic agent (cyclopentolate 1%, scopolamine 0.25%, homatropine 2%, or atropine 1% bid to qid).
- Treat elevations in intraocular pressure as needed, especially glaucomatocyclitic crisis (see Chapter 11); do not use miotic agents.
- Systemic antibiotics for Lyme disease, tuberculosis, syphilis, Whipple's disease, and toxoplasmosis (see Chapter 10).
- Topical antiviral medications (trifluridine [Viroptic] 9 times/day) for herpes simplex infections with concomitant corneal epithelial involvement.
- Systemic antiviral medications (acyclovir 800 mg 5 times/day for 10 days) for herpes zoster.
- Consider oral steroids (prednisone 60-100 mg po qd); check purified protein derivative (PPD), blood glucose, and chest radiographs before starting systemic steroids.
- Add H_2-blocker (ranitidine [Zantac] 150 mg po bid) or proton pump inhibitor when administering systemic steroids.
- Consider sub-Tenon steroid injection (triamcinolone acetonide 40 mg/mL) or intravitreal steroid injection (triamcinolone acetonide 4 mg/0.1 mL). Both biodegradable and nonerodable sustained release steroid implants are in clinical testing and may supplant steroid injections.
- If the uveitis becomes steroid dependent, then consider a stepladder approach to treat with steroid-sparing agents that would eventually allow the tapering or minimal use of topical and systemic corticosteroid:
  1. **Nonsteroidal antiinflammatory drugs:** diclofenac (Voltaren) 75 mg po bid or diflunisal (Dolobid) 250 mg po bid. Other nonsteroidal antiinflammatory agents that can be used as a second line of therapy include indomethacin (Indocin SR) 75 mg po bid or naproxen (Naprosyn) 250 mg po bid. In patients with a known history of gastritis or peptic ulceration, the use of COX-2 inhibitors should be considered: celecoxib (Celebrex) 100 mg po bid or rofecoxib (Vioxx) 25 mg po qd.
  2. **Immunosuppressive chemotherapy:** this form of treatment should be managed by a uveitis specialist or in coordination with a medical specialist familiar with these medications; indications for these agents include Behçet's disease, sympathetic ophthalmia, Vogt-Koyanagi-Harada syndrome, rheumatoid necrotizing scleritis or peripheral ulcerative keratitis, Wegener's granulomatosis, polyarteritis nodosa, relapsing polychondritis, juvenile rheumatoid arthritis, or sarcoidosis unresponsive to conventional therapy.
     - **Antimetabolites:** azathioprine 1-3 mg/kg/day, methotrexate 0.15 mg/kg/day, mycophenolate mofetil 1 gm po qd ("off-label" use for autoimmune ocular inflammatory diseases).
     - **Alkylating agents:** cyclophosphamide 1-3 mg/kg/day, chlorambucil 0.1 mg/kg/day.
     - **Adjuvants:** colchicine 0.6 mg po bid for Behçet's disease is controversial.
     - **Other agents:** cyclosporine 2.5-5.0 mg/kg/day, FK506 (tacrolimus [Prograf]) 0.1-0.15 mg/kg/day, dapsone 25-50 mg bid or tid.
- Lens extraction for phacoanaphylactic endophthalmitis.

Prognosis

Depends on etiology; most are benign. Poor if sequelae of chronic inflammation exist including cataract, glaucoma, posterior synechiae, band keratopathy, iris atrophy, cystoid macular edema, retinal detachment, retinal vasculitis, optic neuritis, neovascularization, hypotony, phthisis.

Uveitis-Glaucoma-Hyphema Syndrome

Definition

Triad of findings found in patients with closed-loop and rigid anterior chamber, iris-supported, or loose sulcus IOLs secondary to trauma to angle structures, iris, or ciliary body.

Symptoms

Pain, photophobia, red eye, and decreased vision.

Signs

Decreased visual acuity, increased intraocular pressure, anterior chamber cells and flare, hyphema, IOL implant; may have corneal edema.

Differential Diagnosis

Neovascular glaucoma, trauma.

Evaluation

* Complete ophthalmic history and eye examination with attention to cornea, tonometry, anterior chamber, gonioscopy, iris, and ophthalmoscopy.

Management

* Intraocular pressure control as needed (see Chapter 11; do not use miotic agents).
* Topical steroid (prednisolone acetate 1% up to q1h then taper slowly over weeks to months) and cycloplegic agent (scopolamine 0.25% tid or atropine 1% bid).
* Usually requires surgery for IOL removal or exchange, and possibly subsequent glaucoma surgery.

Prognosis

Poor.

Chapter

7

IRIS AND PUPILS

Trauma

Definition

Angle Recession

Tear in ciliary body between longitudinal and circular muscle fibers; associated with hyphema; 10% develop glaucoma if more than two thirds of angle involved.

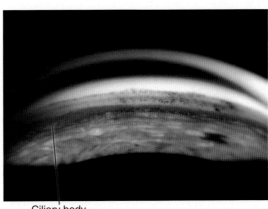

Figure 7-1 • Gonioscopic view of angle recession demonstrating deepened angle and blue-gray face of the ciliary body.

Ciliary body

Cyclodialysis

Disinsertion of ciliary body from scleral spur.

Iridodialysis

Disinsertion of iris root from ciliary body; appears as peripheral iris hole; usually related to trauma and associated with hyphema at time of injury.

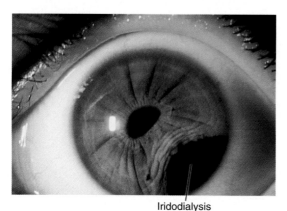

Figure 7-2 • Iridodialysis. The iris is disinserted for approximately 90 degrees (from the 3 o'clock to 6 o'clock position).

Iridodialysis

Sphincter Tears

Small radial iris tears at pupillary margin; usually due to blunt trauma; associated with hyphema at time of injury; may result in permanent pupil dilation (traumatic mydriasis).

Symptoms

Pain, photophobia, red eye, and decreased vision.

Signs

Normal or decreased visual acuity, conjunctival injection, subconjunctival hemorrhage, anterior chamber cells and flare, hyphema, unusually deep anterior chamber, iris tears, abnormal pupil, angle tears, iridodonesis; may have other signs of ocular trauma including lid or orbital trauma, dislocated lens, phacodonesis, cataract, vitreous hemorrhage, commotio retinae, retinal tear or detachment, choroidal rupture, or traumatic optic neuropathy; may have signs of glaucoma with increased intraocular pressure, optic nerve cupping, and visual field defects.

Differential Diagnosis

See above, distinguish by careful gonioscopy; also, surgical iridectomy or iridotomy, essential iris atrophy, Reiger's anomaly.

Evaluation

- Complete ophthalmic history and eye examination with attention to cornea, tonometry, iris, lens, and ophthalmoscopy.
- Check gonioscopy and employ scleral depression if globe is intact and there is no hyphema.
- B-scan ultrasonography if unable to visualize the fundus; consider ultrasound biomicroscopy to evaluate angle structures and localize the injury.
- Rule out open globe and intraocular foreign body (see Chapter 4).

Management

- **Angle recession:** Observe patients for angle-recession glaucoma.
- **Cyclodialysis:** Consider surgical or laser reattachment for persistent hypotony.
- **Iridodialysis:** Consider cosmetic contact lens or surgical repair for disabling glare or diplopia.
- **Sphincter tears:** No treatment required; consider cosmetic contact lens or surgical repair of dilated nonreactive pupil.
- May require treatment of increased intraocular pressure (see Chapter 11).
- Treat other traumatic injuries as indicated.

Prognosis

Depends on amount of damage; poor when associated with angle recession glaucoma or chronic hypotony.

Corectopia

Definition

Displaced or ectopic pupil.

Symptoms

Asymptomatic; may have decreased vision.

Signs

Normal or decreased visual acuity, distorted pupil.

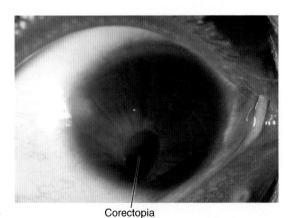

Figure 7-3 • Corectopia demonstrating inferiorly displaced pupil.

Corectopia

Differential Diagnosis

Mesodermal dysgenesis syndromes, iridocorneal endothelial syndromes, chronic uveitis, trauma, postoperative, ectopia lentis et pupillae.

Evaluation

- Complete ophthalmic history and eye examination with attention to cornea, tonometry, anterior chamber, iris, and lens.
- Rule out open globe (peaked pupil after trauma, see Chapter 4).

Management

- No treatment recommended.
- May require treatment (see Chapter 6) of iritis or increased intraocular pressure (see Chapter 11).

Prognosis

Usually benign; depends on etiology.

Seclusio Pupillae

Definition

Posterior synechiae (iris adhesions to the lens) at the pupillary border for 360 degrees. *Note:* different from occlusio pupillae, which is a fibrotic membrane across the pupil.

Symptoms

Asymptomatic; may have pain, red eye, and decreased vision.

Signs

Normal or decreased visual acuity, posterior synechiae, poor or irregular pupil dilation, increased intraocular pressure, acute or chronic signs of iritis, including anterior chamber cells and flare, keratic precipitate, iris atrophy, iris nodules, cataract, and cystoid macular edema.

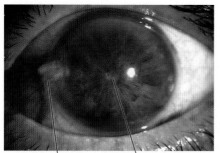

Pterygium   Seclusio pupillae

Figure 7-4 • Seclusio pupillae. The iris is completely bound down to the underlying cataractous lens visible as a white spot through the small pupil.

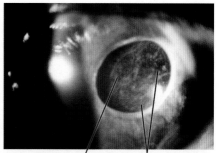

Occlusio pupillae Neovascularization

Figure 7-5 • Occlusio pupillae with thin, white, fibrotic membrane and neovascularization covering the pupil.

Differential Diagnosis

As for anterior uveitis (see Chapter 6).

Evaluation

- Complete ophthalmic history and eye examination with attention to cornea, tonometry, anterior chamber, gonioscopy, iris, and ophthalmoscopy.
- Consider anterior uveitis workup (see Chapter 6).

Management

- Treat active uveitis and angle-closure glaucoma (see Chapter 6) if present.
- Consider laser iridotomy to prevent angle-closure glaucoma.

Prognosis

Depends on etiology; poor if glaucoma has developed.

Peripheral Anterior Synechiae (PAS)

Definition

Peripheral adhesions of iris to the cornea or angle structures; extensive PAS (>60% angle involvement) can cause increased intraocular pressure and angle-closure glaucoma.

Etiology

Peripheral iridocorneal apposition due to previous pupillary block, flat or shallow anterior chamber, or inflammation.

Symptoms

Asymptomatic; may have symptoms of angle-closure glaucoma (see Chapter 6).

Signs

Iris adhesions to Schwalbe's line and cornea; may have increased intraocular pressure.

Angle neovascularization

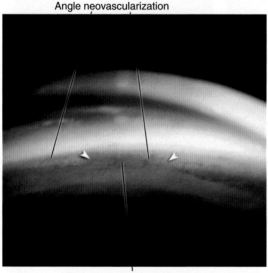

Peripheral anterior synechiae

Figure 7-6 • Peripheral anterior synechiae demonstrating a broad band of iris occluding the angle structures (area between *arrowheads*) as viewed with gonioscopy; also note that this patient has rubeosis with fine neovascularization.

Differential Diagnosis

See above; any cause of angle-closure glaucoma (see Chapter 6).

Evaluation

Complete ophthalmic history and eye examination with attention to cornea, tonometry, anterior chamber, gonioscopy, iris, and ophthalmoscopy.

Management

- May require treatment of increased intraocular pressure (see Chapter 11) or angle-closure glaucoma (see Chapter 6).
- Consider goniosynechiolysis for recent PAS (<12 months).

Prognosis

Usually good; depends on extent of synechial angle closure and intraocular pressure control.

Rubeosis Iridis

Definition

Neovascularization of the iris and angle.

Etiology

Ocular ischemia; most commonly seen with proliferative diabetic retinopathy, central retinal vein occlusion, and carotid occlusive disease; also associated with anterior segment ischemia, chronic retinal detachment, tumors, sickle cell retinopathy, chronic inflammation, and other rarer causes.

Symptoms

Asymptomatic; may have decreased vision or angle-closure symptoms (see Chapter 6).

Signs

Normal or decreased visual acuity, abnormal blood vessels on iris and angle, particularly at pupillary margin and around iridectomies; may have spontaneous hyphema, or retinal lesions; may have signs of angle-closure or neovascular glaucoma with increased intraocular pressure, optic nerve cupping, and visual field defects.

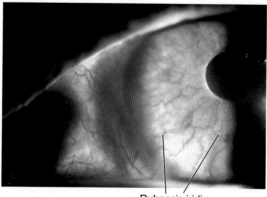

Figure 7-7 • Rubeosis iridis demonstrating florid neovascularization of the iris with large branching vessels.

Rubeosis iridis

Differential Diagnosis

See above.

Evaluation

- Complete ophthalmic history and eye examination with attention to tonometry, gonioscopy, iris, and ophthalmoscopy.
- Consider fluorescein angiogram to narrow differential diagnosis and determine cause of ocular ischemia if not apparent on direct examination.
- Consider medical consultation for systemic diseases including duplex and Doppler scans of carotid arteries to rule out carotid occlusive disease.

Management

- Topical steroid (prednisolone acetate 1% qid) and cycloplegic agent (atropine 1% bid) for inflammation.
- Usually requires laser photocoagulation for retinal ischemia if cornea clear; if cornea cloudy may require peripheral cryotherapy.
- Observe for neovascular glaucoma by monitoring intraocular pressure.
- May require treatment of increased intraocular pressure (see Chapter 11) and neovascular glaucoma (see below).

Prognosis

Poor; the rubeotic vessels may regress with appropriate therapy, but most causes of neovascularization are chronic progressive diseases.

Neovascular Glaucoma

Definition

A form of secondary angle-closure glaucoma in which neovascularization of the iris and angle causes occlusion of the trabecular meshwork.

Etiology

Any cause of rubeosis iridis (see above).

Symptoms

Decreased vision and angle-closure symptoms (see Chapter 6).

Signs

Decreased visual acuity; abnormal blood vessels on iris and angle, particularly at pupillary margin and around iridectomies; increased intraocular pressure, optic nerve cupping, and visual field defects; may have corneal edema, spontaneous hyphema, or retinal lesions.

Differential Diagnosis

As for Rubeosis Iridis (see above).

Evaluation

- Complete ophthalmic history and eye examination with attention to cornea, tonometry, anterior chamber, gonioscopy, iris, and ophthalmoscopy.
- Consider fluorescein angiography to narrow differential diagnosis and determine cause of ocular ischemia if not apparent on direct examination.
- Consider medical consultation for systemic diseases, including duplex and Doppler scans of carotid arteries to rule out carotid occlusive disease.

Management

- Topical steroid (prednisolone acetate 1% qid) and cycloplegic agent (atropine 1% bid) for inflammation.
- Choice and order of topical glaucoma medications depend on many factors, including patient's age, intraocular pressure level and control, and amount and progression of optic nerve cupping and visual field defects. Treatment options are presented in the Primary Open-Angle Glaucoma section (see Chapter 11); more resistant to treatment than primary open-angle glaucoma.
- Usually requires laser photocoagulation for retinal ischemia if cornea clear; if cornea cloudy may require peripheral cryotherapy.
- Neovascular glaucoma with elevated intraocular pressure despite maximal medical therapy may require glaucoma filtering surgery, a glaucoma drainage implant, or a cyclodestructive procedure.

Prognosis

Poor; the rubeotic vessels may regress with appropriate therapy, but most causes of neovascularization are chronic progressive diseases.

Pigment Dispersion Syndrome

Definition

Liberation of pigment from the iris with subsequent accumulation on anterior segment structures.

Etiology

Chafing of posterior iris surface on zonules produces pigment dispersion.

Epidemiology

More common in 20- to 50-year-old white men and in patients with myopia; affected women are usually older; associated with lattice degeneration in 20% of cases and retinal detachment in up to 5% of cases; 25-50% develop pigmentary glaucoma. Mapped to chromosome 7q35-q36 (*GLC1F* gene).

Symptoms

Asymptomatic.

Signs

Radial, midperipheral, iris transillumination defects, pigment on corneal endothelium (Krukenberg spindle), posterior bowing of midperipheral iris, dark pigment band overlying trabecular meshwork, pigment in iris furrows and on anterior lens capsule; may have signs of glaucoma with increased intraocular pressure, optic nerve cupping, and visual field defects (see below); may have pigmented anterior chamber cells, especially following pupil dilation.

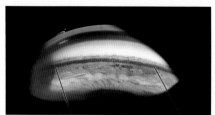

Pigment on TM   Pigment deposition

Figure 7-8 • Pigment dispersion syndrome demonstrating pigment deposition on the trabecular meshwork that appears as a dark brown band when viewed with gonioscopy.

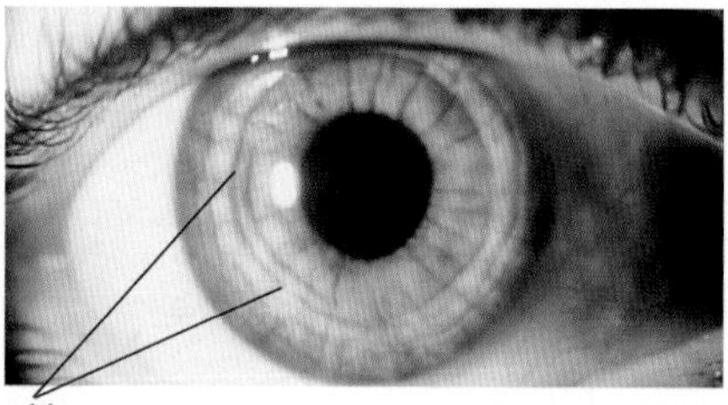

Figure 7-9 • Pigment dispersion syndrome demonstrating pigment deposition in concentric rings on the iris surface.

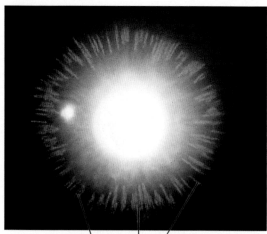

Transillumination defects

Figure 7-10 • Pigment dispersion syndrome demonstrating radial, midperipheral, slit-like iris transillumination defects for 360 degrees.

Differential Diagnosis

Uveitis, albinism, pseudoexfoliation syndrome, iris atrophy.

Evaluation

- Complete ophthalmic history and eye examination, with attention to cornea, tonometry, anterior chamber, the pattern of iris transillumination, gonioscopy, lens, and ophthalmoscopy.
- Check visual fields in patients with elevated intraocular pressure or optic nerve cupping to rule out glaucoma.

Management

- Observe for pigmentary glaucoma by monitoring intraocular pressure.
- May require treatment of increased intraocular pressure (see Chapter 11).

Prognosis

Usually good; poor if pigmentary glaucoma develops.

Pigmentary Glaucoma

Definition

A form of secondary open-angle glaucoma caused by pigment liberated from the posterior iris surface (i.e., a sequela of uncontrolled increased intraocular pressure in pigment dispersion syndrome).

Epidemiology

Develops in 25% to 50% of patients with pigment dispersion syndrome; same associations as in pigment dispersion syndrome (see above). Mapped to chromosome 7q35-q36 (*GLC1F* gene).

Mechanism

Obstruction of the trabecular meshwork by dispersed pigment and pigment-laden macrophages.

Symptoms

Asymptomatic; may have decreased vision or constricted visual fields in late stages; exercise or pupil dilation can cause pigment release with acute elevation of intraocular pressure and symptoms including halos around lights and blurred vision.

Signs

Normal or decreased visual acuity, large fluctuations in intraocular pressure (especially with exercise); similar ocular signs as in pigment dispersion syndrome (see above), optic nerve cupping, nerve fiber layer defects, and visual field defects.

Differential Diagnosis

Primary open-angle glaucoma, other forms of secondary open-angle glaucoma.

Evaluation

* Complete ophthalmic history and eye examination with attention to cornea, tonometry, anterior chamber, gonioscopy, iris, lens, and ophthalmoscopy.
* Check visual fields.
* Stereo-optic nerve photos are useful for comparison at subsequent evaluations.

Management

* Choice and order of topical glaucoma medications depend on many factors, including patient's age, intraocular pressure level and control, and amount and progression of optic nerve cupping and visual field defects. Treatment options are presented in the Primary Open-Angle Glaucoma section (see Chapter 11).
* Consider initial treatment with pilocarpine 1-4% qid to minimize iris contact with lens zonules.
* Laser trabeculoplasty is effective, but action may be short lived.
* If posterior bowing of the iris exists, then consider laser peripheral iridotomy to alter iris configuration and minimize pigment liberation.
* May require glaucoma filtering surgery if medical treatment fails.

Prognosis

Poorer than primary open-angle glaucoma.

Iris Heterochromia

Definition

Heterochromia Iridis

Unilateral; single iris with two colors (iris bicolor).

Heterochromia Iridum

Bilateral; irises are different colors (e.g., one blue, one brown).

Etiology

Congenital

Hypochromic (involved eye lighter)   Congenital Horner's syndrome, Waardenburg's syndrome, Hirschsprung's disease, Perry-Romberg hemifacial atrophy.

Hyperchromic (involved eye darker)   Ocular or oculodermal melanocytosis, iris pigment epithelium hamartoma.

Acquired

Hypochromic   Acquired Horner's syndrome, juvenile xanthogranuloma, metastatic carcinoma, Fuchs' heterochromic iridocyclitis, stromal atrophy (glaucoma or inflammation).

Hyperchromic   Siderosis, hemosiderosis, chalcosis, medication (topical prostaglandin analogues for glaucoma), iris nevus or melanoma, iridocorneal endothelial syndrome, iris neovascularization.

Symptoms

Usually asymptomatic; depends on etiology.

Signs

Iris heterochromia; blepharoptosis, miosis, and anhidrosis in Horner's syndrome; white forelock, premature graying, leucism (cutaneous hypopigmentation), facial anomalies, dystopia canthorum, and deafness in Waardenburg's syndrome; skin, scleral, and choroidal pigmentation in ocular or oculodermal melanocytosis; anterior chamber cells and flare, keratic precipitates, and increased intraocular pressure in uveitis, siderosis, and chalcosis; may have intraocular foreign body (siderosis, chalcosis), old hemorrhage (hemosiderosis), or tumor.

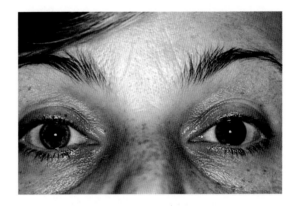

Figure 7-11 • Heterochromia iridum. The patient's right iris is blue and the left iris is hazel.

Differential Diagnosis

See above.

Evaluation

• Complete ophthalmic history and eye examination with attention to cornea, tonometry, anterior chamber, gonioscopy, iris, and ophthalmoscopy.
• Consider B-scan ultrasonography if unable to visualize the fundus.

- Consider orbital computed tomography (CT) or radiographs to rule out intraocular foreign bodies.
- Consider electroretinogram (ERG) to evaluate retinal function in siderosis, hemosiderosis, and chalcosis.
- Consider medical consultation.

Management

- Most forms do not require treatment.
- May require treatment of active uveitis (see Chapter 6), increased intraocular pressure (see Chapter 11), or malignancy (see Tumor section).
- Intraocular foreign body may require surgical removal.

Prognosis

Depends on etiology.

Anisocoria

Definition

Inequality in the size of the pupils.

Etiology

Greater Anisocoria in Dark (Abnormal Pupil is Smaller)

Horner's syndrome, Argyll Robertson pupil, iritis, pharmacologic (miotic agent, narcotic, insecticide).

Greater Anisocoria in Light (Abnormal Pupil is Larger)

Adie's tonic pupil, cranial nerve III palsy, Hutchinson's pupil (uncal herniation with cranial nerve III entrapment in a comatose patient), pharmacologic (mydriatic agent, cycloplegic agent, cocaine), iris damage (traumatic, ischemic, or surgical).

Anisocoria Equal in Light and Dark

Physiologic (difference in pupil size ≤1 mm).

Epidemiology

Up to 20% of population has physiologic anisocoria.

Symptoms

Asymptomatic; may have glare, pain, photophobia, diplopia, or blurred vision, depending on etiology.

Signs

Involved pupil may be larger or smaller, round or irregular, reactive or nonreactive; may have other signs depending on etiology.

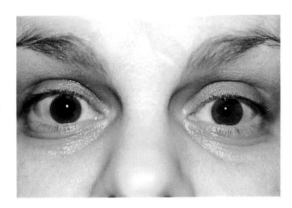

Figure 7-12 • Anisocoria demonstrating larger pupil of the right eye.

Evaluation

- Complete ophthalmic history and eye examination with attention to pupils (size in light and dark, pupil response to light and near), lids, motility, and iris.
- Gonioscopy and tonometry in traumatic cases to assess associated angle structure damage.
- **Greater anisocoria in dark (abnormal pupil is smaller):** Pharmacologic pupil testing (*Note:* testing must be performed before cornea has been manipulated; i.e., before any drops, applanation, or other tests have been performed; otherwise the test will be invalid):

    (1) Topical cocaine 4-10% in each eye: after 40 minutes equal dilation = simple anisocoria; still asymmetric = Horner's syndrome (see below).
    (2) Topical hydroxyamphetamine 1% (Paredrine): equal dilation = central or preganglionic Horner's syndrome; still asymmetric = postganglionic Horner's syndrome.
    Note: tests cannot be performed on the same day or will be invalid.

- **Greater anisocoria in light (abnormal pupil is larger):** Pharmacologic pupil testing:

    (1) Topical pilocarpine 0.1% or methacholine 2.5%: constricts = Adie's tonic pupil (see below); no constriction = go to #2.
    (2) Topical pilocarpine 1%: constricts = cranial nerve III palsy; no constriction = pharmacologic dilation.

- **Lab tests:** Venereal Disease Research Laboratory (VDRL) test, fluorescent treponemal antibody absorption (FTA-ABS) test (Argyll Robertson).
- Lumbar puncture for VDRL, FTA-ABS, total protein, and cell counts to rule out neurosyphilis (Argyll Robertson).
- Consider head, neck, or chest CT scan or magnetic resonance imaging (MRI) to rule out masses and vascular anomalies.

Management

- May require treatment of underlying cause.
- Consider iris repair in traumatic cases.

Prognosis

Often benign; depends on etiology.

Adie's Tonic Pupil

Definition

Idiopathic, benign form of internal ophthalmoplegia due to lesion in ciliary ganglion or short posterior ciliary nerves with aberrant regeneration of ciliary muscle fibers to iris sphincter.

Etiology

Denervation hypersensitivity due to dysfunction of the ciliary ganglion or its neurons.

Epidemiology

Usually occurs in 20- to 40-year-old women (90%); 80% unilateral (may become bilateral over time).

Symptoms

Asymptomatic; may have blurred near vision and photophobia.

Signs

Anisocoria greater in light than dark, dilated pupil with poor light response, segmental palsy with vermiform movements, slow or tonic near response (constriction and redilation), poor accommodation, light-near dissociation; 70% have decreased deep tendon reflexes (Adie's syndrome).

Differential Diagnosis

Sarcoidosis, iris ischemia, diabetes mellitus, botulism, and any cause of light-near dissociation (unilateral total afferent visual loss, Argyll Robertson pupil, dorsal midbrain syndrome, aberrant regeneration of cranial nerve III, diabetes mellitus, amyloidosis).

Evaluation

- Complete ophthalmic history, neurologic examination, and eye examination with attention to pupils (size in light and dark, pupil response to light and near), iris, and deep tendon reflexes.

Pharmacologic testing with topical pilocarpine 0.1% or methacholine 2.5% (see Anisocoria section); Adie's tonic pupil constricts (normal does not) due to cholinergic supersensitivity; false-positive test result may occur in cranial nerve III palsy. (If recent onset, no response to dilute pilocarpine may be seen.)

Management

- No treatment recommended.

Prognosis

Good; accommodative paresis is usually temporary (months).

Argyll Robertson Pupil

Definition

Small, irregular pupil that reacts briskly to near (accommodation), but not to light; usually bilateral and asymmetric; associated with tertiary syphilis.

Symptoms

Asymptomatic.

Signs

Miotic, irregular pupil, normal near response, absent reaction to light (light-near dissociation), poor dilation; may have stigmata of congenital syphilis (e.g., Hutchinson's triad, fundus changes, skeletal deformities).

Differential Diagnosis

Argyll Robertson–like pupils seen in diabetes mellitus, alcoholism, multiple sclerosis, sarcoidosis.

Evaluation

- Complete ophthalmic history, neurologic examination, and eye examination with attention to pupils, iris, and ophthalmoscopy.
- **Lab tests:** VDRL, FTA-ABS.
- Lumbar puncture for VDRL, FTA-ABS, total protein, and cell counts to rule out neurosyphilis.
- Medical consultation.

Management

- If neurosyphilis present, treat with systemic penicillin G (2.4 million U IV q4h for 10-14 days, then 2.4 million U IM q week for 3 weeks); or tetracycline for penicillin-allergic patients.
- Follow serum VDRL to monitor treatment efficacy.

Prognosis

Pupil abnormality itself is benign; poor for untreated tertiary syphilis.

Horner's Syndrome

Definition

Group of findings seen in oculosympathetic paresis. Sympathetic damage may occur anywhere along the three-neuron pathway:

Central

Hypothalamus to ciliospinal center of Budge (C8-T2).

Preganglionic

Spinal cord to superior cervical ganglion.

Postganglionic

Along carotid artery to cranial nerve V and VI to orbit and finally to iris dilator muscle.

Etiology

Failure of sympathetic nervous system to dilate affected pupil and to stimulate Müller's muscle in the lid.

Central

Cerebrovascular accident, neck trauma, tumor, demyelinating disease (rarely causes isolated Horner's syndrome).

Preganglionic

Pancoast's tumor, mediastinal mass, cervical rib, neck trauma, abscess, thyroid tumor, after thyroid or neck surgery.

Postganglionic

Neck lesion, head trauma, migraine, cavernous sinus lesion, carotid dissection, carotid-cavernous fistula, internal carotid artery aneurysm, nasopharyngeal carcinoma, vascular disease, infections (complicated otitis media). Congenital Horner's syndrome usually due to birth trauma (brachial plexus injury during delivery).

Symptoms

Asymptomatic; may have droopy eyelid, blurred vision, pain (especially with vascular postganglionic etiologies), and other symptoms depending on site and cause of lesion (central usually has other neurologic deficits). Initially ipsilateral nasal stuffiness may occur.

Signs

Triad of mild (1-2 mm) ptosis, miosis, and anhidrosis (anhidrosis usually indicates preganglionic lesion); abnormal pupil is smaller and dilates poorly in the dark; upside-down ptosis (lower lid elevation); in congenital or longstanding cases heterochromia iridum (iris on involved side is lighter). Initially, ipsilateral conjunctival hyperemia or reduced intraocular pressure may occur.

Evaluation

- Complete ophthalmic history, neurologic examination, and eye examination, with attention to lids, motility, pupils, and iris.
- **Pharmacologic pupil testing** (*Note:* testing must be performed before cornea has been manipulated; i.e., before any drops, applanation, or other tests have been performed; otherwise the test result will be invalid):

  (1) Topical cocaine 4-10% (place 2 drops in each eye, remeasure pupil after 30 minutes): determines presence of Horner's syndrome (normal pupil dilates; pupil does not dilate as well in patient with Horner's syndrome).
  (2) Topical hydroxyamphetamine 1% (Paredrine): distinguishes between preganglionic (first-order and second-order neurons) and postganglionic (third-order neuron) lesions (central or preganglionic pupil in patient with Horner's syndrome dilates equal to normal pupil; in postganglionic Horner's syndrome pupil does not dilate as well); this test does not determine whether a preganglionic lesion affects the first-order or second-order neuron.

  Note: tests cannot be performed on the same day or will be invalid.

- A young child with Horner's syndrome needs to be evaluated for neuroblastoma with an MRI of sympathetic chain from abdomen to neck, along with checking urine for vanillylmandelic acid and homovanillic acid.
- Horner's syndrome associated with neck pain, shoulder pain, or abnormal taste in the mouth should have an axial MRI of the neck to rule out carotid dissection.
- Smokers should have a chest radiograph to rule out Pancoast tumor.

Management

- Treat underlying cause.
- Consider ptosis repair.

Prognosis

Depends on etiology; postganglionic lesions are usually benign; preganglionic and central lesions are usually more serious.

Relative Afferent Pupillary Defect
▉ (RAPD, Marcus Gunn Pupil)

Definition

Dilation of one pupil in response to light, due to difference in amount of light perceived by the two eyes when swinging flashlight test is performed.

Etiology

Asymmetric optic nerve disease or widespread retinal damage. Most common causes include optic neuropathy, optic neuritis, central retinal vein or artery occlusion, and retinal detachment. Mild relative afferent pupillary defect (RAPD) may rarely be seen with a dense ocular media opacity, including vitreous hemorrhage and cataract; very rarely seen with amblyopia; optic tract lesions can cause a contralateral RAPD (due to more nasal crossing fibers in the chiasm).

Symptoms

Decreased vision, color vision, contrast sensitivity.

Signs

Positive RAPD, decreased visual acuity, visual field defect; may have decreased color vision, swollen or pale optic nerve, or retinal findings.

Differential Diagnosis

See above.

Evaluation

- Complete ophthalmic history and eye examination with attention to visual acuity, color vision, pupils, iris, and ophthalmoscopy.
- **Swinging flashlight test:** Bright light is shined into one eye and then rapidly into the other in an alternating fashion; positive test result is when the pupil that the light is shined into dilates instead of constricts; when the pupil of the involved eye is nonreactive or nonfunctional, observe the fellow, normal eye for a reverse afferent defect (dilation when light is on nonreactive eye, constriction when light is shined on reactive eye).
- Grading system with neutral density filters or 1^+ to 4^+ scale.

Management

- Treat underlying cause.

Prognosis

Depends on etiology.

Leukocoria

Definition

Variety of disorders that cause the pupil to appear white; usually noted in infancy or early childhood.

Symptoms

Decreased vision, white pupil; may notice eye turn or abnormal size of eye.

Signs

Decreased visual acuity, leukocoria; may have positive RAPD, nystagmus, strabismus, buphthalmos, microphthalmos, anterior chamber cells and flare, increased intraocular pressure, cataract, vitritis, retinal detachment, tumor, or other retinal findings; may have systemic findings.

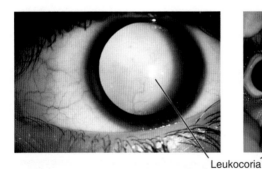

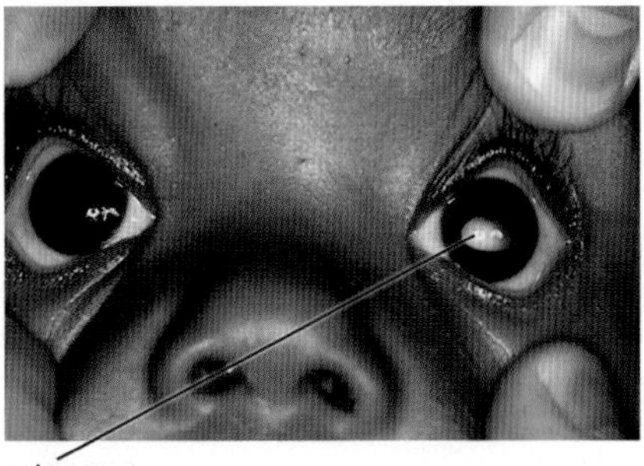

Leukocoria

Figure 7-13 • Leukocoria in a patient with toxocariasis. The large white reflex in the dilated pupil represents the retina; a retinal vessel is visible.

Figure 7-14 • Leukocoria due to retinoblastoma in the left eye. The white pupil in the left eye is strikingly evident in comparison with the normal (black) pupil of the fellow eye.

Differential Diagnosis

Cataract, retinoblastoma, retinopathy of prematurity, persistent hyperplastic primary vitreous, Coats' disease, toxocariasis, toxoplasmosis, coloboma, myelinated nerve fibers, Norrie's disease, retinal dysplasia, cyclitic membrane, retinal detachment, incontinentia pigmenti, retinoschisis, and medulloepithelioma.

Evaluation

• Complete ophthalmic history and eye examination, with attention to retinoscopy, pupils, tonometry, anterior chamber, lens, vitreous cells, and ophthalmoscopy.
• B-scan ultrasonography to evaluate retrolenticular area, vitreous, and retina if unable to visualize the fundus.
• Consider orbital radiograph, and head and orbital CT scans or MRI to rule out foreign body.
• Pediatric consultation.

Management

• Treat underlying cause.

Prognosis

Usually poor, unless due to mature cataract in an adult.

Congenital Anomalies

Aniridia

Absence of iris, except for small, hypoplastic remnant or stump; patients also have photophobia, nystagmus, glare, decreased visual acuity, amblyopia, and strabismus; associated with glaucoma in 28-50%, lens opacities in 50-85%, corneal pannus, and foveal hypoplasia; seen in 1:100,000 births; mapped to chromosome 11p; three forms:

AN 1 (autosomal dominant [AD])   Eighty-five percent of cases; only ocular findings.

AN 2   Thirteen percent of cases; includes Miller's syndrome with both aniridia and Wilms' tumor, and WAGR (Wilms' tumor, aniridia, genitourinary abnormalities, and mental retardation); sporadic, but mapped to chromosome 11p (*PAX6* gene).

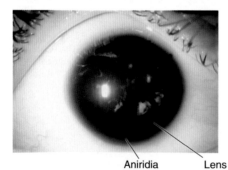
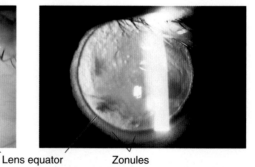

Aniridia   Lens equator   Zonules

Figure 7-15 • Aniridia with entire cataractous lens visible. The inferior edge of the lens is visible.

Figure 7-16 • Aniridia with the lens equator and zonules visible on retroillumination.

AN 3 (autosomal recessive [AR])   Two percent of cases; associated with mental retardation and cerebellar ataxia (Gillespie's syndrome); do not develop Wilms' tumor.

- May require treatment of increased intraocular pressure (see Chapter 11).
- May require cyclocryotherapy or glaucoma filtering surgery if medical treatment fails.
- Lensectomy if visually significant cataract develops; consider use of artificial iris segments.
- Consider painted contact lens to decrease photophobia or glare.

Coloboma

Iris sector defect due to failure of embryonic fissure to close completely; usually seen inferiorly; may have other colobomata (lid, lens, retina, choroid, optic nerve); associated with multiple genetic syndromes, including trisomy 22 (cat-eye syndrome), trisomy 18, trisomy 13, and chromosome 18 deletion.

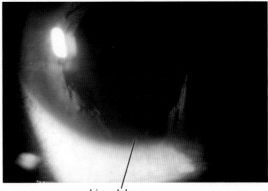

Figure 7-17 • Coloboma of inferior iris.

Iris coloboma

Persistent Pupillary Membrane

Benign, embryonic, mesodermal remnants (tunica vasculosa lentis) that appear as thin iris strands bridging the pupil; most common ocular congenital anomaly; occurs in 80% of dark eyes and 35% of light eyes; two types:

Type 1   Attached only to the iris.

Type 2   Iridolenticular adhesions.

- No treatment required.
- If iris strands cross visual axis and are affecting vision, consider Nd:YAG (neodymium: yttrium-aluminum-garnet) laser treatment.

Plateau Iris (Configuration or Syndrome)

Atypical iris configuration (flat contour with steep insertion due to anteriorly rotated ciliary processes; anterior chamber is deep centrally and shallow peripherally); familial, more

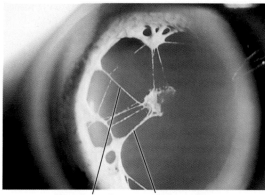

Figure 7-18 • Persistent pupillary membrane type 2 demonstrating multiple iris strands adhering to the anterior lens surface.

Type 2 persistent pupillary membrane

common in young, myopic women; 5-8% develop angle-closure glaucoma (plateau iris syndrome) (see Chapter 6).

• May require treatment of increased intraocular pressure (see Chapter 11).
• Consider miotic agents (pilocarpine 1% qid) or iridoplasty.

Mesodermal Dysgenesis Syndromes

Definition

Group of bilateral, congenital, hereditary disorders involving anterior segment structures. Originally thought to be due to faulty cleavage of angle structures and, therefore, termed *angle cleavage syndromes.*

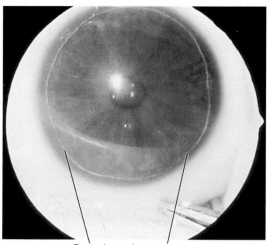

Figure 7-19 • Posterior embryotoxon can be clearly seen as a white ring in the peripheral cornea.

Posterior embryotoxon

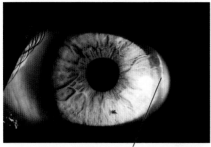

Posterior embryotoxon

Figure 7-20 • Axenfeld's anomaly with abnormal iris (extensive stromal atrophy) and posterior embryotoxon.

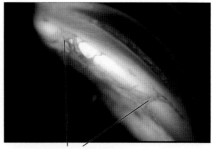

Iris processes

Figure 7-21 • Gonioscopy view of Axenfeld's anomaly demonstrating iris adhesions to the cornea.

Axenfeld's Anomaly (AD)

Posterior embryotoxon (anteriorly displaced Schwalbe's line that appears as a prominent, white, corneal line inside the limbus); found in 15% of normal individuals) and prominent iris processes; associated with secondary glaucoma in 50% of patients; mapped to chromosome 4q25 (*PITX2* gene), 6p25 (*FOXC1* gene), 13q14 (*RIEG2* gene).

Alagille's Syndrome

Axenfeld's anomaly and pigmentary retinopathy, corectopia, esotropia, and systemic abnormalities, including absent deep tendon reflexes, abnormal facies, pulmonic valvar stenosis, peripheral arterial stenosis, and skeletal abnormalities. Abnormal electroretinogram and electro-oculogram; mapped to chromosome 20p12, mutation in the *JAG1* gene, a NOTCH receptor ligand.

Rieger's Anomaly

Axenfeld's anomaly and iris hypoplasia with holes; associated with secondary glaucoma in 50% of patients; mapped to chromosome 4q25 (*PITX2* gene), 6p25 (*FOXC1* gene), 13q14 (*RIEG2* gene).

Rieger's Syndrome (AD)

Combination of Rieger's anomaly with mental retardation and systemic abnormalities, including dental, craniofacial, genitourinary, and skeletal problems; mapped to chromosome 4q25 (*PITX2* gene), 6p25 (*FOXC1* gene), 13q14 (*RIEG2* gene).

Peters' Anomaly

Corneal leukoma (due to central defect in Descemet's membrane and absence of endothelium) and iris adhesions with or without cataract; usually sporadic; 80% bilateral; associated with secondary glaucoma in 50% of patients, congenital cardiac defects, cleft lip or palate, craniofacial dysplasia, and skeletal abnormalities; mapped to chromosome 11p (*PAX6* gene).

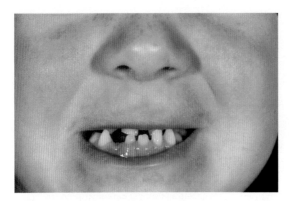

Figure 7-22 • Dental abnormalities in patient with Rieger's syndrome.

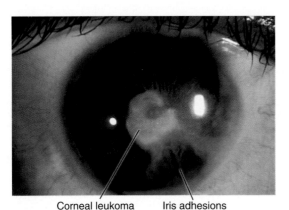

Figure 7-23 • Peters' anomaly demonstrating central, white, corneal opacity (leukoma).

Corneal leukoma   Iris adhesions

Symptoms

Asymptomatic; may have decreased vision or iris abnormalities or a white spot on eye.

Signs

Normal or decreased visual acuity; may have systemic abnormalities and signs of glaucoma, including increased intraocular pressure, optic nerve cupping, and visual field defects.

Differential Diagnosis

Iridocorneal endothelial syndromes, posterior polymorphous dystrophy, aniridia, coloboma, ectopia lentis et pupillae.

Evaluation

• Complete ophthalmic history and eye examination with attention to cornea, tonometry, anterior chamber, gonioscopy, iris, lens, and ophthalmoscopy.

- Check visual fields in patients with elevated intraocular pressure or optic nerve cupping to rule out glaucoma.
- B-scan ultrasonography in Peters' anomaly if unable to visualize the fundus.

Management

- Often no treatment necessary.
- May require treatment of increased intraocular pressure (see Chapter 11).
- May require penetrating keratoplasty, cataract extraction, and treatment of amblyopia for Peter's anomaly.

Prognosis

Poor for Peters' anomaly or when associated with glaucoma; otherwise fair.

Iridocorneal Endothelial (ICE) Syndromes

Definition

Unilateral, nonhereditary, slowly progressive abnormality of the corneal endothelium causing a spectrum of diseases with features including corneal edema, iris distortion, and secondary angle-closure glaucoma.

Essential Iris Atrophy (Progressive Iris Atrophy)

Iris atrophy with holes and corectopia, ectropion uveae, and focal stromal effacement.

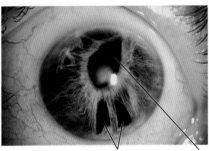

Iris atrophy   Corectopia   Iris atrophy

Figure 7-24 • Essential iris atrophy demonstrating iris atrophy and corectopia.

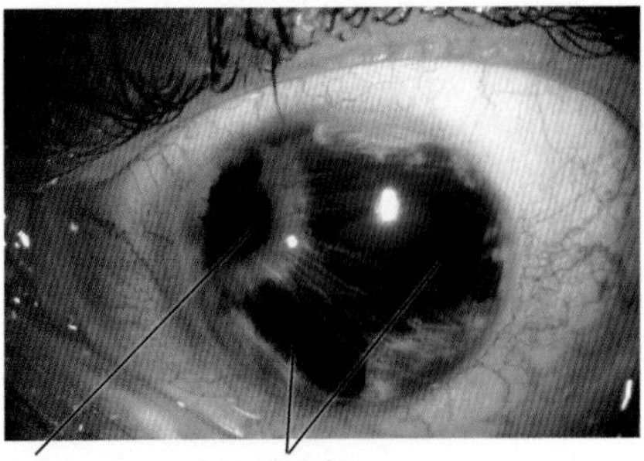

Figure 7-25 • Advanced essential iris atrophy demonstrating marked pupil displacement nasally and extreme atrophy with frank iris holes.

Chandler's Syndrome

Variant of essential iris atrophy with mild or no iris changes, corneal edema common, intraocular pressure may not be elevated.

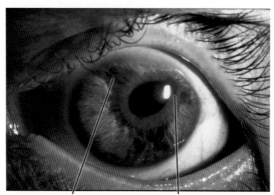

Figure 7-26 • Chandler's syndrome with mild corectopia and moderate iris atrophy.

Iris atrophy　　　Corectopia

Iris Nevus (Cogan-Reese) Syndrome

Pigmented iris nodules, flattening of iris stroma, pupil abnormalities, and ectropion uveae.

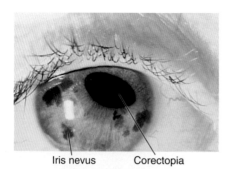

Iris nevus　　Corectopia

Figure 7-27 • Iris nevus (Cogan-Reese) syndrome demonstrating iris nevi, iris atrophy, and corectopia.

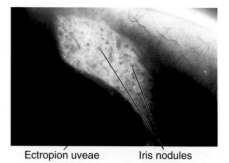

Ectropion uveae　　　Iris nodules

Figure 7-28 • Iris nevus (Cogan-Reese) syndrome with small, pigmented iris nodules and ectropion uveae.

Mechanism

Altered, abnormal corneal endothelium proliferates across the angle and onto the iris, forming a membrane that obstructs the trabecular meshwork, distorts the iris, and may form nodules by contracting around the iris stroma.

Epidemiology

Mostly young or middle-aged women; increased risk of secondary angle-closure glaucoma.

Symptoms

Asymptomatic; may have decreased vision, glare, monocular diplopia or polyopia; may notice iris changes.

Signs

Normal or decreased visual acuity, beaten metal appearance of corneal endothelium, corneal edema, increased intraocular pressure, peripheral anterior synechiae, iris changes (see above).

Differential Diagnosis

Posterior polymorphous dystrophy, mesodermal dysgenesis syndromes, Fuchs' endothelial dystrophy, iris nevi or melanoma, aniridia, iridodialysis, iridoschisis.

Evaluation

- Complete ophthalmic history and eye examination with attention to cornea, tonometry, anterior chamber, gonioscopy, iris, lens, and ophthalmoscopy.
- Check visual fields in patients with elevated intraocular pressure or optic nerve cupping to rule out glaucoma.

Management

- Often no treatment necessary.
- May require treatment of increased intraocular pressure (see Chapter 11).
- May require penetrating keratoplasty or glaucoma surgery.

Prognosis

Chronic, progressive process; poor when associated with glaucoma. Essential iris atrophy and iris nevus syndrome may have worse glaucoma than Chandler's syndrome.

Tumors

Cyst

Can be primary (more common; usually peripheral from stroma or iris pigment epithelium) or secondary (usually posttraumatic or surgical due to ingrowth of surface epithelium); may cause segmental elevation of iris and angle-closure; rarely detaches and becomes free-floating in anterior chamber; may also form at pupillary margin from long-term use of strong miotic medications; complications include distortion of pupil, occlusion of visual axis, and secondary glaucoma.

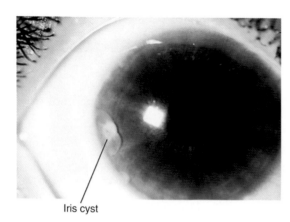

Figure 7-29 • Peripheral iris cyst seen as translucent round lesion at the iris periphery.

Iris cyst

- May require treatment of increased intraocular pressure (see Chapter 11).
- Consider surgical excision if vision is affected or secondary glaucoma exists.

Iris Nevus

Single or multiple, flat, pigmented, benign lesions; pigment spots or freckles occur in 50% of population; rare before 12 years of age; nevus differentiated from melanoma by size (<3 mm in diameter), thickness (<1 mm thick), and the absence of vascularity, ectropion uveae, secondary cataract, secondary glaucoma, and signs of growth.

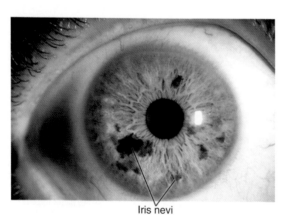

Figure 7-30 • Variably pigmented, small, flat, iris nevi are seen diffusely scattered over the anterior iris surface.

Iris nevi

- Serial anterior segment photographs to document any evidence of growth.
- Follow closely for evidence of elevation of intraocular pressure.
- Consider iris fluorescein angiogram to differentiate between nevus and melanoma: nevus has filigree filling pattern that becomes hyperfluorescent early and leaks late or is angiographically silent; melanoma has irregular vessels that fill late.

Iris Nodules

Collections of cells on iris surface; several different types:

Brushfield spots   Ring of small, white-gray, peripheral iris spots associated with Down's syndrome; occurs in 24% of normal individuals (Kunkmann Wolffian bodies).

Lisch nodules   Bilateral, lightly pigmented, gelatinous, melanocytic hamartomas seen in 92% of patients with neurofibromatosis type 1 (NF-1); very rare in NF-2; usually involve inferior half of iris; do not involve iris stroma.

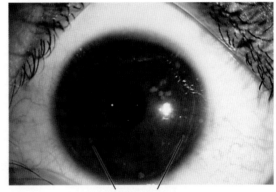

Figure 7-31 • Lisch nodules in a patient with neurofibromatosis appear as small, round, lightly colored nodules.

Lisch nodules

Inflammatory nodules   Composed of monocytes and inflammatory debris seen in granulomatous uveitis; two types:

   Busacca Nodules   Nodules on anterior iris surface.

   Koeppe Nodules   Nodules at pupillary border.

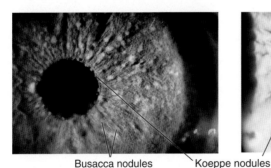

Busacca nodules   Koeppe nodules

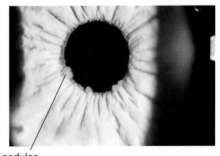

Figure 7-32 • Busacca and Koeppe nodules are small, lightly colored collections of inflammatory cells.

Figure 7-33 • Koeppe nodules.

Iris Pigment Epithelium Tumors

Very rare tumors of the iris pigment epithelium (adenoma or adenocarcinoma); appear as darkly pigmented, friable nodules.

• Treatment with chemotherapy, radiation, and surgical excision, which should be performed by a tumor specialist.

Juvenile Xanthogranuloma

Yellow iris lesions composed of histiocytes; may bleed, causing spontaneous hyphema.

Malignant Melanoma

Dark or amelanotic (pigmentation variable), elevated lesion that usually involves inferior iris and replaces the iris stroma; may be diffuse (associated with heterochromia and secondary glaucoma), tapioca (dark tapioca appearance), ring-shaped, or localized; some have feeder vessels; may involve angle structures; may cause sectoral cataract, hyphema, or secondary glaucoma; 1-3% of all malignant melanomas of the uveal tract involve the iris; predilection for whites and patients with light irides, rare in blacks; many patients have history of nevus that undergoes growth; prognosis good; 4% mortality.

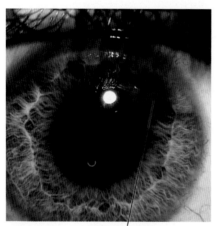

Malignant melanoma

Figure 7-34 • Malignant melanoma is seen as a hazy brown confluent patch on this blue iris.

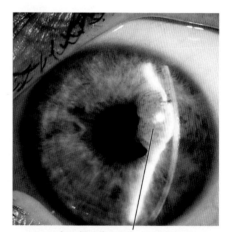

Amelanotic malignant melanoma

Figure 7-35 • Amelanotic melanoma is visible as a large, pedunculated, vascular mass with obvious elevation as depicted by the bowed appearance of the slit-beam light over the iris surface.

• Consider B-scan ultrasonography or ultrasound biomicroscopy to rule out ciliary body involvement.
• Treatment with chemotherapy, radiation, surgical excision, and enucleation; should be performed by a tumor specialist.

• May require treatment of increased intraocular pressure (see Chapter 11); glaucoma filtering surgery is not recommended.

Metastatic Tumors

Rare; usually amelanotic, and from primary carcinoma of the breast, lung, or prostate; often found after primary lesion is discovered.

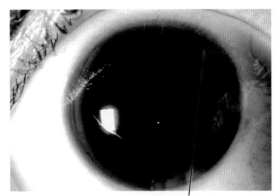

Figure 7-36 • Metastatic carcinoid appearing as an orange-brown peripheral iris lesion.

Metastatic carcinoid

• Treatment with chemotherapy, radiation, and surgical excision, which should be performed by a tumor specialist.
• May require treatment of increased intraocular pressure (see Chapter 11); glaucoma filtering surgery is not recommended.

8   *C h a p t e r*

LENS

▎ Congenital Anomalies

Definition

Coloboma

Focal inferior lens flattening due to ciliary body coloboma with focal absence of zonular support (not a true coloboma); other ocular colobomata (iris) usually exist; ciliary body tumors may cause a secondary lens "coloboma."

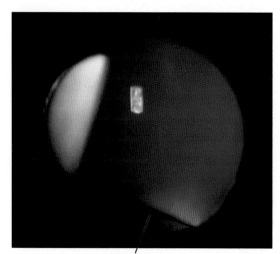

Figure 8-1 • Lens coloboma appears as inferior flattening or truncation of lens due to lack of zonular attachments when viewed with retroillumination.

Lens coloboma

256

Lenticonus

Cone-shaped lens due to bulging from a thin lens capsule; either anteriorly or posteriorly, rarely in both directions.

Anterior Usually males; bilateral; may be associated with Alport's syndrome (autosomal dominant [AD]) (basement membrane disease associated with acute hemorrhagic nephropathy, deafness, anterior lenticonus, anterior polar or cortical cataracts, and albipunctatus-like spots in the fundus).

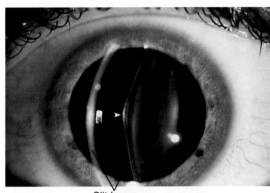

Figure 8-2 • Anterior lenticonus in a patient with Alport's syndrome; note peaked slit beam as it crosses anterior lens surface (arrowhead).

Slit-beam

Posterior More common; slight female predilection; may have associated cortical lens opacities.

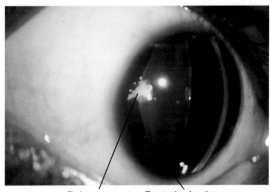

Figure 8-3 • Posterior lenticonus with polar cataract.

Polar cataract   Posterior lenticonus

Lentiglobus

Globe-shaped lens caused by bulging from thin lens capsule; rare.

Microsprerophakia

Small spheric lens; isolated anomaly or part of various syndromes (Weill-Marchesani syndrome, Lowe's syndrome).

Mittendorf Dot

A small white spot on the posterior lens capsule that represents a remnant of the posterior tunica vasculosa lentis where the former hyaloid artery attached.

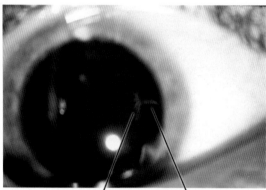

Figure 8-4 • Mittendorf dot demonstrating a small white spot on the posterior lens capsule that represents a remnant of the posterior tunica vasculosa lentis.

Mittendorf dot   Cloquet's canal

Symptoms

Asymptomatic (Mittendorf dot, coloboma); may have decreased vision (lenticonus, lentiglobus, and microspherophakia), diplopia, or angle-closure symptoms (microspherophakia).

Signs

Normal or decreased visual acuity; may have amblyopia, strabismus, nystagmus; myopia, and an "oil-droplet" fundus reflex on retroillumination in lenticonus and lentiglobus; may have dislocated lens and increased intraocular pressure in microspherophakia.

Differential Diagnosis

See above.

Evaluation

• Complete ophthalmic history and eye examination with attention to cycloplegic refraction, retinoscopy, gonioscopy, lens, and ophthalmoscopy.

Management

- Correct any refractive error.
- Patching or occlusion therapy for amblyopia (see Chapter 12).
- Microspherophakia causing pupillary block is treated with a cycloplegic agent (scopolamine 0.25% tid or atropine 1% bid); may also require laser iridotomy or lens extraction.

Prognosis

Usually good; poorer if amblyopia exists.

■ Congenital Cataract

Definition

Congenital opacity of the crystalline lens usually categorized by etiology or location.

Capsular

Opacity of the lens capsule, usually anteriorly.

Lamellar or Zonular

Central, circumscribed opacity surrounding the nucleus; "sand dollar" appearance.

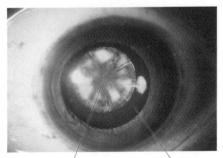

Figure 8-5 • Congenital zonular cataract.

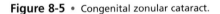

Congenital cataract   Clear lens

Lenticular or Nuclear

Opacity of the lens nucleus.

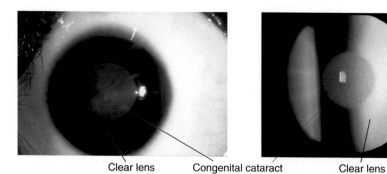

Clear lens   Congenital cataract   Clear lens

Figure 8-6 • Congenital nuclear cataract with central white discoid appearance.

Figure 8-7 • Same patient as in Fig. 8-6. Congenital nuclear cataract as viewed with retroillumination.

Polar

Central opacity located near the lens capsule, anteriorly or posteriorly.

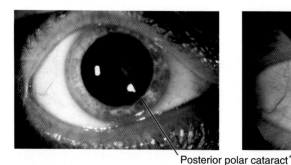
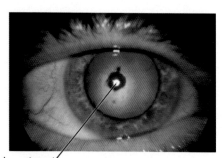

Posterior polar cataract

Figure 8-8 • Congenital posterior polar cataract.

Figure 8-9 • Same patient as Figure 8-8 demonstrating congenital polar cataract in retroillumination.

Sutural

Opacity of the Y-shaped sutures in the center of the lens.

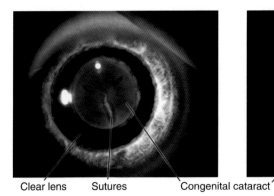 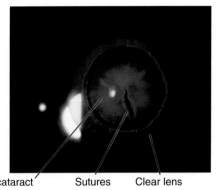

Clear lens   Sutures   Congenital cataract   Sutures   Clear lens

Figure 8-10 • Congenital cataract with prominent suture lines.

Figure 8-11 • Same patient as Figure 8-10 demonstrating congenital sutural cataract in retroillumination.

Etiology

Hereditary or Syndromes

Without chromosomal abnormalities   AD, autosomal recessive (AR), X-linked.

With chromosomal abnormalities   Down's syndrome (snowflake cataract), Turner's syndrome, and others.

Other syndromes   Craniofacial, central nervous system, skin.

Intrauterine Infections

Congenital rubella syndrome   Cataracts, glaucoma, microcornea, microphthalmos, iris hypoplasia, and retinopathy with characteristic fine, granular, salt-and-pepper appearance (most common finding); other complications include prematurity, mental retardation, neurosensory deafness, congenital heart disease, growth retardation, hepatosplenomegaly, interstitial pneumonitis, and encephalitis.

Congenital varicella syndrome   Cataract, chorioretinitis, optic nerve atrophy or hypoplasia, nystagmus, and Horner's syndrome; systemic findings include hemiparesis, bulbar palsies, dermatomal cicatricial skin lesions, developmental delay, and learning difficulties.

Metabolic

Galactosemia   Bilateral, oil-droplet cataracts from accumulation of galactose metabolites (galactitol) due to hereditary enzymatic deficiency; usually galactose-1-phosphate uridyltransferase, also galactokinase; associated with mental retardation, hepatosplenomegaly, cirrhosis, malnutrition, and failure to thrive.

Lowe's oculocerebrorenal syndrome (x-linked)   Small discoid lens, posterior lenticonus, and glaucoma; systemic findings include acidosis, aminoaciduria, renal rickets, hypotonia, mental retardation; female carriers have posterior, white, punctate cortical opacities and subcapsular, plaquelike opacities.

Also, hypoglycemia, hypocalcemia (diffuse lamellar punctate opacities), Alport's syndrome (anterior polar cataract), Fabry's disease (spokelike cataract in 25%), mannosidosis (posterior spokelike opacity).

Ocular Disorders

Persistent hyperplastic primary vitreous, Peter's anomaly, Leber's congenital amaurosis, retinopathy of prematurity, aniridia, posterior lenticonus, tumors.

Other

Birth trauma, idiopathic, and maternal drug ingestion.

Epidemiology

Congenital cataracts occur in approximately 1 of 2000 live births. Roughly one third are isolated, one third are familial (usually dominant), and one third are associated with a syndrome; most unilateral cases are not metabolic or genetic in origin.

Symptoms

Decreased vision; may notice white pupil and eye turn.

Signs

Decreased visual acuity, leukocoria, amblyopia; may have strabismus (usually with unilateral cataracts), nystagmus (usually does not appear until 2-3 months of age; rarely when cataracts develop after age 6 months).

Differential Diagnosis

See Leukocoria in Chapter 7.

Evaluation

- Complete ophthalmic history with attention to family history of eye disease, trauma, maternal illnesses during pregnancy, systemic diseases in the child, and birth problems.
- Complete eye examination with attention to cycloplegic refraction, retinoscopy, gonioscopy, lens (size and density of the opacity as viewed with retroillumination), and ophthalmoscopy.
- May require examination under anesthesia.
- Keratometry and A-scan biometry when intraocular lens (IOL) implantation is anticipated.
- **Lab tests:** TORCH titers (toxoplasmosis, other infections [syphilis], rubella, cytomegalovirus, and herpes simplex), fasting blood sugar (hypoglycemia), urine reducing substances after milk feeding (galactosemia), calcium (hypocalcemia), and urine amino acids (Lowe's syndrome).
- B-scan ultrasonography if unable to visualize the fundus (can perform through the lids of a crying child).
- Pediatric consultation.

Management

- Dilation (tropicamide 1% [Mydriacyl] with or without phenylephrine 2.5% [Mydfrin] tid) may be used as a temporary measure before surgery to allow light to pass around the cataract; however, surgery should not be delayed.
- If the cataract obscures the visual axis (media opacity >3 mm) or is causing secondary ocular disease (glaucoma or uveitis), cataract extraction should be performed within days to a week after diagnosis in infants because delay may lead to amblyopia; postoperatively, the child requires proper aphakic correction with contact lens or spectacles if bilateral; depending on age and etiology, IOL implantation should be considered.
- If the cataract is not causing amblyopia, glaucoma, or uveitis, the child is observed closely for progression.
- Patching or occlusion therapy for amblyopia (see Chapter 12).
- Almost all patients with visually significant, unilateral, congenital cataracts have strabismus and may require muscle surgery after cataract extraction.
- Restrict dietary galactose in galactosemia.

Prognosis

Depends on age and duration of visually significant cataract prior to surgery; poor if amblyopia exists.

Acquired Cataract

Definition

Lenticular opacity usually categorized by etiology or location.

Cortical Degeneration

Caused by swelling and liquefaction of the younger cortical fiber cells; various types.

Spokes and vacuoles Asymmetrically located, radial, linear opacities and punctate dots.

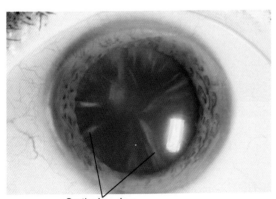

Figure 8-12 • Cortical cataract demonstrating white cortical spoking.

Cortical spokes

Mature cataract   Completely white lens; no red reflex visible from fundus.

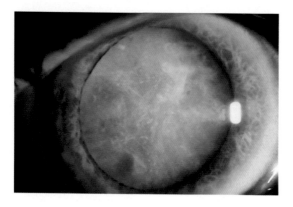

Figure 8-13 • Mature cataract with white, liquefied cortex.

Morgagnian cataract   Dense nucleus displaced inferiorly in completely liquefied, white cortex.

Hypermature cataract   After morgagnian cataract formation, the lens shrinks, the capsule wrinkles, and calcium deposits can form; proteins may leak into the anterior chamber causing phacolytic glaucoma.

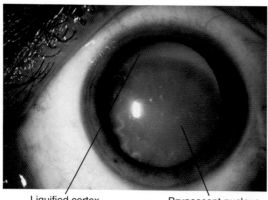

Liquified cortex   Brunescent nucleus

Figure 8-14 • Hypermature (morgagnian) cataract demonstrating a dense, brown nucleus sinking inferiorly in a white, liquefied cortex.

Nuclear Sclerosis

Centrally located lens discoloration (yellow-green or brown [brunescent]); caused by deterioration of the older fiber cells near the center of the lens.

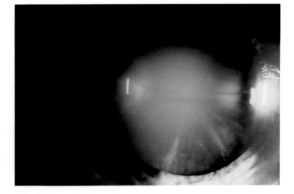

Figure 8-15 • Cataract with 2⁺ yellow-brown nuclear sclerosis.

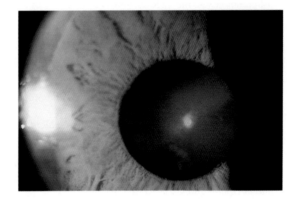

Figure 8-16 • Brunescent nuclear sclerotic cataract.

Subcapsular Cataract

Anterior subcapsular   Central fibrous plaque caused by metaplasia of the central zone lens epithelial cells beneath the anterior lens capsule. Medications can cause anterior subcapsular stellate changes; acute angle-closure attacks can cause anterior subcapsular opacities (glaukomflecken) due to lens epithelial necrosis.

Posterior subcapsular   Asymmetric granular opacities at the posterior surface of the lens; caused by posterior migration of epithelial cells and formation of bladder (Wedl) cells.

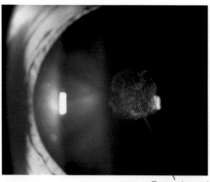

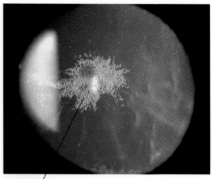

Posterior subcapsular cataract

Figure 8-17 • Posterior subcapsular cataract demonstrating typical white, hazy appearance.

Figure 8-18 • Posterior subcapsular cataract due to topical steroid use, as viewed with retroillumination.

Etiology

Most commonly senile; also secondary to a variety of causes.

Systemic Disease

Many different systemic diseases can cause cataracts, including:

Diabetes mellitus   "Sugar" cataracts are cortical or posterior subcapsular opacities that occur earlier in diabetic patients than in age-matched controls, progress rapidly, and are related to poor glucose control more than duration of disease.

Hypocalcemia   Lens opacities are usually small white dots but can aggregate into larger flakes.

Myotonic dystrophy   Central, polychromatic, iridescent, cortical crystals (Christmas tree cataract); may develop a posterior subcapsular cataract later (see Chronic Progressive External Ophthalmoplegia section in Chapter 2).

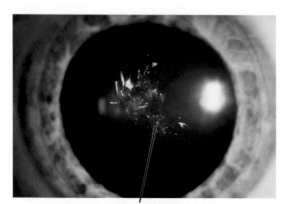

Figure 8-19 • Polychromatic, refractile, cholesterol deposits within the crystalline lens.

"Christmas tree" cholesterol cataract

Wilson's disease Sunflower cataract due to copper deposition (chalcosis lentis); green-brown surface opacity in the central lens with short stellate processes rather than the full flower petal pattern seen in chalcosis (copper foreign body).

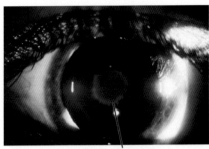

Sunflower cataract

Figure 8-20 • Sunflower cataract in a patient with Wilson's disease.

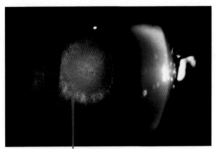

Chalcosis lentis

Figure 8-21 • Sunflower cataract (chalcosis lentis) with green-brown central opacities in the lens (same patient as in Figure 5-73 with Kayser-Fleischer ring).

Others Fabry's disease, atopic dermatitis (anterior subcapsular shieldlike plaque), NF-2 (posterior subcapsular), and ectodermal dysplasia.

Other Eye Diseases

Uveitis, angle-closure glaucoma (glaukomflecken), retinal detachment, myopia, intraocular tumors, retinitis pigmentosa (posterior subcapsular cataracts), Refsum's disease (posterior subcapsular cataracts), Stickler's syndrome (cortical cataracts), phthisis bulbi.

Toxic

Steroids (posterior subcapsular cataracts), miotic agents, phenothiazines, amiodarone, busulfan; ionizing (x-rays, gamma rays, and neutrons), infrared, ultraviolet, microwave, and shortwave radiation; electricity, and chemicals.

Figure 8-22 • Anterior subcapsular star-pattern cataract due to phenothiazine use.

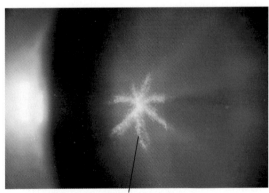

Anterior subcapsular cataract

Trauma

Blunt or penetrating; intraocular foreign bodies (iron, copper); and postoperative.

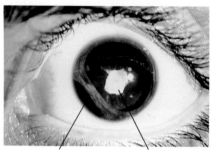

Iridodialysis   Traumatic cataract

Figure 8-23 • Dense, white, central cataract due to trauma; also note iridodialysis *(arrow)*.

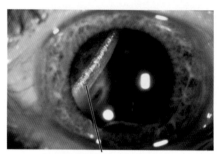

Intralenticular foreign body

Figure 8-24 • Intralenticular foreign body.

Epidemiology

Senile cataracts represent senescent lens changes related, in part, to ultraviolet B radiation. In the Framingham Eye Study, the prevalence of senile cataracts was 4.5% in adults 52-64 years old, 18.0% in 65-74 year olds, and 45.9% in 75-85 year olds. Black men and women were more likely to have cataracts in every age category. Cataracts *are* the leading cause of blindness worldwide.

Symptoms

Painless, progressive loss of vision, decreased contrast and color sensitivity, glare; rarely monocular diplopia.

Signs

Decreased visual acuity (distance vision usually affected more than near vision in nuclear sclerosis, and near vision affected more than distance vision in posterior subcapsular), focal or diffuse lens opacification (yellow, green, brown, or white; often best appreciated with retroillumination), induced myopia; intumescent cataracts may cause the iris to bow forward and lead to secondary angle closure (see Chapter 6); hypermature cataracts may leak lens proteins and cause phacolytic glaucoma (see Lens-Induced Secondary Glaucoma section).

Differential Diagnosis

See above; senile cataract is a diagnosis of exclusion; rule out secondary causes.

Evaluation

- Complete ophthalmic history with attention to systemic diseases, medications, prior use of steroids, trauma, radiation treatment, other ocular diseases, congenital problems, and functional visual status.
- Complete eye examination with attention to refraction, cornea, gonioscopy, lens, and ophthalmoscopy.
- Consider brightness acuity tester (BAT) and potential acuity meter (PAM) testing (the latter is used to estimate visual potential, especially when posterior segment pathology exists).
- B-scan ultrasonography if unable to visualize the fundus.
- Keratometry and A-scan biometry to calculate the IOL implant power before cataract surgery; also consider specular microscopy and pachymetry if cornea guttata or corneal edema exists.

Management

- Cataract extraction and insertion of an IOL is indicated when visual symptoms interfere with daily activities and the patient desires improved visual function, when the cataract causes other ocular diseases (e.g., phacolytic glaucoma, uveitis), or when the cataract prevents examination or treatment of a preexisting ocular condition (e.g., diabetic retinopathy, glaucoma).
- Dilation (tropicamide 1% [Mydriacyl] with or without phenylephrine 2.5% [Mydfrin] tid) may help the patient see around a central opacity in those rare instances when the patient cannot undergo or declines cataract surgery.

Prognosis

Very good; success rate for routine cataract surgery is over 95%.

Posterior Capsular Opacification (Secondary Cataract)

Definition

Clouding of the posterior lens capsule after extracapsular cataract extraction.

Epidemiology

After cataract extraction, up to 50% of adult patients may develop posterior capsule opacification; increased incidence in children and patients with uveitis (approaches 100%). Newer IOL materials and designs have reduced the incidence of posterior capsular opacification to less than 10%.

Etiology

Epithelial cell proliferation (Elschnig's pearls) and fibrosis of the capsule.

Symptoms

Asymptomatic or may have decreased vision and glare.

Signs

Posterior capsule opacification.

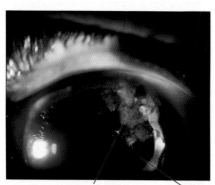

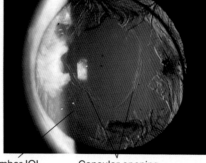

Elschnig's pearls   Posterior chamber IOL   Capsular opening

Figure 8-25 • Secondary cataract composed of Elschnig's pearls.

Figure 8-26 • Posterior capsule opening following Nd:YAG laser capsulotomy when viewed with retroillumination. Jagged edges or leaflets of the larger anterior capsulotomy are visible as is the superior edge of the intraocular lens optic from the 12 o'clock to 3 o'clock position.

Evaluation

• Complete ophthalmic history and eye examination with attention to refraction, cornea, tonometry, gonioscopy, IOL position and stability, posterior capsule, and ophthalmoscopy.

Management

• If visually significant, treat with neodymium:yttrium-aluminum-garnet (Nd:YAG) laser posterior capsulotomy.
    • *Procedure parameters:* a contact lens is used to stabilize the eye and produce smaller focus diameter of the beam; the goal is to create a central 3-4 mm opening in the posterior capsule; pupil dilation is usually performed but is not always necessary. Laser energy setting is typically 1-3 mJ and is titrated according to tissue response.
• In young children, a primary posterior capsulotomy and anterior vitrectomy are performed at the time of cataract surgery.

Prognosis

Very good; complications of Nd:YAG capsulotomy are rare but include increased intraocular pressure, IOL damage or dislocation, corneal burn, retinal detachment, cystoid macular edema, and hyphema.

■ Aphakia

Definition

Absence of crystalline lens; usually secondary to surgery, rarely traumatic (total dislocation of crystalline lens [Figure 8-36]), or very rarely congenital.

Symptoms

Loss of accommodation and decreased *uncorrected* vision.

Signs

Decreased *uncorrected* visual acuity (usually very high hyperopia), no lens, iridodonesis; may have a visible surgical wound, peripheral iridectomy, vitreous in anterior chamber, complications from surgery (bullous keratopathy, increased intraocular pressure, iritis, posterior capsule opacification, cystoid macular edema), or evidence of ocular trauma (see appropriate sections).

Evaluation

- Complete ophthalmic history and eye examination with attention to refraction, tonometry, gonioscopy, iris, lens, and ophthalmoscopy.
- Consider specular microscopy and pachymetry if cornea guttata or corneal edema exists.

Management

- Proper aphakic correction with contact lens; consider aphakic spectacles if bilateral.
- Consider secondary IOL implantation.
- Treat complications if present.

Prognosis

Usually good; increased risk of retinal detachment, especially for high myopes and if posterior capsule is not intact.

▉ Pseudophakia

Definition

Presence of IOL implant after crystalline lens has been removed; may be inserted primarily or secondarily.

Symptoms

Asymptomatic; may have decreased vision, loss of accommodation, edge glare, monocular diplopia or polyopia, or induced myopia with decentered IOL.

Signs

IOL implant (may be in anterior chamber, iris plane, capsular bag, or ciliary sulcus with or without suture fixation to iris or sclera); may have a visible surgical wound, peripheral iridectomy, complications from surgery (bullous keratopathy, iris capture, decentered IOL, increased intraocular pressure, iritis, hyphema, opacified posterior capsule, cystoid macular edema).

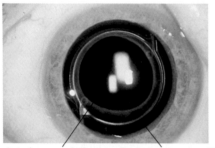

Anterior capsulorhexis   Posterior chamber IOL   Anterior chamber IOL   Pupil

Figure 8-27 • Pseudophakia demonstrating posterior chamber intraocular lens (IOL) well centered in the capsular bag. The anterior capsulorhexis edge has fibrosed and is visible as a white circle overlying the IOL optic; the edges of the IOL haptics where they insert into the optic are also seen.

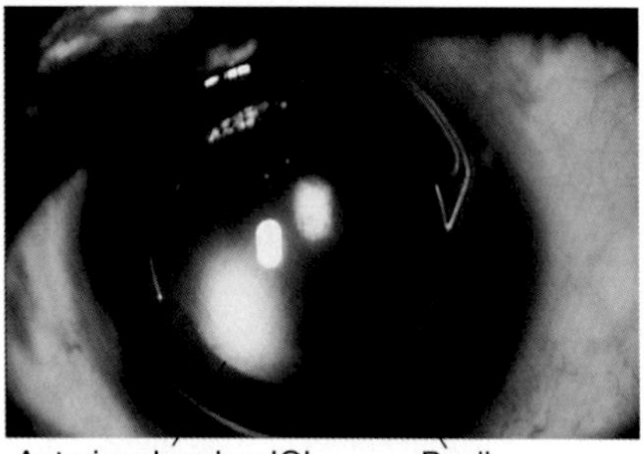

Figure 8-28 • Pseudophakia demonstrating anterior chamber intraocular lens in good position above the iris.

Evaluation

• Complete ophthalmic history and eye examination with attention to refraction, cornea, gonioscopy, IOL position and stability, posterior capsule integrity and clarity, and ophthalmoscopy.

Management

• May require correction of refractive error (usually reading glasses).
• Treat complications if present.

Prognosis

Usually good; increased risk of retinal detachment, especially for high myopes.

Exfoliation

Definition

True exfoliation is delamination, or schisis, of the anterior lens capsule into sheetlike lamellae.

Epidemiology

Rare; caused by infrared and thermal radiation, classically seen in glass blowers; also senile form.

Symptoms

Asymptomatic.

Signs

Splitting of anterior lens capsule, appears as scrolls; may have posterior subcapsular cataract.

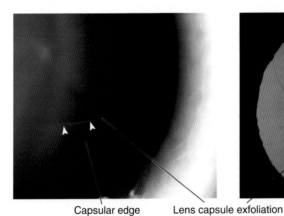
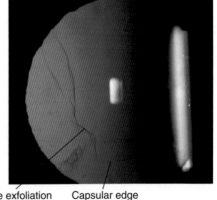

Capsular edge   Lens capsule exfoliation   Capsular edge

Figure 8-29 • True lens exfoliation demonstrating scrolling of split anterior lens capsule *(arrowheads)*.

Figure 8-30 • Same patient as shown in Figure 8-29, demonstrating appearance of lens capsule exfoliation as viewed with retroillumination.

Differential Diagnosis

Pseudoexfoliation syndrome.

Evaluation

• Complete ophthalmic history and eye examination with attention to lens.

Management

• No treatment recommended.
• Prevention by use of protective goggles.
• May require cataract extraction.

Prognosis

Good.

Pseudoexfoliation Syndrome

Definition

Pseudoexfoliation is a generalized basement membrane disorder that causes abnormal accumulation of small, gray-white fibrillar aggregates (resembling amyloid) on the lens capsule, iris, anterior segment structures, and systemically; may involve the skin, heart, and lungs.

Epidemiology

Pseudoexfoliation is often unilateral; usually asymmetric; found in all racial groups, common in Scandinavians, South African blacks, Navaho Indians, and Australian aborigines; almost absent in Eskimos; age related, rare in individuals under 50 years old, incidence increases after 60 years of age (4-6% in patients over 60 years old); up to 60% develop ocular hypertension or glaucoma (see below); in the United States, 20% have elevated intraocular pressure at initial examination, and 15% develop it within 10 years.

Symptoms

Asymptomatic.

Signs

Loss of pupillary ruff, iris transillumination defects, pigment deposits on the iris, trabecular meshwork, and anterior to Schwalbe's line (Sampaolesi's line); target pattern of exfoliative material on lens capsule (central disc and peripheral ring with intervening clear area); white exfoliation material is also seen on zonules, anterior hyaloid, iris, and pupillary margin; shallow anterior chamber due to forward migration of lens-iris diaphragm; may have phacodonesis, cataract (40%), or increased intraocular pressure.

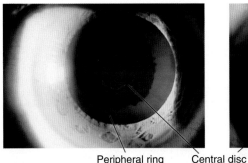 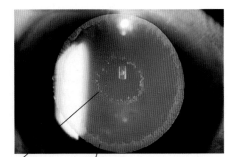

Peripheral ring   Central disc   Peripheral ring

Figure 8-31 • Exfoliative material on the anterior lens surface in typical pattern of central disc and peripheral ring in a patient with pseudoexfoliation syndrome.

Figure 8-32 • Central disc and peripheral ring of exfoliative material as seen with retroillumination.

Evaluation

- Complete ophthalmic history and eye examination with attention to tonometry, gonioscopy, iris, lens, and ophthalmoscopy.
- Consider visual fields in patients with elevated intraocular pressure or optic nerve cupping to rule out glaucoma.

Management

- Observe for pseudoexfoliation glaucoma by monitoring intraocular pressure.
- May require treatment of increased intraocular pressure (see Chapter 11).

Prognosis

Good; poorer if glaucoma exists; increased incidence of complications at cataract surgery due to weak zonules and increased lens mobility.

■ Pseudoexfoliation Glaucoma

Definition

A form of secondary open-angle glaucoma associated with the pseudoexfoliation syndrome.

Epidemiology

Most common cause of secondary open-angle glaucoma; 2% of U.S. population over 50 years old; up to 60% with pseudoexfoliation syndrome develop ocular hypertension or glaucoma;

50% bilateral, often asymmetric; age related (rare in individuals under 50 years old, increases after age 60 years).

Mechanism

Trabecular meshwork dysfunction due to dispersion of pigment or exfoliative material.

Symptoms

Asymptomatic; may have decreased vision or visual field defects in late stages.

Signs

Intraocular pressure elevation can be very high and asymmetric; similar ocular signs as pseudoexfoliation syndrome (see above).

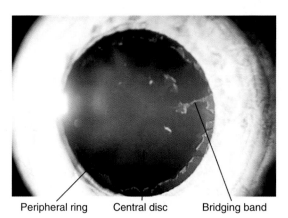

Figure 8-33 • Patient with pseudoexfoliation glaucoma demonstrating peripheral ring of exfoliative material on the lens surface with bridging band connecting to the central disc.

Peripheral ring　Central disc　Bridging band

Differential Diagnosis

Primary open-angle glaucoma, other secondary forms of open-angle glaucoma.

Evaluation

• Complete ophthalmic history and eye examination with attention to cornea, tonometry, anterior chamber, gonioscopy, iris, lens, and ophthalmoscopy.

- Check visual fields.
- Stereo-optic nerve photos are useful for comparison at subsequent evaluations.

Management

- Choice and order of topical glaucoma medications depend on many factors, including patient's age, intraocular pressure level and control, and amount and progression of optic nerve cupping and visual field defects. Treatment options are presented in the Primary Open-Angle Glaucoma section (see Chapter 11); more resistant to treatment than primary open-angle glaucoma.
- Laser trabeculoplasty is effective, but action may be short lived.
- May require glaucoma filtering procedure if medical treatment fails.

Prognosis

Poorer than primary open-angle glaucoma; increased incidence of angle-closure; lens removal has no effect on progression of disease; increased incidence of complications at cataract surgery due to weak zonules and increased lens mobility.

Lens-Induced Secondary Glaucoma

Definition

Secondary glaucoma due to lens-induced abnormalities.

Mechanism

Lens Particle

Retained cortex or nucleus after cataract surgery or penetrating trauma causes inflammatory reaction and obstructs trabecular meshwork; more anterior segment inflammation than phacolytic.

Phacolytic

Lens proteins from hypermature cataract leak through intact capsule and are ingested by macrophages; can occur with intact, dislocated lens; lens proteins and macrophages obstruct trabecular meshwork.

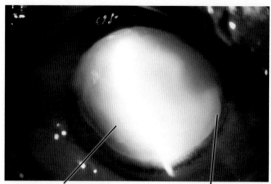

Figure 8-34 • Phacolytic glaucoma demonstrating mature white cataract with anterior chamber inflammation.

Hypermature cataract   Shallow chamber

Phacomorphic

Enlarged, cataractous lens pushes the iris forward, causing secondary angle-closure (see Chapter 6).

Corneal edema

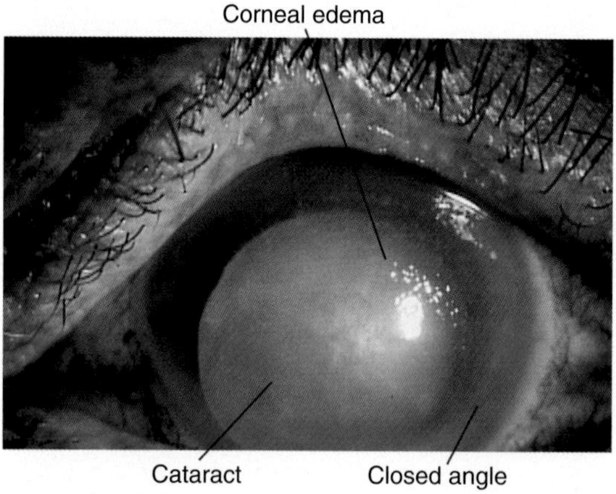

Figure 8-35 • Phacomorphic angle-closure glaucoma due to intumescent cataract pushing the iris forward and thereby obstructing the trabecular meshwork.

Cataract   Closed angle

Symptoms

Decreased vision, pain, photophobia, red eye; may have halos around lights and signs of angle-closure (see Chapter 6).

Signs

Decreased visual acuity, increased intraocular pressure, ciliary injection, anterior chamber cells and flare, peripheral anterior synechiae, cataract or residual lens material, signs of recent surgery or trauma including surgical wounds, sutures, and signs of an open globe (see Chapter 4).

Differential Diagnosis

See above; other secondary forms of glaucoma, uveitis, endophthalmitis.

Evaluation

- Complete ophthalmic history and eye examination with attention to cornea, tonometry, anterior chamber, gonioscopy, iris, lens, and ophthalmoscopy.
- B-scan ultrasonography if unable to visualize the fundus.
- Topical steroid (prednisolone acetate 1% up to q1h) and cycloplegic agent (cyclopentolate 1% or scopolamine 0.25% bid to tid).
- Definitive treatment consists of surgical lens extraction or removal of retained lens fragments.
- May require glaucoma filtering procedure.

> ### Management
>
> - Medical treatment of increased intraocular pressure. Treatment options are presented in the Primary Open-Angle Glaucoma and Angle-Closure Glaucoma sections (see Chapters 11 and 6, respectively).

Prognosis

Good if definitive treatment is performed early and pressure control is achieved.

■ Dislocated Lens (Ectopia Lentis)

Definition

Congenital, developmental, or acquired displacement of the crystalline lens; may be incomplete (subluxation) or complete (luxation) dislocation of the lens into the anterior chamber or vitreous.

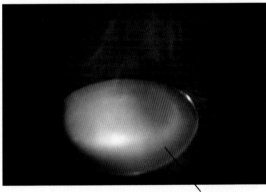

Figure 8-36 • Dislocated crystalline lens resting on the retina.

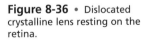

Dislocated crystalline lens

Etiology

Ectopia Lentis et Pupillae (AR)

Associated with oval or slitlike pupils; pupil displacement is in opposite direction of the lens displacement.

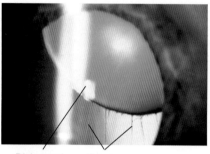

Dislocated   Zonules
crystalline lens

Figure 8-37 • Subluxed lens (up and out) due to trauma; note broken inferior zonular fibers.

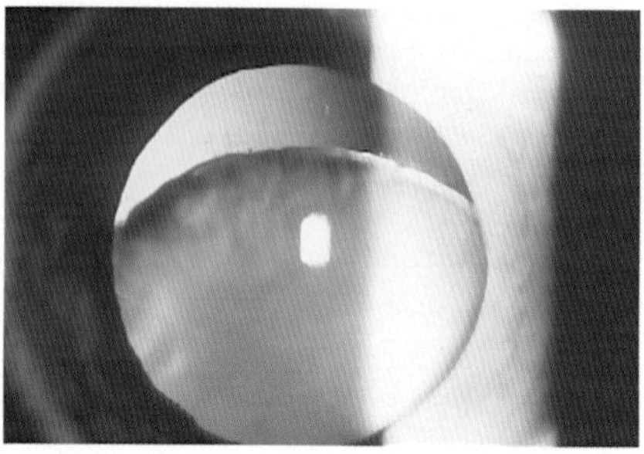

Figure 8-38 • Lens subluxed (downward) due to trauma.

Homocystinuria (AR)

Lens dislocation is not present at birth; progressive thereafter, typically in a down and inward direction; more than 90% have dislocated lenses by the third decade; enzymatic disorder of methionine metabolism with elevated levels of homocystine and methionine; patients develop seizures, osteoporosis, mental retardation, and thromboembolism.

Hyperlysinemia

Inability to metabolize lysine; lens subluxation, muscular hypotony, and mental retardation.

Marfan's Syndrome (AD)

Usually bilateral; occurs in about two thirds of Marfan's patients due to a defective zonular apparatus; direction of lens displacement is typically up and out; other signs include marfanoid habitus with disproportionate growth of extremities, arachnodactyly, joint laxity, pectus deformities, scoliosis, and increasing dilation of the ascending aorta with aortic insufficiency (may cause death); mapped to chromosome 15q.

Microspherophakia

Small spheric lens seen as isolated anomaly or as part of various syndromes (dominant spherophakia, Weill-Marchesani syndrome, Lowe's syndrome).

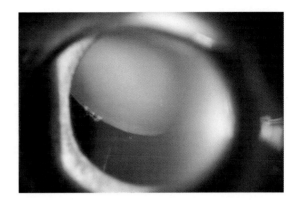

Figure 8-39 • Lens subluxed (upward) in a patient with Marfan's syndrome.

Simple Ectopia Lentis (AD)

Often present at birth; lens is small and spheric (microphakic and spherophakic); direction of lens displacement is typically up and out.

Sulfite Oxidase Deficiency (AR)

Error of sulfur metabolism with ectopia lentis, seizures, and mental retardation.

Other

Aniridia, Ehlers-Danlos syndrome, trauma, syphilis, megalocornea.

Epidemiology

Most common cause of lens subluxation or luxation is trauma (22-50%); associated with cataract and rhegmatogenous retinal detachment; most frequent cause of heritable lens dislocation is Marfan's syndrome.

Symptoms

Asymptomatic; may have decreased vision, diplopia, symptoms of angle-closure.

Signs

Normal or decreased visual acuity, subluxated or luxated lens, phacodonesis, iridodonesis; may have increased intraocular pressure, anterior chamber cells and flare, vitreous in anterior chamber, iris transillumination defects, angle abnormalities, and other signs of ocular trauma.

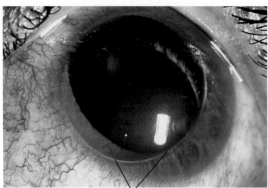

Figure 8-40 • Dislocated lens in the anterior chamber. The edge of the clear lens is visible overlying the iris.

Dislocated crystaline lens

Differential Diagnosis

See above.

Evaluation

- Complete ophthalmic history and eye examination with attention to refraction, corneal diameter, tonometry, gonioscopy, iris, and lens.
- Consider B-scan ultrasonography if unable to visualize the fundus.
- **Lab tests:** Venereal Disease Research Laboratory test, fluorescent treponema antibody absorption test, and lumbar puncture if syphilis suspected.
- Medical consultation for systemic diseases.
- Microspherophakia causing pupillary block is treated with a cycloplegic agent (scopolamine 0.25% tid or atropine 1% bid); may also require laser iridotomy.
- Treat underlying disorder (e.g., dietary restriction in homocystinuria, IV penicillin for syphilis).

Management

- Correct any refractive error.
- Consider lens extraction.
- May require treatment of angle-closure (see Chapter 6); miotic agents may exacerbate a pupillary block and should be avoided.

Prognosis

Depends on etiology.

Chapter 9

VITREOUS

Amyloidosis

Localized or systemic disease with abnormal protein deposition in various organs, classified into primary, myeloma-associated, and secondary amyloidosis. The vitreous and eyelids are common sites of involvement, but the disease can involve other ocular structures including the orbit, extraocular muscles, lacrimal gland, conjunctiva, cornea, iris, retina, choroid, optic nerve, and higher visual pathways. Vitreous opacities have a granular, glass-wool appearance with strands attached to the retina. Other findings include yellow waxy eyelid papules, purpuric lesions of the eyelids, lacrimal gland, caruncle, or conjunctiva; ptosis, proptosis, ophthalmoplegia, dry eye, corneal deposits, iris stromal infiltrates, retinal vascular occlusions, cotton-wool spots, retinal neovascularization, and compressive optic neuropathy (see Chapter 3).

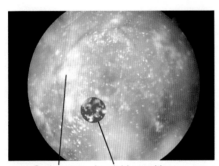

Optic nerve Amyloid opacities

Figure 9-1 • Amyloidosis demonstrating the characteristic granular, glass-wool opacities in the midvitreous cavity that obscure the view of the retina. The optic nerve is barely visible.

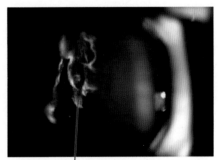

Amyloid opacities in anterior vitreous

Figure 9-2 • Amyloidosis demonstrating the characteristic granular, glass-wool opacities in the anterior vitreous cavity as seen with slit lamp.

- Medical consultation for systemic workup.
- Biopsy is gold standard for diagnosis.
- No treatment recommended for vitreous involvement unless opacities significantly reduce vision, then consider pars plana vitrectomy; should be performed by a vitreoretinal specialist.
- Recurs even after vitrectomy.

Asteroid Hyalosis

Multiple, yellow-white, round, birefringent particles composed of calcium phosphate soaps attached to the vitreous framework. Common degenerative process seen in elderly patients over 60 years of age (0.5% of population). Usually asymptomatic, does not cause floaters or interfere with vision, but does affect view of fundus; usually unilateral (75%); associated with diabetes mellitus (30%); good prognosis.

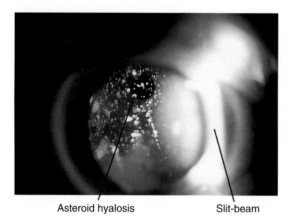

Figure 9-3 • The yellow-white particles of asteroid hyalosis are seen in the anterior vitreous cavity behind the lens. They are best seen using a fine slit beam at an oblique angle.

Asteroid hyalosis   Slit-beam

- No treatment usually recommended.
- Consider pars plana vitrectomy if particles become so severe that they affect vision or interfere with the diagnosis or treatment of retinal disorders; should be performed by a vitreoretinal specialist.

Persistent Hyperplastic Primary Vitreous

Definition

Sporadic, unilateral (90%), developmental anomaly with abnormal regression of the tunica vasculosa lentis (hyaloid artery) and primary vitreous.

Symptoms

Decreased vision; may have eye turn (lazy eye).

Signs

Leukocoria, strabismus, microphthalmos, nystagmus, pink-white retrolenticular or intravitreal membrane often with radiating vessels; lens is clear early but becomes cataractous; associated with shallow anterior chamber (more shallow with age), elongated ciliary processes extending toward membrane, large radial blood vessels that often cover iris; may have angle-closure (see Chapter 6), vitreous hemorrhage, or retinal detachment.

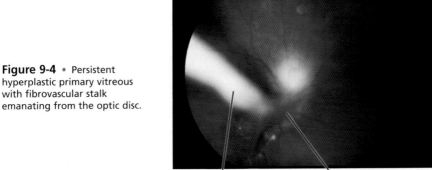

Figure 9-4 • Persistent hyperplastic primary vitreous with fibrovascular stalk emanating from the optic disc.

Fibrovascular stalk   Optic nerve

Differential Diagnosis

Leukocoria (see Chapter 7).

Evaluation

- Complete ophthalmic history and eye examination with attention to tonometry, lens, and vitreous; Hruby lens, noncontact biomicroscopic or contact lens fundus examination.
- B-scan ultrasonography if unable to visualize the fundus.
- Check orbital computed tomography (CT) scan for intraocular calcifications.

Management

- Correct any refractive error.
- Retinal surgery with pars plana vitrectomy, lensectomy, and membrane peel advocated early (within first few months of life); should be performed by a vitreoretinal specialist.
- Patching or occlusion therapy for amblyopia (see Chapter 12).

Prognosis

Poor prognosis without treatment secondary to glaucoma, recurrent vitreous hemorrhages, and eventually phthisis; earlier treatment improves prognosis.

Posterior Vitreous Detachment

Definition

Syneresis (liquefaction) of the vitreous gel that causes dehiscence of the posterior hyaloid from the retina (internal limiting membrane) and collapse of the vitreous toward the vitreous base away from the macula and optic disc. Can be localized, partial, or total.

Epidemiology

Most commonly caused by aging (53% by 50 years old, 65% by 65 years old); by age 70, majority of the posterior vitreous is liquefied (synchesis senilis); female predilection; occurs earlier after trauma, vitritis, cataract surgery, neodymium:yttrium-aluminum-garnet (Nd:YAG) laser posterior capsulotomy, and in patients with myopia, diabetes mellitus, hereditary vitreoretinal degenerations, and retinitis pigmentosa.

Symptoms

Acute onset of floaters and photopsias, especially with eye movement.

Signs

Circular vitreous condensation often over disc (Weiss ring), anterior displacement of the posterior hyaloid, vitreous opacities, vitreous pigment cells (tobacco dust), focal intraretinal, preretinal, or vitreous hemorrhage.

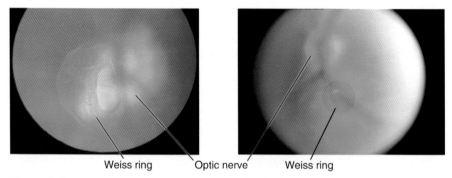

Weiss ring   Optic nerve   Weiss ring

Figure 9-5 • Circular Weiss ring seen over the optic nerve in the midvitreous cavity.

Figure 9-6 • Horseshoe-shaped posterior vitreous detachment seen over the optic nerve in the midvitreous cavity.

Differential Diagnosis

Vitreous hemorrhage (see below), vitritis, fungal cyst.

Evaluation

* Complete ophthalmic history and eye examination with attention to anterior vitreous; Hruby lens, noncontact biomicroscopic or contact lens fundus examination, and careful depressed peripheral retinal examination to identify any retinal tears or holes.

Management

- No treatment recommended.
- Instruct patient on retinal detachment warning signs: photopsias, increased floaters, and shadow or shade in peripheral vision or visual field defect; instruct patient to return immediately if warning signs occur to rule out retinal tear or detachment.
- Repeat dilated retinal examination 1-3 months after acute posterior vitreous detachment to rule out asymptomatic retinal tear or detachment.
- Treat retinal breaks if present (see Chapter 10).

Prognosis

Good; 10-15% risk of retinal break in acute, symptomatic posterior vitreous detachments; 70% risk of retinal break if vitreous hemorrhage is present.

Synchesis Scintillans

Golden brown, refractile crystals that are freely mobile within vitreous cavity; associated with liquid vitreous, so the crystals settle in the most dependent area of the vitreous body; rare syndrome that occurs after chronic vitreous hemorrhage, uveitis, or trauma; composed of cholesterol crystals.

Vitreous Hemorrhage

Definition

Blood in the vitreous space.

Etiology

Retinal break, posterior vitreous detachment, ruptured retinal arterial macroaneurysm, juvenile retinoschisis, familial exudative vitreoretinopathy, Terson's syndrome (blood dissects through the lamina cribrosa into the eye due to subarachnoid hemorrhage and elevated intracranial pressure, often bilateral with severe headache), trauma, retinal angioma, retinopathy of blood disorders, Valsalva retinopathy, and neovascularization from various disorders including diabetic retinopathy, Eales' disease, hypertensive retinopathy, radiation retinopathy, sickle cell retinopathy, and retinopathy of prematurity.

Symptoms

Sudden onset of floaters and decreased vision.

Signs

Decreased visual acuity, vitreous cells (red blood cells), poor or no view of fundus, poor or absent red reflex; old vitreous hemorrhage appears gray-white.

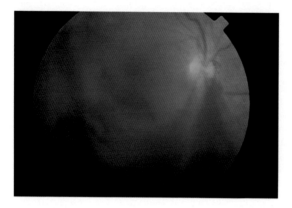

Figure 9-7 • Vitreous hemorrhage obscures the view of the retina in this diabetic patient. Gravity has layered the blood inferiorly.

Differential Diagnosis

Vitritis, asteroid hyalosis, pigment cells, pars planitis.

Evaluation

- Complete ophthalmic history and eye examination with attention to visual acuity, tonometry, noncontact biomicroscopic or contact lens fundus examination, and careful depressed peripheral retinal examination to identify any retinal tears or holes.
- B-scan ultrasonography to rule out retinal tear or detachment if unable to visualize the fundus.

Management

- Conservative treatment and follow for resolution of vitreous hemorrhage, unless associated with a retinal tear or hole which needs to be treated immediately (see Chapter 10).
- Bedrest and elevation of head of bed may settle hemorrhage inferiorly to allow visualization of fundus.
- Avoid aspirin, aspirin-containing products, and other anticoagulants.
- Consider pars plana vitrectomy if there is persistent *idiopathic* vitreous hemorrhage for more than 6 months, nonclearing diabetic vitreous hemorrhage for more than 1 month, intractable increased intraocular pressure (ghost cell glaucoma), decreased vision in fellow eye, retinal tear or hole, or retinal detachment; should be performed by a vitreoretinal specialist.
- Treat underlying medical condition.

Prognosis

Usually good.

▇ Trauma

Choroidal Rupture

Tear in choroid, Bruch's membrane, and retinal pigment epithelium (RPE) usually seen after blunt trauma. Acutely, the rupture site may be obscured by hemorrhage. Anterior ruptures are usually parallel to the ora serrata; posterior ruptures are usually crescent-shaped and concentric to the optic nerve. Patient may have decreased vision if commotio retinae or subretinal hemorrhage is present or if rupture is located in the macula; increased risk of developing a choroidal neovascular membrane (CNV). Prognosis is good if macula is not involved, poor if fovea is involved.

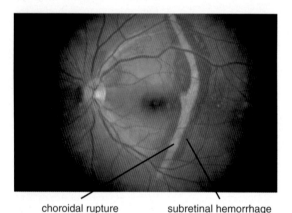

Figure 10-1 • Crescent-shaped, choroidal rupture that is concentric to the optic nerve with surrounding subretinal hemorrhage.

choroidal rupture   subretinal hemorrhage

- No treatment recommended unless CNV occurs.
- Laser photocoagulation of juxtafoveal and extrafoveal CNV; consider photodynamic therapy (PDT) for subfoveal CNV (experimental).
- Monitor for CNV with Amsler grid.

Commotio Retinae (Berlin's Edema)

Gray-white discoloration of the outer retina due to photoreceptor outer segment disruption following blunt eye trauma; can affect any area of the retina and may be accompanied by hemorrhages or choroidal rupture; can cause acute decrease in vision if located within the macula that resolves as the retinal discoloration disappears; may cause permanent loss of vision if fovea is damaged.

- **Fluorescein angiogram:** Early blocked fluorescence in the areas of commotio retinae.
- No treatment recommended.

Purtscher's Retinopathy

Multiple patches of retinal whitening, large cotton-wool spots, and hemorrhages that surround the optic disc following multiple long bone fractures with fat emboli or severe compressive injuries to the chest or head. May have optic disc edema and a positive relative afferent pupillary defect (RAPD). Usually resolves over weeks to months.

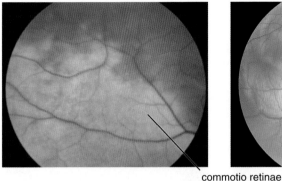

commotio retinae   subretinal hemorrhage

Figure 10-2 • Gray-white discoloration of the outer retina in a patient with commotio retinae.

Figure 10-3 • Commotio retinae following blunt trauma demonstrating retinal whitening; note subretinal hemorrhage from underlying choroidal rupture.

Figure 10-4 • Multiple patches of retinal whitening, cotton-wool spots, and intraretinal hemorrhages secondary to Purtscher's retinopathy.

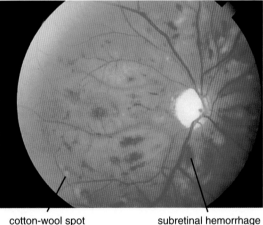

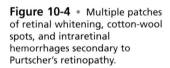

cotton-wool spot   subretinal hemorrhage

In the absence of trauma, a Purtscher-like retinopathy may be associated with acute pancreatitis, collagen-vascular disease, and amniotic fluid embolus.

• No treatment recommended.

Retinal Break

Full-thickness tear in the retina, often horseshoe-shaped, that usually occurs along the vitreous base, posterior border of lattice degeneration, or at cystic retinal tufts (areas with strong vitreoretinal adhesions). Giant retinal tears (tears >90 degrees in circumferential extent or >3 clock hours), avulsion of vitreous base, and retinal dialysis (circumferential separation of the retina at the ora serrata, usually in superonasal quadrant) are more common after trauma.

Associated with pigmented vitreous cells ("tobacco-dust"), vitreous hemorrhages, operculum (often located over the break), and posterior vitreous detachment. Patients usually report photopsias and floaters that shift with eye movement. Liquefied vitreous can pass through the tear into the subretinal space, causing a retinal detachment even months to years after the tear forms; chronic tears have a ring of pigment around the break.

horseshoe tear   retinal vessel   giant retinal tear

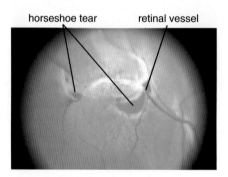
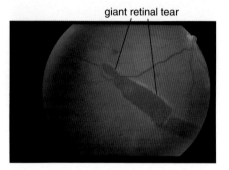

Figure 10-5 • Two horseshoe-shaped retinal tears with a bridging retinal vessel seen across the larger tear.

Figure 10-6 • Very posterior giant retinal tear that extends for more than 3 clock hours.

- If asymptomatic, close follow-up.
- If symptomatic (photopsias and floaters), treatment with cryopexy along edge of tear (do not treat bare retinal pigment epithelium) or two or three rows of laser photocoagulation demarcation around the tear.
- Retinal surgery is required if retinal detachment, retinal dialysis, avulsion of the vitreous base, or giant retinal tear exists; should be performed by a retina specialist.

Hemorrhages

Preretinal Hemorrhage

Hemorrhage located between retina and posterior vitreous face (subhyaloid) or under internal limiting membrane of the retina (sub-ILM). Often amorphous or boat-shaped, with flat upper border and curved lower border that obscures the underlying retina; caused by trauma, retinal neovascularization (diabetic retinopathy, radiation retinopathy, breakthrough bleeding from a choroidal neovascular membrane), hypertensive retinopathy, Valsalva retinopathy, posterior vitreous detachment, shaken-baby syndrome, or retinal breaks, and less frequently by vascular occlusion, retinopathy of blood disorders, and leukemia.

Intraretinal Hemorrhage

Bilateral intraretinal hemorrhages are associated with systemic disorders (e.g., diabetes mellitus and hypertension); unilateral intraretinal hemorrhages generally occur in venous occlusive diseases.

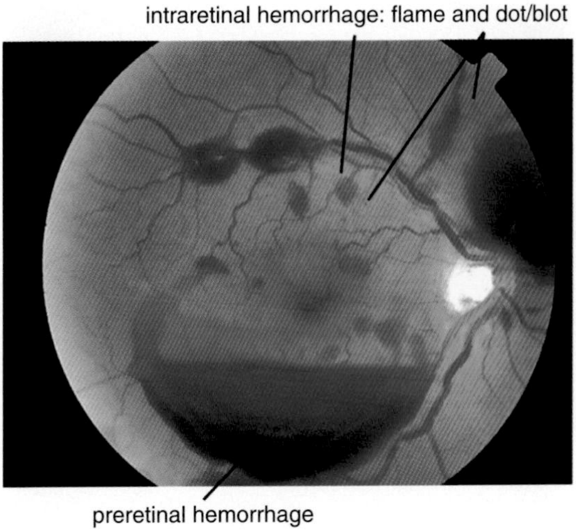

intraretinal hemorrhage: flame and dot/blot

Figure 10-7 • Diabetic retinopathy demonstrating intraretinal and preretinal (boat-shaped configuration due to attached hyaloid containing the blood) hemorrhages.

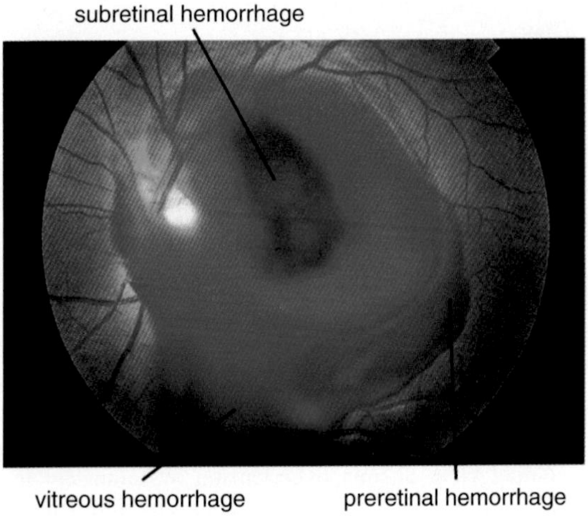

preretinal hemorrhage

subretinal hemorrhage

Figure 10-8 • Valsalva retinopathy demonstrating vitreous, preretinal, and subretinal hemorrhages.

vitreous hemorrhage   preretinal hemorrhage

Flame-shaped hemorrhage   Located in the superficial retina oriented with the nerve fiber layer; feathery borders; usually seen in hypertensive retinopathy and vein occlusion; may be peripapillary in glaucoma, especially in normal-tension glaucoma (called *splinter hemorrhage*) and disc edema.

Dot/blot hemorrhage   Located in the outer plexiform layer, confined by the antero-posterior orientation of the photoreceptor, bipolar, and Müller's cells; round dots or larger blots; usually seen in diabetic retinopathy.

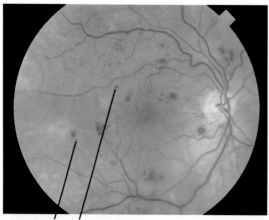

Figure 10-9 • Intraretinal dot and blot hemorrhages in a patient with nonproliferative diabetic retinopathy.

dot/blot intraretinal hemorrhage

Roth spot   Hemorrhage with white center that represents an embolus with lymphocytic infiltration; classically associated with subacute bacterial endocarditis (seen in 1-5% of such patients); also occurs in leukemia, severe anemia, sickle cell disease, collagen-vascular diseases, diabetes mellitus, multiple myeloma, and acquired immunodeficiency syndrome (AIDS) (see Figs. 10-35 and 10-38).

Subretinal Hemorrhage

Amorphous hemorrhage located under the neurosensory retina or RPE; appears dark and is deep to the retinal vessels; associated with trauma, subretinal and choroidal neovascular membranes, and macroaneurysms (see Fig. 10-61).

All three types of hemorrhage may occur together in several disorders including age-related macular degeneration (AMD), acquired retinal macroaneurysms, Eales' disease, and capillary hemangioma.

Cotton-Wool Spot (CWS)

Asymptomatic, yellow-white, fluffy lesions in the superficial retina (see Fig. 10-4); believed to result from focal retinal ischemia; nonspecific finding seen in several systemic diseases including AIDS, anemia, hypertension, leukemia, collagen-vascular diseases, cardiac valvular diseases, acute pancreatitis, and diabetes mellitus (most common cause); also associated with vascular occlusions, radiation retinopathy, and high-altitude retinopathy.

• Treat underlying medical condition (identified in 95% of cases).

Branch Retinal Artery Occlusion (BRAO)

Definition

Disruption of the vascular perfusion in a branch of the central retinal artery (BRAO), leading to focal retinal ischemia. The site of the obstruction is usually at the bifurcation of retinal arteries.

Etiology

Mainly due to embolism from cholesterol (Hollenhorst's plaques), calcifications (heart valves), platelet-fibrin plugs (ulcerated atheromatous plaques due to arteriosclerosis); rarely due to leukoemboli (vasculitis, Purtscher's retinopathy), fat emboli (long bone fractures), amniotic fluid emboli, tumor emboli (atrial myxoma), or septic (heart valve vegetations seen in bacterial endocarditis or IV drug abuse). May result from vasospasm (migraine), compression, or coagulopathies.

Epidemiology

Usually occurs in elderly patients (seventh decade); associated with hypertension (67%), carotid occlusive disease (25%), diabetes mellitus (33%), and cardiac valvular disease (25%). Central retinal artery occlusion (CRAO) more common (57%) than BRAO (38%) or cilioretinal artery occlusion (5%) (in 32% of eyes, a cilioretinal artery is present).

Symptoms

Sudden, unilateral, painless, partial loss of vision, with a visual field defect depending on the location of the occlusion. May have history of amaurosis fugax (fleeting episodes of loss of vision), prior cerebrovascular accident (CVA), or transient ischemic attacks (TIAs).

Signs

Visual field defect with normal or decreased visual acuity; focal, wedge-shaped area of retinal whitening within the distribution of a branch arteriole; 90% involve temporal retinal vessels; emboli (visible in 62% of cases) or Hollenhorst's plaques may be seen at retinal vessel bifurcations. Retinal whitening resolves over several weeks, and visual acuity can improve.

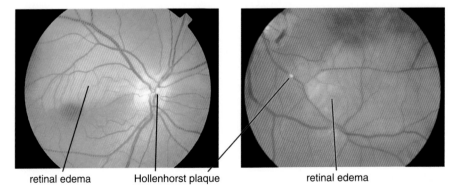

retinal edema   Hollenhorst plaque   retinal edema

Figure 10-10 • Superior branch artery occlusion with retinal edema extending in a wedge-shaped pattern from the artery occluded by the Hollenhorst plaque.

Figure 10-11 • Inferior branch retinal artery occlusion with Hollenhorst plaque and wedge-shaped retinal edema.

Differential Diagnosis

Commotio retinae, central retinal vein occlusion.

Evaluation

- Complete ophthalmic history and eye examination with attention to pupils, 78/90 diopter or contact lens fundus examination, and ophthalmoscopy (retinal vasculature and arteriole bifurcations).
- Check blood pressure.
- **Lab tests:** Fasting blood glucose (FBS) and complete blood count (CBC) with differential; consider platelets, prothrombin time/partial thromboplastin time (PT/PTT), protein C, protein S, antithrombin III, homocysteine, antinuclear antibody (ANA), rheumatoid factor (RF), antiphospholipid antibody, serum protein electrophoresis, hemoglobin electrophoresis, Venereal Disease Research Laboratory (VDRL) test, and fluorescent treponemal antibody absorption (FTA-ABS) test. In patients >50 years old, check erythrocyte sedimentation rate (ESR) to rule out temporal arteritis. If positive, start temporal arteritis treatment immediately (see Chapter 11).
- **Fluorescein angiogram:** Delayed or absent retinal arterial filling in a branch of the central retinal artery; delayed arteriovenous transit time; capillary nonperfusion in wedge-shaped area supplied by the branch artery; staining of occlusion site and vessel wall in late views. When occlusion dissolutes, retinal blood flow usually restored.
- Consider B-scan ultrasonography or orbital computed tomography (CT) to rule out compressive lesion if history suggests compression.
- Medical consultation for complete cardiovascular evaluation including electrocardiogram, echocardiogram (may require transthoracic echocardiogram to rule out valvular disease), and carotid Doppler studies.

Management

- Same treatment as CRAO (see below) if foveal circulation affected, but this is controversial due to good prognosis and questionable benefit of treatment.

Prognosis

Retinal pallor fades and circulation is restored over several weeks. Good prognosis if fovea spared; 80% have ≥20/40 vision, but most have some degree of permanent visual field loss.

Central Retinal Artery Occlusion (CRAO)

Definition

Disruption of the vascular perfusion in the central retinal artery leading to global retinal ischemia.

Etiology

Due to emboli (only visible in 20-40% of cases) or thrombus at the level of the lamina cribrosa; other causes include temporal arteritis, leukoemboli in collagen-vascular diseases, fat emboli, trauma (through compression, spasm, or direct vessel damage), hypercoagulation disorders, syphilis, sickle cell disease, amniotic fluid emboli, mitral valve prolapse, particles (talc) from IV drug abuse, and compressive lesions; associated with optic nerve drusen, papilledema, prepapillary arterial loops, and primary open-angle glaucoma.

Epidemiology

Usually occurs in elderly patients; associated with hypertension (67%), carotid occlusive disease (25%), diabetes mellitus (33%), and cardiac valvular disease (25%). CRAO more common (57%) than BRAO (38%) or cilioretinal artery occlusion (5%) (in 32% of eyes, a cilioretinal artery is present). Bilateral involvement rare.

Symptoms

Sudden, unilateral, painless, profound loss of vision. May have history of amaurosis fugax (fleeting episodes of loss of vision), prior cerebrovascular accident (CVA), or transient ischemic attacks (TIAs).

Signs

Decreased visual acuity in the count fingers (CF) to light perception (LP) range; positive relative afferent pupillary defect (RAPD); diffuse retinal whitening and arteriole constriction with segmentation ("boxcar-ing") of blood flow; visible emboli (20-40%) rarely seen in central retinal artery or a branch; cherry-red spot in the macula (thin fovea allows visualization of the underlying choroidal circulation). In ciliary retinal artery–sparing CRAO (25%), small wedge-shaped area of perfused retina may be present temporal to the optic disc (10% spare the foveola, in which case visual acuity improves to 20/50 or better in 80%). *Note:* Ophthalmic artery obstruction usually does not produce a cherry-red spot due to underlying choroidal ischemia.

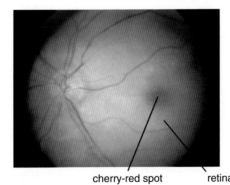
cherry-red spot

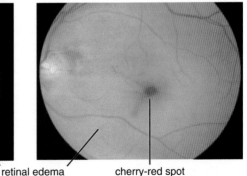
retinal edema   cherry-red spot

Figure 10-12 • Central retinal artery occlusion with cherry-red spot in the fovea and surrounding retinal edema.

Figure 10-13 • Central retinal artery occlusion with cherry-red spot.

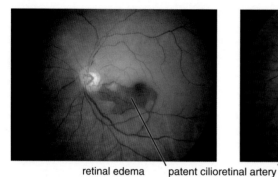

retinal edema | patent cilioretinal artery | absent flow

Figure 10-14 • Cilioretinal artery-sparing central retinal artery occlusion with patent cilioretinal artery allowing perfusion (thus no edema) in a small section of the macula.

Figure 10-15 • Fluorescein angiogram of same patient in Figure 10-14 demonstrating no filling of retinal vessels except in cilioretinal artery and surrounding branches.

Differential Diagnosis

Ophthalmic artery occlusion, commotio retinae, cherry-red spot due to inherited metabolic or lysosomal storage diseases.

Evaluation

- Complete ophthalmic history and eye examination with attention to pupils, 78/90 diopter or contact lens fundus examination, and ophthalmoscopy (retinal vasculature).
- Check blood pressure.
- **Lab tests:** Fasting blood glucose (FBS) and complete blood count (CBC) with differential; consider platelets, prothrombin time/partial thromboplastin time (PT/PTT), protein C, Protein S, antithrombin III, homocysteine, antinuclear antibody (ANA), rheumatoid factor (RF), antiphospholipid antibody, serum protein electrophoresis, hemoglobin electrophoresis, Venereal Disease Research Laboratory (VDRL) test, and fluorescent treponemal antibody absorption (FTA-ABS) test. In patients >50 years old, check erythrocyte sedimentation rate (ESR) to rule out arteritic ischemic optic neuropathy.
- **Fluorescein angiogram:** Delayed retinal arterial filling and arteriovenous transit time with normal choroidal filling and perfusion of optic nerve from ciliary branches; prolonged arteriovenous circulation times; extensive capillary nonperfusion.
- **Electrophysiologic testing:** ERG (reduced b-wave amplitude, normal a wave).
- Consider B-scan ultrasonography or orbital computed tomography (CT) to rule out compressive lesion if history suggests compression.
- Medical consultation for complete cardiovascular evaluation including electrocardiogram, echocardiogram (may require transthoracic echocardiogram to rule out valvular disease), and carotid Doppler studies.

Management

OPHTHALMIC EMERGENCY

- Treatment controversial due to poor prognosis and questionable benefit of treatment.

Management—cont'd

- Treatment controversial due to poor prognosis and questionable benefit of treatment.
- Treat immediately before starting workup (if patient presents within 24 hours of visual loss).
- Digital ocular massage to try and dislodge emboli.
- Systemic acetazolamide (Diamox 500 mg IV or po).
- Topical ocular hypotensive drops: β-blocker (timolol 0.5% 1 gtt q15min × 2, repeat as necessary).
- Anterior chamber paracentesis.
- Consider admission to hospital for carbogen treatment (95% oxygen, 5% carbon dioxide for 10 minutes q2h for 24-48 hours) to attempt to increase oxygenation and induce vasodilation.
- Unproven treatments include hyperbaric oxygen, antifibrinolytic drugs, retrobulbar vasodilators, and sublingual nitroglycerine.
- If arteritic ischemic optic neuropathy (see Chapter 11) is suspected: systemic steroids (methylprednisolone 1 g IV qd in divided doses for 3 days, then prednisone 60-100 mg po qd with a slow taper; decrease by no more than 2.5-5.0 mg/wk).

Prognosis

Retinal pallor fades and circulation is restored over several weeks. Poor prognosis; most have persistent severe visual loss with constricted retinal arterioles and optic atrophy (positive APD). Rubeosis (20%) and disc or retinal neovascularization (2-3%) can occur. Presence of visible embolus associated with increased mortality.

Ophthalmic Artery Occlusion

Definition

Vascular obstruction at the level of the ophthalmic artery that affects both the retinal and choroidal circulation leading to ischemia more severe than CRAO.

Etiology

Usually due to emboli or thrombus but can be caused by any of the etiologies listed for CRAO.

Epidemiology

Usually occurs in elderly patients; associated with hypertension (67%), carotid occlusive disease (25%), diabetes mellitus (33%), and cardiac valvular disease (25%). CRAO more common (57%) than BRAO (38%) or cilioretinal artery occlusion (5%) (in 32% of eyes, a cilioretinal artery is present). Bilateral involvement rare.

Symptoms

Sudden, unilateral, painless, profound loss of vision up to the level of light perception or even no light perception.

Signs

Marked constriction of the retinal vessels; marked retinal edema often without a cherry-red spot (although it may be present); may have afferent pupillary defect; later, optic atrophy, retinal vascular sclerosis, and diffuse pigmentary changes.

Differential Diagnosis

Central retinal artery occlusion, commotio retinae, cherry-red spot due to inherited metabolic or lysosomal storage diseases.

Evaluation

- Complete ophthalmic history and eye examination with attention to pupils, 78/90 diopter or contact lens fundus examination, and ophthalmoscopy.
- Check blood pressure.
- **Lab tests:** Fasting blood glucose (FBS) and complete blood count (CBC) with differential; consider platelets, prothrombin time/partial thromboplastin time (PT/PTT), protein C, protein S, antithrombin III, homocysteine, antinuclear antibody (ANA), rheumatoid factor (RF), antiphospholipid antibody, serum protein electrophoresis, hemoglobin electrophoresis, Venereal Disease Research Laboratory (VDRL) test, and fluorescent treponemal antibody absorption (FTA-ABS) test. In patients >50 years old, check erythrocyte sedimentation rate (ESR) to rule out arteritic ischemic optic neuropathy.
- **Fluorescein angiogram:** Delayed or absent choroidal and retinal vascular filling, extensive capillary nonperfusion.
- **Electrophysiologic testing:** ERG (reduced a- and b-wave amplitudes).
- Medical consultation for complete cardiovascular evaluation including electrocardiogram, echocardiogram (may require transthoracic echocardiogram to rule out valvular disease), and carotid Doppler studies.

Management

OPHTHALMIC EMERGENCY

- Treatment controversial due to poor prognosis and questionable benefit of treatment.
- Treat immediately before starting workup (if patient presents within 24 hours of visual loss).
- Digital ocular massage to try and dislodge emboli.
- Systemic acetazolamide (Diamox 500 mg IV or po).
- Topical ocular hypotensive drops: β-blocker (timolol 0.5% 1 gtt q15min × 2, repeat as necessary).
- Anterior chamber paracentesis.
- Consider admission to hospital for carbogen treatment (95% oxygen, 5% carbon dioxide for 10 minutes q2h for 24-48 hours) to attempt to increase oxygenation and induce vasodilation.
- Unproven treatments include hyperbaric oxygen, antifibrinolytic drugs, retrobulbar vasodilators, and sublingual nitroglycerine.
- If arteritic ischemic optic neuropathy (see Chapter 11) is suspected: systemic steroids (methylprednisolone 1 g IV qd in divided doses for 3 days, then prednisone 60-100 mg po qd with a slow taper; decrease by no more than 2.5-5.0 mg/wk).

Prognosis

Severe visual loss is usually permanent.

Branch Retinal Vein Occlusion (BRVO)

Definition

Occlusion of a branch retinal vein (BRVO); usually caused by a thrombus at arteriovenous crossings where a thickened artery compresses the underlying venous wall.

Etiology

Associated with hypertension, coronary artery disease, diabetes mellitus, and peripheral vascular disease; rarely associated with hypercoagulable states (e.g., macroglobulinemia, cryoglobulinemia), hyperviscosity states (polycythemia vera, Waldenström's macroglobulinemia), systemic lupus erythematosus, syphilis, sarcoidosis, homocystinuria, malignancies (e.g., multiple myeloma, polycythemia vera, leukemia), optic nerve drusen, and external compression. In younger patients, associated with oral contraceptive pills, collagen-vascular disease, AIDS, protein S/protein C/antithrombin III deficiency, or activated protein C resistance (factor V Leiden polymerase chain reaction [PCR] assay).

Epidemiology

Usually seen in elderly patients, 60-70 years old; associated with hypertension (50-70%), cardiovascular disease, diabetes mellitus, increased body mass index, and open-angle glaucoma; slight male and hyperopic predilection. Two types: nonischemic (64%) and ischemic (defined as ≥5 disc areas of capillary nonperfusion on fluorescein angiography). Second most common vascular disease after diabetic retinopathy. Risk of another BRVO in same eye is 3% and in fellow eye is 12%.

Symptoms

Sudden, unilateral, painless, visual field defect. Patients may have normal vision, especially when macula is not involved.

Signs

Quadrantic visual field defect; dilated, tortuous retinal veins with superficial, retinal hemorrhages and cotton-wool spots in a wedge-shaped area radiating from an arteriovenous crossing (usually arterial overcrossing where an arteriole and venule share a common vascular sheath). More common superotemporally (60%) than inferotemporally (40%; rare nasally, since usually asymptomatic). The closer the obstruction is to the optic disc, the greater the area of retina involved and more serious the complications. Microaneurysms or macroaneurysms, macular edema (50%), epiretinal membranes (20%), retinal and/or iris or angle neovascularization (very rare), and vitreous hemorrhage may develop. Neovascular glaucoma is rare.

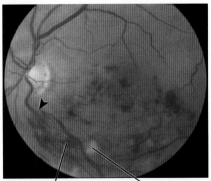

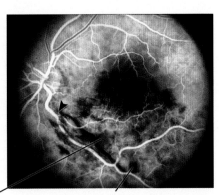

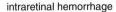
intraretinal hemorrhage   cotton-wool spots   intraretinal hemorrhage

Figure 10-16 • Inferior branch retinal vein occlusion demonstrating wedge-shaped area of intraretinal hemorrhages and cotton-wool spots.

Figure 10-17 • Fluorescein angiogram of same patient in Figure 10-16 demonstrating lack of perfusion in inferior retinal vein with blocking defects from the intraretinal hemorrhages. Arrowhead indicates site of occlusion.

Differential Diagnosis

Venous stasis retinopathy, ocular ischemic syndrome, hypertensive retinopathy, leukemic retinopathy, retinopathy of anemia, diabetic retinopathy, papilledema, papillophlebitis (in young patients).

Evaluation

- Complete ophthalmic history and eye examination with attention to pupils, tonometry, gonioscopy, 78/90 diopter or contact lens fundus examination, and ophthalmoscopy.
- Check visual fields.
- Check blood pressure.
- **Lab tests:** Fasting blood glucose, glycosylated hemoglobin; consider CBC with differential, platelets, PT/PTT, ANA, RF, angiotensin converting enzyme (ACE), ESR, serum protein electrophoresis, lipid profile, hemoglobin electrophoresis in blacks, sedimentation rate, VDRL and FTA-ABS, depending on clinical situation. In a patient <40 years old and in whom a hypercoagulable state is being considered: check human immunodeficiency virus (HIV) status, functional protein S assay, functional protein C assay, functional antithrombin III assay (type II heparin-binding mutation), antiphospholipid antibody titer, lupus anticoagulant, anticardiolipin antibody titer (IgG and IgM), homocysteine level (if elevated test for folate, B12, and creatinine), and activated protein C resistance (factor V Leiden PCR assay); if these tests are normal and clinical suspicion for a hypercoagulable state still exists: add plasminogen antigen assay, heparin cofactor II assay, thrombin time, reptilase time, and fibrinogen functional assay.
- **Fluorescein angiogram:** Delayed retinal venous filling in a branch of the central retinal vein, increased transit time in affected venous distribution, blocked fluorescence in areas of retinal hemorrhages, and capillary nonperfusion (ischemic defined as ≥5 disc areas of capillary nonperfusion) in the area supplied by the involved retinal vein. Retinal edema with cystic changes is not present acutely but appears later.
- Medical consultation for complete cardiovascular evaluation.

Management

- Quadrantic scatter laser photocoagulation (500 µm spots) when rubeosis (≥2 clock hours of iris or any angle neovascularization), disc or retinal neovascularization, or neovascular glaucoma develops (Branch Vein Occlusion Study [BVOS] conclusion); prophylactic laser was not evaluated in BVOS, but is not recommended.
- Macular grid/focal photocoagulation (50-100 µm spots) when macular edema lasts >3 months and vision is worse than 20/40 (BVOS conclusion).
- Experimental options include intravitreal 4mg triamcinolone acetonide [Kenalog] for macular edema and arteriovenous sheathotomy.
- Discontinue oral contraceptives.
- Consider aspirin (80-325 mg po qd).
- Treat underlying medical conditions.

Prognosis

Good; 50% have ≥20/40 vision unless foveal ischemia or chronic macular edema is present.

Central/Hemiretinal Vein Occlusion (CRVO/HRVO)

Definition

Occlusion of the central retinal vein (CRVO) usually caused by a thrombus in the area of the lamina cribrosa; hemiretinal occlusion (HRVO) occurs when the superior and inferior retinal drainage does not merge into a central retinal vein (20%) and is occluded (more like CRVO than BRVO).

Etiology

Associated with hypertension (60%), coronary artery disease, diabetes mellitus, peripheral vascular disease, and primary open-angle glaucoma (40%); rarely associated with hypercoagulable states (e.g., macroglobulinemia, cryoglobulinemia), hyperviscosity states especially in bilateral cases (polycythemia vera, Waldenström's macroglobulinemia), systemic lupus erythematosus, syphilis, sarcoidosis, homocystinuria, malignancies (e.g., multiple myeloma, polycythemia vera, leukemia), optic nerve drusen, and external compression. In younger patients, associated with oral contraceptive pills, collagen-vascular disease, AIDS, protein S/protein C/antithrombin III deficiency, or activated protein C resistance (factor V Leiden polymerase chain reaction [PCR] assay).

Epidemiology

Usually seen in elderly patients (90% are >50 years old); slight male predilection. Two types: nonischemic (67%) and ischemic (defined as ≥10 disc areas of capillary nonperfusion on fluorescein angiography). Ischemic disease is more common in patients with cardiovascular disease. Younger patients can get inflammatory condition, termed *papillophlebitis,* or benign retinal vasculitis with benign clinical course.

Symptoms

Sudden, unilateral loss of vision or less frequently history of transient obscuration of vision with complete recovery. Some report pain and present initially with neovascularization of the iris and neovascular glaucoma following a loss of vision 3 months earlier ("90-day glaucoma"). Patients may have normal vision, especially when macula is not involved.

Signs

Decreased visual acuity ranging from 20/20 to hand motion (HM) with most worse than 20/200; dilated, tortuous retinal veins with superficial, retinal hemorrhages, and cotton-wool spots in all four quadrants extending to periphery; optic disc hyperemia, disc edema, and macular edema common; positive relative afferent pupillary defect (RAPD), degree of defect correlates with amount of ischemia; ischemic disease can produce rubeosis (20% in CRVO, rare in BRVO), disc or retinal neovascularization (border of perfused/nonperfused retina), neovascular glaucoma, and vitreous hemorrhages. Collateral optociliary shunt vessels between retinal and ciliary circulations (50%) occur late. Impending CRVO may have absence of spontaneous venous pulsations (but this also occurs in normal individuals). Transient patchy ischemic retinal whitening may occur early in nonischemic CRVO.

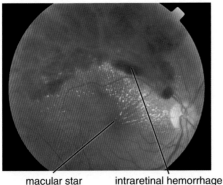

Figure 10-18 • Hemiretinal vein occlusion with exudates forming partial macular star.

macular star   intraretinal hemorrhage

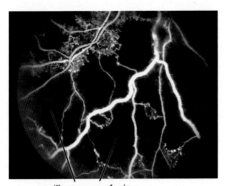

Figure 10-19 • Fluorescein angiogram of a patient with a retinal vein occlusion demonstrating peripheral capillary nonperfusion.

capillary nonperfusion

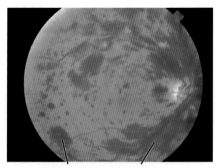

intraretinal hemorrhages

Figure 10-20 • Central retinal vein occlusion demonstrating hemorrhages in all four quadrants.

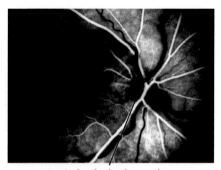

central retinal vein occulus

Figure 10-21 • Fluorescein angiogram demonstrating no filling of the central retinal vein.

Figure 10-22 • Optociliary shunt vessels in a patient with an old central retinal vein occlusion.

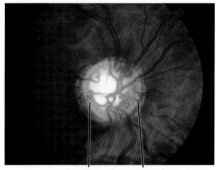

optociliary shunt vessels

Differential Diagnosis

Venous stasis retinopathy, ocular ischemic syndrome, hypertensive retinopathy, leukemic retinopathy, retinopathy of anemia, diabetic retinopathy, and papilledema.

Evaluation

- Complete ophthalmic history and eye examination with attention to pupils, tonometry, gonioscopy, 78/90 diopter or contact lens fundus examination, and ophthalmoscopy.
- Check blood pressure.
- **Lab tests:** Fasting blood glucose, glycosylated hemoglobin; consider CBC with differential, platelets, PT/PTT, ANA, RF, angiotensin converting enzyme (ACE), ESR, serum protein electrophoresis, lipid profile, hemoglobin electrophoresis in blacks, sedimentation rate, VDRL, and FTA-ABS, depending on clinical situation. In a patient <40 years old and in whom a hypercoagulable state is being considered: check HIV status, functional protein S assay, functional protein C assay, functional antithrombin III assay (type II heparin-binding mutation), antiphospholipid antibody titer, lupus anticoagulant,

anticardiolipin antibody titer (IgG and IgM), homocysteine level (if elevated test for folate, B12, and creatinine), and activated protein C resistance (factor V Leiden PCR assay); if these tests are normal and clinical suspicion for a hypercoagulable state still exists: add plasminogen antigen assay, heparin cofactor II assay, thrombin time, reptilase time, and fibrinogen functional assay.

• **Fluorescein angiogram:** Delayed retinal venous filling, increased transit time (>20 seconds increases risk of rubeosis), extensive capillary nonperfusion (ischemic defined as ≥10 disc areas of capillary nonperfusion), staining of vascular walls, and blocking defects due to retinal hemorrhages; retinal edema with cystic changes are not present acutely but appear later.

• **Electrophysiologic testing:** ERG (reduced b-wave amplitude, reduced b:a wave ratio [<1 associated with increased risk of ischemia and neovascularization], prolonged b-wave implicit time).

• Medical consultation for complete cardiovascular evaluation.

Management

• Panretinal laser photocoagulation (PRP) (500 μm spots) when rubeosis (≥2 clock hours of iris or any angle neovascularization), disc or retinal neovascularization, or neovascular glaucoma develops; no benefit to prophylactic PRP (Central Retinal Vein Occlusion Study [CVOS] conclusion).

• Focal laser photocoagulation decreases macular edema but has no effect on visual acuity (CVOS conclusion); trend in CVOS for focal laser to work in younger patients. Experimentally, intravitreal 4 mg triamcinolone acetonide [Kenalog] has been shown to decrease macular edema and transiently improve visual acuity.

• Creation of chorioretinal venous anastomosis by intentional rupture of Bruch's membrane with high intensity laser photocoagulation or surgical blade is successful in one third of cases but still experimental.

• Other experimental surgical options include radial optic neurotomy (RON), intravenous injection of tissue plasminogen activator (tPA) into the lumen of the central retinal vein, and intravitreal 4 mg triamcinolone acetonide (Kenalog).

• Discontinue oral contraceptives and change diuretics to an alternate antihypertensive.

• Consider aspirin (80-325 mg po qd).

• Treat underlying medical conditions.

Prognosis

Clinical course is variable; evaluate monthly for first 6 months. Nonischemic has better prognosis. Risk of neovascularization depends on amount of ischemia (CVOS conclusion); two thirds of patients with ischemic disease develop neovascular complications; one third of nonischemic patients develop ischemic disease, especially older patients.

▌ Venous Stasis Retinopathy

Milder form of nonischemic central retinal vein occlusion (CRVO) representing patients with better perfusion; dot/blot/flame hemorrhages, dilated/tortuous vasculature, and microaneurysms are seen, usually bilateral; more benign course; associated with hyper-viscosity syndromes including polycythemia vera, multiple myeloma, and Waldenström's macroglobulinemia.

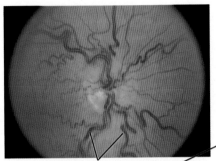

dilated, tortuous vasculature

Figure 10-23 • Dilated, tortuous, retinal vessels in a patient with hyperviscosity syndrome.

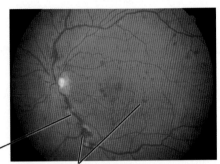

intraretinal hemorrhages

Figure 10-24 • Intraretinal hemorrhages in a patient with venous stasis retinopathy.

Ocular Ischemic Syndrome

Definition

Widespread ischemia of the eye due to ipsilateral carotid occlusive disease (less frequently, obstruction of the ipsilateral ophthalmic artery).

Etiology

Ninety percent or greater occlusion of ipsilateral carotid artery or rarely ophthalmic artery.

Epidemiology

Usually seen in patients 50-70 years old; 80% unilateral; male predilection (2:1); associated with atherosclerosis, heart disease, hypertension, and diabetes mellitus.

Symptoms

Gradual loss of vision (90%) over weeks with accompanying dull eye pain or headache (40%); patients may also report amaurosis fugax or a prolonged recovery of vision after exposure to bright light.

Signs

Decreased visual acuity ranging from 20/20 to no light perception (NLP); retinal arterial narrowing and venous dilation without tortuosity, retinal hemorrhages (80% midperipheral), microaneurysms, cotton-wool spots, disc or retinal neovascularization (37%), and spontaneous pulsations of the retinal arteries; anterior segment signs including episcleral injection, corneal edema, anterior chamber (AC) cells and flare, iris atrophy, and rubeosis (66%) are common. Intraocular pressure may be elevated.

Differential Diagnosis

CRVO, venous stasis retinopathy, diabetic retinopathy, hypertensive retinopathy, aortic arch disease.

Evaluation

- Complete ophthalmic history and eye examination with attention to pupils, tonometry, anterior chamber, gonioscopy, 78/90 diopter or contact lens fundus examination, and ophthalmoscopy.
- Check blood pressure.
- **Fluorescein angiogram:** Delayed or patchy choroidal filling, arterial vascular staining, and increased arteriovenous transit time.
- **Electrophysiologic testing:** ERG (reduced or absent a-wave and b-wave amplitude).
- Medical consultation for complete cardiovascular evaluation including duplex and Doppler scans of carotid arteries: (≥90% obstruction of the ipsilateral internal or common carotid arteries).

Management

- Panretinal laser photocoagulation (PRP) (500 μm spots) when anterior or posterior segment neovascularization develops.
- Consider carotid endarterectomy if carotid obstruction exists; more beneficial if performed before rubeosis develops.
- Ocular hypotensive (glaucoma) medications if elevated intraocular pressure present.

Prognosis

Poor prognosis; 5-year mortality rate is 40% with the leading cause of death being cardiovascular disease. 60% of patients have count fingers or worse vision at 1-year follow-up; only 25% have better than 20/50 vision.

▮ Retinopathy of Prematurity (ROP)

Definition

Abnormal retinal vasculature development in premature infants, especially after supplemental oxygen therapy.

Epidemiology

Premature birth (<36 weeks' gestation), low birth weight (<750 g: 90% develop ROP and 16% develop threshold disease; 1000-1250 g: 45% develop ROP and 2% develop threshold disease), supplemental oxygen therapy (>50 days), and a complicated hospital course.

Symptoms

Asymptomatic; later may have decreased vision; may notice white pupil and/or eye turn.

Signs

Shallow anterior chamber, corneal edema, iris atrophy, poor pupillary dilation, posterior synechiae, ectropion uveae, leukocoria, vitreous hemorrhage, retinal detachment, and retrolental fibroplasia. Usually bilateral.

International classification of ROP describes the retinal changes in five stages:

Stage 1   Thin, circumferential, flat, white, demarcation line develops between posterior vascularized and peripheral avascular retina (beyond line).

Stage 2   Demarcation line becomes elevated and organized into a pink-white ridge; no fibrovascular growth seen.

Stage 3   Extraretinal fibrovascular proliferation from surface of the ridge.

Stage 4   Dragging of vessels and subtotal traction retinal detachment (4A is macula attached; 4B involves macula).

Stage 5   Total retinal detachment (almost always funnel detachment).

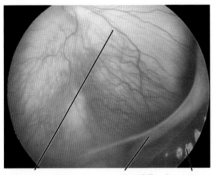

dragged vessels   traction RD   laser spots

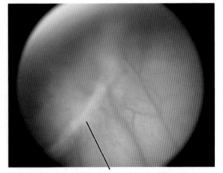

extraretinal fibrovascular proliferation

Figure 10-25 • Retinopathy of prematurity (ROP) demonstrating dragged vessels, traction retinal detachment, and laser spots anterior to the regressed fibrovascular proliferation (stage 4a ROP).

Figure 10-26 • Retinopathy of prematurity (ROP) demonstrating extraretinal fibrovascular proliferation along the ridge (stage 3 ROP).

International classification of ROP also describes the extent of retina involved by number of clock hours and location by zone (centered on optic disc, not the fovea, because retinal vessels emanate from disc).

Zone 1   Inner zone (posterior pole) corresponding to the area enclosed by a circle around the optic disc with radius equal to twice the distance from the disc to the macula (diameter of 60 degrees).

Zone 2   The area between zone 1 and a circle centered on the optic disc and tangent to the nasal ora serrata.

Zone 3   Remaining temporal crescent of retina (last area to become vascularized). Finally, international classification of ROP defines "plus" disease:

"Plus" disease   Shunted blood causes vascular engorgement in the posterior pole, with tortuous arteries, dilated veins, pupillary rigidity due to iris vascular engorgement, and vitreous haze.

Differential Diagnosis

Coats' disease, Eales' disease, familial exudative vitreoretinopathy, sickle cell retinopathy, juvenile retinoschisis, persistent hyperplastic primary vitreous, incontinentia pigmenti (Bloch-Sulzberger syndrome), and leukocoria (see Chapter 7).

Evaluation

- Screen all premature infants at 4-6 weeks' chronologic age who weighed <1250-1750 g at birth, as well as larger premature infants on supplemental oxygen for >50 days.
- Complete ophthalmic history with attention to birth history and birth weight.
- Complete eye examination with attention to iris, lens, and ophthalmoscopy (retinal vasculature and retinal periphery with scleral depression).
- Pediatric consultation.

Management

- Treat with ablation of avascular retina when patient reaches "threshold" disease defined as stage 3 plus disease with at least five contiguous or eight noncontiguous, cumulative clock hours involvement in zone 1 or 2.
- Indirect argon green or diode laser photocoagulation (500 μm spots) to entire avascular retina in zone 1 and peripheral zone 2; laser is at least as effective as cryotherapy (Laser-ROP study conclusion) or
- Cryotherapy to entire avascular retina in zone 2, but not ridge (Cryotherapy for ROP [CRYO-ROP] study conclusion)
- Tractional retinal detachment or rhegmatogenous retinal detachment (cicatricial ROP, stages 4 and 5) require vitreoretinal surgery with pars plana vitrectomy, with or without lensectomy, membrane peel, and possible scleral buckle; should be performed by a retina specialist trained in pediatric retinal disease.
- Follow very closely (every 1-2 weeks depending on location and severity of the disease) until extreme periphery is vascularized, then monthly thereafter. Beware of "rush" disease, defined as plus disease in zone 1 or posterior zone 2. "Rush" disease has a significant risk of rapid progression to stage 5 within a few days.

Prognosis

Depends on the amount and stage of ROP; 80-90% will spontaneously regress; may develop amblyopia, macular dragging, strabismus; stage 5 disease carries a poor prognosis (functional success in only 3%); may develop high myopia, glaucoma, cataracts, keratoconus, band keratopathy, and retinal detachment.

Coats' Disease/Leber's Miliary Aneurysms

Unilateral (80%), idiopathic, progressive, developmental retinal vascular abnormality (telangiectatic and aneurysmal vessels with a predilection for the macula); usually occurs in young males (10:1) <20 years old. Retinal microaneurysms (MA), lipid exudation, "light-bulb" vascular dilations, capillary nonperfusion, and occasionally neovascularization are seen primarily in the temporal quadrants, especially on fluorescein angiogram where micro-aneurysm leakage is common. May present with poor vision, strabismus, or leukocoria. Spectrum of disease, from milder form seen in older patients with equal sex predilection and often bilateral (Leber's miliary aneurysms) to severe form with localized exudative retinal detachments and yellowish subretinal masses; included in the differential diagnosis of leuko-coria (Coats' disease). Clinical course varies but generally progressive. Rarely associated with systemic disorders including Alport's disease, fascioscapulohumeral dystrophy, muscular dystrophy, tuberous sclerosis, Turner's syndrome, and Senior-Loken syndrome.

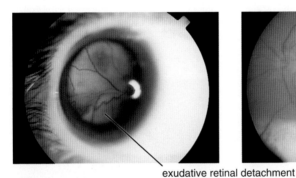 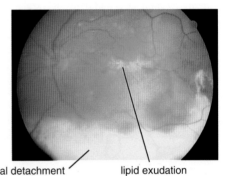

exudative retinal detachment   lipid exudation

Figure 10-27 • Coats' disease demonstrating leukocoria due to exudative retinal detachment.

Figure 10-28 • Coats' disease with massive exudative retinal detachment.

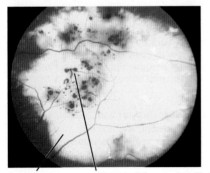 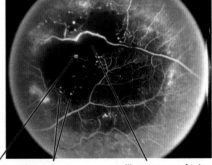

lipid exudate   "light-bulb" vascular dilations   microaneurysms   capillary non-perfusion

Figure 10-29 • Leber's miliary aneurysms demonstrating dilated arterioles with terminal "light bulbs."

Figure 10-30 • Fluorescein angiogram of same patient as Figure 10-29 demonstrating capillary nonperfusion, microaneurysms, and "light-bulb" vascular dilations. Note line points to same site in both pictures.

- **Fluorescein angiogram:** Capillary nonperfusion, microaneurysms, light-bulb vascular dilations, leakage from telangiectatic vessels, and macular edema.
- Scatter laser photocoagulation to posterior or cryotherapy to anterior areas of abnormal vasculature and areas of nonperfusion when symptomatic. May require multiple treatment sessions. Goal is to ablate areas of vascular leakage and to allow resorption of exudate.

Eales' Disease

Bilateral, idiopathic, peripheral obliterative vasculopathy seen in healthy, young adults 20-30 years old; male predilection. Patients usually notice floaters and decreased vision and have areas of perivascular sheathing, vitreous cells, peripheral retinal nonperfusion, microaneurysms, intraretinal hemorrhages, white sclerotic ghost vessels, disc (NVD)/iris (NVI)/retinal (NVE) neovascularization, and vitreous hemorrhages. Fibrovascular proliferation may lead to tractional retinal detachments. May have signs of ocular inflammation with keratic precipitates, anterior chamber cells and flare, and cystoid macular edema; variable prognosis. Diagnosis of exclusion. Must exclude other causes of inflammation or neovascularization including BRVO, diabetic retinopathy, sickle cell retinopathy, multiple sclerosis, sarcoidosis, tuberculosis, SLE, and other collagen-vascular diseases.

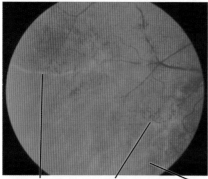 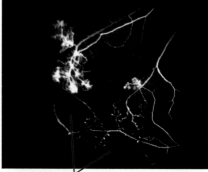

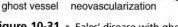
ghost vessel   neovascularization   peripheral non-perfusion

Figure 10-31 • Eales' disease with ghost vessels, peripheral capillary nonperfusion, and neovascularization.

Figure 10-32 • Fluorescein angiogram of patient with Eales' disease demonstrating extensive peripheral nonperfusion and neovascularization.

- **Fluorescein angiogram:** Midperipheral retinal nonperfusion with well-demarcated boundary between perfused and nonperfused areas; microaneurysms and neovascularization.
- Scatter laser photocoagulation to nonperfused retina when neovascularization develops. If vitreous hemorrhage obscures view of retina, peripheral cryotherapy can be applied to ablate peripheral avascular retina.
- Consider periocular or systemic steroids for inflammatory component.

Idiopathic Juxtafoveal Retinal Telangiectasia (JXT)

Group of retinal vascular disorders with abnormal perifoveal capillaries confined to the juxtafoveal region (1-199 μm from center of fovea). Several forms:

Type 1A (Unilateral Congenital Parafoveal Telangiectasia)

Seen in men 40-50 years old; yellow exudate seen at outer edge of telangiectasis usually temporal to the fovea and one to two disc diameters in area; decreased vision ranging from 20/25 to 20/40 from macular edema and exudate. May represent mild presentation of Coats' disease in an adult.

- **Fluorescein angiogram:** Unilateral cluster of telangiectatic vessels with variable leakage; macular edema often with petalloid leakage.
- Consider focal laser photocoagulation to leaking, nonsubfoveal vessels.

Type 1B (Unilateral Idiopathic Parafoveal Telangiectasia)

Seen in middle-aged men; minimal exudate usually confined to one clock hour at the edge of the foveal avascular zone; usually asymptomatic with vision better than 20/25.

- **Fluorescein angiogram:** Unilateral cluster of telangiectatic vessels with variable leakage; macular edema often with petalloid leakage.
- No treatment recommended.

Type 2 (Bilateral Acquired Parafoveal Telangiectasia)

Onset of symptoms in the fifth to sixth decades with equal sex distribution; symmetric, bilateral, right-angle venules within one disc diameter of the central fovea; usually found temporal to the fovea but may surround the fovea; mild blurring of central vision early, slowly progressive loss of central vision over years; blunting or grayish discoloration of the foveal reflex, right-angle retinal venules, and characteristic stellate retinal pigment epithelial hyperplasia/atrophy; leakage from telangiectatic vessels, but no exudates; associated with choroidal neovascular membranes (CNV), hemorrhagic macular detachments, and retinochoroidal anastomosis. May be caused by chronic venous stasis in the macula from unknown reasons.

- **Fluorescein angiogram:** Bilateral, right-angle venules with variable leakage; macular edema often with petalloid leakage; choroidal neovascularization can develop.
- No treatment recommended unless CNV develops because focal laser photocoagulation to leaking, nonsubfoveal vessels does not prevent visual loss.
- Consider focal laser photocoagulation of juxtafoveal and extrafoveal CNV, and photodynamic therapy (PDT) for subfoveal CNV (experimental).

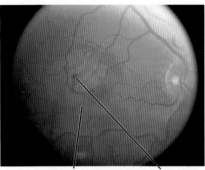

RPE hyperplasia   intraretinal hemorrhage   vascular leakage

Figure 10-33 • Juxtafoveal telangiectasia type 2 with abnormal foveal reflex, intraretinal hemorrhages and retinal pigment epithelium (RPE) changes.

Figure 10-34 • Fluorescein angiogram of patient shown in Figure 10-33 demonstrating hyperfluorescent leakage from telangiectatic vessels and blockage from the hemorrhages.

Type 3 (Bilateral Perifoveal Telangiectasis with Capillary Obliteration)

Rare form; seen in adults in the fifth decade; slowly progressive loss of vision due to the marked aneurysmal dilation and obliteration of the perifoveal telangiectatic capillary network; no leakage from telangiectasis; associated with optic nerve pallor, hyperactive deep tendon reflexes, and other central nervous system symptoms.

• **Fluorescein angiogram:** Aneurysmal dilation of capillary bed with minimal to no leakage; extensive, progressive macular capillary nonperfusion, choroidal neovascularization can develop.
• No treatment recommended unless CNV develops.
• Consider focal laser photocoagulation of juxtafoveal and extrafoveal CNV, and photo-dynamic therapy (PDT) for subfoveal CNV (experimental).
• Neurology consultation to rule out central nervous system disease.

Retinopathies Associated with Blood Abnormalities

Retinopathy of Anemia

Superficial, flame-shaped, intraretinal hemorrhages, cotton-wool spots, and rarely exudates, retinal edema, and vitreous hemorrhage in patients with anemia (hemoglobin <8 g/100 mL). Retinopathy is worse when associated with thrombocytopenia. Roth spots are seen in pernicious anemia and aplastic anemia.

• Resolves with treatment of anemia.
• Medical or hematology consultation.

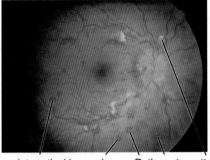

intraretinal hemorrhage   Roth spots cotton-wool spots   flame hemorrhage

Figure 10-35 • Retinopathy of anemia demonstrating intraretinal hemorrhage, cotton-wool spots, and Roth spots.

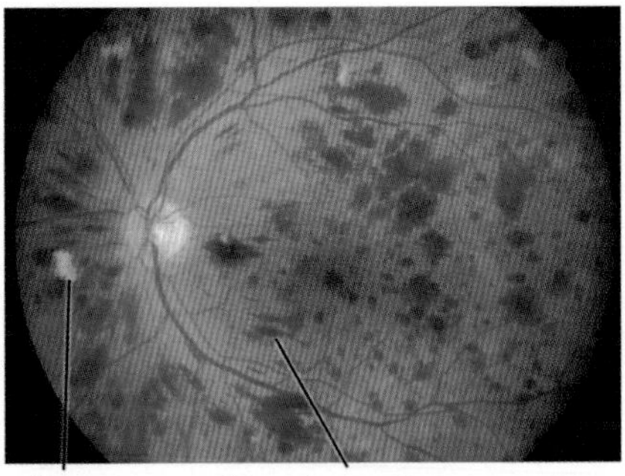

Figure 10-36 • Retinopathy of anemia demonstrating intraretinal hemorrhage and cotton-wool spots.

Leukemic Retinopathy

Ocular involvement in leukemia is common (80%). Patients are usually asymptomatic. Characterized by superficial, flame-shaped, intraretinal (24%), preretinal, and vitreous hemorrhages (2%), microaneurysms, Roth spots (11%), cotton-wool spots (16%), dilated/tortuous vessels, perivascular sheathing, and disc edema; rarely, direct leukemic infiltrates (3%); direct choroidal involvement appears with choroidal infiltrates, choroidal thickening, and an overlying serous retinal detachment. Sea fan–shaped retinal neovascularization can occur late. Retinopathy is due to the associated anemia, thrombocytopenia, and hyperviscosity. Opportunistic infections are also seen in patients with leukemia but are not considered part of leukemic retinopathy.

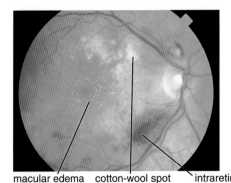

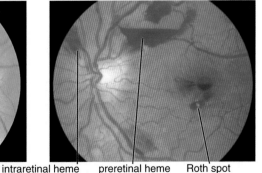

macular edema   cotton-wool spot   intraretinal heme   preretinal heme   Roth spot

Figure 10-37 • Leukemic retinopathy with macular edema, cotton-wool spots, and intraretinal hemorrhages.

Figure 10-38 • Leukemic retinopathy with intraretinal and preretinal hemorrhages, cotton-wool spots, and Roth spots.

- **Lab tests:** CBC, platelets, bone marrow biopsy.
- Resolves with treatment of underlying hematologic abnormality.
- Treat direct leukemic infiltrates with systemic chemotherapy to control the underlying problem and/or ocular radiation therapy if systemic therapy fails; should be performed by an experienced tumor specialist.
- Medical or oncology consultation.

Sickle Cell Retinopathy

Nonproliferative and proliferative vascular changes due to the sickling hemoglobinopathies. Results from mutations in hemoglobin (Hb) where the valine is substituted for glutamate at the 6th position in the polypeptide chain (linked to 11p15), altering Hb conformation and deformability in erythrocytes. This leads to poor flow through capillaries. Proliferative changes (response to retinal ischemia) are more common with Hb SC (most severe) and Hb SThal variants; Hb SS associated with angioid streaks; Hb AS and Hb AC mutations rarely cause ocular manifestations; patients are usually asymptomatic, but may have decreased vision, visual field defects, floaters, photopsias, scotomas, and dyschromatopsia; more common in people of African and Mediterranean descent. Follows orderly progression.

Stage I   Background (nonproliferative) stage with venous tortuosity, "salmon patch" hemorrhages (pink intraretinal hemorrhages), iridescent spots (schisis cavity with refractile elements), cotton-wool spots, hairpin vascular loops, macular infarction, angioid streaks, black "sunburst" chorioretinal scars, comma-shaped conjunctival and optic nerve head vessels, and peripheral arteriole occlusions.

Stage II   Arteriovenous (AV) anastomosis stage with peripheral "silver-wire" vessels and shunt vessels between arterioles and medium-sized veins at border of perfused and non-perfused retina.

Stage III   Neovascular (proliferative) stage with sea-fan peripheral neovascularization (spontaneously regresses in 60% of cases due to autoinfarction); sea-fans grow along retinal surface in a circumferential pattern and have a predilection for superotemporal quadrant (develops approximately 18 months after formation of AV anastomosis).

Stage IV   Vitreous hemorrhage stage with vitreous traction bands contracting around the sea-fans, causing vitreous hemorrhages (most common in SC variant, 21-23%; SS, 2-3%).

Stage V   Retinal detachment stage with tractional and rhegmatogenous retinal detachments from contraction of the vitreous traction bands.

- **Lab tests:** Sickle cell prep, hemoglobin electrophoresis (hemoglobin C disease and sickle cell trait may have negative sickle cell prep).
- **Fluorescein angiogram:** Capillary nonperfusion near hairpin loops, enlarged foveal avascular zone, peripheral nonperfusion, arteriovenous anastomosis, and sea-fan neovascularization.
- When active peripheral neovascularization develops, scatter laser photocoagulation (500 μm spots) to nonperfused retina.
- If neovascularization persists, then complete panretinal photocoagulation and consider adding direct laser photocoagulation to neovascularization or feeder vessels (increases risk of complications, including vitreous hemorrhage).
- The use of triple freeze-thaw cryotherapy for peripheral neovascularization is controversial; should be performed by a retinal specialist.

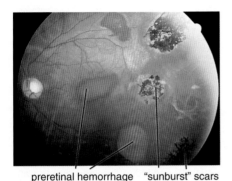

preretinal hemorrhage   "sunburst" scars

Figure 10-39 • Nonproliferative sickle cell retinopathy demonstrating salmon patch hemorrhages, iridescent spots, and black sunbursts.

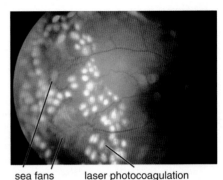

sea fans   laser photocoagulation

Figure 10-40 • Proliferative sickle cell retinopathy demonstrating sea-fans following laser treatment.

- Retinal surgery for traction retinal detachment and nonclearing, vitreous hemorrhage (>6 months); should be performed by a retinal specialist; consider exchange transfusion preoperatively (controversial); avoid scleral buckling to prevent ocular ischemia.
- Medical or hematology consultation.

Diabetic Retinopathy (DR)

Definition

Retinal vascular complication of diabetes mellitus classified into nonproliferative (NPDR) and proliferative (PDR) forms.

Epidemiology

Leading cause of blindness in US population 20-64 years old.

Insulin-Dependent Diabetes (IDDM; type I)

Juvenile onset, usually occurs before 30 years of age; most patients are free of retinopathy during first 5 years after diagnosis; 95% of patients with IDDM get DR after 15 years; 72% will develop PDR, and 42% will develop CSME; severity worsens with increasing duration of diabetes mellitus.

Non-Insulin-Dependent Diabetes (NIDDM; type II)

Adult onset, usually diagnosed after 30 years of age; more common form (90%) with optimal control without insulin; DR commonly exists at the time of diagnosis (60%) in NIDDM, with 3% having PDR or CSME at diagnosis of diabetes; 30% will have retinopathy in 5 years and 80% in 15 years. Risk of DR increases with hypertension, chronic hyperglycemia, renal disease, hyperlipidemia, and pregnancy.

Symptoms

Asymptomatic, may have decreased or fluctuating vision. Advanced retinopathy can lead to complete blindness.

Signs

Nonproliferative Diabetic Retinopathy (NPDR)

Grading of NPDR (Box 10-1) and risk of progression to PDR depends on the amount and location of hard and soft exudates, intraretinal hemorrhages, microaneurysms (MA), venous beading and loops, and intraretinal microvascular abnormalities (IRMA). Cotton-wool spots, dot and blot hemorrhages, posterior subcapsular cataracts, and induced myopia or hyperopia (from lens swelling due to high blood sugar) are common. Usually bilateral.

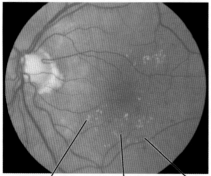

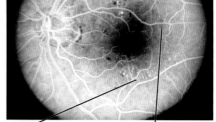

lipid exudate dot hemorrhage   microaneurysm   dot hemorrhage

Figure 10-41 • Moderate nonproliferative diabetic retinopathy with intraretinal hemorrhages, microaneurysms, and lipid exudate.

Figure 10-42 • Fluorescein angiogram of same patient as Figure 10-41 demonstrating tiny blocking defects from the intraretinal hemorrhages and spots of hyperfluorescence due to microaneurysms.

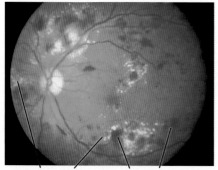

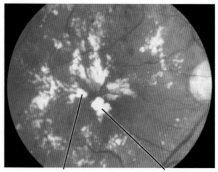

lipid exudate   intraretinal hemorrhages   diffuse macular edema and exudate

Figure 10-43 • Severe nonproliferative diabetic retinopathy with extensive hemorrhages, microaneurysms, and exudates.

Figure 10-44 • Severe nonproliferative diabetic retinopathy with diffuse macular edema and lipid exudate.

Proliferative Diabetic Retinopathy (PDR)

Findings of NPDR often present in addition to neovascularization of the disc (NVD) or elsewhere in the retina (NVE), preretinal and vitreous hemorrhages, fibrovascular proliferation on posterior vitreous surface or extending into the vitreous cavity, and tractional retinal detachments; may develop neovascularization of the iris (NVI) and subsequent neovascular glaucoma (NVG). Usually asymmetric but eventually bilateral.

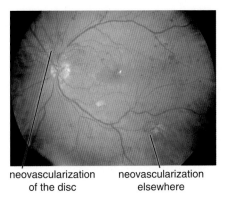

neovascularization   neovascularization
  of the disc   elsewhere

Figure 10-45 • Proliferative diabetic retinopathy demonstrating florid neovascularization of the disc and elsewhere.

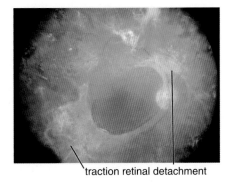

traction retinal detachment

Figure 10-46 • Proliferative diabetic retinopathy demonstrating neovascularization, fibrosis, and traction retinal detachment.

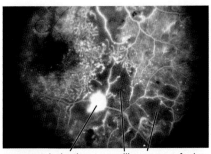

neovascularization   capillary nonperfusion

Figure 10-47 • Fluorescein angiogram of a patient with proliferative diabetic retinopathy showing extensive capillary nonperfusion, neovascularization elsewhere, and vascular leakage.

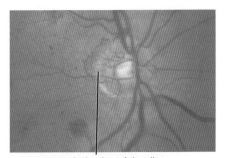

neovascularization of the disc

Figure 10-48 • Proliferative diabetic retinopathy demonstrating neovascularization of the disc.

Differential Diagnosis

Hypertensive retinopathy, CRVO, BRVO, ocular ischemic syndrome, radiation retinopathy, retinopathy associated with blood disorders, Eales' disease.

Evaluation

- Complete ophthalmic history and eye examination with attention to tonometry, gonioscopy (NVG), iris (NVI), lens, 78/90 diopter or contact lens fundus examination, and ophthalmoscopy (retinal vascular abnormalities, optic disc [NVD], and midperiphery [NVE]).
  - IDDM (type I): examine 5 years after onset of diabetes mellitus, then annually if no retinopathy is seen.
  - NIDDM (type II): examine at diagnosis of diabetes mellitus, then annually if no retinopathy is seen.
  - During pregnancy: examine before pregnancy, each trimester, and 3-6 months postpartum.
- **Lab tests:** Fasting blood glucose, hemoglobin A_1C, blood urea nitrogen (BUN), and creatinine
- **Fluorescein angiogram:** Capillary nonperfusion, microaneurysms, macular edema, and disc or retinal neovascularization.
- **Optical coherence tomography:** Increased retinal thickness, cysts, and subretinal fluid in cases of macular edema; can highlight the presence of posterior hyaloidal traction and traction macular detachment.
- **B-scan ultrasonography:** Used to rule out tractional retinal detachment in eyes when dense vitreous hemorrhage obscures view of fundus.
- Medical consultation with attention to blood pressure, cardiovascular system, renal status, and glycemic control.

Management

- Tight control of blood glucose levels (Diabetes Control and Complications Trial [DCCT] conclusion for type I diabetics and United Kingdom Prospective Diabetes Study [UKPDS] conclusion for type II diabetics).
- Tight blood pressure control (UKPDS conclusion for type II diabetics).
- Laser photocoagulation using transpupillary delivery and argon green (focal/panretinal photocoagulation) or krypton red laser (panretinal photocoagulation when vitreous hemorrhage or cataract is present), depending on stage of diabetic retinopathy:
- **Clinically significant macular edema (CSME; see Box 10-1):** macular grid photocoagulation (50-100 μm spots) to areas of diffuse leakage and focal treatment to focal leaks regardless of visual acuity (Early Treatment Diabetic Retinopathy Study [ETDRS] conclusion). If foveal avascular zone is enlarged (macular ischemia) on fluorescein angiography, then light treatment away from the foveal ischemia can be considered.
- **High-risk (HR) PDR (see Box 10-1):** scatter panretinal photocoagulation (PRP), 1200-1600 burns, one burn width apart (500 μm gray-white spots) in two or three sessions (Diabetic Retinopathy Study [DRS] conclusion). Treat inferior and nasal quadrants first to allow further treatment in case of subsequent vitreous hemorrhage during treatment and to avoid worsening macular edema.
- Additional indications for panretinal photocoagulation: rubeosis, neovascular glaucoma, widespread retinal ischemia on fluorescein angiogram, NVE alone in IDDM, poor patient compliance, and severe NPDR in a fellow eye or patient with poor outcome in first eye.

Management—cont'd

- Patients approaching high-risk PDR should have focal treatment to macular edema before panretinal photocoagulation to avoid worsening of macular edema with PRP; if high-risk characteristics exist, do not delay panretinal photocoagulation for focal treatment.
- Pars plana vitrectomy, endolaser, and removal of any fibrovascular complexes in patients with nonclearing vitreous hemorrhage for 6 months or vitreous hemorrhage for >1 month in IDDM (diabetic retinopathy vitrectomy study [DRVS] conclusions); other indications for vitreoretinal surgery include monocular patient with vitreous hemorrhage, bilateral vitreous hemorrhage, diabetic macular edema due to posterior hyaloidal traction, tractional retinal detachment (TRD) with rhegmatogenous component, TRD involving macula, progressive fibrovascular proliferation despite complete PRP, dense premacular hemorrhage or if ocular media are not clear enough for adequate view of fundus to perform PRP; should be performed by a retina specialist.
- Experimental pharmaceutical treatments for refractory, diffuse macular edema include posterior sub-Tenon's injection of 40 mg triamcinolone acetonide, intravitreal 4 mg triamcinolone acetonide, Bausch and Lomb's Retisert sustained-release (1000 day) implant with fluocinolone acetonide, Occulex biodegradable dexamethasone implant, protein kinase C-β inhibitors, and intravitreal antivascular endothelial growth factors (VEGF) injections.
- Experimental surgical treatment of refractory, diffuse macular edema includes pars plana vitrectomy with peeling of posterior hyaloid with or without removal of the internal limiting membrane especially with the presence of a taut, posterior hyaloid exerting traction on the macula.

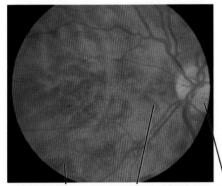 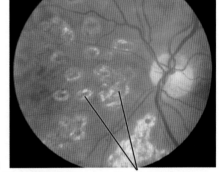

neovascularization elsewhere   neovascularization of the disc   laser spots

Figure 10-49 • Proliferative diabetic retinopathy before laser treatment.

Figure 10-50 • Same patient as Figure 10-49 demonstrating quiescent proliferative diabetic retinopathy following panretinal photocoagulation. Note absence of neovascularization.

Box 10-1   Diabetic Retinopathy Definitions

Clinically significant macular edema (CSME)

Retinal thickening ≤500 μm from center of fovea *or*
Hard exudates ≤500 μm from center of fovea with adjacent thickening *or*
Retinal thickening ≥1 disc area in size ≤1 disc diameter from center of fovea

High-risk (HR) characteristics of proliferative diabetic retinopathy (PDR)

Neovascularization of the disc (NVD) ≥ standard photo 10A used in DRS (one quarter to one
   third disc area) *or*
Any NVD *and* vitreous hemorrhage (VH) or preretinal hemorrhage *or*
Neovascularization elsewhere (NVE) ≥ standard photo 7 (one half disc area) *and* VH or
   preretinal hemorrhage

Severe nonproliferative diabetic retinopathy (NPDR) 4:2:1 rule

Diffuse intraretinal hemorrhages and microaneurysms in 4 quadrants *or*
Venous beading in 2 quadrants *or*
Intraretinal microvascular abnormalities (IRMA) in 1 quadrant

Prognosis

Early treatment allows better control. Prognosis is good for NPDR without CSME. After
adequate treatment, diabetic retinopathy often becomes quiescent for extended periods. Focal
laser photocoagulation improves vision in 17% of cases (ETDRS conclusion). Complications
include cataracts (often posterior subcapsular) and neovascular glaucoma.

Hypertensive Retinopathy

Definition

Retinal vascular changes secondary to chronic or acutely (malignant) elevated systemic blood
pressure.

Epidemiology

Hypertension defined as blood pressure >140/90 mm Hg; 60 million Americans over 18 years
of age have hypertension; more prevalent in blacks.

Symptoms

Asymptomatic; rarely, decreased vision.

Signs

Retinal arteriole narrowing and straightening, copper or silver-wire arteriole changes (arteriolosclerosis), arteriovenous crossing changes (nicking), cotton-wool spots, microaneurysms, flame hemorrhages, hard exudates (may be in a circinate or macular star pattern), Elschnig spots (yellow [early] or hyperpigmented [late] patches of retinal pigment epithelium overlying infarcted choriocapillaris lobules), Siegrist streaks (linear hyperpigmented areas over choroidal vessels), arterial macroaneurysms, and disc hyperemia or edema with dilated tortuous vessels (in malignant hypertension).

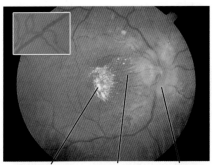

macular star   retinal folds   disc edema

Figure 10-51 • Hypertensive retinopathy with disc edema, macular star, and retinal folds in a patient with acute, malignant hypertension. Inset shows arteriovenous nicking.

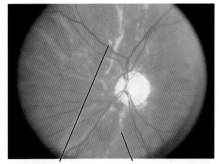

Elschnig spots   Siegrist streaks

Figure 10-52 • Hypertensive retinopathy demonstrating attenuated arterioles, choroidal ischemia, Elschnig spots, and Siegrist streaks.

Differential Diagnosis

Diabetic retinopathy, radiation retinopathy, vein occlusion, leukemic retinopathy, retinopathy of anemia, collagen-vascular disease.

Evaluation

* Complete ophthalmic history and eye examination with attention to 78/90 diopter or contact lens fundus examination and ophthalmoscopy (retinal vasculature and arteriovenous crossings).
* Check blood pressure.
* **Fluorescein angiogram:** Retinal arteriole narrowing and straightening, microaneurysms, capillary nonperfusion, and macular edema.
* Medical consultation with attention to cardiovascular and cerebrovascular systems.

Management

* Treat underlying hypertension.

Prognosis

Usually good.

Toxemia of Pregnancy

Severe hypertension, proteinuria, edema (preeclampsia), and seizures (eclampsia) seen in 2-5% of obstetric patients in the third trimester; patients have decreased vision, photopsias, and floaters usually just before or after delivery; signs include focal arteriolar narrowing, cotton-wool spots, retinal hemorrhages, hard exudates, Elschnig spots (RPE changes from choroidal infarction), bullous exudative retinal detachments, neovascularization, and disc edema; all due to hypertensive-related changes.

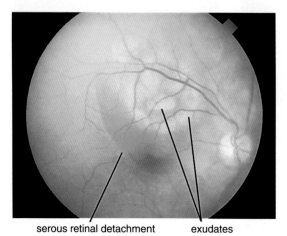

Figure 10-53 • Toxemia of pregnancy with serous retinal detachment and yellow-white patches.

serous retinal detachment   exudates

- **Fluorescein angiogram:** Poor choroidal filling, capillary nonperfusion, optic disc leakage, and neovascularization.
- Usually resolves without sequelae after treating hypertension and delivery.
- Emergent obstetrics consultation if presenting to ophthalmologist.

Acquired Retinal Arterial Macroaneurysm (RAM)

Focal dilation of retinal artery (>100 μm) often at bifurcation or crossing site; more common in women >60 years old with hypertension (50-70%) or atherosclerosis. Usually asymptomatic, unilateral, and solitary; may cause sudden loss of vision from vitreous hemorrhage; macroaneurysms nasal to the optic disc are less likely to cause symptoms. Subretinal, intraretinal, preretinal, or vitreous hemorrhages (multilevel hemorrhages) from rupture of aneurysm, and surrounding circinate exudates are common. May spontaneously sclerose, forming a Z-shaped kink at old aneurysm site.

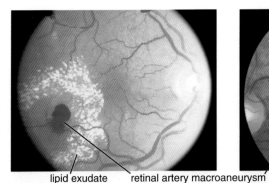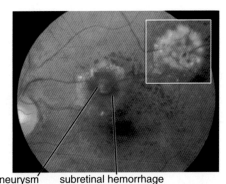

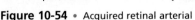
lipid exudate   retinal artery macroaneurysm   subretinal hemorrhage

Figure 10-54 • Acquired retinal arterial macroaneurysm with circinate exudate.

Figure 10-55 • Acquired retinal arterial macroaneurysm before laser photocoagulation. Inset shows the same lesion after laser treatment.

- **Fluorescein angiogram:** Immediate uniform, focal filling of the macroaneurysm early with late leakage.
- **Indocyanine green angiography:** Uniform, focal filling of the macroaneurysm; very useful to identify RAM in the presence of intraretinal and preretinal hemorrhage.
- Most require no treatment, especially in the absence of loss of vision.
- Low intensity, longer duration, argon green or yellow laser photocoagulation to microvascular changes around leaking aneurysm if decreased acuity is present (direct treatment controversial because it may cause a vitreous hemorrhage, distal ischemia, or a BRAO).
- Consider pars plana vitrectomy with surgical evacuation of subretinal hemorrhage (with or without injection of subretinal tissue plasminogen activator) in cases of massive, subfoveal hemorrhage < 10 days old (experimental).
- Medical consultation for hypertension.

Radiation Retinopathy

Definition

Alteration in retinal vascular permeability after receiving local ionizing radiation, usually from external beam radiotherapy or plaque brachytherapy.

Etiology

Vascular endothelial cell DNA damage secondary to the radiation, leading to progressive cell death and damage to the retinal blood vessels.

Epidemiology

Usually requires >30-35 Gy (3000-3500 rads) total radiation dose; appears 1-2 years after ionizing radiation; diabetics and patients receiving chemotherapy have a lower threshold.

Symptoms

Often asymptomatic until retinopathy involves macula; decreased vision.

Signs

Microaneurysms, telangiectasias, cotton-wool spots, hard exudates, retinal hemorrhages, macular edema, vascular sheathing, disc edema, retinal/disc/iris neovascularization.

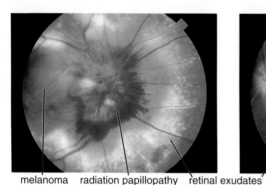

melanoma   radiation papillopathy   retinal exudates   sclerotic vessels   melanoma

Figure 10-56 • Radiation papillopathy. Note regressed malignant melanoma temporally.

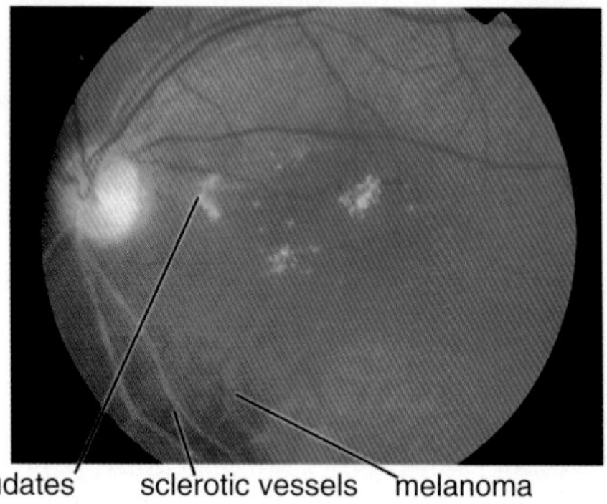

Figure 10-57 • Radiation retinopathy with sclerotic vessels overlying regressed malignant melanoma.

Differential Diagnosis

Diabetic retinopathy, sickle cell retinopathy, hypertensive retinopathy, retinal vascular occlusion.

Evaluation

- Complete radiation history with attention to radiated field, total dose delivered, and fractionation schedule.
- Complete eye examination with attention to tonometry, gonioscopy, iris, lens, 78/90 diopter or contact lens fundus examination, and ophthalmoscopy.
- **Fluorescein angiogram:** Capillary nonperfusion, macular edema, and neovascularization.

Management

- Treatment based on similar principles used in diabetic retinopathy.
- Focal grid laser photocoagulation (50-100 μm spots) to areas of macular edema.
- Panretinal photocoagulation with 1200-1600 applications (500 μm spots) if neovascular complications develop.

Prognosis

Fair; complications include cataract, macular edema/ischemia, optic atrophy, vitreous hemorrhage, and neovascular glaucoma; two thirds of patients maintain vision better than 20/200.

Age-Related Macular Degeneration (AMD)

Definition

Progressive degenerative disease of the retinal pigment epithelium, Bruch's membrane, and choriocapillaris. Generally classified into two types: (1) nonexudative, or "dry," AMD, characterized by drusen and pigmentary changes (90%), and (2) exudative, or "wet," AMD, characterized by choroidal neovascularization (CNV) and eventually disciform scarring (10%).

Epidemiology

Leading cause of blindness in U.S. population in patients over 65 years of age, as well as the most common cause of blindness in the Western world; 6.4% of patients 65-74 years of age and 19.7% of patients >75 years of age had signs of AMD in the Framingham Eye Study; more prevalent in whites; slight female predilection. Risk factors include increasing age (>75 years of age), positive family history, cigarette smoking, hyperopia, light iris color, hypertension, hypercholesterolemia, female gender, and cardiovascular disease; nutritional factors and light toxicity also play a role in pathogenesis. There may also be a genetic component to AMD.

Nonexudative (Dry) Macular Degeneration

Symptoms

Initially asymptomatic or possibly decreased vision, metamorphopsia early. Advanced atrophic form may have central or pericentral scotoma.

Signs

Normal or decreased visual acuity; abnormal Amsler grid (central/paracentral scotomas or metamorphopsia); small, hard drusen, larger, soft drusen, geographic atrophy of the retinal pigment epithelium (RPE), RPE clumping, and blunted foveal reflex.

 Box 10-2   Age-Related Eye Disease Study Definitions

Category 1: Less than 5 small (<63 microns) drusen.
Category 2 (Mild AMD): Multiple small drusen *or* single or nonextensive intermediate-size (63-124 microns) drusen; or pigment abnormalities.
Category 3 (Intermediate AMD): Extensive intermediate-size drusen *or* 1 or more large (>125 microns) drusen; or noncentral geographic atrophy.
Category 4 (Advanced AMD): Vision loss (<20/32) due to AMD in 1 eye (either due to central/subfoveal geographic atrophy or exudative macular degeneration).

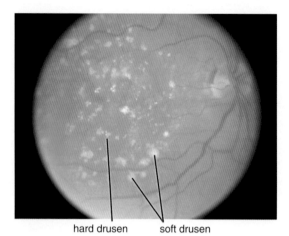

Figure 10-58 • Dry, age-related macular degeneration demonstrating drusen and pigmentary changes (category 3).

hard drusen   soft drusen

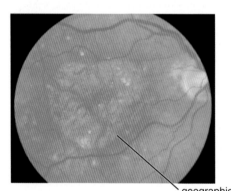

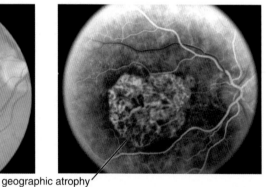

geographic atrophy

Figure 10-59 • Advanced atrophic, nonexudative, age-related macular degeneration demonstrating subfoveal geographic atrophy (category 4).

Figure 10-60 • Fluorescein angiogram of same patient as Figure 10-59 demonstrating well-defined window defect corresponding to the area of geographic atrophy.

Differential Diagnosis

Dominant drusen, pattern dystrophy, Best's disease, Stargardt's disease, cone dystrophy, and drug toxicity.

Evaluation

• Complete ophthalmic history and eye examination with attention to Amsler grid and 78/90 diopter or contact lens fundus examination.

- **Fluorescein angiogram:** Window defects from geographic atrophy and punctate hyperfluorescent staining of drusen (no late leakage).

Management

- Follow with Amsler grid qd and examine every 6 months; examine sooner if patient has a change in vision, metamorphopsia, or change in Amsler grid.
- Supplement with high dose antioxidants and vitamins (vitamin C, 500 mg; vitamin E, 400 IU; and beta carotene, 15 mg, zinc, 80 mg and copper, 2 mg) for patients with category 3 (extensive intermediate-size drusen, one large drusen, or noncentral geographic atrophy), or category 4 (vision loss due to AMD in one eye); **Warning:** smokers should not take beta carotene at such high doses due to increased risk of lung cancer (Age-Related Eye Disease Study [AREDS] conclusion).
- Consider supplement with lower dose antioxidants (e.g.. Centrum Silver, iCaps, Occuvite Extra) for patients with category 1 (few small drusen), category 2 (extensive small drusen or few intermediate-size drusen), and patients with strong family history.
- Supplementation with other vitamins including lutein and bilberry still unproved.
- Low power, grid, laser photocoagulation to cause resorption of drusen and improve visual acuity (experimental).
- Low vision aids may benefit patients with bilateral central visual loss due to geographic atrophy.

Prognosis

Usually good unless patient develops central geographic atrophy or exudative AMD. Severe visual loss (defined as loss of >6 lines of vision) occurs in 12% of nonexudative cases; presence of large, soft drusen and focal RPE hyperpigmentation increases risk of developing exudative form (MPS conclusion). Risk of advanced AMD over 5 years varies depending on category: categories 1 and 2 (1.8%), category 3 (18%), category 4 (43%) (AREDS conclusion).

Exudative (Wet) Macular Degeneration

Symptoms

Metamorphopsia, central scotoma , rapid visual loss.

Signs

Gray-green choroidal neovascular membrane (CNV), lipid exudates, subretinal or intraretinal hemorrhage or fluid, pigment epithelial detachment (PED), retinal pigment epithelial tears, and fibrovascular disciform scars.

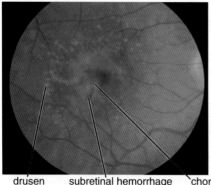

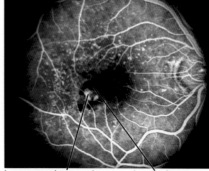

drusen   subretinal hemorrhage   choroidal neovascular membrane   hemorrhage

Figure 10-61 • Exudative age-related macular degeneration demonstrating subretinal hemorrhage from classic choroidal neovascular membrane.

Figure 10-62 • Fluorescein angiogram of same patient as Figure 10-61 demonstrating leakage from the CNV and blocking from the surrounding subretinal blood.

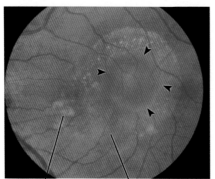

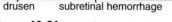

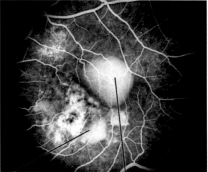

drusen   choroidal neovascular membrane   serous pigment epithelial detachment

Figure 10-63 • Exudative age-related macular degeneration demonstrating drusen, pigmentary changes, and an occult choroidal neovascular membrane with associated serous pigment epithelial detachment *(arrowheads)*.

Figure 10-64 • Fluorescein angiogram of same patient as Figure 10-63 demonstrating hyperfluorescent staining of pigmentary changes and drusen, leakage from the CNV and pooling of fluorescein dye within the serous PED.

Differential Diagnosis

Dominant drusen, pattern dystrophy, Best's disease, central serous retinopathy, Stargardt's disease, cone dystrophy, drug toxicity, and choroidal neovascularization from other causes, including presumed ocular histoplasmosis syndrome, angioid streaks, myopic degeneration, traumatic choroidal rupture, retinal dystrophies, inflammatory choroidopathies, and optic nerve drusen.

Evaluation

• Complete ophthalmic history and eye examination with attention to Amsler grid and 78/90 diopter or contact lens fundus examination.

- **Fluorescein angiogram:** Leakage from CNV defined as two forms: (1) classic leakage, defined as lacy network of bright fluorescence during early choroidal filling views that increases in fluorescence throughout the angiogram and leaks beyond its borders in late views; (2) occult leakage. There are two forms of occult leakage: type 1, or fibrovascular PED, defined as stippled nonhomogeneous hyperfluorescence at the level of the RPE (best seen on stereoscopic views) that persists in late views with leakage that is not as bright/pronounced as classic lesions; and type 2, or late leakage of undetermined origin, where the early views show no apparent leakage, but as the angiogram progresses, there is hyperfluorescent stippling at the level of the RPE in late views.
- **Indocyanine green angiogram:** Useful when the CNV is poorly demarcated or obscured by hemorrhage on fluorescein angiogram or if fibrovascular pigment epithelial detachment is present (to identify areas of focal neovascularization); focal hotspots likely represent retinal angiomatous proliferation (RAP); CNV also appears as plaque of late hyperfluorescence.
- **Optical coherence tomography:** After photodynamic therapy, when the fluorescein angiogram is equivocal between leakage and staining of the CNV, OCT is useful to delineate the presence and extent of intraretinal and subretinal fluid, as well as the presence of a PED.

Management

- Focal laser photocoagulation with argon green/yellow or krypton red laser and a transpupillary delivery system to form confluent (200-500 μm spots) white burns over the entire CNV depending on size, location, and visual acuity based on the results of the Macular Photocoagulation Study (MPS). *(Note:* only patients with a classic, well-defined CNV met eligibility criteria for the MPS study.)
  Extrafoveal: 200 to 2500 μm from center of foveal avascular zone (FAZ).
  - Treat entire CNV and 100 μm beyond all boundaries.
  Juxtafoveal: 1 to 199 μm from center of FAZ or choroidal neovascular membrane (CNV) 200 to 2500 μm from center of FAZ with blood or blocked fluorescence within 1 to 199 μm of FAZ center.
  - Treat entire CNV and 100 μm beyond on nonfoveal side and up to CNV border on foveal side. Lesions that are "barely" juxtafoveal or where laser treatment may damage the center of vision should be considered for photodynamic therapy (PDT). *(Note:* TAP [see below] enrollment criteria included subfoveal lesions only, but there was a small subgroup with barely juxtafoveal lesions who responded well to PDT.)
  Subfoveal: Under geometric center of FAZ.
- Although laser photocoagulation was shown to be beneficial, its use in subfoveal lesions has been supplanted by PDT. Photodynamic therapy with verteporfin (Visudyne) has been shown to prevent visual loss in subfoveal, predominantly classic lesions (>50% of the entire lesion is composed of classic CNV) (Treatment of AMD with Photodynamic Therapy Study, TAP Study conclusion) and in occult lesions with no classic lesions (especially if the lesion is <4 MPS disc areas in size or baseline vision is worse than 20/50) (Verteporfin in Photodynamic Therapy Study, VIP Study conclusion). Fluorescein angiograms must be performed within 7 days of PDT treatment to determine lesion size for treatment. PDT retreatment applied as often as every 3 months if fluorescein leakage found from CNV (average, 3.4 treatments in year 1, 2.2 in year 2; TAP conclusion). Patient should avoid direct sunlight or bright indoor halogen lights for at least 48 hours after each treatment (drug labeling states 5 days).

Continued

Management—cont'd

- There is no effective treatment for minimally classic CNV at this time.
- In certain select cases, submacular surgery for removal of CNV or macular translocation performed by an experienced vitreoretinal surgeon may be considered (experimental).
- Low vision aids and registration with blind services for patients who are legally blind (<20/200 best corrected visual acuity or <20 degree visual field in better seeing eye)
- Treatments being evaluated in clinical trials include radiation therapy, transpupillary thermal therapy, modulating (feeder) vessel laser photocoagulation, different timing and doses of verteporfin PDT, and antiangiogenic or angiostatic agents with or without PDT.

Prognosis

Usually poor prognosis; severe visual loss (defined as loss of >6 lines of vision) occurs in 88% of cases. Chance of severe visual loss is decreased with laser treatment (except in subfoveal group) and PDT. CNV may recur or persist after PDT or laser treatment; risk of fellow eye developing CNV is 4-12% annually.

▌ Myopic Degeneration/Pathologic Myopia

Progressive retinal degeneration seen in high myopia (≥-6.00 diopters, axial length >26.5 mm) and pathologic myopia (≥-8.00 diopters, axial length >32.5 mm) with scleral thinning, posterior staphyloma, lacquer cracks (irregular, yellow streaks), peripapillary, atrophic temporal crescent, tilted optic disc, Fuchs' spots (dark spots due to RPE hyperplasia in macula), "tigroid" fundus due to thinning of RPE allowing visualization of larger choroidal vessels, subretinal hemorrhage (especially near lacquer cracks), and chorioretinal atrophy; increased incidence of posterior vitreous detachment, premature cataract formation, glaucoma, lattice degeneration, giant retinal tears, retinal detachments, macular hole, and CNV. Visual field defects may be present.

- **Fluorescein angiogram:** To evaluate for CNV if suspected clinically, atrophic areas appear as window defects; lacquer cracks are hyperfluorescent linear areas that stain in late views.
- Correct any refractive error; contact lenses help reduce image minification and prismatic effect.
- Recommend polycarbonate safety glasses for sports (increased risk of choroidal rupture with minor trauma).
- Follow for signs of complications (CNV, retinal detachment, retinal breaks, macular holes, glaucoma, and cataracts).
- Treat CNV with focal laser photocoagulation per MPS guidelines in extrafoveal lesions (see Age-Related Macular Degeneration section) or photodynamic therapy for juxtafoveal (since laser scar enlargement ["scar creep"] is common in pathologic myopia after laser treatment) and subfoveal lesions (Verteporfin in Photodynamic Therapy Pathologic Myopia Study [VIP-PM] conclusion).
- Treat retinal detachment and macular holes with vitreoretinal surgery performed by a retina specialist.

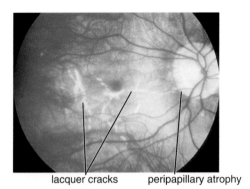

lacquer cracks   peripapillary atrophy

Figure 10-65 • Myopic degeneration with lacquer cracks.

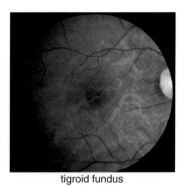

tigroid fundus

Figure 10-66 • "Tigroid" fundus due to thinning of RPE allowing visualization of larger choroidal vessels.

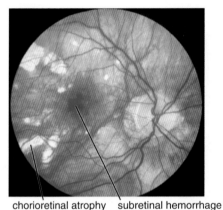

chorioretinal atrophy   subretinal hemorrhage

Figure 10-67 • Myopic degeneration with peripapillary and chorioretinal atrophy, and subretinal hemorrhage from CNV.

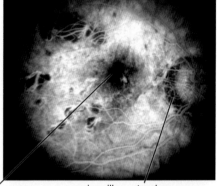

peripapillary atrophy

Figure 10-68 • Fluorescein angiogram of same patient as Figure 10-67 demonstrating blocking defect from subretinal hemorrhage and window defects from chorioretinal and peripapillary atrophy.

Angioid Streaks

Definition

Full-thickness breaks in calcified, thickened Bruch's membrane with disruption of overlying RPE.

Etiology

Idiopathic or associated with systemic diseases (50% of cases) including pseudoxanthoma elasticum (PXE, 60%; redundant skin folds in the neck, gastrointestinal bleeding, hypertension), Paget's disease (8%; extraskeletal calcification, osteoarthritis, deafness, vertigo, increased serum alkaline phosphatase and urine calcium levels), senile elastosis, calcinosis, abetalipoproteinemia, sickle cell disease (5%), thalassemia, hereditary spherocytosis, and Ehlers-Danlos syndrome (blue sclera, hyperextendable joints, elastic skin); also associated with optic nerve drusen, Bassen-Kornzweig syndrome, acromegaly, lead poisoning, Marfan's syndrome, and retinitis pigmentosa.

Symptoms

Usually asymptomatic; may have decreased vision, metamorphopsia if choroidal neovascular membrane develops. Minor trauma can cause rupture of Bruch's membrane leading to hemorrhage or CNV.

Signs

Normal or decreased visual acuity; linear, irregular, deep, dark red-brown streaks radiating from the optic disc in a spokelike pattern; often have "peau d'orange" retinal pigmentation, peripheral salmon spots, "histo-like" scars, and pigmentation around the streaks; may have subretinal hemorrhage or fluid, retinal pigment epithelial detachments, macular degeneration, and central or paracentral scotomas if CNV develops.

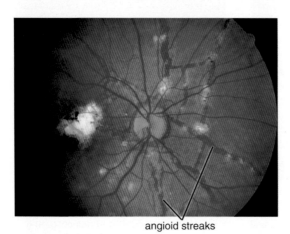

Figure 10-69 • Angioid streaks appear as dark red branching lines radiating from the optic nerve.

angioid streaks

Differential Diagnosis

Age-related macular degeneration, lacquer cracks, myopic degeneration, choroidal rupture, choroidal folds.

Evaluation

- Complete ophthalmic history and eye examination with attention to 78/90 diopter or contact lens fundus examination, and ophthalmoscopy.
- Check Amsler grid to rule out CNV.
- **Lab tests:** Sickle cell prep, hemoglobin electrophoresis (sickle cell disease), serum alkaline phosphatase, serum lead levels, urine calcium, stool guaiac, skin biopsy.
- **Fluorescein angiogram:** To evaluate for CNV if suspected clinically, usually occur along the track of an angioid streak that has granular pattern of hyperfluorescence.
- Medical consultation to rule out systemic diseases including skin biopsy and radiographs.

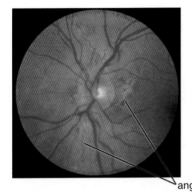 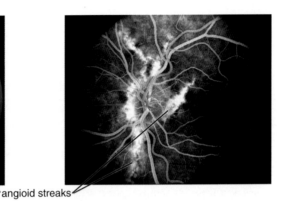

angioid streaks

Figure 10-70 • Angioid streaks radiating from the optic nerve.

Figure 10-71 • Fluorescein angiogram of same patient as shown in Figure 10-70, demonstrating hyperfluorescent window defects corresponding to the angioid streaks.

Management

- Treat CNV with focal photocoagulation similar to MPS guidelines in juxtafoveal and extrafoveal lesions or photodynamic therapy for subfoveal lesions (see Age-Related Macular Degeneration section).
- Polycarbonate safety glasses because mild blunt trauma can cause subretinal hemorrhages or choroidal rupture.
- Treat underlying medical condition.

Prognosis

Good unless CNV develops (high recurrence rates).

Central Serous Chorioretinopathy (CSR)/Idiopathic Central Serous Choroidopathy (ICSC)

Definition

Idiopathic leakage of fluid from the choroid into the subretinal space (94%), under the RPE (3%), or both (3%) presumably due to RPE or choroidal dysfunction.

Epidemiology

Idiopathic. Usually occurs in males (10:1) 20-50 years of age; in women, tends to occur at a slightly older age; more common in whites, Hispanics, and Asians; rare in blacks; associated with type-A personality, stress, hypochondriasis; also associated with pregnancy, steroid use, hypertension, Cushing's syndrome, systemic lupus erythematosus, and organ transplantation.

Symptoms

Decreased vision, micropsia, metamorphopsia, central scotoma, and mild dyschromatopsia; may be asymptomatic; usually unilateral but can be bilateral,

Signs

Normal or decreased visual acuity ranging from 20/20 to 20/200 (visual acuity improves with pinhole or plus lenses); induced hyperopia, abnormal Amsler grid (central or paracentral scotomas or metamorphopsia); single or multiple, round or oval-shaped, shallow, serous retinal detachment or pigment epithelial detachment (PED) with deep yellow spots at the level of the retinal pigment epithelium; areas of retinal pigment epithelium atrophy may be seen at sites of previous episodes. Subretinal fibrin suggests active leakage. Rarely associated with CNV and subretinal fluid.

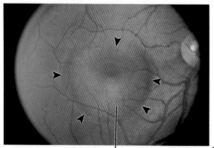

pigment epithelial detachment   "smokestack" leakage

Figure 10-72 • Idiopathic central serous retinopathy with large serous retinal detachment.

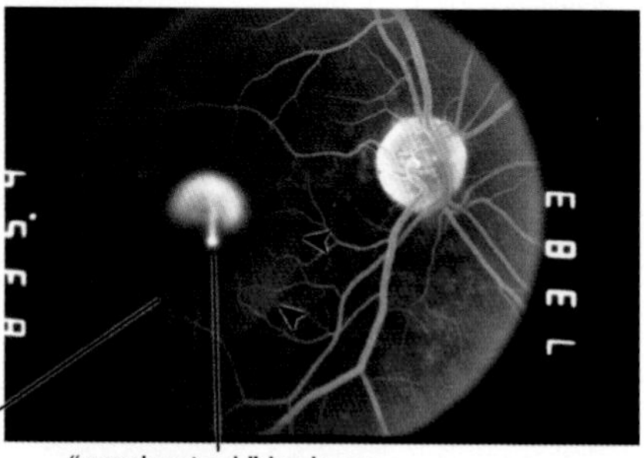

Figure 10-73 • Fluorescein angiogram of same patient as shown in Figure 10-72 demonstrating classic smokestack appearance.

Differential Diagnosis

Age-related macular degeneration (especially in patients >50 years of age), Vogt-Koyanagi-Harada syndrome or other inflammatory choroidal disorders, uveal effusion syndrome, toxemia of pregnancy, optic nerve pit, choroidal tumors, vitelliform macular detachment, PED from other causes including neovascular membranes.

Evaluation

- Complete ophthalmic history and eye examination with attention to Amsler grid, 78/90 diopter or contact lens fundus examination, and ophthalmoscopy.
- **Fluorescein angiogram:** Focal dot of hyperfluorescence early that leaks in a characteristic smokestack pattern (10%) or gradually pools into a pigment epithelial detachment (90%); more than one site may be present simultaneously (30%); often see punctate window defects in other areas in both eyes; recurrent leakage sites are often close to original sites.
- **Indocyanine green angiogram:** Choroidal hyperpermeability.
- **Optical coherence tomography:** Serous retinal detachment and/or pigment epithelial detachment; useful to monitor for resolution of leakage.

Management

- No treatment required in most cases. Usually resolves over 6 weeks
- Focal laser photocoagulation considered for patients who require quicker visual rehabilitation for occupational reasons (monocular, pilots), poor vision in fellow eye due to central serous retinopathy, no resolution of fluid after 4 to 6 months, recurrent episodes with poor vision, or in severe forms of central serous retinopathy known to have a poor prognosis.
- Low-intensity, direct laser photocoagulation to leakage site (must be >500 μm from center of macula) shortens duration by 2 months but has no effect on final acuity. There have been some reports that photocoagulation reduces the recurrence rate, but other authors have observed no difference.
- Photodynamic therapy may be beneficial (experimental).

Prognosis

Good; 94% regain ≥20/30 acuity; 95% of pigment epithelial detachments resolve spontaneously in 3-4 months, acuity improves over 21 months; recurrences are common (45%) and usually occur within a year; prognosis worse with recurrent disease; recovery of visual acuity is faster after laser treatment, but recovery of contrast sensitivity is prolonged and may ultimately be reduced; 5% develop subretinal neovascular membranes. Prognosis is worse for patients with recurrent disease, multiple areas of detachment, or chronic course.

◼ Cystoid Macular Edema (CME)

Definition

Accumulation of extracellular fluid in the macular region with characteristic cystoid spaces in the outer plexiform layer.

Etiology

After surgery (especially in older patients and if the posterior capsule is violated with vitreous loss; CME after cataract surgery is called Irvine-Gass syndrome and usually presents 3-4 weeks postoperatively), after laser treatment (neodymium:yttrium-aluminum-garnet [Nd:YAG] laser capsulotomy, especially if performed within 3 months of cataract surgery), uveitis, diabetic retinopathy, juxtafoveal retinal telangiectasia, vein occlusions, retinal vasculitis, epiretinal membrane, hereditary retinal dystrophies (dominant CME, retinitis pigmentosa), drug toxicity (epinephrine in aphakic patients, dipivefrin, and prostaglandin analogues), hypertensive retinopathy, ARMD, occult rhegmatogenous detachment, intraocular tumors, collagen-vascular diseases, hypotony, and chronic inflammation.

Symptoms

Decreased or washed-out vision.

Signs

Decreased visual acuity, loss of foveal reflex, thickened fovea, foveal folds, intraretinal cystoid spaces, epiretinal membrane, lipid exudates; may have signs of uveitis or surgical complications including open posterior capsule, vitreous to the wound, peaked pupil, and iris incarceration in wound.

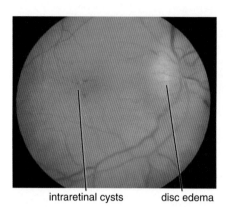

intraretinal cysts   disc edema

Figure 10-74 • Cystoid macular edema with decreased foveal reflex, cystic changes in fovea, and intraretinal hemorrhages.

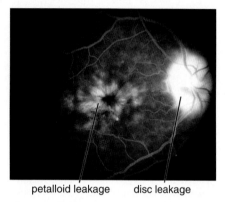

petalloid leakage   disc leakage

Figure 10-75 • Fluorescein angiogram of same patient as shown in Figure 10-74 demonstrating characteristic petalloid appearance with optic nerve leakage.

cystoid macular edema

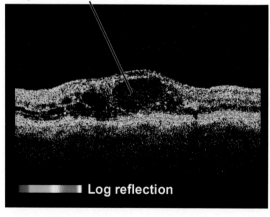

Log reflection

Figure 10-76 • Optical coherence tomography of cystoid macular edema demonstrating intraretinal cystoid spaces and dome-shaped configuration of fovea.

Differential Diagnosis

Macular hole (stage 1), foveal retinoschisis, central serous retinopathy, choroidal neovascular membrane, pseudocystoid macular edema (no leakage on fluorescein angiography).

Evaluation

- Complete ophthalmic history and eye examination with attention to cornea, anterior chamber, iris, lens, 78/90 diopter or contact lens fundus examination, and ophthalmoscopy.
- **Fluorescein angiogram:** Early, perifoveal, punctate hyperfluorescence and characteristic late leakage in a petalloid pattern. *Note:* No leakage seen in pseudocystoid macular edema from juvenile retinoschisis, nicotinic acid (niacin) maculopathy, Goldmann-Favre disease, and some forms of retinitis pigmentosa.
- **Optical coherence tomography:** Increased retinal thickness with cystoid spaces and loss of normal foveal contour with or without subsensory fluid.

Management

- Treat the underlying disorder if possible.
- Discontinue topical epinephrine, dipivefrin, or prostaglandin analogue drops and nicotinic acid–containing medications. Rarely, diuretics and oral contraceptive pills can cause an atypical CME that resolves on discontinuing medication.
- Topical nonsteroidal antiinflammatory drops ([NSAIDs], Voltaren or Acular qid) and/or topical steroid (prednisolone acetate 1% qid for 1 month, then taper slowly).
- Consider posterior sub-Tenon's steroid injection (triamcinolone acetonide 40 mg/mL) in patients who do not respond to topical medications.
- If no response, consider oral NSAIDs (indomethacin 25 mg po tid for 6-8 weeks), oral steroids (prednisone 40-60 mg po qd for 1-2 weeks, then taper slowly), and/or oral acetazolamide (Diamox 250 mg po bid); all are unproven.
- In refractory cases consider intravitreal injection of 0.1 mL (4 mg) triamcinolone acetonide (experimental).
- If vitreous is present to the wound and vision is <20/80, consider Nd:YAG laser vitreolysis or perform pars plana vitrectomy with peeling of posterior hyaloid (Vitrectomy-Aphakic Cystoid Macular Edema Study conclusion).

Prognosis

Usually good; spontaneous resolution in weeks to months (after surgery); prognosis poorer for chronic CME (>6 months); may develop macular hole.

Macular Hole

Definition

Retinal hole in the fovea.

Etiology

Idiopathic; other risk factors are cystoid macular edema, vitreomacular traction, trauma, and after surgery, laser treatment, and inflammation.

Epidemiology

Senile (idiopathic) macular holes (83%) usually occur in women (3:1) 60-80 years of age; traumatic holes are rare (5%); 25-30% bilateral.

Symptoms

Decreased vision, metamorphopsia, and, less commonly, central scotoma.

Signs

Decreased visual acuity ranging from 20/40 in stage 1 to 20/200 in stages 3 and 4; fundus findings can be classified into four stages.

Stage 1   Premacular hole (impending hole) with foveal detachment, absent foveal reflex, macular cyst (1A = yellow spot, 100-200 μm in diameter, 1B = yellow ring, 200-300 μm in diameter).

Stage 2   Early, small, full-thickness hole either centrally within the ring or eccentrically at the ring's margin.

Stage 3   Full-thickness hole (≥400 μm) with yellow deposits at level of retinal pigment epithelium (Klein's tags), absence of a Weiss ring, operculum, cuff of subretinal fluid, cystoid macular edema, and positive Watzke-Allen sign (subjective interruption of slit beam on biomicroscopy).

Stage 4   Stage 3 and posterior vitreous detachment (PVD).
Retinal detachments rare except in high myopes.

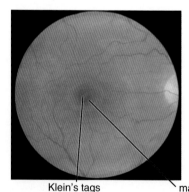

Klein's tags   macular hole

Figure 10-77 • Macular hole with multiple yellow spots (Klein's tags) at the base of the hole.

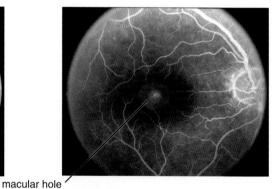

Figure 10-78 • Fluorescein angiogram of same patient in Figure 10-76 demonstrating early hyperfluorescence of the hole that does not leak in late views.

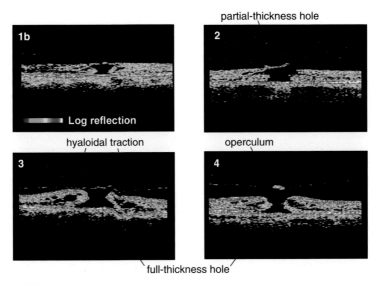

Figure 10-79 • Optical coherence tomography scans demonstrating cross sectional image of all stages of macular hole formation and the full-thickness retinal defect characteristic of stages 3 and 4 holes.

Differential Diagnosis

Epiretinal membrane with pseudo-hole, solar retinopathy, central serous retinopathy, ARMD, vitreomacular traction syndrome, cystoid macular edema, solitary druse, lamellar hole.

Evaluation

- Complete ophthalmic history and eye examination with attention to visual acuity, Amsler grid, Watzke-Allen test, 78/90 diopter or contact lens fundus examination, and ophthalmoscopy.
- **Optical coherence tomography:** Full-thickness defect in retina with or without traction on edges of hole; can differentiate lamellar holes, pseudoholes, and cysts from true macular holes; useful for staging holes.
- **Fluorescein angiogram:** Hyperfluorescent window defect in the central fovea.

Management

- No treatment recommended for stage 1 holes because spontaneous hole closure can occur.
- Pars plana vitrectomy, membrane peel, air-fluid exchange, and gas injection with 7-14 days of prone positioning for stages 2 to 4 holes of recent onset (<1 year) and reduced visual acuity in the range of 20/40 to 20/400; use of adjuvant agents including autologous serum, platelets, and tissue glue is still controversial; should be performed by a retina specialist.

Prognosis

Good for recent-onset holes; surgery has successful anatomic results in 60-90% depending on duration, of which 73% have improved acuity; preoperative visual acuity is inversely correlated with the absolute amount of visual improvement; poor prognosis for holes older than 1 year.

▮ Epiretinal Membrane/Macular Pucker

Definition

Cellular proliferation along the internal limiting membrane and retinal surface. Contraction of this membrane causes the retinal surface to become wrinkled (pucker or cellophane maculopathy).

Etiology

Risk factors include prior retinal surgery, intraocular inflammation, retinal vascular occlusion, sickle cell retinopathy, vitreous hemorrhage, trauma, macular holes, intraocular tumors such as angiomas and hamartomas, telangiectasis, retinal arteriolar macroaneurysms, retinitis pigmentosa, laser photocoagulation, and cryotherapy; often idiopathic.

Epidemiology

Incidence increases with increasing age; occurs in 2% of population >50 years old and in 20% >75 years old; 20-30% bilateral although often asymmetric; slight female predilection (3:2); diabetes has been found to be associated with idiopathic ERMs.

Symptoms

Asymptomatic with normal or near-normal vision; mild distortion or blurred vision; less commonly, macropsia, central photopsia, or monocular diplopia if macular pucker exists.

Signs

Normal or decreased visual acuity; abnormal Amsler grid; thin, translucent membrane appears as mild sheen (cellophane) along macula; may have dragged or tortuous vessels, retinal striae, pseudo-holes, foveal ectopia, and cystoid macular edema. Occasionally multiple punctate hemorrhages occur in the inner retina.

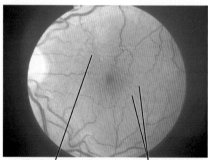

cellophane membrane   retinal striae

Figure 10-80 • Cellophane epiretinal membrane and macular pucker with retinal striae.

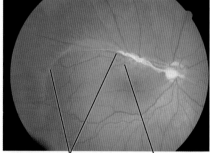

epiretinal membrane   dragged vessels

Figure 10-81 • Epiretinal membrane with macular pucker and dragged vessels.

Differential Diagnosis

Traction retinal detachment from diabetic retinopathy, sickle cell retinopathy, or radiation retinopathy; choroidal folds.

Evaluation

• Complete ophthalmic history and eye examination with attention to 78/90 diopter or contact lens fundus examination, and ophthalmoscopy.

Management

• Treatment rarely required unless visual symptoms become symptomatic.
• Pars plana vitrectomy and membrane peel in patients with reduced acuity (e.g., <20/60) or intractable symptoms; should be performed by a retina specialist.

Prognosis

Good; 75% of patients have improvement in symptoms and acuity after surgery.

Myelinated Nerve Fibers

Abnormal myelination of ganglion cell axons anterior to the lamina cribrosa; appears as yellow-white patches with feathery borders in the superficial retina (nerve fiber layer); typically unilateral (80%) and occurs adjacent to the optic nerve but can be located anywhere in the posterior pole; obscures underlying retinal vasculature and can be confused with cotton-wool spots, astrocytic hamartomas, commotio retinae, or rarely retinal artery occlusion if extensive. Patients are usually asymptomatic, but scotomas corresponding to the areas of myelination can be demonstrated on visual fields; slight male predilection.

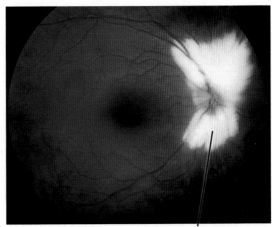

Figure 10-82 • Myelinated nerve fibers demonstrating fluffy white appearance extending from optic nerve and partially obscuring disc margins and retinal vessels.

myelinated nerve fibers

* No treatment required.
* Consider visual fields.

Solar/Photic Retinopathy

Bilateral decreased vision (20/40 to 20/100), metamorphopsia, photophobia, dyschromatopsia, after-images, scotomas, headaches, and orbital pain 1-4 hours after unprotected, long-term sun gazing. Retinal damage ranges from no changes to yellow spot with surrounding pigmentary changes in the foveolar region in the early stages. Late changes include lamellar holes or depressions in the fovea. Vision can improve over 3-6 months, with residual scotomas and metamorphopsia. Similar problems may occur from lasers, welding arcs, and extended exposure to operating-room microscope lights (unilateral).

* No effective treatment.

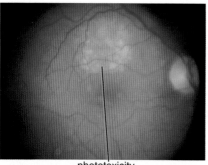

phototoxicity

Figure 10-83 • Photic retinopathy demonstrating retinal edema secondary to operating-room microscope overexposure.

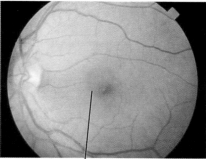

solar retinopathy

Figure 10-84 • Solar retinopathy. Note pigmentary changes in the macula.

Toxic/Drug Maculopathies

Aminoglycosides (Gentamicin, Tobramycin, Amikacin)

Acute, severe, permanent visual loss after intraocular injection of toxic doses. Retinal toxic reaction with marked retinal whitening (especially in macula) and retinal hemorrhages seen after injecting 0.1 mg of gentamicin (also described after diffusion through cataract wound from subconjunctival injection). Optic atrophy and pigmentary changes occur later. Visual prognosis is poor.

* **Fluorescein angiogram:** Sharp zones of capillary nonperfusion corresponding to the areas of ischemic retina.
* No effective treatment.

Canthaxanthine

Usually asymptomatic or produces mild metamorphopsia and decreased vision while this oral tanning agent is being taken. Refractile yellow spots in a wreathlike pattern around the fovea (gold-dust retinopathy). Seen with cumulative doses >35 g.

- Check visual fields (central 10 degrees).
- Decrease or discontinue the medication if toxicity develops.

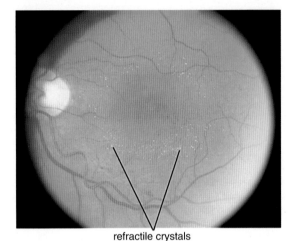

Figure 10-85 • Crystalline maculopathy due to canthaxanthine.

refractile crystals

Chloroquine (Aralen)/Hydroxychloroquine (Plaquenil)

First used as an antimalarial agent in World War II, and now used to treat systemic lupus erythematosus, rheumatoid arthritis, short-term pulse treatment for graft versus host disease, and amebiasis, these medications produce central or paracentral scotomas, blurry vision, nyctalopia, photopsias, dyschromatopsia, photophobia, and in late stages constriction of visual fields. Early changes include loss of foveal reflex and abnormal macular pigmentation (reversible); "bull's-eye" maculopathy (not reversible), peripheral bone spicules, vasculature attenuation, and disc pallor appear later; late stages can appear similar to end-stage retinitis pigmentosa. May also develop eyelash whitening and whorl-like subepithelial corneal deposits (corneal verticillata, vortex keratopathy). Doses >3.5 mg/kg/day or 300 g total (chloroquine), and >6.5 mg/kg/day (<400 mg/day appears safe) or 700 g total (hydroxy-chloroquine) may produce the maculopathy; total daily dose seems more critical than total cumulative dose; often progresses after medications are discontinued because the drug concentrates in the eye. Hydroxychloroquine appears safer because it does not readily cross the blood-retinal barrier (toxicity rarely seen with use < 7 years).

- Differential diagnosis of "bull's-eye" maculopathy includes cone dystrophy, ARMD, Stargardt's disease/fundus flavimaculatus, Spielmeyer-Vogt disease, albinism, fenestrated sheen macular dystrophy, central areolar choroidal dystrophy, benign concentric annular macular dystrophy, clofazimine toxicity, fucosidosis.

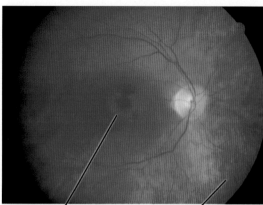

Figure 10-86 • "Bull's-eye" maculopathy due to chloroquine toxicity.

bull's-eye maculopathy   peripheral atrophy

- Check red Amsler grid and visual fields (central 10 degrees with red test object) every 6 months (chloroquine) or 12 months (hydroxychloroquine) while patient is taking medications; color fundus photographs and color vision are optionally checked; patients with drug use >5 years with high fat level body habitus, renal or liver disease, and age >60 years are at higher risk of developing toxicity and should be checked more frequently.
- **Fluorescein angiogram:** Hypofluorescence with ring of hyperfluorescence corresponding to the bull's-eye lesion, often visible before fundus lesion.
- **Electrophysiologic testing:** Electrooculogram (EOG) (normal early, reduced [<1.6] light-to-dark [Arden] ratio later).
- Decrease or discontinue the medication if toxicity develops.

Talc

Refractile yellow deposits near or in arterioles seen in IV drug abusers; similar picture occurs in IV drug abusers injecting suspensions of crushed methylphenidate (Ritalin) tablets.

- No effective treatment.

Tamoxifen

Used to treat breast carcinoma, produces mild decreases in vision. Refractile yellow-white crystals scattered throughout the posterior pole in a donut-shaped pattern, mild cystoid macular edema, and retinal pigmentary changes later; may develop whorl-like, white, subepithelial corneal deposits. Seen with doses >30 mg/day, at the initial higher dosage levels crystals often occur, but can resolve with lowering dose.

- Decrease or discontinue the medication if toxicity develops.

Sildenafil (Viagra)

Used to treat impotence; produces a bluish tint or haze of vision within 1-2 hours of ingestion of the drug. May modify the transduction cascade in photoreceptors; seen in 3% of patients taking a dose of 25-50 mg, 11% of patients taking 100 mg dose, and in 50% taking >100 mg; no permanent visual effects have been reported; long-term effects not known.

- Decrease or discontinue the medication if toxicity develops.
- **Electrophysiologic testing:** Electroretinogram (ERG) mildly reduced during acute episode, reverts back to normal over time; no permanent effects seen.

Thioridazine (Mellaril)

Introduced in 1952 for treatment of psychoses; produces nyctalopia, decreased vision, ring or paracentral scotomas, and brown discoloration of vision. Pigment granularity and clumping in the midperiphery appears first (reversible), then progresses and coalesces into large areas of pigmentation (salt-and-pepper pigment retinopathy) or chorioretinal atrophy with short-term, high-dose use. A variant, termed *nummular retinopathy,* with chorioretinal atrophy posterior to the equator, occurs with chronic use. Late stages can appear similar to end-stage retinitis pigmentosa. Doses >800 mg/day (300 mg recommended) can produce retinopathy; total daily dose seems more critical than total cumulative dose; may progress after medication is withdrawn because the drug is stored in the eye.

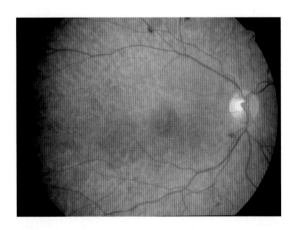

Figure 10-87 • Diffuse pigmentary retinopathy in end-stage thioridazine toxicity.

- Check vision, color vision, and visual fields every 6 months while on medication.
- **Electrophysiologic testing:** Electroretinogram (ERG) (normal early; reduced amplitude and abnormal dark adaptation later).
- **Fluorescein angiography:** Salt-and-pepper pattern of hypofluorescent spots and hyperfluorescent window defects; nummular pattern produces large areas of RPE loss.
- Decrease or discontinue the medication if toxicity develops

▮ Lipid Storage Diseases

Sphingolipid storage diseases cause accumulation of endogenous lipids in lysosomes, especially in retinal ganglion cells, giving a characteristic cherry-red spot in the macula.

Farber's Disease (Lipogranulomatosis) (Autosomal Recessive [AR])

Mild cherry-red spot, failure to thrive, subcutaneous nodules, hoarse cry, progressive arthropathy, and early mortality by 6-18 years of age.

Mucolipidosis (Mucopolysaccharidoses) (AR)

Cherry-red spot, nystagmus, myoclonus, corneal clouding, optic atrophy, cataracts, Hurler-like facies, hepatosplenomegaly, and failure to thrive.

Niemann-Pick Disease (AR)

Prominent cherry-red spot, corneal stromal opacities, splenomegaly, bone marrow foam cells, and hyperlipidemia.

Sandhoff's Disease (Gangliosidosis Type II) (AR)

Prominent cherry-red spot and optic atrophy with associated lipid storage problems in the kidney, liver, pancreas, and other gastrointestinal organs.

Tay-Sachs Disease (Gangliosidosis Type I) (AR)

Prominent cherry-red spot, blindness, deafness, convulsions; mainly seen in Ashkenazi Jewish children.

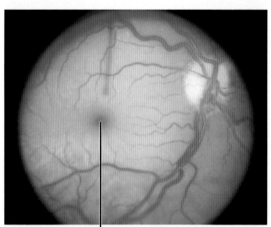

Figure 10-88 • Cherry-red spot in an infant with Tay-Sachs disease.

cherry-red spot

Peripheral Retinal Degenerations

Lattice Degeneration

Occurs in 8-10% of general population; more common in myopes; oval, circumferential area of retinal thinning and overlying vitreous liquefaction found anterior to the equator. Appears as criss-crossing, white lines (sclerotic vessels) with variable overlying retinal pigmentation. Atrophic holes (25%) common; retinal tears can occur with posterior vitreous separation pulling on the atrophic, thinned retina; increased risk of retinal detachment.

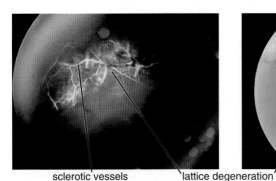 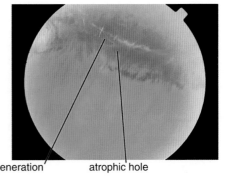

sclerotic vessels   lattice degeneration   atrophic hole

Figure 10-89 • Lattice degeneration demonstrating RPE changes and characteristic linear branching pattern.

Figure 10-90 • Atrophic retinal holes within an area of lattice degeneration.

- Asymptomatic lattice degeneration, atrophic holes, and retinal tears do not require treatment; consider prophylactic treatment in patients with high myopia, aphakia, history of retinal detachment in the fellow eye, or strong family history of retinal detachment. Prophylactic treatment before cataract extraction is controversial.
- Symptomatic lesions (photopsias/floaters) should receive prophylactic treatment with either cryopexy (anterior lesions) or two or three rows of laser photocoagulation around tears or holes (posterior lesions).

Paving Stone/Cobblestone Degeneration

Occurs in 22-27% of general population; round, discrete, yellow-white lesions with darkly pigmented borders found anterior to the equator; correspond to areas of thinned outer retina with loss of choriocapillaris and retinal pigment epithelium; usually found inferiorly; normal vitreous over lesions. May protect against retinal detachment due to adherence of thinned retina and choroid.

- No treatment recommended.

Figure 10-91 • Yellow-white, paving stone lesions with pigmented borders characteristic of peripheral cobblestone degeneration.

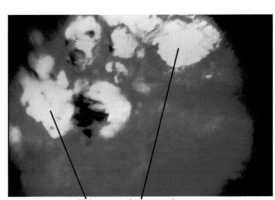

cobblestone degeneration

Peripheral Cystoid Degeneration

Clusters of tiny intraretinal cysts (in the outer plexiform layer) just posterior to ora serrata; retinoschisis precursor; no increased risk of retinal detachment.

• No treatment recommended.

Snail Track Degeneration

Chains of fine, white dots seen circumferentially in the peripheral retina; associated with myopia; atrophic holes may develop in the areas of degeneration, increasing the risk of retinal detachment.

• Asymptomatic snail track degeneration, atrophic holes, and tears do not require treatment; consider prophylactic treatment in patients with high myopia, aphakia, history of retinal detachment in the fellow eye, or strong family history of retinal detachment. Prophylactic treatment before cataract extraction is controversial.
• Symptomatic lesions (photopsias/floaters) should receive prophylactic treatment with either cryopexy (anterior lesions) or two or three rows of laser photocoagulation around tears or holes (posterior lesions)

▮ Retinoschisis

Definition

Splitting of the retina. Two types:

Acquired   Senile, degenerative process with splitting between the inner nuclear and outer plexiform layers.

Juvenile   Congenital process with splitting of the nerve fiber layer.

Epidemiology

Acquired   More common; seen in 4-7% of general population especially in patients >50 years old; 75% bilateral; also associated with hyperopia.

Juvenile (x-linked recessive)   Onset in first decade of life; may be present at birth.
Genetics: Mapped to *XLRS1*/Retinoschisin gene on chromosome Xp22 that codes proteins necessary for cell-cell adhesion; rarely autosomal; 98% bilateral.

Symptoms

Acquired   Usually asymptomatic; may have visual field defect with sharp borders.

Juvenile   Decreased vision (often due to vitreous hemorrhage) or may be asymptomatic; may have eye turn.

Signs

Acquired Bilateral, smooth, convex, elevated schisis cavity usually in inferotemporal quadrant; height of elevation constant, even with change in head position; white dots—"snowflakes" or "frosting"—and retinal vessels (sclerotic in periphery) are seen in the elevated inner retinal layer; outer layer breaks are common; inner layer breaks, vitreous hemorrhage, and rhegmatogenous retinal detachments are rare; cystoid degeneration at the ora serrata; absolute scotoma.

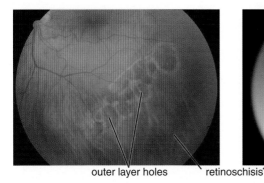

outer layer holes   retinoschisis   demarcation line

Figure 10-92 • Acquired retinoschisis with outer layer breaks.

Figure 10-93 • Acquired retinoschisis with evident demarcation line at edge of elevated schisis cavity.

Juvenile Slowly progressive decreased visual acuity (ranging from 20/25 to 20/80), nystagmus, and strabismus are often seen; foveal schisis with fine, radiating folds from fovea (seen in 100% of cases), spokelike foveal cysts, pigment mottling, and microcystic foveal elevation (looks like cystoid macular edema but does not stain on FA) common; may have vitreous hemorrhage, vitreous veils, retinal vessels bridging inner and outer layers; peripheral retinoschisis (50%) with peripheral pigmentation and loss of retinal vessels, especially in inferotemporal quadrant, often seen.

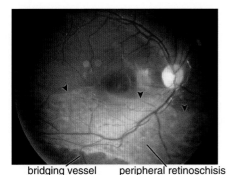

bridging vessel   peripheral retinoschisis

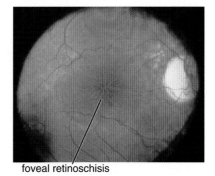

foveal retinoschisis

Figure 10-94 • Juvenile retinoschisis with foveal and peripheral schisis; note bridging retinal vessel.

Figure 10-95 • Foveal retinoschisis with fine, radiating folds and spokelike cysts in a patient with juvenile retinoschisis.

Differential Diagnosis

Retinal detachment, Goldmann-Favre disease, hereditary macular disease.

Evaluation

- Complete ophthalmic history and eye examination with attention to color vision, 78/90 diopter or contact lens fundus examination, ophthalmoscopy, and depressed peripheral retinal examination.
- Check visual fields (absolute scotomas corresponding to areas of schisis).
- **Electrophysiologic testing (in juvenile cases):** Electroretinogram (ERG) (select decrease in b-wave amplitude, normal a-wave; Schubert-Bornsheim tracing or electronegative ERG), electrooculogram (EOG) (normal in mild cases to subnormal in advanced cases), and dark adaptation (normal to subnormal).
- **Color vision:** Initial tritan defect followed by deutan-tritan defect (less severe than for cone-rod dystrophy).
- **Fluorescein angiogram:** Macular cysts seen in foveal schisis do not leak fluorescein.
- **B-scan ultrasonography:** No shifting fluid (serous RD); does not decrease in size on scleral depression.

Management

- No treatment recommended; follow closely if breaks are identified.
- If symptomatic retinal detachment occurs, may require retinal surgery to repair.
- If vitreous hemorrhage occurs, treat conservatively (occlusive patching in child); rarely, pars plana vitrectomy required.

Prognosis

Good; usually stationary for years.

▌Retinal Detachment (RD)

Separation of the neurosensory retina from the retinal pigment epithelium

Rhegmatogenous Retinal Detachment (RRD)

Definition

From Greek *rhegma* = rent; retinal detachment due to full-thickness retinal break (tear, hole, or dialysis) that allows vitreous fluid access to subretinal space.

Etiology

Lattice degeneration (30%), posterior vitreous detachment (especially with vitreous hemorrhage), myopia, trauma (5-10%), and previous ocular surgery (especially with vitreous loss) increase risk of rhegmatogenous retinal detachments; retinal dialysis and giant retinal tears (>3 clock hours in extent) common after trauma.

Symptoms

Acute onset of photopsias, floaters ("shade" or "cob-webs"), shadow or curtain across visual field, decreased vision; may be asymptomatic.

Signs

Undulating, mobile, convex, with corrugated folds; clear subretinal fluid that does not shift with body position; retinal break usually seen; may have "tobacco-dust" (Shafer's sign: pigment cells in the vitreous), vitreous hemorrhage, or operculum; usually lower intraocular pressure in the affected eye and may have positive relative afferent pupillary defect (RAPD); chronic rhegmatogenous retinal detachments may have pigmented demarcation lines, intraretinal cysts, fixed folds, or subretinal precipitates.
Configuration of detachment helps localize retinal break:

(1) Superotemporal/nasal detachment: break within 1-1.5 clock hours of highest border.
(2) Superior detachment that straddles 12-o'clock position: break between 11- and 1-o'clock positions.
(3) Inferior detachment with one higher side: break within 1-1.5 clock hours of highest border.
(4) Inferior detachment equally high on either side: break between 5- and 7-o'clock positions.

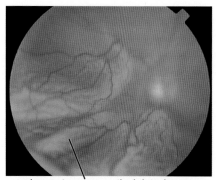

rhegmatogenous retinal detachment

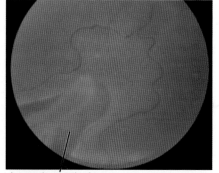

horseshoe retinal tear

Figure 10-96 • Rhegmatogenous retinal detachment demonstrating corrugated folds.

Figure 10-97 • Same patient as shown in Figure 10-96 demonstrating peripheral horseshoe tear that caused the rhegmatogenous retinal detachment.

Differential Diagnosis

Retinoschisis, choroidal detachment, serous retinal detachment, tractional retinal detachment, central serous chorioretinopathy.

Evaluation

• Complete ophthalmic history and eye examination with attention to visual acuity, pupils, ophthalmoscopy, and depressed peripheral retinal examination to identify any retinal breaks.
• **B-scan ultrasonography:** If unable to visualize the fundus; smooth, convex, freely mobile; retina appears as highly reflective echo in the vitreous cavity that is attached at the optic nerve head and ora serrata; retinal tears can be visualized in the periphery. Detachment will diminish in size with scleral depression (in contrast to retinoschisis).

Management

- **Asymptomatic, not threatening macula:** Most should be treated (see below); rarely followed closely by retina specialist; consider wall-off laser photocoagulation.
- **Symptomatic:** Pneumatic retinopexy or retinal surgery with scleral buckle and cryotherapy, with or without pars plana vitrectomy, drainage of subretinal fluid, endolaser, and/or other surgical maneuvers. Macular threatening ("Mac on") rhegmatogenous retinal detachment is treated emergently (within 24 hours); if macula is already detached ("Mac off"), treat urgently (within 48 to 96 hours).

Prognosis

Variable (depends on underlying condition); 5-10% of rhegmatogenous retinal detachment repairs develop proliferative vitreoretinopathy (PVR).

Serous/Exudative Retinal Detachment (SRD)

Definition

Nonrhegmatogenous retinal detachment (not secondary to a retinal break) due to subretinal transudation of fluid from tumor, inflammatory process, vascular lesions, or degenerative lesions.

Etiology

Vogt-Koyanagi-Harada syndrome, Harada's disease, idiopathic uveal effusion syndrome, choroidal tumors, central serous retinopathy, posterior scleritis, hypertensive retinopathy, Coats' disease, optic nerve pit, retinal coloboma, and toxemia of pregnancy.

Symptoms

Usually asymptomatic until serous retinal detachment involves macula; may have acute onset of photopsias, floaters ("shade" or "cob-webs"), shadow across visual field, or decreased vision.

Signs

Smooth, serous elevation of retina; subretinal fluid shifts with changing head position; there is no retinal break by definition; may have mild RAPD.

Differential Diagnosis

Retinoschisis, choroidal detachment, rhegmatogenous retinal detachment, central serous chorioretinopathy.

Evaluation

- Complete ophthalmic history and eye examination with attention to visual acuity, pupils, ophthalmoscopy, and depressed peripheral retinal examination to identify any retinal breaks.
- **B-scan ultrasonography:** If unable to visualize the fundus, smooth, concave, freely mobile echoes that shift with changing head position; retina appears as highly reflective echo in the vitreous cavity that is attached at the optic nerve head and ora serrata.

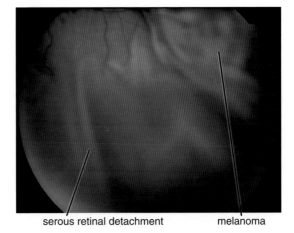

Figure 10-98 • Exudative retinal detachment secondary to malignant melanoma.

serous retinal detachment   melanoma

Management

- Treat underlying condition; rarely requires or responds to surgical intervention.

Prognosis

Variable (depends on underlying condition).

Traction Retinal Detachment (TRD)

Definition

Nonrhegmatogenous retinal detachment (not secondary to a retinal break) due to fibrovascular or fibrotic proliferation and subsequent contraction, pulling retina up.

Etiology

Diabetic retinopathy, sickle cell retinopathy, retinopathy of prematurity, proliferative vitreoretinopathy, toxocariasis, and familial exudative vitreoretinopathy.

Symptoms

May be asymptomatic if traction retinal detachment does not involve macula; acute onset of photopsias, floaters ("shade" or "cob-webs"), shadow across visual field, or decreased vision.

Signs

Smooth, concave, usually localized, does not extend to the ora serrata; usually with fibrovascular proliferation; may have pseudo-holes or true holes in a combined traction-rhegmatogenous detachment that progresses more rapidly than TRD alone; if a retinal tear develops, detachment may become convex. May have mild RAPD.

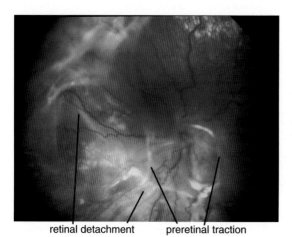

Figure 10-99 • Traction retinal detachment due to proliferative vitreoretinopathy following penetrating ocular trauma.

retinal detachment   preretinal traction

Differential Diagnosis

Retinoschisis, choroidal detachment, rhegmatogenous retinal detachment.

Evaluation

- Complete ophthalmic history and eye examination with attention to visual acuity, pupils, ophthalmoscopy, and depressed peripheral retinal examination to identify any retinal breaks.
- **B-scan ultrasonography:** If unable to visualize the fundus; usually has tented appearance with vitreous adhesions; retina appears as highly reflective echo in the vitreous cavity that is attached at the optic nerve head and ora serrata.

Management

- Observation unless traction retinal detachment threatens the macula or becomes a combined traction-rhegmatogenous detachment.
- Vitreoretinal surgery to release the vitreoretinal traction, depending on clinical situation, should be performed by vitreoretinal specialist.

Prognosis

Variable (depends on underlying condition).

◼ Choroidal Detachment

Smooth, bullous, orange-brown elevation of retina and choroid; usually extends 360 degrees around the periphery in a lobular configuration; the ora serrata can be seen without scleral depression.

Choroidal Effusion

Often asymptomatic with decreased intraocular pressure; may have shallow anterior chamber; associated with acute ocular hypotony, after surgery (excessive filtration through filtering bleb, wound leak, cyclodialysis cleft, postscleral buckling surgery), posterior scleritis, Vogt-Koyanagi-Harada syndrome, trauma (open globe), intraocular tumors, or uveal effusion syndrome.

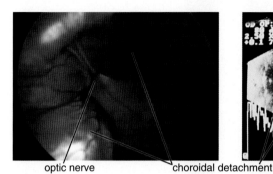

optic nerve   choroidal detachment

Figure 10-100 • Choroidal detachment demonstrating smooth elevations of eye wall.

Figure 10-101 • B-scan ultrasound demonstrating choroidal detachment.

Choroidal Hemorrhage

Causes pain (often severe), decreased vision, red eye, intraocular inflammation, and increased intraocular pressure; classically occurring acutely during anterior segment surgery but may be delayed up to 1-7 days after surgery or trauma, especially in patients with hypertension or taking anticoagulants.

- **B-scan ultrasonography:** Smooth, convex, elevated membrane limited in the equatorial region by the vortex veins and anteriorly by the scleral spur; appears thicker and less mobile than retina.
- Treat intraoperative choroidal hemorrhage with immediate closure of surgical wound and, if massive hemorrhage, perform sclerotomies to allow drainage of blood, to close surgical wound; total intraoperative drainage is usually not possible.
- Topical cycloplegic (atropine 1% bid) and steroid (prednisolone acetate 1% qid).
- May require treatment of increased intraocular pressure (see Chapter 11).
- Consider surgical drainage when appositional or "kissing" (temporal and nasal choroid touch), severe intraocular pressure elevation despite maximal medical treatment, or corneal decompensation; visual results in appositional choroidal hemorrhage is very poor.
- Treat underlying condition.

▪ Proliferative Vitreoretinopathy (PVR)

Fibrotic membranes composed of retinal pigment epithelial, glial, and inflammatory cells that form after retinal detachment or retinal surgery (8-10%); the membranes contract and pull on the retinal surface (6-8 weeks after surgery); may be preretinal or subretinal; primary cause of redetachment after successful retinal detachment surgery. Risk factors include previous retinal surgery, vitreous hemorrhage, choroidal detachment, giant retinal tears, multiple retinal breaks, penetrating trauma, excessive cryotherapy, and failure to reattach the retina at primary surgery. Final anatomic reattachment rates 72-96%; visual prognosis variable (14-37% achieve >20/100 vision).

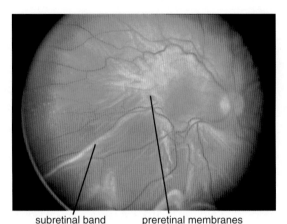

Figure 10-102 • Retinal detachment with proliferative vitreoretinopathy demonstrating retinal folds and dragged vessels.

subretinal band   preretinal membranes

• Retinal surgery to remove preretinal and subretinal fibrotic membranes and reattach retina using silicon oil or intraocular C_3F_8 gas injection (The Silicon Oil Study conclusions); occasionally requires retinectomy to reattach retina; should be performed by a retina specialist.

Intermediate Uveitis/Pars Planitis

Definition

Intermediate uveitis is an inflammation primarily limited to the vitreous cavity that usually involves the pars plana and ciliary body of unknown etiology. Pars planitis is a form of intermediate uveitis, classically with vitritis, pars plana exudate, and peripheral retinal vasculitis.

Epidemiology

Occurs in children and young adults; average age, 23-28 years; 75-90% bilateral; associated with multiple sclerosis (up to 15%) and sarcoidosis; no sex predilection; rare in blacks and Asians; represents roughly 5-8% of all uveitis cases, with an incidence between 2 and 5:100,000.

Symptoms

Decreased vision, floaters; no red eye, pain, or photophobia.

Signs

Decreased visual acuity, fibrovascular exudates especially along the inferior pars plana ("snow-banking"), extensive vitreous cells (100% of cases), vitreous cellular aggregates ("snowballs") inferiorly, minimal anterior chamber cells and flare, posterior vitreous detachment, peripheral vasculitis, and cystoid macular edema (85% of cases); may develop neovascularization and vitreous hemorrhage in the pars plana exudate.

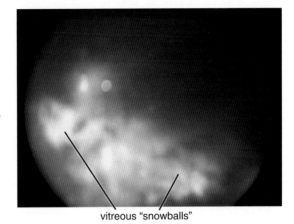

Figure 10-103 • Pars planitis demonstrating "snowballs" in the vitreous cavity.

vitreous "snowballs"

Differential Diagnosis

Sarcoidosis, multiple sclerosis, Lyme disease, Behçet's disease, masquerade syndromes (especially lymphoma), syphilis, posterior uveitis, amyloidosis, familial exudative vitreoretinopathy, Irvine-Gass syndrome (cystoid macular edema after cataract extraction), toxocariasis, toxoplasmosis, candidiasis, fungal endophthalmitis, Eales' disease, VKH, and retinoblastoma.

Evaluation

- Complete ophthalmic history and eye examination with attention to anterior chamber, anterior vitreous, 78/90 diopter or contact lens fundus examination, and ophthalmoscopy (cystoid macular edema and retinal periphery).
- **Fluorescein angiogram:** Petalloid leakage from cystoid macular edema seen in late views.
- **Lab tests:** Rule out other causes from differential diagnosis, although HLA-DR2 sometimes associated. ACE, chest radiographs, and serum lysozyme to rule out sarcoidosis, CBC to rule out masquerade syndromes, VDRL, FTA-ABS, Lyme titers, and toxocariasis and toxoplasmosis IgG and IgM serology to rule out infection.
- CT scan of the chest to rule out mediastinal lymphadenopathy.

Management

- Posterior sub-Tenon's steroid injection (triamcinolone acetonide 40 mg/mL) when vision is affected by cystoid macular edema or severe inflammation.

Continued

Management—cont'd

- Oral steroids (prednisone 1 mg/kg po qd pulse with rapid taper to 10-15 mg/day) if unable to tolerate injections or in severe bilateral cases. Check PPD, blood glucose, and chest radiographs before starting systemic steroids.
- Add H2-blocker (ranitidine [Zantac] 150 mg po bid) or proton pump inhibitor when taking systemic steroids.
- Consider topical steroids (prednisolone acetate 1% q2-6h) and cycloplegic (scopolamine 0.25% bid to qid) if severe inflammation or macular edema exists (minimal effect).
- Cryotherapy to the peripheral retina reserved for neovascularization. Pars plana vitrectomy is gaining acceptance to treat difficult cases.
- Consider immunosuppressive agents Cyclosporine (Neoral), Azathioprine, Methotrexate, Cytoxan for recalcitrant cases (see Posterior Uveitis management section).

Prognosis

Fifty-one percent of patients will achieve 20/30 vision; 10-20% may have self-limited or 40-60% will have a smoldering, chronic course with episodic exacerbations and remissions. Macular edema generally determines visual outcome. Zero tolerance to inflammation and aggressive treatment of active inflammation is a key factor in determining a good outcome.

Neuroretinitis/Leber's Idiopathic Stellate Neuroretinitis

Definition

Optic disc edema and macular star formation with no other systemic abnormalities.

Etiology

Due to pleomorphic gram-negative bacillus *Bartonella henselae* (formerly known as *Rochalimaea*); associated with cat-scratch disease.

Symptoms

Mild, unilateral decreased vision, rarely pain with eye movement; may have viral prodrome (52%) with fever, malaise, lymphadenopathy, upper respiratory tract, gastrointestinal, or urinary tract infection.

Signs

Decreased visual acuity, visual field defects (cecocentral or central scotomas), positive relative afferent pupillary defect (RAPD), optic disc edema with macular star, peripapillary exudative retinal detachment, vitreous cells, rare anterior chamber cells and flare, yellow-white lesions at level of retinal pigment epithelium.

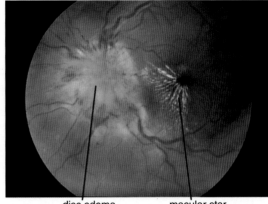

Figure 10-104 • Leber's idiopathic stellate neuroretinitis demonstrating optic disc edema and partial macular star.

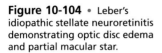

disc edema   macular star

Differential Diagnosis

Hypertensive retinopathy, diabetic retinopathy, anterior ischemic optic neuropathy (AION), retinal vein occlusion, syphilis, diffuse unilateral subacute neuroretinitis (DUSN), acute macular neuroretinopathy, viral retinitis, sarcoidosis, toxocariasis, toxoplasmosis, tuberculosis, papilledema.

Evaluation

- Complete ophthalmic history and eye examination with attention to pupils, 78/90 diopter and contact lens fundus examination, and ophthalmoscopy.
- **Fluorescein angiogram:** Leakage from optic disc capillaries, no perifoveal leakage.
- **Lab tests:** Venereal Disease Research Laboratory test (VDRL), fluorescent treponemal antibody absorption test (FTA-ABS), purified protein derivative (PPD), indirect fluorescent antibody test for *Bartonella henselae (Rochalimaea)*.
- Check blood pressure.

Management

- No treatment recommended.
- Use of systemic antibiotics (doxycycline, tetracycline, ciprofloxacin, trimethoprim [Bactrim]) and steroids is controversial.

Prognosis

Good; 67% regain >20/20 vision, and 97% >20/40 vision; usually spontaneous recovery; disc edema resolves over 8-12 weeks, macular star over 6-12 months; optic atrophy may develop.

▉ Posterior Uveitis: Infections

Acute Retinal Necrosis (ARN)

Fulminant retinitis and vitritis due to the herpes zoster virus (HZV), herpes simplex virus (HSV), or, rarely, cytomegalovirus (CMV) seen in healthy, as well as immunocompromised, patients. Slight male predilection (2:1); patients have pain, decreased vision, and floaters after a recent herpes simplex or zoster infection. Starts with small, well-demarcated areas of retinal necrosis outside the vascular arcades that spread rapidly and circumferentially into large, confluent areas of white, retinal necrosis with retinal vascular occlusions and small satellite lesions; 36% bilateral (BARN); associated with granulomatous anterior uveitis and retinal vasculitis. In the cicatricial phase (1-3 months later), retinal detachments (50-75%) with multiple holes and giant tears are common; poor visual prognosis (only 30% achieve >20/200 vision).

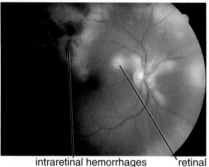

intraretinal hemorrhages   retinal necrosis

Figure 10-105 • Acute retinal necrosis demonstrating hemorrhage and yellow-white patches of necrosis.

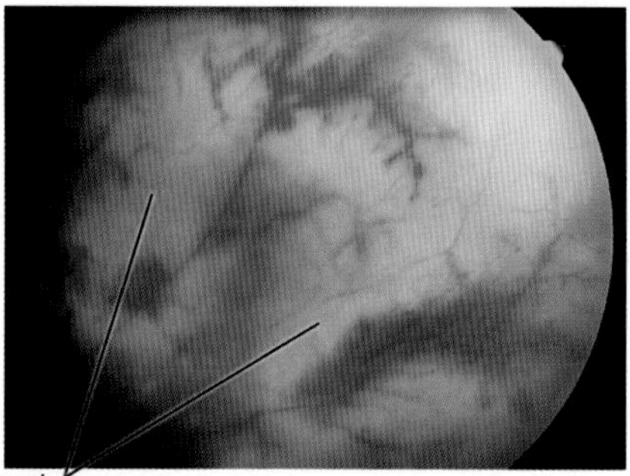

Figure 10-106 • Same patient as shown in Figure 10-105, 2 days later demonstrating rapid progression with confluence of lesions.

- **Lab tests:** HZV and HSV (types 1 and 2) immunoglobulin G and M titers.
- Systemic antivirals (acyclovir 5-10 mg/kg IV in three divided doses qd until resolution of the retinitis, and then 800 mg acyclovir po 5×/day for 1-2 months) or 1 g valacyclovir po tid; follow blood urea nitrogen (BUN) and creatinine levels for nephrotoxicity.
- 24 hours after acyclovir started, oral steroids (prednisone 60-100 mg po qd for 1-2 months with slow taper); check PPD, blood glucose, and chest radiographs before starting systemic steroids.
- Add H2-blocker (ranitidine [Zantac] 150 mg po bid) or proton pump inhibitor when giving systemic steroids.
- Topical steroid (prednisolone acetate 1% should be tailored to anterior segment inflammation) and cycloplegic (homatropine 5% bid) in the presence of active inflammation.
- If treatment fails, fulminant course, or patient is HIV-positive, then consider IV ganciclovir and/or foscarnet, as well as intravitreal ganciclovir injections (see doses in Cytomegalovirus section).
- Role of anticoagulation is controversial.
- Consider three or four rows of laser photocoagulation to demarcate active areas of retinitis and necrosis to prevent retinal breaks and retinal detachments (controversial).

- Laser demarcation or retinal surgery for retinal detachments; usually requires use of silicon oil.
- Medical consultation.

Candidiasis

Endogenous endophthalmitis caused by fungal *Candida* species (*C. albicans* or *C. tropicalis*) with white, fluffy, chorioretinal infiltrates and overlying vitreous haze; vitreous "puff-balls," anterior chamber cells and flare, hypopyon, Roth spots, and hemorrhages occur less often. Occurs in IV drug abusers and debilitated or immunocompromised patients who have decreased vision and floaters.

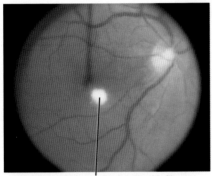

Candida albicans chorioretinal infiltrate

Figure 10-107 • Candidiasis demonstrating white, fluffy, chorioretinal infiltrate.

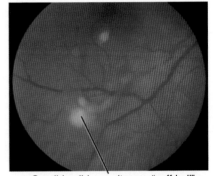

Candida albicans vitreous "puff-ball"

Figure 10-108 • Vitreous "puff-ball" due to *Candida albicans* endogenous endophthalmitis.

- **Lab tests:** Sputum, urine, blood, and stool cultures for fungi.
- Systemic antifungal (fluconazole 100 mg po bid or amphotericin B 0.25-1.0 mg/kg IV over 6h) if disseminated disease is present.
- If moderate to severe inflammation, pars plana vitrectomy and intraocular injection of antifungal (amphotericin B 0.005 mg/0.1 mL) and steroid (dexamethasone 0.4 mg/0.1 mL).
- Topical steroid (prednisolone acetate 1% qid) and cycloplegic (scopolamine 0.25% bid to qid).
- Medical consultation to treat systemic source of infection.

Cysticercosis

Subretinal or intravitreal, round, mobile, translucent, yellow-white cyst due to *Cysticercus cellulosae*, the larval form of the tapeworm *Taenia solium*; asymptomatic until the parasite grows and causes painless, progressive, decreased vision and visual field defects. Worm death may incite an inflammatory response. Can also have central nervous system (CNS) involvement with seizures, hydrocephalus, and headaches.

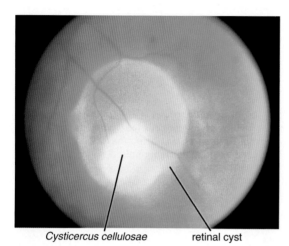

Figure 10-109 • Cysticercosis with cyst surrounding the tapeworm.

Cysticercus cellulosae   retinal cyst

- **B-scan ultrasonography:** Highly reflective echoes from the cyst walls and often the worm within the cystic space.
- **Lab tests:** Enzyme-linked immunosorbent assay (ELISA) for anticysticercus immunoglobulin G.
- No antihelminthic medication is effective for intraocular infection.
- Consider direct laser photocoagulation of worm.
- Pars plana vitrectomy for removal of intravitreal *Cysticercus.*
- Neurology consultation to rule out CNS involvement.

Cytomegalovirus (CMV)

Hemorrhagic retinitis with thick, yellow-white retinal necrosis, vascular sheathing (severe sheathing with frosted-branch appearance may occur outside of area of retinitis), mild anterior chamber cells and flare, vitreous cells, and retinal hemorrhages. Brush-fire appearance with indolent, granular, yellow advancing border and peripheral, atrophic region is also common. Less commonly, CMV retinitis may present with a clinical picture of frosted-branch angiitis. Retinal detachments (15-50%) with multiple, small, peripheral breaks commonly occur in atrophic areas. Patients are usually asymptomatic but may have floaters, paracentral scotomas, metamorphopsia, and decreased acuity. Bilateral on presentation in 40%; 15-20% become bilateral after treatment. Most common retinal infection in AIDS (15-46%), especially when CD4 <50 cells/mm^3.

- **Lab tests:** HIV antibody test, CD4 count, HIV viral load, urine for CMV; consider CMV polymerase chain reaction (PCR) assay.
- If first episode, induction therapy with either:
  - Ganciclovir (Cytovene 5-7.5 mg/kg IV bid for 2-4 weeks, then maintenance with 5-10 mg/kg IV qd); follow CBC for neutropenia (worsened by zidovudine [formerly AZT]) and thrombocytopenia; if bone marrow suppression is severe, add recombinant granulocyte colony stimulating factor (G-CSF) (filgrastim [Neupogen]) or recombinant granulocyte-macrophage colony stimulating factor (GM-CSF) (sargramostim [Leukine]).

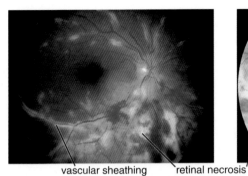
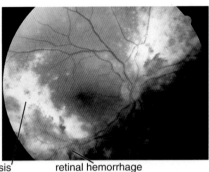

vascular sheathing   retinal necrosis   retinal hemorrhage

Figure 10-110 • Cytomegalovirus retinitis demonstrating patchy necrotic lesions, hemorrhage, and vascular sheathing.

Figure 10-111 • Cytomegalovirus retinitis with larger areas of necrosis and hemorrhage.

- Foscarnet (Foscavir, 90 mg/kg IV bid or 60 mg/kg IV tid for 2 weeks, then maintenance with 90-120 mg/kg IV qd); infuse slowly with 500-1000 mL normal saline or 5% dextrose; push liquids to avoid dehydration; follow electrolytes (potassium, phosphorus, calcium, and magnesium), BUN, and creatinine for nephrotoxicity; avoid other nephrotoxic medications.
- *Note:* Foscarnet-Ganciclovir CMV Retinitis Trial showed equal efficacy between foscarnet and ganciclovir; possible survival advantage with IV foscarnet.
- Cidofovir (Vistide, 3-5 mg/kg IV every week for 2 weeks, then maintenance with 3-5 mg/kg IV q2wk) and probenecid (1 g po before infusion, 2 mg po after infusion); does not work in patients with ganciclovir resistance; follow BUN and creatinine for nephrotoxicity.
- Alternatively, combination of intravitreal surgical implantation of a ganciclovir pellet (releases 1 µg per hour, lasts ~6-8 months) and oral ganciclovir (1000-2000 mg po tid) for systemic CMV prophylaxis; good choice in new onset, unilateral cases; do not use in recurrent cases; should be performed by retina specialist.
- Recurrence or progression can be reinduced with same regimen or new drug regimen (mean time to relapse ~60 days in Foscarnet-Ganciclovir CMV Retinitis Trial). In the era of Highly Active Antiretroviral Therapy (HAART), much longer period of remission before reactivation.
- Treatment failures should be induced with new drug or a combination of drugs (use lower dosages due to the higher risk of toxic side effects); combination treatment is effective against disease progression (Cytomegalovirus Retreatment Trial conclusion).
- Intravitreal injections can be used if there is an intolerance to antiviral therapy or progressive retinitis despite systemic treatment (should be performed by retina specialist):
  - Ganciclovir (Cytovene, 200-2000 µg/0.1 mL 2 to 3 times a week for 2-3 weeks, then maintenance with 200-2000 µg/0.1 mL once a week).
  - Foscarnet (Foscavir, 2.4 mg/0.1 mL or 1.2 mg/0.05 mL 2 to 3 times a week for 2-3 weeks, then maintenance with 2.4 mg/0.1 mL 1 to 2 times a week).
  - Vitravene (165-330 µg every week for 3 weeks, then every 2 weeks for maintenance).
- Follow monthly with serial photography (60-degree, nine peripheral fields) to document inactivity or progression.

- Retinal detachments that threaten the macula with no macular retinitis may be treated with pars plana vitrectomy, endolaser, and silicon oil tamponade; peripheral shallow detachments may be followed closely (especially inferiorly) or demarcated with two or three rows of laser photocoagulation.
- Medical consultation.

Diffuse Unilateral Subacute Neuroretinitis (DUSN)

Unilateral, indolent, multifocal, diffuse pigmentary changes with gray-yellow outer retinal lesions that reflect the movement of a subretinal nematode: *Ancylostoma caninum* (dog hookworm, 400-1000 µm, endemic in southeastern United States, South America, and the Caribbean) or *Baylisascaris procyonis* (raccoon intestinal worm, 400-2000 µm, endemic in northern and midwestern United States). Movement of worm felt to cause destruction of photoreceptor outer segments. Usually minimal intraocular inflammation; occurs in healthy patients with decreased vision (often out of proportion to retinal findings); may have a positive relative afferent pupillary defect (RAPD). Chronic infection causes irreversible poor vision (20/200 or worse), visual field defects, optic nerve pallor, chorioretinal atrophy, and narrowed retinal vessels in a retinitis pigmentosa–like pattern. Poor prognosis without treatment; variable prognosis with treatment if worm can be killed.

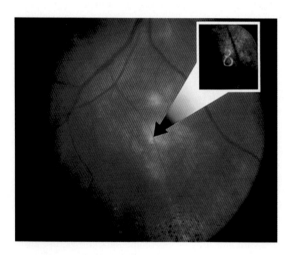

Figure 10-112 • Diffuse unilateral subacute neuroretinitis demonstrating subretinal nematode (inset).

- Complete history with attention to travel and animal exposure.
- **Fluorescein angiogram:** Lesions hypofluorescent early and stain late, perivascular leakage, and disc staining; more advanced disease shows widespread window defects.
- **Lab tests:** Stool for ova and parasites, CBC with differential (eosinophilia sometimes present); LDH and SGOT sometimes elevated.
- **Electrophysiologic testing:** ERG (subnormal, loss of b-wave) helps differentiate from optic nerve abnormalities.

- Most effective treatment is direct laser photocoagulation of the worm. Surgical subretinal removal of the worm is controversial.
- Systemic antihelminthic medications (thiabendazole, diethylcarbamazine, pyrantel pamoate) are controversial and often not effective; steroids usually added because worm death may increase inflammation.

Human Immunodeficiency Virus (HIV)

Asymptomatic, nonprogressive, microangiopathy characterized by multiple cotton-wool spots (50-70%), Roth spots (40%), retinal hemorrhages, and microaneurysms in the posterior pole that resolves without treatment within 1-2 months. Seen in up to 50% of patients.

- **Lab tests:** HIV antibody test, CD4 count, HIV viral load.
- No treatment necessary.
- Medical consultation.

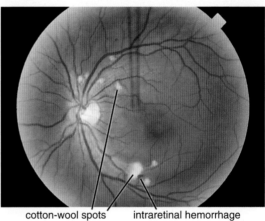

Figure 10-113 • Human immunodeficiency virus retinopathy demonstrating cotton-wool spots and one intraretinal hemorrhage.

cotton-wool spots   intraretinal hemorrhage

Pneumocystis Carinii Choroidopathy

Asymptomatic, unifocal or multifocal, round, creamy, yellow choroidal infiltrates located in the posterior pole caused by disseminated infection from the opportunistic organism *Pneumocystis carinii*; enlarge slowly with minimal vitreous inflammation; may be bilateral; resolution takes weeks to months after therapy is initiated; has become very rare with the elimination of aerosolized pentamidine prophylaxis.

- **Lab tests:** Induced sputum or bronchoalveolar lavage (BAL) for histopathologic staining.
- **Fluorescein angiogram:** Early hypofluorescence with late staining of lesions.
- Systemic antibiotics (trimethoprim 20 mg/kg and sulfamethoxazole 100 mg/kg divided equally IV qid) or pentamidine isethionate (slow infusion 4 mg/kg IV qd) for 14-21 days.
- Medical consultation.

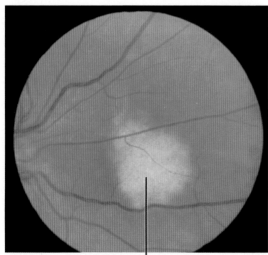

Figure 10-114 • Round, creamy, yellow choroidal infiltrate from *Pneumocystis carinii* choroidopathy.

Pneumocystis carinii infiltrate

Presumed Ocular Histoplasmosis Syndrome (POHS)

Small, round, yellow-brown, punched-out chorioretinal lesions ("histo spots") in mid-periphery and posterior pole, and juxtapapillary atrophic changes caused by the dimorphic fungus, *Histoplasma capsulatum*; endemic in the Ohio and Mississippi river valleys; no vitritis; histo spots occur in 2-3% of population in endemic areas; rare in blacks; usually asymptomatic; macular disciform lesions can occur due to choroidal neovascular membranes (CNV); better visual prognosis than CNV due to age-related macular degeneration, 30% recurrence rate; associated with HLA-B7.

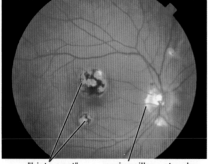

"histo spot"   peripapillary atrophy

Figure 10-115 • Presumed ocular histoplasmosis syndrome demonstrating macular and peripapillary lesions.

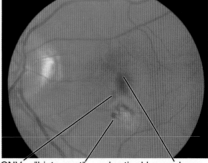

CNV   "histo spot"   subretinal hemorrhage

Figure 10-116 • Presumed ocular histoplasmosis syndrome demonstrating CNV and "histo" spot.

- Check Amsler grid.
- **Fluorescein angiogram:** Early hypofluorescence and late staining of histo spots, also identifies CNV if present.
- **Lab tests:** Histoplasmin antigen skin testing (not necessary).
- Extrafoveal and juxtafoveal CNV (see section on age-related macular degeneration) can be treated with focal laser photocoagulation (MPS-OHS conclusion). Subfoveal CNV should not be treated with laser (14% regress spontaneously).
- Subfoveal CNV should be treated with ocular photodynamic therapy (Visudyne in Ocular Histoplasmosis [VOH] Study conclusion).
- Removal of CNV with subretinal surgery is being evaluated in the Subretinal Surgery Trials (group H); however, up to 50% recur within 1 year (experimental).
- Consider intravitreal 4 mg triamcinolone acetonide either alone or combined with PDT (experimental) for subfoveal CNV.
- Oral steroid treatment (prednisone 60-100 mg po qd with slow taper) and/or intravitreal steroids (4 mg triamcinolone acetonide) are controversial.

Progressive Outer Retinal Necrosis Syndrome (PORN)

Multifocal, patchy, retinal opacification that starts in the posterior pole and spreads rapidly to involve the entire retina due to the herpes zoster virus (HZV); minimal anterior chamber cells and flare, vitreous cells, or retinal vasculitis (differentiates from acute retinal necrosis); occurs in severely immunocompromised patients; poor response to therapy; may develop retinal detachments.

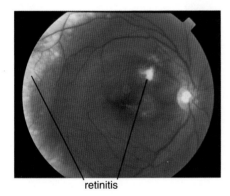

retinitis

Figure 10-117 • Progressive outer retinal necrosis with multifocal retinal opacification.

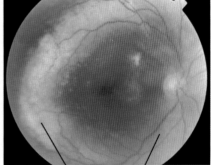

progressive outer retinal necrosis

Figure 10-118 • Same patient as shown in Figure 10-117, 7 days later with a massive increase in retinal necrosis. The posterior pole lesion has become atrophic.

- **Lab tests:** HZV immunoglobulin G and M titers.
- Systemic antivirals (acyclovir 5-10 mg/kg IV in divided doses tid until resolution of retinitis, then 800 mg po 5×/d for 1-2 months); follow BUN and creatinine for nephrotoxicity.
- 24 hours after acyclovir started, oral steroids (prednisone 60-100 mg po qd for 1-2 months with slow taper); check PPD, blood glucose, and chest radiographs before starting systemic steroids.

- Add H2-blocker (ranitidine [Zantac] 150 mg po bid) or proton pump inhibitor when giving systemic steroids.
- Frequency of topical steroids (prednisolone acetate 1%) should be tailored to the severity of inflammation; cycloplegic (scopolamine 0.25% bid to qid) while inflamed.
- If treatment fails or fulminant course, consider IV ganciclovir and/or foscarnet, as well as intravitreal ganciclovir injections (see CMV section for doses).
- Laser demarcation or retinal surgery for retinal detachments; usually requires use of silicon oil.
- Medical consultation.

Rubella

Congenital syndrome classically characterized by congenital cataracts, glaucoma, and rubella retinopathy with salt-and-pepper pigmentary changes; also associated with microphthalmia, iris transillumination defects, bilateral deafness, congenital heart disease, growth retardation, and bone and dental abnormalities; 80% bilateral; vision is generally good (20/25); may rarely develop choroidal neovascular membrane (CNV).

- **Fluorescein angiogram:** Mottled hyperfluorescence.

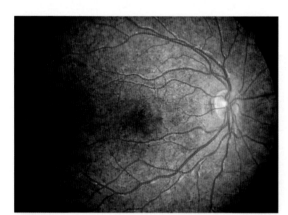

Figure 10-119 • Rubella retinopathy demonstrating salt-and-pepper fundus appearance.

Syphilis (Luetic Chorioretinitis)

Extensive iritis, retinitis, and vitritis (panuveitis) seen in secondary syphilis (6 weeks to 6 months after primary infection) due to the spirochete *Treponema pallidum*. Signs include anterior chamber cells and flare, keratic precipitates, vitritis, multifocal, yellow-white chorioretinal infiltrates, salt-and-pepper pigmentary changes, flame-shaped retinal hemorrhages, and vascular sheathing; called "great mimic," since it can resemble many other retinal diseases; associated with sectoral interstitial keratitis, papillitis, and rarely CNV. Variant called *acute syphilitic posterior placoid chorioretinitis (ASPPC),* with large, placoid, yellow lesions with faded centers. Mucocutaneous manifestations of secondary syphilis are often evident.

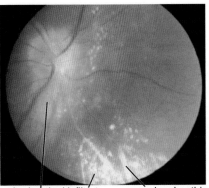

chorioretinal infiltrates   vascular sheathing

Figure 10-120 • Multifocal, yellow-white
chorioretinal infiltrates and vascular
sheathing in a patient with luetic
chorioretinitis.

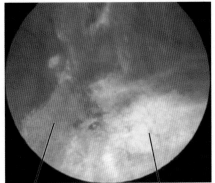

pigmentary changes   chorioretinal infiltrate

Figure 10-121 • Late luetic chorioretinitis
with pigmentary changes and resolving
chorioretinal infiltrate.

- **Lab tests:** Rapid Plasma Reagin (RPR, reflects current activity) or Venereal Disease Research Laboratory test (VDRL, reflects current activity), and fluorescent treponemal antibody absorption test (FTA-ABS) or microhemagglutination for *Treponema pallidum* (MHA-TP).
- Lumbar puncture for VDRL, FTA-ABS, total protein, and cell counts to rule out neurosyphilis.
- Penicillin G (2.4 million U IV q4h for 10-14 days then 2.4 million U IM every week for 3 weeks); tetracycline if patient is allergic to penicillin.
- Long-term tetracycline (250-500 mg po qd) or doxycycline (100 mg po qd) in HIV-positive or immunocompromised patients.
- Follow serum RPR or VDRL to monitor treatment efficacy.
- Medical consultation.

Toxocariasis

Unilateral, multifocal, subretinal, yellow-white granulomas; associated with papillitis, serous and traction retinal detachments, dragged macula and retinal vessels, vitritis, dense vitreous infiltrates, and chronic endophthalmitis; caused by the second-stage larval form of the round-worm *Toxocara canis*. Gray-white chorioretinal scars remain after active infection. Usually occurs in children (included in differential diagnosis of leukocoria) and young adults; associated with pica (eating dirt) and close contact with puppies; children with visceral larva migrans do not develop ocular involvement.

- **Lab tests:** ELISA for *Toxocara* antibody titers.
- Topical steroid (prednisolone acetate 1% q2-6h) and cycloplegic (scopolamine 0.25% bid to qid) for active anterior segment inflammation.
- Posterior sub-Tenon's steroid injection (triamcinolone acetonide 40 mg/mL) and oral steroids (prednisone 60-100 mg po qd) for severe inflammation. Check PPD, blood glucose, and chest radiographs before starting systemic steroids.

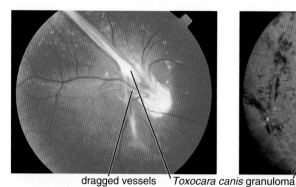

dragged vessels   *Toxocara canis* granuloma   chorioretinal scars

Figure 10-122 • Toxocariasis demonstrating fibrous attachment of peripheral granuloma to optic nerve with dragged retina and vessels.

Figure 10-123 • End stage infection with *Toxocara canis* demonstrating diffuse chorioretinal scarring, dragged vessels, and granuloma.

- Add H2-blocker (ranitidine [Zantac] 150 mg po bid) or proton pump inhibitor when giving systemic steroids.
- Systemic antihelminthic medications (thiabendazole, diethylcarbamazine, pyrantel pamoate) controversial, since worm death may increase inflammation.
- Retinal surgery for retinal detachment (successful in 70-80%)

Toxoplasmosis

Acquired (eating poorly cooked meat) or congenital (transplacental transmission) necrotizing retinitis caused by the parasite *Toxoplasma gondii*. Congenital toxoplasmosis appears as an atrophic, chorioretinal scar (often located in the macula) with gray-white punctate peripheral lesions; associated with microphthalmia, nystagmus, strabismus, intracranial calcifications, microcephaly, and hydrocephalus. Acquired toxoplasmosis (especially in immunocompromised patients) and reactivated congenital lesions present with decreased vision, photophobia, floaters, vascular sheathing, full-thickness retinal necrosis, fluffy, yellow-white retinal lesion adjacent to old scars, overlying vitreous reaction, and anterior chamber cells and flare. May have peripapillary form with disc edema and no chorioretinal lesions (simulating optic neuritis). Treatment is usually reserved for vision-threatening lesions.

- **Lab tests:** ELISA or indirect immunofluorescence assay (IFA) for *Toxoplasma* immunoglobulin G or M (definitive test) except in immunocompromised patients.
- **Posterior pole lesions (involving macula and optic nerve):** sulfadiazine (2 g po loading dose, then 1 g po qid for maintenance), pyrimethamine (Daraprim, 75-100 mg po loading dose then 25 mg po qd for maintenance), and folinic acid (leucovorin 5 mg po 2-3 times a week); give plenty of fluids to prevent sulfadiazine renal crystals.
- **Peripheral lesions:** clindamycin (300 mg po qid) and sulfadiazine (2 g po loading dose, then 1 g po qid for maintenance) or trimethoprim-sulfamethoxazole (Bactrim, 1 double-strength tablet po bid). Note: Immunocompetent patients may not require treatment.
- Treat with antibiotic combinations for 4-6 weeks; immunocompromised patients may require indefinite treatment and should be treated regardless of location of lesion.

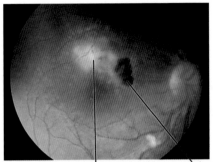 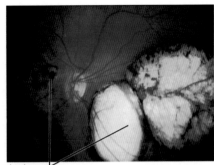

Toxoplasma gondii retinitis   chorioretinal scar

Figure 10-124 • Toxoplasmosis demonstrating active, fluffy white lesion adjacent to old, darkly pigmented scar.

Figure 10-125 • Congenital toxoplasmosis demonstrating inactive chorioretinal macular and peripheral scars.

- If lesion is near the optic disc, in posterior pole, or if there is intense vitritis, may add oral steroid (prednisone 20-80 mg po qd for 1 week, then taper) 24 hours after starting antimicrobial therapy (never start steroids alone); check PPD, blood glucose, and chest radiographs before starting systemic steroids.
- Add H2-blocker (ranitidine [Zantac] 150 mg po bid) or proton pump inhibitor when giving systemic steroids.

Tuberculosis

Multifocal (may be focal), light-colored choroidal granulomas caused by the bacilli *Mycobacterium tuberculosis;* may present as endophthalmitis; usually associated with constitutional symptoms including malaise, night sweats, and pulmonary symptoms.

Figure 10-126 • Tuberculosis with choroidal tubercle appearing as a large white subretinal mass.

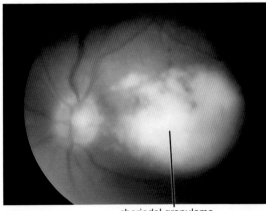

choriodal granuloma

- **Lab tests:** Positive purified protein derivative (PPD) skin test and chest radiographs.
- Isoniazid (INH, 300 mg po qd) and rifampin (600 mg po qd) for 6-9 months; follow liver function tests for toxicity.
- Consider adding pyrazinamide (25-35 mg/kg po qd) for first 2 months.
- Medical consultation for systemic evaluation.

Posterior Uveitis: White Dot Syndromes

Group of inflammatory disorders that produce discrete yellow-white retinal lesions mainly in young adults; differentiated by history, appearance, laterality, and fluorescein angiogram findings.

Acute Macular Neuroretinopathy

Acute onset of paracentral scotomas usually in 20- to 30-year-old women (89%) following a viral prodrome (68%). Vision is often normal but may be decreased. Usually presents with bilateral (68%) cloverleaf or wedge-shaped, brown-red lesions in the posterior pole with no vitreous cells. Recovery of visual field defect is rare.
- Check Amsler grid.
- **Fluorescein angiogram:** Minimal hypofluorescence of the lesions.
- No effective treatment.

Acute Posterior Multifocal Placoid Pigment Epitheliopathy (APMPPE)

Rapid loss of central or paracentral vision in 20- to 30-year-old (mean, 29 years) healthy adults after a viral prodrome; no sex predilection; usually bilateral, but asymmetric; multiple, round, discrete, large, flat gray-yellow, placoid lesions scattered throughout the posterior pole at the level of retinal pigment epithelium that later develop into well-demarcated retinal pigment epithelium scars; minimal vitreous cell; may have associated disc edema, cerebral vasculitis, headache, dysacousia, and tinnitus. Spontaneous resolution with late visual recovery within 1-6 months (80% regain ≥20/40 vision); recurrences rare.

APMPPE lesions

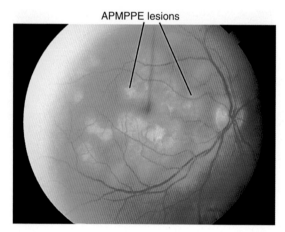

Figure 10-127 • Acute posterior multifocal placoid pigment epitheliopathy demonstrating multiple posterior pole lesions.

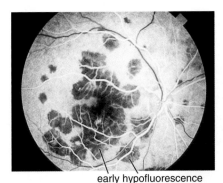

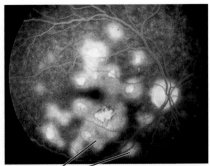

early hypofluorescence   late staining

Figure 10-128 • Fluorescein angiogram of same patient as shown in Figure 10-127 demonstrating early hypofluorescence of the lesions.

Figure 10-129 • Fluorescein angiogram of same patient as shown in Figure 10-128 demonstrating late staining of the lesions.

- **Fluorescein angiogram:** Early hypofluorescence and late staining of the placoid lesions.
- No treatment necessary.

Acute Retinal Pigment Epitheliitis/Krill's Disease

Rare cause of acute, moderate, visual loss in young adults; no sex predilection; no viral prodrome. Discrete clusters of hyperpigmented spots (300-400 μm) with hypopigmented halos at the level of the retinal pigment epithelium in the perifoveal region. Usually unilateral with no vitritis. Spontaneous resolution with recovery of visual acuity within 7-10 weeks; recurrences possible.

- **Fluorescein angiogram:** Blockage from the central spot and hyperfluorescence corresponding to the halo.
- No effective treatment.

Birdshot Choroidopathy/Vitiliginous Chorioretinitis

Multiple, small, discrete, ovoid, creamy yellow-white spots—scattered like a birdshot blast from a shotgun—in the midperiphery (spares macula); often in a vascular distribution; associated with mild vitritis, mild anterior chamber cells and flare (in 25% of cases), cystoid macular edema, and disc edema; usually bilateral; occurs in 50- to 60-year-old women (70%) and almost exclusively in whites. Patients have mild blurring of vision and floaters. Chronic, slowly progressive, recurring disease with variable visual prognosis; choroidal neovascular membranes, epiretinal membranes, and macular cysts or holes are late complications; associated with HLA-A29 (90-98%).

- **Fluorescein angiogram:** Mild hyperfluorescence, early and late staining of lesions; active lesions may hypofluoresce early. Late views show profuse vascular incompetence with leakage and secondary retinal staining.
- **Electrophysiologic testing:** ERG (subnormal) and EOG (subnormal); can monitor course of disease with serial ERG and can be used to monitor systemic immunomodulatory therapy.

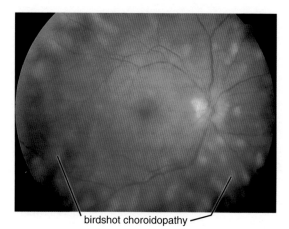

Figure 10-130 • Birdshot choroidopathy/vitiliginous chorioretinitis demonstrating scattered fundus lesions.

birdshot choroidopathy

- Treatment is reserved for patients with decreased visual acuity, significant inflammation, or complications including cystoid macular edema.
- Despite historically poor responses to steroids, initial improvement can be seen with oral steroids (prednisone 60-100 mg po qd). Check PPD, blood glucose, and chest radiographs before starting systemic steroids.
- Add H2-blocker (ranitidine [Zantac] 150 mg po bid) or proton pump inhibitor when giving systemic steroids.
- Consider sub-Tenon's steroid injection (triamcinolone acetonide 40 mg/mL) in patients with severe inflammation or cystoid macular edema.
- Cyclosporine (2-5 mg/kg/d) can dramatically improve vitritis and cystoid macular edema; should only be administered by a specialist trained in inflammatory diseases

Multifocal Choroiditis and Panuveitis (MCP)/ Subretinal Fibrosis and Uveitis Syndrome

Spectrum of disorders causing blurred vision, metamorphopsia, paracentral scotomas, and photopsias; mainly occurs in 30- to 40-year-old (mean, 36 years), healthy, white (86%), women (3:1 over men). Usually unilateral symptoms with bilateral (80%) fundus findings including small (100-200 μm), round, discrete, yellow-white spots and minimal signs of intraocular inflammation. Lesions develop into atrophic scars or subretinal fibrosis; choroidal neovascular membranes and macular edema are late complications; poor visual prognosis; recurrences common. Etiology unknown.

- **Fluorescein angiogram:** Early hyperfluorescence and late staining of the lesions.
- Treatment with steroids is controversial.

Punctate Inner Choroidopathy

Acute onset of blurred vision, metamorphopsia, paracentral scotomas, and photopsias; mainly occurs in 20- to 30-year-old (mean, 27 years), healthy, myopic (mean -6 diopters) women (>90%). Usually unilateral symptoms with bilateral fundus findings including small

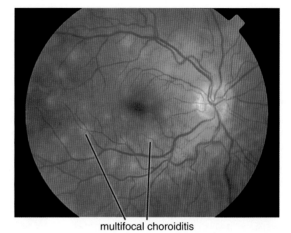

Figure 10-131 • Multifocal choroiditis demonstrating small, deep spots in the macula.

multifocal choroiditis

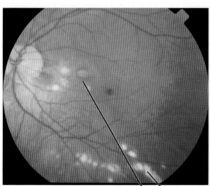

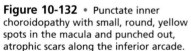

punctate inner choroidopathy

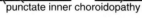

Figure 10-132 • Punctate inner choroidopathy with small, round, yellow spots in the macula and punched out, atrophic scars along the inferior arcade.

Figure 10-133 • Fluorescein angiogram of the same patient as shown in Figure 10-132 demonstrating hyperfluorescence of the active lesions and window defects of the atrophic scars.

(100-200 μm), round, discrete, yellow-white spots and minimal to no signs of intraocular inflammation. Lesions develop into atrophic scars over 1 month; scars progressively pigment and enlarge; choroidal neovascular membranes and macular edema are common, late complications; good visual prognosis unless CNV or macular edema occur; recurrences common. Unknown etiology.

- **Fluorescein angiogram:** Early hyperfluorescence and late staining of the lesions.
- Treatment with steroids is controversial.

Multiple Evanescent White Dot Syndrome (MEWDS)

Sudden, unilateral, acute visual loss with paracentral or central scotomas and photopsias mainly occurs in 20- to 30-year-old (mean, 2 8 years), healthy women (4:1 over men) after a viral prodrome (seen in 50% of cases). Cause unknown. Multiple, small (100-200 μm), discrete, gray-white spots at the level of the retinal pigment epithelium in the posterior pole sparing the fovea (spots appear and disappear quickly). May have positive relative afferent pupillary defect (RAPD), foveal granularity, mild vitritis, mild anterior chamber cells and flare, optic disc edema, and an enlarged blind spot. Spontaneous resolution with recovery of vision in 3-10 weeks; white dots disappear first, followed by improvement in vision; recurrences rare (10%).

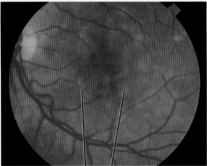

multiple evanescent white dot syndrome

Figure 10-134 • Multiple evanescent white dot syndrome demonstrating faint white spots.

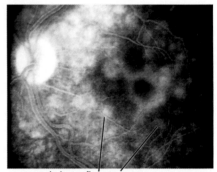

early hyperfluorescence

Figure 10-135 • Same patient as shown in Figure 10-134 demonstrating early fluorescein angiogram appearance.

* Check Amsler grid or visual fields (central 10 degrees).
* **Fluorescein angiogram:** Early, punctate hyperfluorescence in a wreathlike pattern and late staining of the lesions.
* **Electrophysiologic testing:** ERG (reduced a-wave).
* No treatment recommended.

Acute Idiopathic Blind Spot Enlargement Syndrome (AIBSE)

Subset of MEWDS (see above) seen in young women with enlargement of the blind spot and no optic disc edema and no visible fundus lesions; may represent MEWDS after lesions have faded; usually no RAPD exists.

* Check Amsler grid or visual fields (central 10 degrees).
* No treatment recommended.

Posterior Uveitis: Other Inflammatory Disorders

Behçet's Disease

Triad of aphthous oral ulcers, genital ulcers, and bilateral nongranulomatous uveitis; also associated with erythema nodosum, arthritis, vascular lesions, HLA-B5 (subtypes Bw51 and B52) and HLA-B12. The uveitis (see Chapter 6) is severe and recurring, causing hypopyon, iris atrophy, posterior synechiae, optic disc edema, attenuation of arterioles, severe vitritis, cystoid macular edema, and an occlusive retinal vasculitis with retinal hemorrhages and edema. Patients have photophobia, pain, red eye, and decreased vision. Lab tests are positive for antinuclear antibody (ANA), elevated erythrocyte sedimentation rate (ESR), C-reactive protein, acute phase reactants, and serum proteins, but are not diagnostic. Visual prognosis is poor; frequent relapses are common; ischemic optic neuropathy is a late complication.

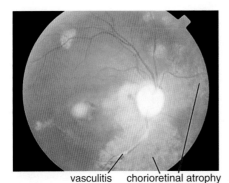

vasculitis   chorioretinal atrophy

Figure 10-136 • Behçet's disease demonstrating old vasculitis with sclerosed vessels and chorioretinal atrophy.

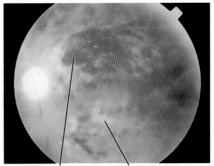

retinal hemorrhages   retinal edema

Figure 10-137 • Behçet's disease demonstrating acute vasculitis with hemorrhage.

Figure 10-138 • Behçet's disease demonstrating aphthous oral ulcers on tongue.

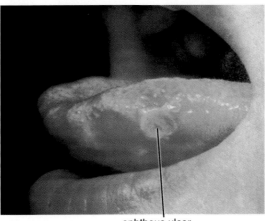

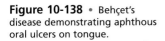

aphthous ulcer

- **Fluorescein angiogram:** Extensive vascular leakage early with late staining of vessel walls.
- **Lab tests:** Behçetine skin test (prick skin with sterile needle; formation of a pustule within a few minutes is a positive result), ESR, ANA, C-reactive protein, serum haplotyping.
- Topical steroid (prednisolone acetate 1% q2-6h).
- Colchicine (600 mg po bid) is controversial.
- **Mild:** oral steroid (prednisone 60-100 mg po qd); check PPD, blood glucose, and chest radiographs before starting systemic steroids.
- Add H2-blocker (ranitidine [Zantac] 150 mg po bid) or proton pump inhibitor when giving systemic steroids.
- **Severe:** sub-Tenon's steroid injection (triamcinolone acetonide 40 mg/mL), oral steroid (prednisone 60-100 mg po qd), and either chlorambucil (0.1 mg/kg/d), cyclophosphamide (1-2 mg/kg/d IV), or cyclosporine (2-7 mg/kg/d) should be administered by a specialist trained in inflammatory diseases.
- Medical consultation.

Idiopathic Uveal Effusion Syndrome

Bullous serous retinal detachment (with shifting fluid), serous choroidal and ciliary body detachments, mild vitritis, leopard spot retinal pigment epithelium pigmentation, and dilated conjunctival vessels. Patients have decreased vision, metamorphopsia, and scotomas. Occurs in healthy, middle-aged men. Chronic, recurrent course.

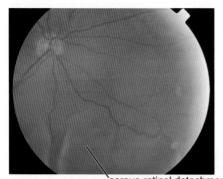

serous retinal detachment

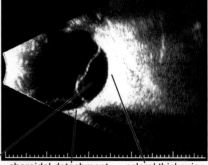

choroidal detachment   scleral thickening

Figure 10-139 • Bullous serous retinal detachment in a patient with idiopathic uveal effusion syndrome that shifts with changes in head position.

Figure 10-140 • B-scan ultrasound of same patient as shown in Figure 10-139 demonstrating serous retinal detachment with shifting fluid, shallow peripheral choroidal detachment, and diffuse scleral thickening.

- **B-scan ultrasonography:** Thickening of the sclera.
- **Fluorescein angiogram:** No discrete leak under serous retinal detachment.
- Steroids and antimetabolites are not effective.
- Consider decompression of vortex veins and scleral resection in nanophthalmic eyes.
- Surgery to create partial-thickness scleral windows is controversial.

Masquerade Syndromes

Systemic and ophthalmologic diseases can mimic uveitis. These should always be considered in the differential diagnosis of uveitis because they can be life threatening. The masquerade syndromes can be classified according to etiology: malignancy, endophthalmitis, and noninfectious/nonmalignant.

Malignancy

Intraocular Lymphoma   This rare and lethal malignancy is commonly a non-Hodgkin's large B cell lymphoma of the eye and the CNS. It commonly occurs in late adulthood (median age, 50 to 60 years), and the sex distribution is not clear. The most common symptoms are blurred vision and floaters associated with vitritis. The vitreous has large clumps of cells, and the fundus examination is significant for multifocal, large, yellow, subretinal infiltrative lesions.

- A high level of suspicion is essential to make the diagnosis.
- Thorough neurologic evaluation should be performed in search of CNS involvement, including MRI and CNS cytology
- Diagnostic pars plana vitrectomy in cases where diagnosis is in doubt. An undilute vitreous biopsy should be performed in the eye with vitritis and sent for cytology, flow-cytometry analysis for B and T cell markers and kappa/lambda light chains. Other ancillary tests include the measurement of IL-6 and IL-10 (high IL-10 and high ratio of IL-10 to IL-6 are suggestive of intraocular lymphoma).
- The treatment of intraocular lymphoma is still controversial, but in cases where CNS involvement is present, the use of combined chemotherapy and radiation treatment is indicated.
- Medical consultation required.

Other Malignancies   Other malignancies that can present as a masquerade uveitis include leukemia, malignant melanoma, retinoblastoma, and metastatic tumors.

Endophthalmitis   The diagnosis and treatment of endophthalmitis is covered in Chapter 6; however, it is important to remember that chronic postoperative endophthalmitis and endogenous endophthalmitis can present as a masquerade syndrome.

Nonmalignant/noninfectious   These forms of masquerade syndromes are a group of disorders characterized by the presence of intraocular cells secondary to noninflammatory conditions. Although rare, the following disorders should be considered: rhegmatogenous retinal detachment, retinitis pigmentosa, intraocular foreign body, ocular ischemic syndrome, and juvenile xanthogranuloma.

Posterior Scleritis

Orange-red elevation of choroid and retinal pigment epithelium by the thickened sclera with overlying serous retinal detachments, choroidal folds, vitritis, and optic disc edema; scleral thickening can cause induced hyperopia, proptosis, limitation of ocular motility, and angle-closure glaucoma (anterior rotation of ciliary body with forward displacement of the lens-iris diaphragm); usually occurs in 20- to 30-year-old women; 20-30% bilateral; patients have pain, photophobia, and decreased vision; associated with collagen-vascular diseases, rheumatoid arthritis, relapsing polychondritis, inflammatory bowel disease, Wegener's granulomatosis, and syphilis.

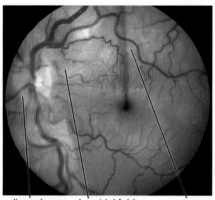

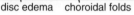

disc edema   choroidal folds   serous retinal detachment   punctate hyperfluorescence

Figure 10-141 • Posterior scleritis with orange-red choroidal elevation superiorly, serous retinal detachments, vitritis, and mild optic disc edema.

Figure 10-142 • Fluorescein angiogram of same patient as shown in Figure 10-141 demonstrating punctate hyperfluorescence and early pooling into the serous retinal detachments.

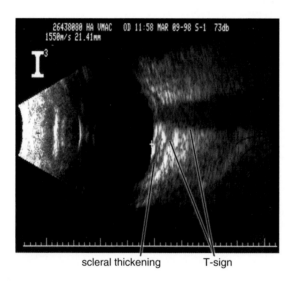

scleral thickening   T-sign

Figure 10-143 • B-scan ultrasound of same patient as shown in Figure 10-141 demonstrating scleral thickening and the characteristic peripapillary T-sign.

- **B-scan ultrasonography:** Diffuse scleral thickening (echolucent space between choroid and Tenon's capsule) and edema with medium reflectivity in Tenon's space; T-sign in peripapillary region from scleral thickening around echolucent optic nerve.
- **Fluorescein angiogram:** Punctate hyperfluorescence early with pooling late within serous retinal detachments.
- Oral steroid (prednisone 60-100 mg po qd); if severe, consider high-dose IV steroids; check PPD, blood glucose, and chest radiographs before starting systemic steroids.
- Oral nonsteroidal antiinflammatory drugs (NSAIDs; indomethacin 25-50 mg po tid).

- Add H2-blocker (ranitidine [Zantac] 150 mg po bid) or proton pump inhibitor when giving systemic steroids or NSAIDs.
- Sub-Tenon's steroid injection (triamcinolone acetonide 40 mg/mL) sometimes required.
- Consider immunosuppressive therapy (azathioprine, cyclosporine) in refractory cases; should be administered by a specialist trained in inflammatory diseases.
- Medical consultation.

Sarcoidosis

Granulomatous panuveitis with retinal vasculitis, vascular sheathing, periphlebitis (candle wax drippings), vitreous snowballs or string of pearls, yellow-white retinal/choroidal granulomas, anterior chamber cells and flare, mutton fat keratic precipitates, Koeppe and Busacca iris nodules, and macular edema. Disc or retinal neovascularization (often in sea-fan configuration) and epiretinal membranes are late complications. The disease is more severe in young blacks (incidence 82:100,000); however, sarcoidosis can occur in elderly, white women. Bimodal age distribution with peaks at 20-30 years and 50-60 years. Chronic, relapsing course (72%). Ocular findings occur in 25-75% of patients with sarcoidosis, and 94% have lung findings; patients present first with ocular complaints in only 2-3% of cases, 15-40% present with respiratory complaints; blacks are more likely to develop ocular complications. Systemic findings include hilar adenopathy, pulmonary parenchymal involvement, pulmonary fibrosis, erythema nodosum, subcutaneous nodules, lupus pernio (purple lupus), lymphadenopathy; may also have involvement of CNS, bone, connective tissue, heart, kidney, and sinuses. Pathologic hallmark is noncaseating granulomas. Most patients are asymptomatic; however, can have chronic, potentially fatal course.

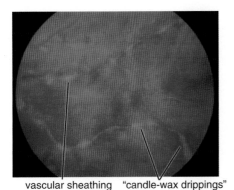 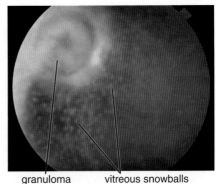

vascular sheathing "candle-wax drippings"   granuloma   vitreous snowballs

Figure 10-144 • Sarcoidosis with periphlebitis and vascular sheathing.

Figure 10-145 • Sarcoidosis demonstrating peripheral granuloma with overlying vitritis and vitreous snowballs.

- **Fluorescein angiogram:** Early hyperfluorescence and late leakage from vascular permeability and macular edema.
- **Lab tests:** Angiotensin converting enzyme (ACE), chest radiographs, serum lysozyme, sickle cell prep and hemoglobin electrophoresis (to rule out sickle cell anemia); consider CT scan of the chest to rule out mediastinal lymphadenopathy; consider gallium scan, Kneim-Silzbach skin test/reaction.

- Oral steroid (prednisone 60-100 mg po qd); check PPD, blood glucose, and chest radiographs before starting systemic steroids.
- Add H2-blocker (ranitidine [Zantac] 150 mg po bid) or proton pump inhibitor when giving systemic steroids.
- Sub-Tenon's steroid injection (triamcinolone acetonide 40 mg/mL) when macular edema is severe; topical steroids reserved for only anterior disease.
- Laser photocoagulation to areas of capillary nonperfusion when neovascularization persists or progresses after steroid treatment.
- Consider immunosuppressive therapy (hydroxychloroquine; methotrexate; chlorambucil; azathioprine) in refractory cases; should only be administered by a specialist trained in inflammatory diseases.
- Medical consultation.

Serpiginous Choroidopathy/Geographic Helicoid Peripapillary Choroidopathy (GHPC)

Bilateral, asymmetric uveitis with active lesions that appear as peripapillary, well-circumscribed, gray-white lesions. The lesions extend centrifugally from the disc in a pseudopodal, serpiginous pattern, leaving chorioretinal scars in areas of previous infection; skip lesions common; mild vitritis; may develop choroidal neovascular membranes (25%); usually bilateral, slight male predilection, and occurs in the fifth to seventh decades. Patients have paracentral scotomas and decreased vision; chronic, recurrent disease with good visual prognosis (severe visual loss rare); etiology unknown; associated with HLA-B7.

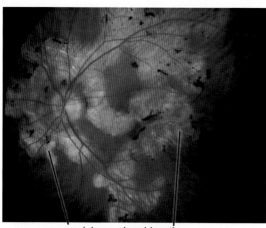

serpiginous choroidopathy

Figure 10-146 • Serpiginous choroidopathy demonstrating typical pattern of atrophic scarring extending from the optic nerve.

- **Fluorescein angiogram:** Hypofluorescence early and late staining beginning at the borders of the lesion and spreading centrally.
- Oral steroids (prednisone 1 mg/kg/day po) and sub-Tenon's steroid injection (triamcinolone acetonide 40 mg/mL) are controversial (consider when macula threatened).
- Consider immunosuppressive therapy (azathioprine 5 mg/kg/day, cyclosporine 1.5 mg/kg/day) in refractory cases; should only be administered by a specialist trained in inflammatory diseases.

• Laser photocoagulation or photodynamic therapy for CNV, depending on location in relation to the fovea.

Sympathetic Ophthalmia (SO)

Rare, bilateral, immune-mediated, mild to severe granulomatous uveitis seen 2 weeks to 3 months (80%) after penetrating trauma or surgery. Scattered, multifocal, yellow-white subretinal infiltrates (Dalen-Fuchs nodules, 50%) with overlying serous retinal detachments, vitritis, and papillitis. Associated with inflammation in sympathizing (fellow) eye and worsened inflammation in exciting (injured) eye (keratic precipitates are an ominous sign); may have meningeal signs, poliosis, and alopecia (as in Vogt-Koyanagi-Harada syndrome). Patients have transient obscuration of vision, photophobia, pain, and blurred vision. Male predilection (probably reflects increased incidence of trauma in this group); chronic, recurring course; prognosis good (65% achieve >20/60 vision after treatment); associated with HLA-A11.

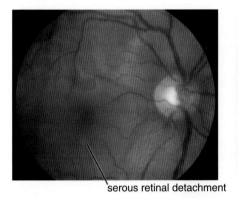

serous retinal detachment

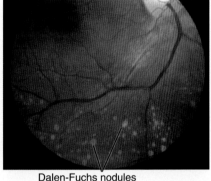

Dalen-Fuchs nodules

Figure 10-147 • Early sympathetic ophthalmia demonstrating serous retinal detachment.

Figure 10-148 • Dalen-Fuchs nodules in a patient with sympathetic ophthalmia.

• Check for previous history of penetrating surgery or trauma.
• **Fluorescein angiogram:** Pinpoint areas of hyperfluorescence with central hypofluorescence and patchy areas of choriocapillaris hypoperfusion, leakage late from optic nerve.
• Moderate to high-dose oral steroids (prednisone 60-200 mg po qd); check PPD, blood glucose, and chest radiographs before starting systemic steroids.
• Add H2-blocker (ranitidine [Zantac] 150 mg po bid) or proton pump inhibitor when giving systemic steroids.
• Sub-Tenon's steroid injection (triamcinolone acetonide 40 mg/mL).
• Topical steroids (prednisolone acetate 1% q2-6h) and cycloplegic (scopolamine 0.25% bid to qid).
• Consider immunosuppressive therapy (azathioprine, methotrexate, chlorambucil); should be administered by a specialist trained in inflammatory diseases.
• No proven benefit in enucleating exciting eye, but this option should be considered in eyes with no light perception (NLP) vision, since removal of the eye within 2 weeks of injury may prevent sympathetic ophthalmia.

Vogt-Koyanagi-Harada Syndrome (VKH)/Harada's Disease

Bilateral inflammatory disorder with yellow-white exudates at the level of the retinal pigment epithelium, bullous serous retinal detachments (75%, shifting fluid often present), and focal retinal pigment epithelial detachments; associated with anterior chamber cells and flare, mutton fat keratic precipitates, posterior synechiae, vitritis, choroidal folds, choroidal thickening, Dalen-Fuchs-like nodules, optic disc hyperemia, and systemic manifestations including meningeal signs (headache, nausea, stiff neck), dysacousis (deafness, tinnitus), and skin changes (alopecia, vitiligo, and poliosis); if only eye findings, then Harada's disease; late retinal pigment epithelial changes result in yellow-orange ("sunset glow") fundus. Occurs in pigmented individuals (Native Americans, blacks, Asians, and Hispanics) 20-40 years old; slight female predilection (60%); patients have decreased vision and photophobia; associated with HLA-DR4, HLA-DRw53, HLA-DQw7, HLA-DQw3, and HLA-Bw54; recurrences common; visual prognosis good.

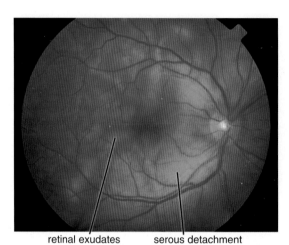

Figure 10-149 • Vogt-Koyanagi-Harada syndrome with multiple serous retinal detachments.

retinal exudates   serous detachment

- **B-scan ultrasonography:** Low reflectivity and choroidal thickening with overlying serous retinal detachment.
- **Fluorescein angiogram:** Pinpoint areas of hyperfluorescence and delayed choroidal fluorescence.
- Moderate- to high-dose oral steroids (prednisone 60-200 mg po qd, then taper slowly); check PPD, blood glucose, and chest radiographs before starting systemic steroids.
- Add H2-blocker (ranitidine [Zantac] 150 mg po bid) or proton pump inhibitor when giving systemic steroids.
- Topical steroid (prednisolone acetate 1% q2-6h) and cycloplegic (scopolamine 0.25% bid to qid) if anterior uveitis present.
- Sub-Tenon's steroid injection (triamcinolone acetonide 40 mg/mL) sometimes required.
- Cyclosporine (2-7 mg/kg/d) or immunosuppressive agents for refractory cases; should be administered by a specialist trained in inflammatory diseases.

Posterior Uveitis Evaluation/Management

Evaluation

- Consider workup as clinical examination and history dictate (see below)
- **Lab tests** (basic testing recommended for posterior uveitis with a negative history, review of systems and medical examination): complete blood count (CBC), erythrocyte sedimentation rate (ESR), Rapid Plasma Reagin (RPR; syphilis) or Venereal Disease Research Laboratory test (VDRL; syphilis), microhemagglutination for *Treponema pallidum* (MHA-TP; syphilis) or treponemal antibody absorption test (FTA-ABS; syphilis), Lyme titer, purified protein derivative (PPD; tuberculosis) and controls, serum lysozyme, angiotensin converting enzyme (ACE; sarcoidosis).
- **Other lab tests** (ordered according to history and/or evidence of granulomatous inflammation): ANA, RF (juvenile rheumatoid arthritis), ELISA for Lyme immunoglobulin M (IgM) and immunoglobulin G (IgG), HIV antibody test, chest radiographs (sarcoidosis, tuberculosis), sacroiliac radiographs (ankylosing spondylitis), gallium scan (sarcoidosis), urinalysis.
- **Special diagnostic lab tests:** HLA typing (HLA-A29; birdshot choroidopathy), in the presence of vasculitis: ANCA (Wegener's granulomatosis, polyarteritis nodosa), Raji cell and C1q binding assays for circulating immune complexes (SLE, systemic vasculitides), complement proteins: C3, C4, total complement (SLE, cryoglobulinemia, glomerulonephritis), soluble IL-2 receptor.
- Medical consultation.

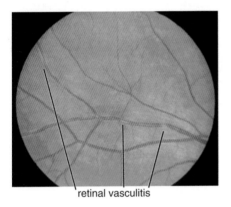

retinal vasculitis

Figure 10-150 • Retinal vasculitis with sheathing of retinal vessels.

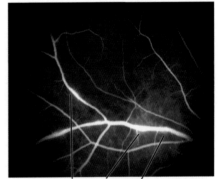

leakage from vessels

Figure 10-151 • Fluorescein angiogram of same patient as shown in Figure 10-150 demonstrating retinal vascular leakage.

Management

- Consider oral steroids (prednisone 60-100 mg po qd); check PPD, blood glucose, and chest radiographs before starting systemic steroids.
- Add H2-blocker (ranitidine [Zantac] 150 mg po bid) or proton pump inhibitor when giving systemic steroids.

Continued

Management—cont'd

- Consider sub-Tenon's steroid injection (triamcinolone acetonide 40 mg/mL) or intravitreal steroid injection (triamcinolone acetonide 4 mg/ 0.1 mL).
- If the uveitis becomes steroid dependent then consider a step-ladder approach to treat with steroid-sparing agents that would eventually allow the tapering or minimal use of topical and systemic corticosteroids:

  1. Nonsteroidal antiinflammatory drugs
  - Diclofenac (Voltaren) 75 mg po bid or diflunisal (Dolobid) 250 mg po bid. Other NSAIDs that can be used as a second line of therapy include indomethacin (Indocin SR) 75 mg po bid or naproxen (Naprosyn) 250 mg po bid. In patients with a known history of gastritis or peptic ulceration, the use of COX-2 inhibitors should be considered (celecoxib [Celebrex] 100 mg po bid or rofecoxib [Vioxx] 25 mg po qd).

  2. Immunosuppressive chemotherapy
  - This form of treatment should be managed by a uveitis specialist or in coordination with a medical specialist familiar with these medications; indications for these agents include Behçet's disease, sympathetic ophthalmia, VKH, rheumatoid necrotizing scleritis and/or peripheral ulcerative keratitis (PUK), Wegener's granulomatosis, polyarteritis nodosa, relapsing polychondritis, JRA, or sarcoidosis unresponsive to conventional therapy.
  - **Antimetabolites:** azathioprine 1-3 mg/kg/day, methotrexate 0.15 mg/kg/day, mycophenolate mofetil 1 g po qd ("off-label" use for autoimmune ocular inflammatory diseases).
  - **Alkylating agents:** cyclophosphamide 1-3 mg/kg/day, chlorambucil 0.1 mg/kg/day.
  - **Adjuvants:** colchicine 0.6 mg po bid for Behçet's disease is controversial.
  - **Other agents:** cyclosporine 2.5-5.0 mg/kg/day, FK506 (tacrolimus [Prograf]) 0.1-0.15 mg/kg/day, dapsone 25-50 mg bid-tid.

▊ Hereditary Chorioretinal Dystrophies

Central Areolar Choroidal Dystrophy (AD)

Starts as mild, nonspecific retinal pigment epithelial granularity and mottling in the fovea and progresses to a round, well-defined area of geographic atrophy, with loss of the choriocapillaris; the area of atrophy slowly enlarges, with large choroidal vessels visible underneath. Symptoms appear in third to fifth decades with decreased vision (20/25-20/200). Usually bilateral and symmetric.

- **Genetics:** Linked to *RDS*/perpherin gene on chromosome 6p and CACD on chromosome 17p13.
- **Color vision:** Moderate protan-deutan defect.
- **Electrophysiologic testing:** Photopic ERG (normal to slightly subnormal), scotopic ERG (normal), EOG (normal to slightly subnormal), and dark adaptation (normal).
- **Fluorescein angiogram:** Early lesions may show faint RPE transmission defects within the fovea; later, well-circumscribed hyperfluorescent window defects that correspond to the areas of atrophy.

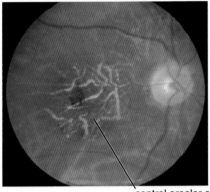

central areolar choroidal dystrophy

Figure 10-152 • Central geographic atrophy in a patient with central areolar choroidal dystrophy.

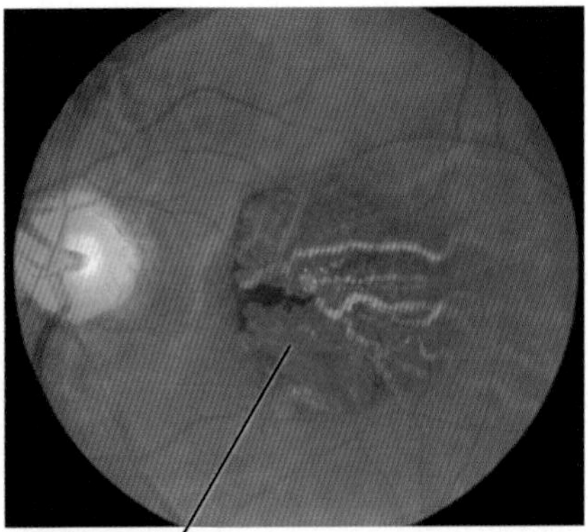

Figure 10-153 • Left eye of same patient as shown in Figure 10-152 demonstrating similar central geographic atrophy.

- **Visual field:** Large central scotoma in late stages.
- No effective treatment.

Choroideremia (X-linked)

Progressive, bilateral, diffuse atrophy of the choriocapillaris and overlying retinal pigment epithelium with scalloped edges and large choroidal vessels visible underneath; spares macula until late. Affected males have nyctalopia, photophobia, and constricted visual fields in late childhood. Female carriers have normal vision, visual fields, color vision, and ERG but may show pigmentary retinal changes; poor prognosis with legal blindness by 50-60 years of age.

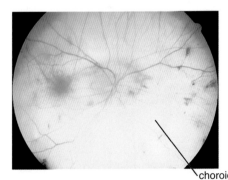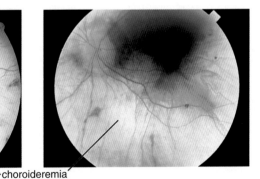

choroideremia

Figure 10-154 • Choroideremia demonstrating late stage with complete atrophy of the RPE and visible choroidal vessels.

Figure 10-155 • Choroideremia demonstrating scalloped border of atrophic changes near macula. Radial choroidal vessels are easily seen inferiorly.

- **Genetics:** Mapped to chromosome Xq21.
- Check color vision.
- **Electrophysiologic testing:** ERG (markedly reduced).
- **Fluorescein angiogram:** Absent choroidal flush with large choroidal vessels visible underneath with scalloped borders.
- Visual fields: Constricted.
- No effective treatment.

Congenital Stationary Night Blindness (CSNB)

Group of bilateral, nonprogressive disorders with reduced night vision (rods) and normal day vision (cones). Patients have normal acuity, color vision, and full visual fields but have reduced acuity with low light levels (nyctalopia), paradoxic pupillary response, absent Purkinje shift, and reduced rod ERG by first decade. Two categories:

Without fundus changes

Nougaret's Disease (AD) Night blindness but no reduction in central vision. Onset at birth. Retina totally normal ophthalmoscopically.

- **Genetics:** Associated with *GNAT1* gene on chromosome 3p21.
- **Electrophysiologic testing:** Photopic ERG (normal), scotopic ERG (subnormal, no rod a-wave), EOG (normal).

Riggs Type (AR) Rare; some residual rod function, no myopia. Retina totally normal ophthalmoscopically.

- **Electrophysiologic testing:** Photopic ERG (normal), scotopic ERG (subnormal, some rod a-wave detectable), EOG (normal).

Schubert-Bornschein Type (X-Linked Recessive) No rod function (type 1, complete form) or some residual rod function (type 2, incomplete form); nonprogressive. May have nystagmus; distinguished from dominant Nougaret type by presence of myopia and by mode of inheritance; carriers are asymptomatic. Retina usually normal, but may show myopic changes, some pigment washout, and some fine pigmentary changes in the periphery.

- **Genetics:** Type 1 (complete) linked to *NYX* gene on chromosome Xp11.4; type 2 (incomplete) linked to *CACNA1F* gene on chromosome Xp11.23.
- **Electrophysiologic testing:** Photopic ERG (normal), scotopic ERG (minimal to no rod function depending on type), and dark adaptation (may be abnormal).
- **Fluorescein angiogram:** Usually normal but may show minor window transmission defects.

With fundus changes

Fundus Albipunctatus (AR) Distinctive, discrete, yellow-white (50 μm) deep dots located in the midperipheral retina, sparing the macula. Not all lesions fluoresce on fluorescein angiogram (unlike drusen); stationary, unlike retinitis punctata albescens.

- **Genetics:** Associated with *RDH5* gene on chromosome 12q13-q14; gene encodes 11-*cis* retinol dehydrogenase 5, an RPE microsomal enzyme involved in photoreceptor transduction.

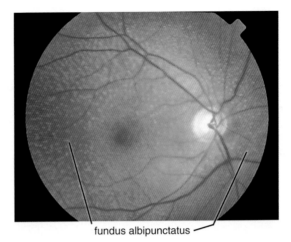

Figure 10-156 • Fundus albipunctatus demonstrating small white spots in the posterior pole sparing the central macula.

fundus albipunctatus

- **Electrophysiologic testing:** ERG (delayed cone and rod adaptation; a- and b-wave amplitudes increase slowly with dark adaptation and reach normal levels after about 3 hours).

Kandori's Flecked Retina Syndrome (AR)   Irregularly shaped, deep yellow spots usually seen in the equatorial region. Fewer and larger spots than fundus albipunctatus (may be variant).

Oguchi's Disease (AR)   Diffuse golden-brown/yellow or gray retinal discoloration in light that returns to normal retinal color (orange-red) with prolonged (2-12 hours) dark adaptation (Mizuo phenomenon). Onset at birth.

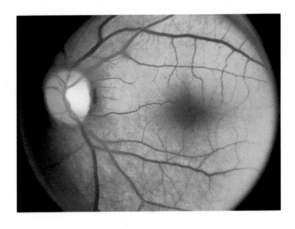

Figure 10-157 • Oguchi's disease demonstrating characteristic golden retinal sheen.

- **Genetics:** Mapped to Oguchi1/Arrestin/*SAG* gene on chromosome 2q37.1 and Oguchi2 on chromosome 13q34 encoding rhodopsin kinase (RHOK).
- **Electrophysiologic testing:** Photopic ERG (normal), scotopic ERG (reduced, no b-wave, a-wave increases with dark adaptation time), and dark adaptation (no rod phase).

- **Fluorescein angiogram:** Normal.
- No effective treatment.

Crystalline Retinopathy of Bietti (AR)

Glittering, yellow-white, refractile spots scattered throughout fundus (located in inner and outer layers of retina) with multiple areas of geographic atrophy. Associated with crystals in the perilimbal anterior corneal stroma. Patients have slowly progressive decreased vision beginning in fifth decade.

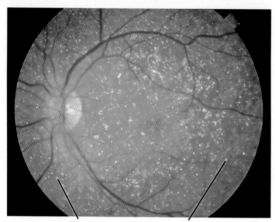

Figure 10-158 • Crystalline retinopathy of Bietti demonstrating refractile fundus lesions.

Bietti's crystalline retinopathy

- **Electrophysiologic testing:** ERG (reduced).
- **Fluorescein angiogram:** Patchy areas of blocked fluorescence and window defects corresponding to the areas of atrophy; crystals hyperfluoresce early.
- No effective treatment.

Gyrate Atrophy (AR)

Progressive, bilateral retinal degeneration with well-circumscribed, scalloped areas of chorioretinal atrophy that enlarge and coalesce starting anteriorly and spreading posteriorly. Patients develop nyctalopia, constricted visual fields, and decreased vision by the second decade. Abnormal laboratory studies including hypolysinemia, hyperornithinuria, and increased plasma ornithine levels (10-20 times normal) due to deficiency of the mitochondrial matrix enzyme, ornithine aminotransferase. Associated with posterior subcapsular cataracts and high myopia.

- **Genetics:** Associated with numerous mutations in *OAT* gene on chromosome 10q26 that encodes ornithine aminotransferase.
- **Lab tests:** Plasma ornithine levels; also consider urine ornithine levels and plasma lysine levels.
- **Electrophysiologic testing:** ERG (reduced) and dark adaptation (prolonged).
- **Fluorescein angiogram:** Window defects corresponding to the areas of atrophy.
- Restrict dietary arginine and protein; vitamin B6 pyridoxine 300-500 mg po qd; therapy may be helpful.

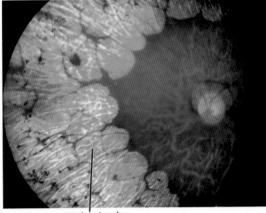

Figure 10-159 • Gyrate atrophy demonstrating coalescence of well-circumscribed atrophic patches.

gyrate atrophy

Progressive Cone Dystrophy (AD>AR>X-linked)

Profound cone dysfunction with normal rod function. Often develop "bull's-eye" macular pigment changes, patchy atrophy in the posterior pole, vascular attenuation, and temporal pallor or optic atrophy. Patients have slowly progressive loss of central vision (worse during day), dyschromatopsia, and photophobia that develops in the first through third decades. Called *cone degeneration* when not inherited. Poor prognosis, with vision deteriorating to the 20/200 level by fourth decade.

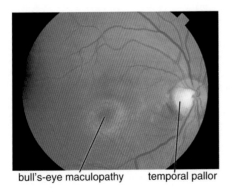

bull's-eye maculopathy   temporal pallor

Figure 10-160 • Progressive cone dystrophy with "bull's-eye" appearance and temporal optic atrophy.

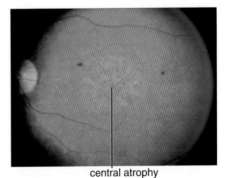

central atrophy

Figure 10-161 • Progressive cone dystrophy with patchy atrophy in the posterior pole.

- **Genetics:** Cone dystrophy mapped to several loci including: *COD1/RPGR* gene on chromosome Xp21.1 encoding retinitis pigmentosa GTPase regulator; *COD2* gene linked to chromosome Xq27; *COD3/GUCA1A/GCAP1* gene on chromosome 6p21.1 encoding guanylate cyclase activating protein.
- **Color vision:** Severe deutan-tritan defect out of proportion to visual acuity; no color perception.

- **Electrophysiologic testing:** Photopic ERG (markedly reduced to nonrecordable), scotopic ERG (can be normal, often subnormal), EOG (normal to subnormal), and dark adaptation (cone segment: abnormal; rod segment: normal [may be subnormal to abnormal later in disease]).
- **Fluorescein angiogram:** Hypofluorescence with ring of hyperfluorescence corresponding to the "bull's-eye" lesion; diffuse, irregular window defects throughout posterior pole and often midperiphery.
- **Visual field:** Central scotomas, peripheral fields usually intact; may get midperipheral relative scotomas late.
- No effective treatment; dark glasses may help photophobia.

Rod Monochromatism (Achromatopsia) (AR)

Total absence of cone function with normal rod function. Patients have poor central vision (20/200), achromatopsia (no color perception), congenital nystagmus, and photophobia from birth. May have normal macula, but often develop similar pigmentary changes as progressive cone dystrophy with granular changes and "bull's-eye" maculopathy; nonprogressive; poor prognosis with vision deteriorating to the 20/200 level by fourth decade.

- **Genetics:** Linked to *ACHM1* gene on chromosome 14; *ACHM2/CNGA3* gene encoding a cone photoreceptor cGMP-gated cation channel alpha subunit; *ACHM3/CNGB3* gene encoding cone cGMP-gated cation channel beta 3 subunit.
- **Color vision:** No color perception; all colors appear as shades of gray.
- **Electrophysiologic testing:** Photopic ERG (absent, nonrecordable), scotopic ERG (usually normal, may be subnormal), flicker fusion frequency (generally below 20 Hz), EOG (normal), dark adaptation (cone segment: abnormal and may be absent; rod segment: normal).
- **Fluorescein angiogram:** Normal, or may show window defects in areas of pigmentary changes.
- **Visual field:** Central scotomas, peripheral fields intact.
- No effective treatment; dark glasses may help photophobia.

■ Hereditary Macular Dystrophies

Adult Foveomacular Vitelliform Dystrophy (AD)

Bilateral, symmetric, round, slightly elevated, yellow-orange lesions with surrounding darker border and pigment clumping. Onset between 30-50 years of age with minimally affected vision and metamorphopsia (often unilateral symptoms, but bilateral disease). Smaller lesions than in Best's disease, no disruption or layering of the yellow pigment, and seen in older patients; good prognosis.

Best's Disease (AD)

Uncommon hereditary macular dystrophy with high phenotypic variability. Usually starts asymptomatic (75% better than 20/40) with yellow, round, subretinal vitelliform macular lesion ("egg-yolk" lesion) in early childhood (5-10 years). Progresses to the "scrambled-egg" stage as the cysts break apart with irregular subretinal spots, then the pseudohypopyon stage as the subretinal material layers with retinal pigment epithelium atrophy, and finally leaves a round atrophic scar. Usually bilateral and seen in whites who are slightly hyperopic; good

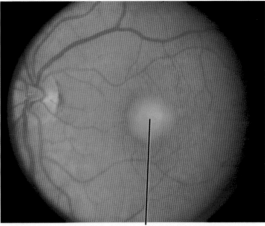

Figure 10-162 • Adult foveomacular vitelliform dystrophy demonstrating central round yellow lesion.

adult foveomacular vitelliform lesion

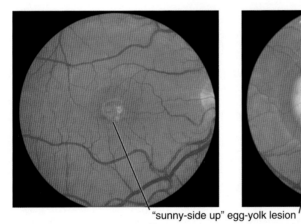

"sunny-side up" egg-yolk lesion

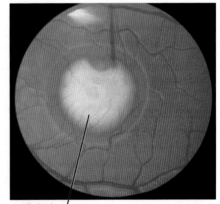

Figure 10-163 • Small egg-yolk lesion in 7-year-old boy with Best's disease.

Figure 10-164 • Left eye of same patient as shown in Figure 10-163 demonstrating characteristic "sunny-side up" egg-yolk lesion.

prognosis, vision deteriorates slowly and may be stable for years (75-88% have >20/40 vision in one eye up to age 50 years); cannot predict visual function from fundus appearance; tritan color deficiency; incidental trauma can lead to visual loss; may develop choroidal neovascular membrane (CNV); good prognosis, with vision ranging from 20/30 to 20/100 unless CNV develops.

- **Genetics:** Mapped to *VMD2*/Bestrophin gene on chromosome 11q13; protein function still unknown.
- **Color vision:** Color defects proportional to degree of visual loss.

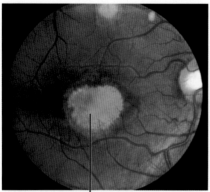

"scrambled egg" stage

Figure 10-165 • Best's disease demonstrating "scrambled egg" lesion in the macula.

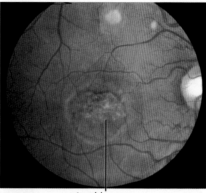

atrophic scar

Figure 10-166 • Same patient as shown in Figure 10-165, 5 years later demonstrating atrophic lesion in central macula.

- **Electrophysiologic testing:** ERG (normal), EOG (markedly abnormal even in otherwise normal-appearing carriers, Arden ratio <1.5 light peak/dark trough), and dark adaptation (normal).
- **Fluorescein angiogram:** Blockage by vitelliform lesion; transmission when cyst ruptures; irregular RPE transmission and staining depending on presence of pigmentary disturbance, choroidal neovascularization, and scarring.
- **Visual field:** Relative central scotoma early; more dense scotomas may be noted after degeneration and organization of lesion.
- No effective treatment.

Butterfly Pattern Dystrophy (AD)

Bilateral, subtle RPE mottling in younger patients; symmetric, gray-yellow, butterfly-shaped lesions in central macula with surrounding halo of depigmentation in older patients. Onset between 20-50 years of age with mild decrease in vision (20/25 to 20/40) and slow progression. May develop choroidal neovascular membrane; relatively good prognosis unless CNV develops.

- **Genetics:** Linked to *RDS*/peripherin gene on chromosome 6p21.1-cen encoding peripherin.
- **Color vision:** Normal.
- **Electrophysiologic testing:** Photopic ERG (normal to subnormal), scotopic ERG (normal to subnormal), EOG (usually normal but can be markedly subnormal), and dark adaptation (normal).
- **Fluorescein angiogram:** Hypofluorescent blocking defects by pigment and lipofuscin, window defects corresponding to the areas of the atrophy; hyperfluorescent leakage from CNV if present.
- **Visual fields:** Relative central scotoma; normal peripheral fields.
- No effective treatment.

Dominant Drusen/Doyne's Honeycomb Dystrophy/Malattia Leventinese (AD)

Asymptomatic, unless degenerative changes occur in the macula. Bilateral, symmetric, round, yellow-white deposits (nodular thickening of the retinal pigment epithelium basement membrane) scattered throughout the posterior pole and nasal to the optic disc. Seen by 20-30 years of age. The lesions coalesce (forming a honeycomb appearance), enlarge, or disappear. May be associated with pigment clumping, RPE pigmentary disturbance, RPE detachment, chorioretinal atrophy, and choroidal neovascular membrane.

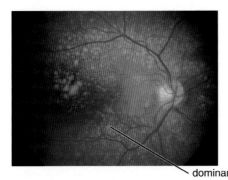 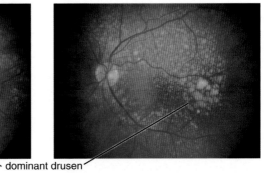

dominant drusen

Figure 10-167 • Dominant drusen demonstrating abundant yellow lesions in the posterior pole.

Figure 10-168 • Left eye of same patient shown in Figure 10-167.

- **Genetics:** Mapped to *EFEMP1* gene on chromosome 2p16-21; produces an extracellular matrix protein.
- **Color vision:** Normal.
- **Electrophysiologic testing:** ERG (normal), EOG (subnormal in late stages), and dark adaptation (normal).
- **Fluorescein angiogram:** Early blockage and late hyperfluorescent staining of drusen; irregular dye transmission, leakage and pooling within macula depending on degree of associated degenerative change; hyperfluorescent leakage from CNV if present.
- **Visual field:** Normal; central scotoma if macular degeneration present.
- No effective treatment.

North Carolina Macular Dystrophy (Lefler-Wadsworth-Sidbury Dystrophy) (AD)

Yellow spots (drusen) appear in early childhood (first decade) and progress to chorioretinal atrophy, macular staphyloma or "colobomas," and peripheral drusen. Normal central vision early unless atrophic macular "coloboma" forms; possible progression to 20/200 vision or worse late in patients who develop choroidal neovascular membranes. Typically nonprogressive. Three grades:

Grade I   Drusen-like lesions and pigment dispersion in fovea.

Grade II   Confluent drusen-like lesions in fovea.

Grade III   Atrophy of RPE and choriocapillaris within central macula.

- **Genetics:** Linked to *MCDR1* gene on chromosome 6q14-q16.2 at same location as clinically distinct dominant progressive bifocal chorioretinal atrophy.
- **Color vision:** Normal.
- **Electrophysiologic testing:** ERG (normal), EOG (normal), dark adaptation (normal).
- **Fluorescein angiogram:** Grades I and II: RPE transmission defects and late staining of drusen-like lesions; grade III: nonperfusion of choriocapillaris.
- **Visual field:** Central scotoma; normal peripheral fields.
- No effective treatment.

Pseudoinflammatory Macular Dystrophy (Sorsby's) (AD)

Bilateral, symmetric, choroidal atrophy with decreased vision, nyctalopia, and tritan color deficiency seen in 40- to 50-year old patients. Three early patterns seen: disciform maculopathy with drusenoid deposits, disciform maculopathy without deposits, and chorioretinal atrophy. All patterns lead to end-stage pattern of progressively enlarging chorioretinal atrophy from the macula outward. May develop choroidal neovascular membrane. Poor prognosis with final vision in hand motion range.

- **Genetics:** Linked to SFD/TIMP-3 gene cloned on chromosome 22q12.1-q13.2 encoding tissue inhibitor of metalloproteinase-3 (TIMP-3).
- Check color vision.
- **Electrophysiologic testing:** ERG (subnormal in advanced stages), EOG (subnormal in advanced stages), and dark adaptation (delayed).
- **Fluorescein angiogram:** Hyperfluorescent window defects in areas of atrophy and hyperfluorescent leakage from CNV if present.
- No effective treatment.

Sjögren Reticular Pigment Dystrophy (AR)

Hyperpigmented fishnet-reticular pattern at the level of the retinal pigment epithelium that starts centrally and spreads peripherally. Usually asymptomatic with good vision.

- **Electrophysiologic testing:** ERG (normal), EOG (lower limit of normal), and dark adaptation (normal).
- **Fluorescein angiogram:** Hypofluorescence of the fishnet-reticulum over normal background fluorescence in early views.
- No effective treatment.

Stargardt's Disease/Fundus Flavimaculatus (AR>AD)

Most common hereditary macular dystrophy. Onset in first to second decades. Bilateral, deep, symmetric, yellow pisciform (fish-tail shaped) flecks (yellow flecks are groups of enlarged RPE cells packed with a granular substance with ultrastructural, autofluorescent, and histochemical properties consistent with lipofuscin) at the level of the retinal pigment epithelium and scattered throughout the posterior pole. Spectrum of disease: fundus flavimaculatus (no macular dystrophy; seen in adults) to Stargardt's disease ("bull's-eye" atrophic maculopathy with "beaten bronze" appearance, patchy areas of atrophy; seen in late childhood and adolescence). Salt-and-pepper pigmentary changes in periphery may develop late; no sex predilection; patients have bilateral decreased vision even before fundus changes appear; poor prognosis with vision deteriorating to the 20/200 level by third decade and stable or continued slowly progressive loss of vision thereafter. Autosomal dominant form has more benign course with milder color and night vision changes, no photophobia, later onset, and generally less severe clinical course.

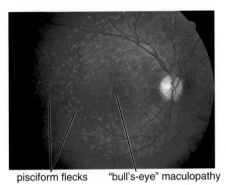

pisciform flecks   "bull's-eye" maculopathy

Figure 10-169 • Stargardt's disease demonstrating pisciform flecks along the vascular arcades and pigmentary changes in the fovea.

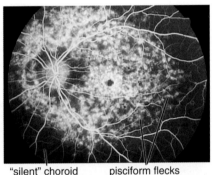

"silent" choroid   pisciform flecks

Figure 10-170 • Fluorescein angiogram of patient shown in Figure 10-169 demonstrating hyperfluorescence of the lesions and the characteristic "silent" choroid.

- **Genetics:** Mapped to *STGD1/ABCA4* gene on chromosome 1p21-22 associated with autosomal recessive Stargardt's disease; autosomal dominant Stargardt's disease linked to *STGD4* gene on chromosome 4p and to *STGD3/ELOVL4* gene on chromosome 6q14 encoding a photoreceptor-specific component of a polyunsaturated fatty acid elongation system; fundus flavimaculatus mapped to *ABCA4* gene on chromosome 1p21-p13.
- **Color vision:** May be abnormal with mild to moderate deutan-tritan defects as disease progresses.
- **Electrophysiologic testing:** ERG (usually normal, but one third may have photopic abnormalities), EOG (normal to subnormal), and dark adaptation (usually normal, mildly elevated in late stages).
- **Fluorescein angiogram:** Generalized decreased choroidal fluorescence (dark or "silent" choroid sign), hyperfluorescent spots that do not correspond to the flecks seen clinically; flecks demonstrate early blockage and late hyperfluorescent staining and window defects corresponding to the areas of the macular atrophy.
- **Visual field:** May be normal, or develop central scotoma late.
- No effective treatment.

Hereditary Vitreoretinal Degenerations

Familial Exudative Vitreoretinopathy (FEVR) (AD)

Rare, slowly progressive, bilateral, peripheral vascular developmental disorder; similar in appearance to retinopathy of prematurity but without premature birth and supplemental oxygen.

Stage 1   Starts with peripheral avascularity, white without pressure, vitreous bands, peripheral cystoid degeneration, microaneurysms, telangiectasia, straightened vessels, and vascular engorgement especially in the temporal periphery; asymptomatic in 73% of cases but may have strabismus and nystagmus. Progression to stage 2 may or may not occur.

Stage 2   Neovascularization, fibrovascular proliferation, subretinal and intraretinal exudation, dragging of disc and macula, falciform retinal folds, and localized retinal detachments. Visual loss after second or third decade is rare unless degeneration progresses to stage 3.

Stage 3   Cicatrization causes traction (rare) and/or rhegmatogenous retinal detachments (10-20%); retinal detachments common in third to fourth decades; retinal detachments difficult to repair (recurrent retinal detachments and proliferative vitreoretinopathy).

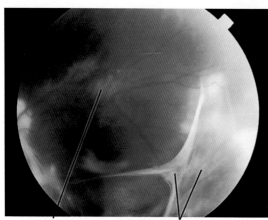

Figure 10-171 • Familial exudative vitreoretinopathy demonstrating fibrovascular proliferation, exudates, and cicatrization.

exudate   fibrovascular proliferation

- **Genetics:** Phenotypes linked to chromosome 11q13-q23 (*EVR1* gene) and chromosome 11p13-p12 (*EVR3* gene).
- **Fluorescein angiogram:** Peripheral nonperfusion past vascularized retina; at border area, arteriovenous anastomoses form and leak fluorescein.
- Prophylactic treatment of the avascular retina is controversial; retinal surgery for retinal detachments.

Enhanced S-Cone Syndrome/Goldmann-Favre Syndrome (AR)

Rare, bilateral vitreotapetoretinal degeneration with foveal and peripheral retinoschisis (similar to juvenile retinoschisis), optically empty vitreous cavity, condensed vitreous veils, attenuation of retinal vessels, peripheral pigmentary (bone spicules) changes, subretinal dotlike flecks in peripheral retina, lattice degeneration, progressive cataracts, and waxy optic disc pallor. No sex predilection (unlike juvenile retinoschisis). Patients have nyctalopia and constricted visual fields from early childhood. Reduced vision becomes evident with age. Goldmann-Favre refers to severe end of spectrum of disease.

- **Genetics:** Phenotypes linked to *NR2E3* or *PNR* gene on chromosome 15q23.
- **Electrophysiologic testing:** Photopic ERG (more sensitive to blue than to red or white stimuli), scotopic ERG (does not reveal any rod-driven responses; large, slow waveforms are detected in response to bright flashes), and EOG (abnormal, reduced light peak; *Note:* helps differentiate from juvenile retinoschisis).
- **Fluorescein angiogram:** No leakage from foveal schisis.
- Consider prophylactic treatment of any retinal breaks or tears.
- Retinal surgery for retinal detachments.

Snowflake Degeneration (AD)

Rare degeneration with yellow-white deposits in peripheral retina associated with white without pressure, sheathing of retinal vessels, vitreous degeneration, and cataracts. Increased risk of retinal detachments.

- No treatment recommended.
- Retinal surgery for rhegmatogenous retinal detachments.

Wagner/Jansen/Stickler Vitreoretinal Dystrophies (AD)

All have optically empty vitreous cavity with thick, transvitreal and preretinal membranes and strands, retinal perivascular pigmentary changes, and lattice degeneration; associated with myopia, glaucoma, and posterior subcapsular cataracts.

Wagner's Disease   No systemic associations and no increased risk of retinal detachments.

- **Genetics:** Linked to *WGN1* gene on chromosome 5q13-q14; additional phenotype linked to mutation in exon 2 of *COL2A1* gene on chromosome 12q13.11-q13.2, the candidate gene for Stickler's syndrome. This exon is present in vitreous collagen mRNAs but absent in cartilage mRNAs, thus accounting for the lack of systemic manifestations associated with Wagner's.

Jansen's Disease   No systemic associations, but patients do have an increased risk of retinal detachments; often bilateral retinal detachments.

Stickler's Syndrome   Associated with systemic abnormalities including marfanoid habitus, facial hypoplasia, cleft palate, neurosensory hearing loss, skeletal abnormalities, and arthritis; patients have increased risk of retinal breaks (75%) and bilateral detachments (42%).

- **Genetics:** Linked to genes encoding collagen precursors including *COL2A1* gene on chromosome 12q13.11-q13.2, *COL11A1* gene on chromosome 1p21 and *COL11A2* gene on chromosome 6p21.3.
- **Electrophysiologic testing:** ERG (reduced) and EOG (normal).
- Retinal surgery for retinal detachments.

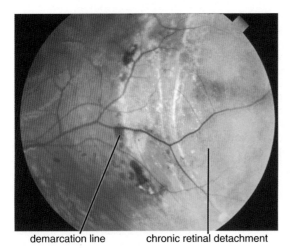

Figure 10-172 • Stickler's vitreoretinal dystrophy with pigmented and hypopigmented demarcation lines from a chronic retinal detachment.

demarcation line   chronic retinal detachment

Leber's Congenital Amaurosis (AR)

Group of disorders with onset at birth or early childhood of severe visual impairment, sluggish pupils, nyctalopia, light sensitivity (50%), and nystagmus. May have range of fundus abnormalities, from no fundus changes (most common, especially early in life) to progressive retinal pigment epithelial granularity, vascular attenuation, tapetal sheen, yellow flecks, salt-and-pepper fundus, macular "colobomas," chorioretinal atrophy, or a retinitis pigmentosa appearance. Associated with high hyperopia, oculodigital sign, mental retardation (37%), deafness, seizures, musculoskeletal and renal abnormalities, posterior subcapsular cataracts, and keratoconus.

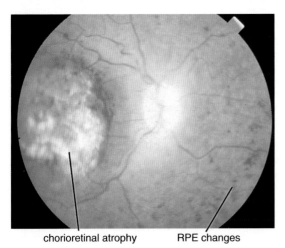

Figure 10-173 • Leber's congenital amaurosis demonstrating granular and RP-like pigmentary changes, attenuated vessels, and a macular scar.

chorioretinal atrophy   RPE changes

• **Genetics:** *RPE65/LCA2* gene on chromosome 1p31 accounts for up to 16% of Leber's congenital amaurosis (LCA), encoding protein essential in vitamin A metabolism; *RPGRIP1* gene on chromosome 14q11 encodes RPGR-interacting protein 1 and accounts for 6% of LCA; *LCA1* and *LCA4* genes on chromosome 17p13.1 encode arylhydrocarbon-interacting receptor protein-like 1 and account for approximately 15% of LCA; *CRX* gene on chromosome 19q13.3 encodes cone-rod otx-like photoreceptor homeobox transcription factor and accounts for 3% of LCA.

- **Color vision:** Abnormal.
- **Electrophysiologic testing:** ERG (markedly reduced, absent); EOG (abnormal).
- **Visual field:** Constricted.
- No effective treatment.

Retinitis Pigmentosa

Definition

Group of hereditary, progressive retinal degenerations (rod-cone dystrophies) that result from abnormal production of photoreceptor proteins. There are more than 29 loci associated with various phenotypes of RP.

Atypical Forms

Retinitis Pigmentosa Inversus

Macula and posterior pole are affected differentially; confused with hereditary macular disorders; central and color vision are reduced earlier than normal, and pericentral ring/central scotomas occur.

Retinitis Pigmentosa Sine Pigmentosa

Descriptive term to describe patients who have symptoms of retinitis pigmentosa but who fail to show pigmentary fundus changes; seen in up to 20% of cases; associated with more pronounced cone dysfunction.

Retinitis Punctata Albescens (AR)

Multiple, punctate white (50-100 μm) spots at the level of the retinal pigment epithelium scattered in the midperiphery with attenuated vessels and bone spicules. Slowly progressive disease (differentiated from fundus albipunctatus).

Sector Retinitis Pigmentosa

Subtype with pigmentary changes limited to one retinal area that generally does not enlarge; usually inferonasal quadrants; relatively good ERG responses.

Forms Associated with Systemic Abnormalities

Abetalipoproteinemia (Bassen-Kornzweig Syndrome) (AR)

Associated with ataxia, steatorrhea, erythrocyte acanthocytosis, growth retardation, neuropathy, and lack of serum betalipoprotein, causing intestinal malabsorption of fat-soluble vitamins (A, D, E, K), triglycerides, and cholesterol; minimal pigmentary changes early.

- **Genetics:** Cloned *MTP* gene on chromosome 4q24 produces microsomal triglyceride transfer protein.
- Treat with vitamin A (15,000 IU po qd), vitamin E (100 IU/kg po qd), vitamin K (0.15 mg/kg po qd), omega-3 fatty acids (0.10 g/kg po qd), and dietary fat restriction.

Alström's Disease (AR)

Associated with cataracts, deafness, obesity, renal failure, acanthosis nigricans, baldness, and hypogenitalism. Early and profound visual loss.

- **Genetics:** Gene *ALMS1* gene cloned on chromosome 2p13.

Cockayne's Syndrome

Associated with band keratopathy, cataracts, dwarfism, deafness, intracranial calcifications, and psychosis.

Kearns-Sayre Syndrome (AR)

Associated with chronic, progressive external ophthalmoplegia, ptosis, cardiac conduction defects (arrhythmias, heart block, cardiomyopathy), and other abnormalities (see Chapter 2). "Ragged red" fibers seen histologically on muscle biopsy.

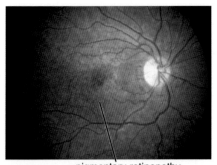

pigmentary retinopathy

Figure 10-174 • Kearns-Sayre syndrome with pigmentary retinopathy.

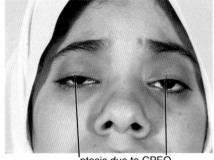

ptosis due to CPEO

Figure 10-175 • Same patient as shown in Figure 10-174 demonstrating chronic progressive external ophthalmoplegia with ptosis. This patient could not move her eyes.

Laurence-Moon/Bardet-Biedl Syndromes (AR)

Bardet-Biedl (polydactyly in 75% and syndactyly in 14%) and Laurence-Moon (spastic paraplegia, no polydactyly/syndactyly). Both include short stature, congenital obesity, hypogenitalism (50%), partial deafness (5%), renal abnormalities, and mental retardation (85%). Minimal pigmentary changes early.

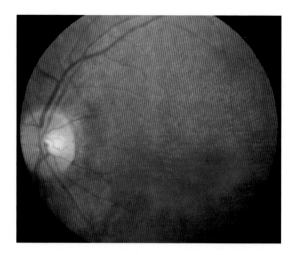

Figure 10-176 • Diffuse pigmentary changes in a patient with Laurence-Moon syndrome.

- **Genetics:** Linked to *BBS1* gene on chromosome 11q13; *BBS2* gene on chromosome 16q21; *BBS3* gene on chromosome 3p13-p12; *BBS4* gene on chromosome 15q22.3-q23; *BBS5* gene on chromosome 2q31; and *BBS6* gene on chromosome 20p12.

Neuronal Ceroid Lipofuscinosis (Batten Disease) (AR)

Associated with seizures, dementia, ataxia, and mental retardation; can have infantile (Hagberg-Santavuori syndrome), juvenile, or adult onset; conjunctival biopsy shows granular inclusions with autofluorescent lipopigments that also accumulate in neurons, causing retinal and CNS degeneration.

Refsum's Disease (AR)

Associated with ichthyosis, electrocardiogram abnormalities, anosmia, deafness, progressive peripheral neuropathy, cerebellar ataxia, hypotonia, hepatomegaly, mental retardation, and elevated CSF protein; minimal pigmentary changes early. Defect in fatty acid metabolism due to phytanic acid oxidase deficiency; causes elevated plasma phytanic acid, pipecolic acid, and very long-chain fatty acid levels.

- **Genetics:** Associated with *PNYH* gene cloned on chromosome 10p15.3-p12.2 that encodes phytanoyl-CoA hydroxylase; infantile Refsum's associated with *PEX1* gene on chromosome 7q21-q22, encoding peroxisome biogenesis factor 1.
- Treat by restricting dietary phytanic acid (animal fats and milk products) and phytol (leafy green vegetables); follow serum phytanic acid levels.

Usher's Syndrome (AR)

Associated with congenital, neurosensory hearing loss. Most common syndrome associated with retinitis pigmentosa (5%). Type I (total deafness with no vestibular function). Type II (partial deafness with normal vestibular function, most common type [67%], better vision). Type III (Hallgren's syndrome: deafness, vestibular ataxia, psychosis). Type IV (deafness and mental retardation). *Note*: controversial whether types III and IV are forms of Usher's syndrome or are separate genetic entities.

- **Genetics:** *USH2A* gene on chromosome 1q41 associated with autosomal recessive Usher's syndrome; produces usherin, a basement membrane protein in the retina and inner ear; numerous additional loci including 10q21-22; 11p15.1; 11q13.5; 14q32; 17q34-35; 21q21.
- Protect ears against loud noises; avoid ototoxic medications.

Epidemiology

Most common hereditary degeneration (1:5000); can have any inheritance pattern: AR (25%), AD (20%, usually with variable penetrance, later onset, milder course), X-linked (9%, more severe, carriers also affected), isolated (38%), and undetermined (8%).

Symptoms

Nyctalopia, dark adaptation problems, photophobia, progressive constriction of visual fields ("tunnel vision"), dyschromatopsia, photopsias, and slowly progressive decreased central vision starting at approximately 20 years of age.

Signs

Decreased visual acuity, constricted visual fields, dyschromatopsia (tritanopic); classic fundus appearance with dark pigmentary clumps in the midperiphery and perivenous areas (bone spicules), attenuated retinal vessels, cystoid macular edema, fine pigmented vitreous cells, and waxy optic disc pallor; associated with posterior subcapsular cataracts (39-72%), high myopia, astigmatism, keratoconus, and mild hearing loss (30%, excluding Usher's patients). 50% of female carriers with X-linked form have golden reflex in posterior pole.

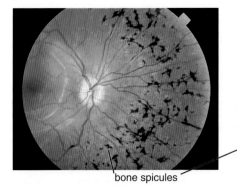

bone spicules

Figure 10-177 • Retinitis pigmentosa demonstrating characteristic bone-spicule pigmentary changes.

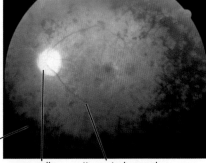

waxy pallor　　attenuated vessels

Figure 10-178 • Retinitis pigmentosa demonstrating dense RPE changes, optic disc pallor, and attenuated retinal vessels.

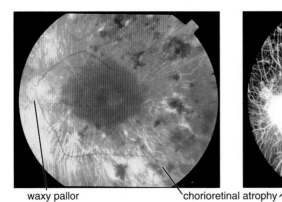

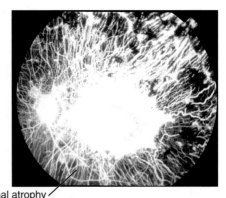

waxy pallor   chorioretinal atrophy

Figure 10-179 • Retinitis pigmentosa with diffuse chorioretinal atrophy and early optic disc pallor.

Figure 10-180 • Fluorescein angiogram of same patient as shown in Figure 10-179 demonstrating the diffuse chorioretinal atrophy.

Differential Diagnosis

Congenital rubella syndrome, syphilis, thioridazine and chloroquine drug toxicity, carcinoma-associated retinopathy, congenital stationary night blindness, vitamin A deficiency, atypical cytomegalovirus or herpes virus chorioretinitis, trauma, diffuse unilateral subacute neuro-retinitis, gyrate atrophy, bear tracks, congenital hypertrophy of the retinal pigment epithelium (CHRPE).

Evaluation

- Complete ophthalmic history with attention to consanguinity, family history, and hearing.
- Complete eye examination with attention to refraction, pupils, cornea, lens, vitreous cells, and ophthalmoscopy.
- **Color vision** (Farnsworth panel D15): Normal except very late in the disease.
- **Electrophysiologic testing:** ERG (markedly reduced or absent; decreases 10% per year, abnormal in 90% of female carriers with X-linked form, subnormal scotopic amplitudes precede reduction of photopic amplitudes), EOG (abnormal), dark adaptation (elevated rod and cone thresholds).
- **Visual fields:** Mid-peripheral ring scotoma; progresses to total loss except for central islands that disappear at the very end of the disease process.
- **Lab tests:** Plasma ornithine levels, fat-soluble vitamin levels (especially vitamin A), serum lipoprotein electrophoresis (Bassen-Kornzweig), serum cholesterol and triglycerides, VDRL, FTA-ABS, peripheral blood smears (acanthocytosis), serum phytanic acid levels (Refsum's).

Management

- No effective treatment except in forms with treatable systemic diseases (abetalipoproteinemia, Refsum's disease).
- Correct any refractive error; prescribe dark glasses.
- Low vision consultation for visual aids.

Continued

Management—cont'd

- For common forms of retinitis pigmentosa (>18 years of age): vitamin A (15,000 IU po qd of palmitate form) slows reduction of ERG amplitudes; avoid vitamin E; follow liver function tests and serum retinol levels annually. *Note:* controversial and not tested in atypical forms of RP. The use of vitamin A in younger patients is even more controversial: age 6-10 years, vitamin A (5000 IU po qd of palmitate form), 10-15 years, vitamin A (10,000 IU po qd of palmitate form); check with pediatrician before starting high dose vitamin A therapy.
- Systemic acetazolamide (Diamox 500 mg IV or po) for cystoid macular edema is controversial.
- Cataract surgery may be indicated depending on retinal function; check potential acuity meter (PAM) test when considering cataract extraction.

Prognosis

Poor, usually legally blind by fourth decade.

Albinism

Ocular Albinism (X-Linked/AR)

Congenital disorder of melanogenesis limited to the eye; decreased number of melanosomes (although each melanosome is fully pigmented). Patients have decreased vision and photophobia; signs include nystagmus, strabismus, high myopia, diffuse iris transillumination, foveal hypoplasia, and fundus hypopigmentation.

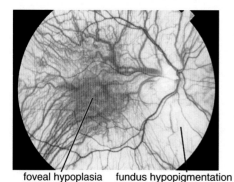

foveal hypoplasia   fundus hypopigmentation

Figure 10-181 • Fundus hypopigmentation in a patient with albinism. The deep choroidal vasculature is clearly visible.

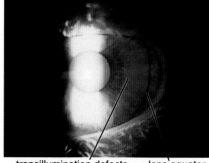

transillumination defects   lens equator

Figure 10-182 • Albinism demonstrating diffuse iris transillumination; note that the equator of the crystalline lens is visible as a dark line near the peripheral iris.

Oculocutaneous Albinism (AR>AD)

Systemic problem with decreased melanin in all melanosomes; two forms: tyrosinase positive (some pigmentation) and tyrosinase negative (no pigmentation). These patients lack pigmentation of the hair, skin, and eyes. Potentially lethal variants of oculocutaneous albinism include Chédiak-Higashi (AR) (reticuloendothelial incompetence with neutropenia, anemia, thrombocytopenia, recurrent infections, leukemia, and lymphoma) and Hermansky-Pudlak (AR) (clotting disorders and bleeding tendencies secondary to platelet abnormalities).

* No effective treatment.
* Medical and hematology consultation to rule out potentially lethal variants.

Phakomatoses

Group of congenital, mainly heritable syndromes with multiple tumorous growths both ocular and systemic; commonly have incomplete penetrance and variable expressivity. *Phako* = "motherspot" (birthmark).

Angiomatosis Retinae (von Hippel–Lindau Disease) (AD)

Bilateral retinal capillary hemangiomas (40-60%), cystic cerebellar hemangioblastoma (60%, most common cause of death), renal cell carcinoma, pheochromocytoma, liver, pancreas, and epididymis cysts (if only retinal findings, then von Hippel disease).

* **Genetics:** Linked to chromosome 3p26-p25; mutation in the VHL tumor suppressor gene.
* Head, upper cervical spinal cord, and abdominal CT scan or MRI.
* Medical consultation if intracranial or systemic lesions exist.

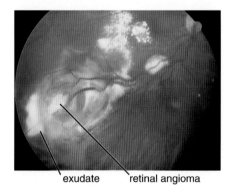
exudate   retinal angioma

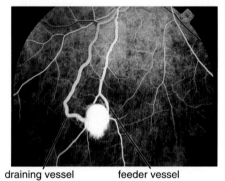
draining vessel   feeder vessel

Figure 10-183 • Angiomatosis retinae (von Hippel–Lindau disease) demonstrating retinal capillary hemangioma with feeder and draining vessels and surrounding exudates.

Figure 10-184 • Fluorescein angiogram of a patient with retinal angioma demonstrating fluorescein filling from feeder vessel and drainage via drainage vessel.

Ataxia Telangiectasia (Louis-Bar Syndrome) (AR)

Progressive cerebellar ataxia (first symptom), telangiectasia of the skin (especially around face, ears, and neck) and bulbar conjunctiva, ocular motility abnormalities; also associated with seborrheic dermatitis, mental retardation, thymus gland hypoplasia with reduced T-cell immunity, high incidence of malignancies (33%) including lymphoma and leukemia, and humoral/cellular immunodeficiency with increased risk of infections, especially chronic respiratory infections; poor prognosis, with death by adolescence.

- **Genetics:** Linked to chromosome 11q22.3; *ATM* gene thought to encode protein vital to DNA repair.
- Medical consultation.

Encephalotrigeminal Angiomatosis (Sturge-Weber Syndrome)

Diffuse, flat, dark red, "tomato catsup" choroidal hemangioma (40-50%), congenital facial hemangioma (nevus flammeus or "port wine stain"), ipsilateral intracranial hemangioma, nevus flammeus involving the eyelid (suspect glaucoma if upper eyelid involved), large anomalous blood vessels in the conjunctiva and episclera, and congenital, ipsilateral glaucoma (30%). May have mental retardation, convulsions, and cerebral calcifications. No hereditary pattern. Variable prognosis depending on CNS involvement.

- **Genetics:** No known locus.
- Head and orbital CT scan.
- May require treatment of increased intraocular pressure (see Chapter 11).
- Neurology consultation if intracranial lesions exist.

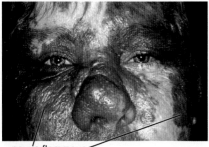

nevus flammeus

Figure 10-185 • Encephalotrigeminal angiomatosis (Sturge-Weber syndrome) demonstrating nevus flammeus.

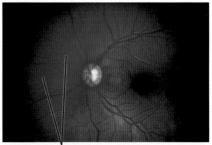

diffuse choroidal hemangioma

Figure 10-186 • Encephalotrigeminal angiomatosis demonstrating tomato-catsup fundus appearance of a diffuse choroidal hemangioma.

Neurofibromatosis (von Recklinghausen's Disease) (AD)

Disorder of the neuroectodermal system. Two forms (see Chapter 3).

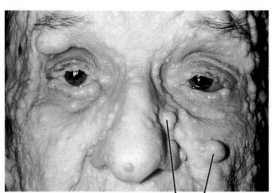

Figure 10-187 • Neurofibromatosis (von Recklinghausen's disease) demonstrating facial neurofibromas.

neurofibromas

Racemose Hemangiomatosis (Wyburn-Mason Syndrome)

Anomalous anastomosis between the arterial and venous systems of the retina, brain (20-30% have intracranial arteriovenous malformations causing mental status changes or hemiparesis; 30% cause visual fields defects including homonymous hemianopsia), orbit, and facial bones (pterygoid fossa, mandible, and maxilla). Usually unilateral (96%) racemose angiomas that appear as intertwined tangles of dilated vessels; may cause visual loss due to retinal or vitreous hemorrhage. Early mortality due to intracranial arteriovenous malformations.

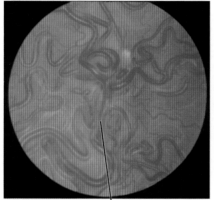 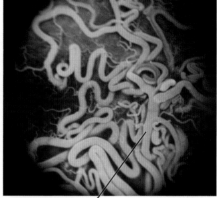

retinal vascular arteriovenous malformation

Figure 10-188 • Racemose hemangiomatosis (Wyburn-Mason syndrome) demonstrating retinal vascular arteriovenous malformation (AVM) with dilated, tortuous vessels.

Figure 10-189 • Fluorescein angiogram of same patient as shown in Figure 10-188 demonstrating the retinal vascular arteriovenous malformation filled with fluorescein dye. *(Note:* line points at same vessel in both pictures.)

- **Genetics:** No known locus.
- Head and orbital CT scan.
- Neurology consultation if intracranial lesions exist.
- Asymptomatic retinal lesions do not require treatment.
- Consider laser photocoagulation around lesions (direct treatment dangerous) if symptomatic.

Tuberous Sclerosis (Bourneville's Disease) (AD)

Triad of seizures (infantile spasms, 80-93%), mental retardation (50-60%), and adenoma sebaceum (85%, a misnomer for angiofibromas, a red-brown papular malar rash). Primary criteria include facial angiofibromas (adenoma sebaceum), subungual angiofibromas, cortical tuber, subependymal hamartomas, and multiple retinal hamartomas. Secondary criteria include infantile spasms (25%), cutaneous shagreen patch (fibromatous skin infiltration especially on lower back and forehead; 25%), ash-leaf spots (hypopigmented skin macules seen best with ultraviolet Wood's lamp; 80%), skin tags (molluscum fibrosum pendulum), bilateral renal angiomyolipomata or cysts (80%), cystic lung disease, cardiac rhabdomyoma, calcified CNS astrocytic hamartomas ("brain stones" in cerebellum, basal ganglia, and posterior fossa), or a first-degree relative with tuberous sclerosis. Poor prognosis, with 75% mortality before age of 20 years.

* **Genetics:** Linked to *TSC1* gene on chromosome 9q34 encoding hamartin and *TSC2* gene on chromosome 16p13.3 encoding tuberin, a GTP-ase activating protein.
* Medical and neurology consultation.

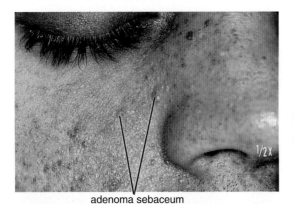

adenoma sebaceum

Figure 10-190 • Tuberous sclerosis (Bourneville's disease) demonstrating adenoma sebaceum.

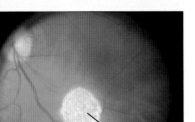

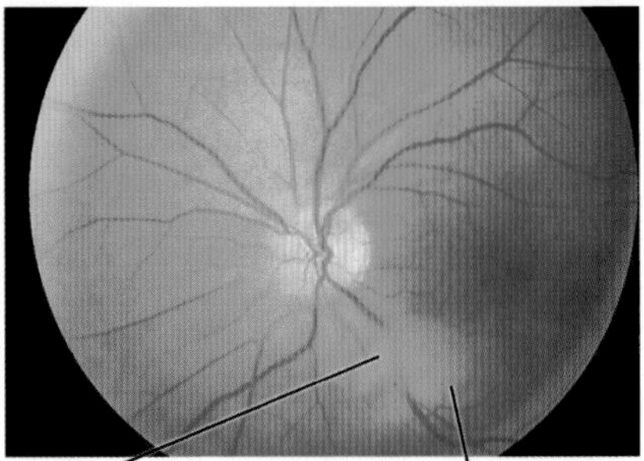

mulberry appearance   astrocytic hamartoma   smooth appearance

Figure 10-191 • Tuberous sclerosis demonstrating astrocytic hamartoma with mulberry appearance.

Figure 10-192 • Tuberous sclerosis demonstrating astrocytic hamartoma with smooth appearance.

Tumors

Benign Choroidal Tumors

Choroidal Hemangioma

Vascular Tumor. Two forms:
(1) Usually unilateral, well-circumscribed, solitary; round, slightly elevated (<3 mm), orange-red lesion located in the posterior pole, often with an overlying serous retinal detachment. Occurs in fourth decade.

(2) Diffuse, reddish, choroidal thickening described as "tomato-catsup" fundus (reddish thickening overlying dark fundus). Occurs in children with Sturge-Weber syndrome (see Fig. 10-186). Usually asymptomatic, but both types can cause exudative retinal detachments (50%).

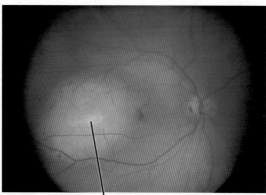

Figure 10-193 • Choroidal hemangioma (discrete type) appearing as an elevated orange lesion in the macula.

choroidal hemangioma

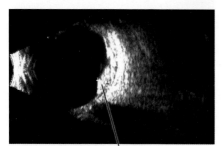

choroidal hemangioma

Figure 10-194 • B-scan ultrasound of same patient as shown in Figure 10-193 demonstrating elevated mass with underlying thickened choroid.

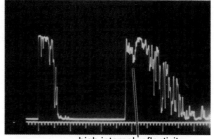

high internal reflectivity

Figure 10-195 • A-scan ultrasound of same patient as shown in Figure 10-193 demonstrating high internal reflectivity.

- **B-scan ultrasonography:** Mass with moderate elevation, thickened choroid, and high internal reflectivity, often with overlying serous retinal detachment.
- **Fluorescein angiogram:** Early filling of the tumor vessels, progressive hyperfluorescence during the transit views, and late leakage (multiloculated pattern).
- **Indocyanine green angiography:** Circumscribed hemangiomas: early hyperfluorescence with relative late hypofluorescence, or "washout" phenomenon. Diffuse hemangioma: early hyperfluorescence with late hypofluorescence of the lesion and persistent hot spots of hyperfluorescence along the vascular channels.
- Observe if asymptomatic.
- Treatment of circumscribed hemangiomas includes grid laser photocoagulation (moderately intense, white reaction on the tumor surface) or iodine 125 plaque brachytherapy if serous retinal detachment threatens fovea; goal of treatment is to decrease serous fluid, not obliterate tumor. Experimental treatments include transpupillary thermotherapy and photodynamic therapy.
- Poor visual acuity results may be expected despite resolution of fluid exudate.

Choroidal Nevus

Dark, gray-brown, pigmented, flat or slightly elevated lesion (<2 mm), often with overlying drusen and a hypopigmented ring around the base. Usually nonprogressive but can grow during puberty. Growth in an adult should be watched carefully. The patient should be reevaluated. Multiple nevi may be seen in patients with neurofibromatosis. Characteristics of suspicious nevi include growth, tumor thickness (>2 mm), presence of visual symptoms, overlying orange pigment, subsensory fluid, and proximity to the optic nerve head. 10% of suspicious nevi progress to malignant melanoma.

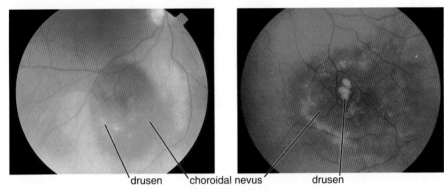

drusen   choroidal nevus   drusen

Figure 10-196 • Large choroidal nevus (nevoma) with overlying drusen.

Figure 10-197 • Flat choroidal nevus with overlying drusen indicating chronicity.

- **B-scan ultrasonography:** Flat to slightly elevated lesion, choroidal discontinuity, and medium to high internal reflectivity.
- Follow with serial photographs, ultrasonography, and clinical examination for any growth that would be suspicious for malignant melanoma at 1, 3, 6, 9, and 12 months, and then on an annual or semi-annual basis if there is no growth.

Choroidal Osteoma

Slightly elevated, well-circumscribed, peripapillary, orange-red (early) to cream-colored (late) benign tumor with small vascular networks on the surface. 80-90% unilateral; growth may occur over years; typically occurs in younger patients who may be asymptomatic or have decreased vision, paracentral scotomas, and metamorphopsia, although well documented in older patients; slight female predilection; consists of mature cancellous bone and may spontaneously resolve; choroidal neovascular membrane common at tumor margins; variable prognosis.

- **B-scan ultrasonography:** Calcification, orbital shadowing, and a high reflective spike from the tumor surface.
- **Fluorescein angiogram:** Irregular hyperfluorescence and late staining of the tumor; the vascular networks may appear hypofluorescent against the hyperfluorescent tumor.
- Orbital radiographs and CT scan show the calcifications within the tumor.
- Treat CNV with laser photocoagulation for juxtafoveal and extrafoveal lesions, often requires multiple sessions; consider photodynamic therapy for subfoveal CNV.

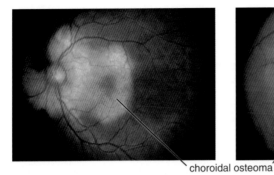

choroidal osteoma   calcification

Figure 10-198 • Choroidal osteoma with orange, placoid appearance.

Figure 10-199 • Choroidal osteoma with calcification.

Benign Retinal Tumors

Astrocytic Hamartoma

Yellow-white, well-circumscribed, elevated lesion that may contain nodular areas of calcification and/or clear cystic spaces; classically has mulberry appearance but may have softer, smooth appearance. Multiple lesions common in tuberous sclerosis. Usually do not grow.

- **Fluorescein angiogram:** Variable vascularization within tumor that leaks in late views.
- No treatment necessary.

Capillary Hemangioma

Benign vascular tumor arising from the inner retina and extending toward the retinal surface. Two forms:

(1) Sporadic, nonhereditary, and unilateral; no systemic associations; usually no feeder vessels.
(2) Hereditary, bilateral (50%), multifocal, and associated with multiple systemic abnormalities (von Hippel–Lindau syndrome); classically has dilated feeder and draining vessels.

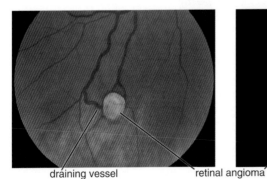

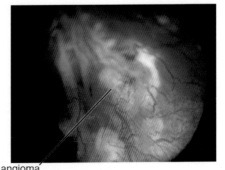

draining vessel   retinal angioma

Figure 10-200 • Retinal angioma with feeder and draining vessels in patient with von Hippel–Lindau syndrome (see Figure 10-184 for fluorescein angiogram).

Figure 10-201 • Capillary hemangioma in a patient with von Hippel disease demonstrating the characteristic pink lesion with a dilated, tortuous, feeder vessel; there is also some surrounding exudate.

Both forms initially appear as a red, pink, or gray lesion that later grows as proliferation of capillary channels within the tumor progresses. These new capillaries leak fluid, leading to exudates and often serous retinal detachments. Associated with preretinal membranes.

- **Fluorescein angiogram:** Early filling of tumor in arterial phase with late leakage.
- No treatment recommended for sporadic tumor unless vision is affected.
- Consider cryotherapy, photocoagulation, and plaque brachytherapy for hereditary tumors; should be performed by an ophthalmic oncologist.
- Medical consultation for hereditary form for evaluation of systemic capillary hemangiomas.

Cavernous Hemangioma

Rare, vascular tumor composed of clumps of saccular, intraretinal aneurysms filled with dark venous blood ("cluster-of-grapes" appearance). Fine, gray epiretinal membranes may cover the tumor. Usually unilateral; occurs between second and third decades and has slight female predilection (60%). No exudation usually seen; retinal and vitreous hemorrhages are rare. Commonly asymptomatic and nonprogressive.

- **Fluorescein angiogram:** Hyperfluorescent saccules with fluid levels.
- No treatment necessary.

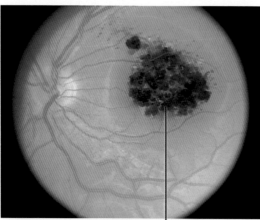

Figure 10-202 • Cavernous hemangioma with "cluster-of-grapes" appearance.

cavernous hemangioma

Congenital Hypertrophy of the Retinal Pigment Epithelium (CHRPE)

Flat or slightly elevated, round, solitary, dark brown-to-black pigmented lesion with sharp borders, scalloped edges, and central hypopigmented lacunae. Vast majority are stationary, although enlargement has been documented. Bilateral, multifocal CHRPE lesions (>4 lesions) seen in familial adenomatous polyposis (Gardner's syndrome [AD]: triad of multiple intestinal polyps, skeletal hamartomas, and soft tissue tumors).

- No treatment necessary if no growth.
- Five reported cases of nodular growth within an area of the CHRPE lesion associated with retina exudates and cystoid macular edema. Consider plaque brachytherapy in these cases (experimental).
- One lesion treated with eye wall resection was documented as low-grade adenocarcinoma.

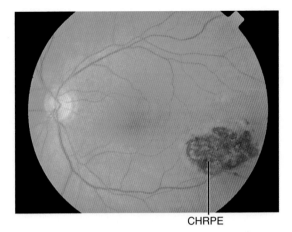

Figure 10-203 • Congenital hypertrophy of the retinal pigment epithelium with hypopigmented lacunae.

CHRPE

Bear Tracks

Multifocal variant of CHRPE clustered in one quadrant with appearance of animal tracks. Polar bear tracks are another variant in which the lesions are hypopigmented. Familial cases have been reported.

• No treatment necessary.

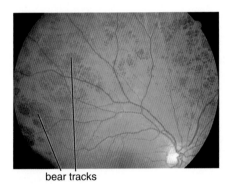

bear tracks

Figure 10-204 • Bear tracks demonstrating multifocal CHRPE clusters.

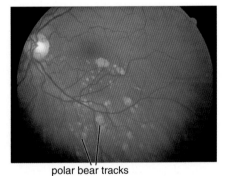

polar bear tracks

Figure 10-205 • Polar bear tracks demonstrating hypopigmented lesions.

Combined Hamartoma of Retinal Pigment Epithelium and Retina

Slightly elevated, dark gray (variable pigmentation) lesion with poorly defined, feathery borders often associated with a fine glial membrane on the surface of the tumor; dilated, tortuous retinal vessels common. Can occur in a peripapillary location (46%) or in the posterior pole; causes decreased vision, metamorphopsia, and strabismus in children and young adults. Choroidal neovascular membrane and subretinal exudation are late complications. Bilateral cases associated with neurofibromatosis type 2 (NF-2); variable prognosis.

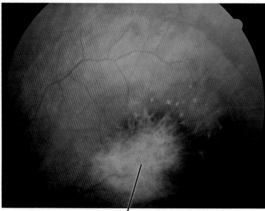

Figure 10-206 • Combined hamartoma of retinal pigment epithelium (RPE) and retina demonstrating gray appearance with feathery borders.

combined hamartoma of RPE and retina

- **Fluorescein angiogram:** Early filling of the dilated, tortuous retinal vessels with late leakage.
- Consider pars plana vitrectomy with membrane peel if epiretinal membrane results in significant visual distortion.
- Laser photocoagulation if CNV develops.

Malignant Tumors

Note: Treatment and workup for tumors of the retina and choroid should be performed by a multidisciplinary team composed of an internist, an oncologist, and an ophthalmic oncology specialist. Therefore, in-depth discussions of management for these tumors is beyond the scope of this book, and treatment is best relegated to the physicians caring for the patient.

Choroidal Malignant Melanoma

Most common primary intraocular malignancy in adults. Focal, darkly pigmented or amelanotic, dome- or collar-button-shaped (break through Bruch's membrane) tumor usually associated with overlying serous retinal detachment and lipofuscin (orange spots); commonly have episcleral sentinel vessels. Collaborative Ocular Melanoma Study (COMS) classified lesions by size: small, medium, and large (see below). Most common sites of metastasis: liver, lung, bone, skin, and central nervous system. Factors predictive of metastasis: presence of epithelioid cells (Callender classification), high number of mitoses, extrascleral extension, increased tumor thickness, ciliary body involvement, tumor growth, and proximity to optic disc.

- Examination: intraocular shadow with transillumination.
- **B-scan ultrasonography:** Collar-button-shaped (27% in COMS) or dome-shaped (60% in COMS) mass >2.5 mm (95%), low to medium (5-60% spike height) internal reflectivity (84% in COMS), regular internal structure, solid consistency, echo attenuation, acoustic hollowness within the tumor, choroidal excavation, and orbital shadowing.
- **Fluorescein angiogram:** May demonstrate double circulation due to intrinsic tumor circulation in large tumors, late staining of lesion with multiple pinpoint hyperfluorescent hot spots; not useful unless the intrinsic circulation is documented.

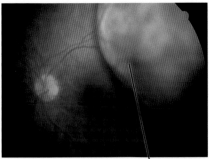

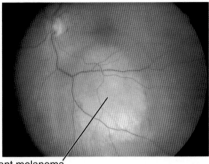

choroidal malignant melanoma

Figure 10-207 • Choroidal malignant melanoma demonstrating elevated dome-shaped tumor.

Figure 10-208 • Choroidal amelanotic melanoma demonstrating hypopigmented subretinal mass.

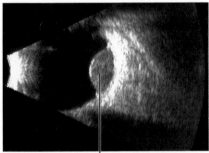

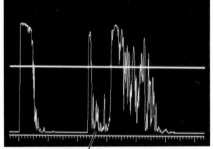

choroidal malignant melanoma

low internal reflectivity

Figure 10-209 • B-scan ultrasound of same patient as shown in Figure 10-208 demonstrating dome-shaped choroidal mass.

Figure 10-210 • A-scan ultrasound of same patient as shown in Figure 10-208 demonstrating low internal reflectivity.

Collaborative Ocular Melanoma Study (COMS) results:

- **Small lesions** (1-3 mm apical height, 5-16 mm basal diameter): 204 patients with tumors not large enough to be randomized were followed in the COMS trial; 6% all-cause mortality at 5 years, 14.9% all-cause mortality at 8 years. 1% melanoma mortality at 5 years, 3.8% at 8 years.
- **Medium lesions** (2.5-10 mm apical height, ≤16 mm longest basal diameter): 1317 patients with medium tumors were randomized to enucleation versus iodine 125 brachytherapy; 34% all-cause mortality for enucleation and 34% all-cause mortality for iodine 125 brachytherapy at 10 years. Metastatic mortality in 17% after enucleation and 17% after iodine 125 brachytherapy at 10 years.
- **Large lesions** (≥2 mm apical height, >16 mm longest basal diameter *or* >10 mm apical height, regardless of basal diameter, *or* >8 mm apical height if <2 mm from the optic disc): 1003 patients with large tumors all received enucleation and were randomized to pre-enucleation external beam radiation (PERT) or not; 61% all-cause mortality for enucleation, 61% all-cause mortality for PERT/enucleation at 10 years. Metastasis in 62% histologically confirmed at time of death; additional 21% suspected on basis of imaging and ancillary testing. Metastatic mortality in 39% after enucleation and 42% after PERT/enucleation at 10 years.

- There is considerable debate over the appropriate management of small tumors. Some authors suggest use of transpupillary thermotherapy for nonfoveal tumors, whereas others advocate radiation treatment or observation. The COMS Study Group is considering evaluating options in a randomized trial.
- Medical and oncology consultation for systemic workup.

Choroidal Metastasis

Most common intraocular malignancy in adults; creamy yellow-white lesions with mottled pigment clumping (leopard spots); low to medium elevation; often with overlying serous retinal detachment; predilection for posterior pole; may be multifocal and bilateral (20%). Most common primary tumors are breast (females, metastasis late), lung (males, metastasis early), and unknown primary; also prostate, renal cell, and cutaneous melanoma; ocular involvement by hematogenous spread; rapid growth; very poor prognosis (median survival is 8.5 months from the time of diagnosis).

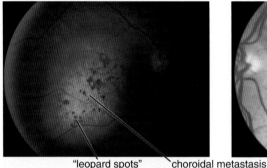

"leopard spots"   choroidal metastasis

Figure 10-211 • Choroidal metastasis with leopard-spot appearance (lung carcinoma).

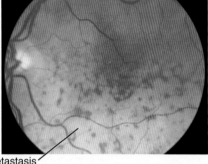

Figure 10-212 • Metastatic breast carcinoma with yellow, creamy posterior pole lesion.

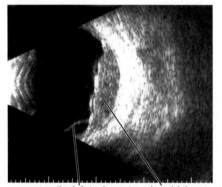

serous retinal detachment   choroidal metastasis

Figure 10-213 • B-scan ultrasound of a patient with choroidal metastasis demonstrating elevated choroidal mass with irregular surface and overlying serous retinal detachment.

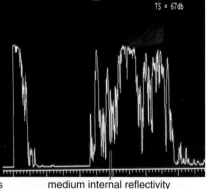

TS = 67db

medium internal reflectivity

Figure 10-214 • A-scan ultrasound of same patient as shown in Figure 10-213 demonstrating medium internal reflectivity.

- **B-scan ultrasonography:** Flat or mildly elevated mass with irregular surface, medium to high internal reflectivity, serous retinal detachment usually visible, no orbital shadowing or acoustically silent zone.
- **Fluorescein angiogram:** Early hypofluorescence with pinpoint hyperfluorescence in the venous phase that increases in later views.
- **Lab tests:** Liver enzymes and chest radiographs.
- Enucleation, laser photocoagulation, radiation therapy, brachytherapy, and chemotherapy are all used; should be performed by an experienced tumor specialist.
- Oncology consultation for metastatic workup if no known primary site.

Primary Intraocular Lymphoma (Reticulum Cell Sarcoma)

Bilateral (80%) anterior uveitis, vitritis, retinal vasculitis, cystoid macular edema, creamy yellow pigment epithelial detachments, hypopigmented retinal pigment epithelial lesions with overlying serous retinal detachments, and disc edema; occurs in sixth to seventh decades; patients have decreased vision and floaters; associated with central nervous system involvement and dementia; poor prognosis, with death within 2 years of diagnosis.

- **Fluorescein angiogram:** Early staining of pigment epithelial detachments with late pooling; window defects seen in areas of atrophy.
- Consider diagnostic pars plana vitrectomy to obtain vitreous biopsy for histopathologic and cytologic analysis.
- Lumbar puncture for cytology.
- Head MRI.
- Treatment with chemotherapy and radiation should be performed by an oncologist.
- Medical and oncology consultation.

Retinoblastoma (RB)

Globular, white-yellow, elevated mass or masses with calcifications that may grow toward the vitreous (endophytic), causing vitreous seeding, toward the choroid (exophytic) causing retinal detachment, or diffusely infiltrating within the retina. Most common primary intraocular malignancy in children (1 in 15-20,000 live births or approximately 300 cases/year in the United States). 90% diagnosed by 5 years of age. 70% are unilateral. Children present with leukocoria (50%), strabismus (18%), intraocular inflammation, and decreased vision. Risk factors for poor prognosis include optic nerve invasion, extraocular extension, and delay in diagnosis. Prognosis is good, with long-term survival approaching 85-90%; 25-30% of children with heritable retinoblastoma may develop a secondary malignancy.

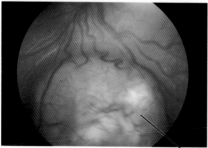

retinoblastoma   serous retinal detachment

Figure 10-215 • Retinoblastoma demonstrating discrete round tumor.

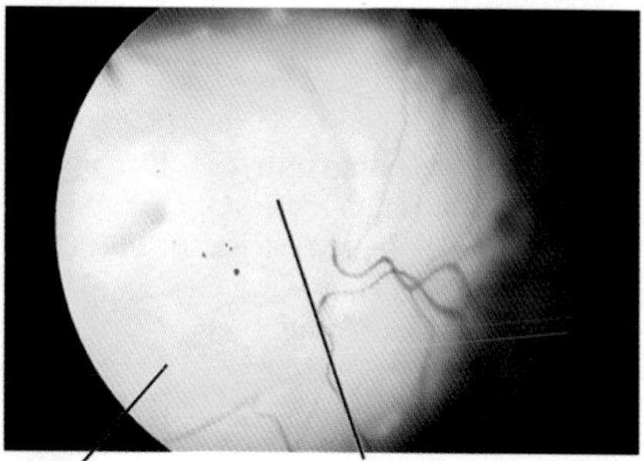

Figure 10-216 • Retinoblastoma demonstrating exophytic growth with a serous retinal detachment.

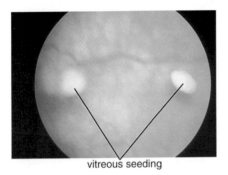

vitreous seeding

Figure 10-217 • Retinoblastoma demonstrating endophytic growth with vitreous seeding.

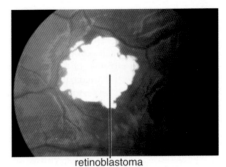

retinoblastoma

Figure 10-218 • Retinoblastoma demonstrating discrete round tumor.

- **Genetics:** 40% heritable, 95% sporadic (25% germinal, 75% somatic), and 5% familial (AD). Mapped to chromosome 13q14.
- Examination under anesthesia required for ophthalmoscopy and treatment.
- B-scan ultrasonography and CT scan to detect calcifications (80%).
- Head and orbital MRI to evaluate for extraocular extension and trilateral retinoblastoma (bilateral with pineal blastoma or parasellar mass).
- Enucleation, cryotherapy, laser photocoagulation, external beam radiation therapy, brachytherapy, and chemotherapy are all used to treat retinoblastoma; should be performed by an experienced ophthalmic oncologist.
- Oncology consultation.

Paraneoplastic Syndromes

Bilateral Diffuse Uveal Melanocytic Proliferation Syndrome (BDUMPS)

Rare paraneoplastic disorder consisting of diffuse uveal thickening with multiple, faint, yellow-orange spots or slightly elevated, pigmented lesions scattered throughout the fundus ("giraffe-skin" fundus). Occurs in elderly patients with a systemic malignancy who have progressive decreased vision; retinal detachment may occur late; poor prognosis, with death within 2 years of diagnosis.

- **B-scan ultrasonography:** Diffuse uveal thickening.
- **Fluorescein angiogram:** Orange spots appear hyperfluorescent.
- **Electrophysiologic testing:** ERG (markedly reduced).
- No effective treatment.
- Oncology consultation.

Carcinoma-Associated Retinopathy (CAR)

Sudden onset of nyctalopia, decreased vision (can progress to no light perception [NLP] over months to years), dyschromatopsia, and visual field changes in patients >50 years of age who have a systemic malignancy (notably small cell lung carcinoma). Patients develop a retinal pigment degeneration with narrowed retinal vessels and vitreous cells; poor prognosis.

- **Electrophysiologic testing:** ERG (markedly reduced).
- No effective treatment.
- Oncology consultation.

Cutaneous Melanoma-Associated Retinopathy (MAR)

Subset of CAR with similar symptoms and fundus findings; paraneoplastic syndrome associated with cutaneous melanoma; antibodies to bipolar cells causes a selective loss of b-wave on ERG.

- **Electrophysiologic testing:** ERG (markedly reduced with selective loss of b-wave).
- No effective treatment.
- Oncology consultation.

OPTIC NERVE AND GLAUCOMA

Papilledema

Definition

Optic disc swelling caused by increased intracranial pressure.

Symptoms

Asymptomatic; may have headache, nausea, emesis, transient visual obscurations (lasting seconds), diplopia, altered mental status, or other neurologic deficits.

Signs

Normal or abnormal visual acuity and color vision (dyschromatopsia), enlarged blind spot, bilateral (rarely unilateral) optic disc edema with blurred disc margins, disc hyperemia, loss of physiologic cup, thickened nerve fiber layer obscuring retinal vessels, peripapillary nerve fiber layer hemorrhages, cotton-wool spots, exudates, and retinal folds (Paton's lines); may have absent venous pulsations (found in 20% of normal individuals) and cranial nerve VI palsy; optic atrophy, visual field defects, vascular attenuation, and decreased visual acuity seen late.

Differential Diagnosis

Intracranial mass, neoplasm, infection (meningitis, encephalitis), or infiltration; subdural or subarachnoid hemorrhage; other causes of optic disc edema including malignant hypertension, idiopathic intracranial hypertension, diabetes mellitus, anemia, central retinal vein occlusion, neuroretinitis, uveitis, optic neuritis (papillitis), anterior ischemic optic neuropathy, Leber's optic neuropathy, hypotony, lymphoma, leukemia, optic nerve mass, Foster-Kennedy syndrome (disc edema with contralateral optic atrophy); pseudopapilledema (e.g., optic nerve drusen).

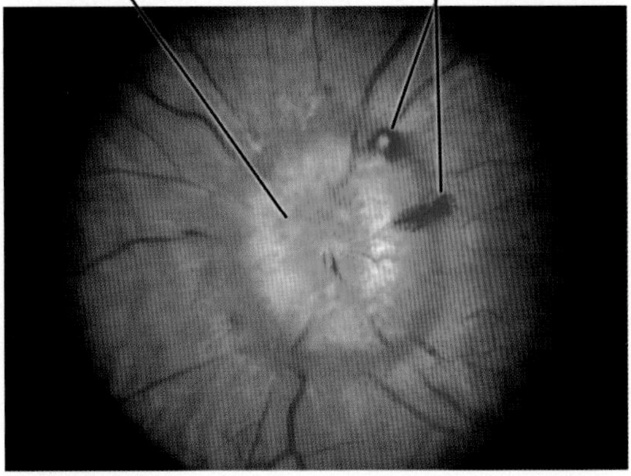

Figure 11-1 • Papilledema due to an intracranial tumor. There is marked edema of the nerve head with blurring of the disc margins 360 degrees and two flame-shaped hemorrhages.

Evaluation

- Complete ophthalmic history, neurologic examination, and eye examination with attention to color vision, pupils, and ophthalmoscopy.
- Check visual fields (enlarged blind spot).
- Emergent head and orbital computed tomography (CT) or magnetic resonance imaging (MRI) to rule out intracranial processes.
- Lumbar puncture to check opening pressure and composition of cerebrospinal fluid.
- **Lab tests:** fasting blood sugar (diabetes mellitus), complete blood count ([CBC] anemia, leukemia, infection), erythrocyte sedimentation rate (ESR).
- Check blood pressure.
- Neuro-ophthalmology consultation.

Management

- Treat underlying cause.

Prognosis

Depends on etiology.

Idiopathic Intracranial Hypertension (Pseudotumor Cerebri)

Definition

Disorder of unknown etiology that meets four criteria: signs and symptoms of increased intracranial pressure (headache, vomiting, papilledema), high cerebrospinal fluid pressure (>250 mm H_2O) with normal composition, normal neuroimaging studies, and normal neurologic examination findings (except cranial nerve VI palsy).

Etiology

Idiopathic; may be associated with vitamin A, tetracycline, oral contraceptive pills, nalidixic acid, lithium, or steroid use or withdrawal; also associated with dural sinus thrombosis, radical neck surgery, middle ear disease, recent weight gain, chronic obstructive pulmonary disease, and pregnancy. Idiopathic intracranial hypertension is a diagnosis of exclusion.

Epidemiology

Usually occurs in obese 20- to 45-year-old females (2:1).

Symptoms

Asymptomatic; patient may have headache, transient visual obscuration (lasting seconds), intracranial noises (whooshing), diplopia, pulsatile tinnitus, dizziness, nausea, and emesis.

Signs

Normal or decreased visual acuity, color vision, and contrast sensitivity; bilateral optic disc edema; may have cranial nerve VI palsy (30%) or visual field defect.

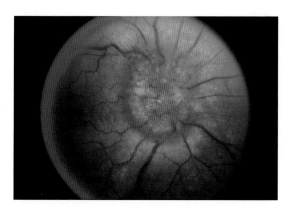

Figure 11-2 • Idiopathic intracranial hypertension demonstrating papilledema.

Differential Diagnosis

Rule out other causes of papilledema and optic disc edema (see Papilledema section).

Evaluation

- Complete ophthalmic history, neurologic examination, and eye examination with attention to color vision, pupils, motility, and ophthalmoscopy.
- Check visual fields (enlarged blind spot, generalized constriction).
- Emergent head and orbital CT scan or MRI to rule out intracranial processes.
- Lumbar puncture to check opening pressure and composition of cerebrospinal fluid.
- Check blood pressure.
- Neurology consultation.

Management

- If the patient is obese, initiate a weight loss program.
- Discontinue vitamin A, tetracycline, oral contraceptive pills, nalidixic acid, lithium, or steroid use.
- No further treatment recommended unless patient exhibits progressive visual loss, visual field defects, or intractable headaches.
- Systemic acetazolamide (Diamox) 500-2000 mg po qd.
- Consider systemic diuretics (furosemide [Lasix] 60-120 mg po divided q6h), follow visual field, visual acuity, and color vision.
- Systemic steroids (prednisone 60-100 mg po qd) are controversial; check purified protein derivative (PPD), blood glucose, and chest radiographs before starting systemic steroids.
- Add H$_2$-blocker (ranitidine [Zantac] 150 mg po bid) or proton pump inhibitor when giving systemic steroids.
- Consider surgery for progressive visual loss despite maximal medical therapy (optic nerve sheath fenestration, lumboperitoneal shunt).

Prognosis

Usually self-limited over 6-12 months; variable if visual loss has occurred.

Optic Neuritis

Definition

Primary demyelination of the optic nerve; type depends on location.

Papillitis

Inflammation is anterior, optic disc swelling present.

Retrobulbar

Inflammation is behind the globe, no optic disc swelling; more common.

Devic's Syndrome

Bilateral optic neuritis with transverse myelitis.

Epidemiology

Usually seen in 15- to 45-year-old females; approximately 55% of patients with multiple sclerosis (MS) develop optic neuritis; initial diagnosis in 20% of MS cases. Stated another way, it is also estimated that 50-60% of patients with isolated optic neuritis will eventually develop MS. *Note:* optic neuritis in children is usually bilateral, postviral, and not associated with MS.

Symptoms

Subacute visual loss (may progress for up to 7 days, then stabilizes and improves), pain on eye movement, dyschromatopsia, decreased brightness sense; may have previous viral syndrome, or phosphenes on eye movement or with loud noises.

Signs

Decreased visual acuity ranging from 20/20 to no light perception; decreased color vision and contrast sensitivity; positive relative afferent pupillary defect (RAPD), central or paracentral scotoma; may have optic disc swelling (35%), mild vitritis, altered depth perception (Pulfrich's phenomenon), and increased latency and decreased amplitude of visual evoked response.

Differential Diagnosis

Idiopathic, viral infection (mumps, measles), intraocular inflammation, malignant hypertension, diabetes mellitus, cat-scratch disease, optic perineuritis, sarcoidosis, syphilis, tuberculosis, collagen vascular disease, Leber's optic neuropathy, optic nerve glioma, orbital tumor, anterior ischemic optic neuropathy, central serous retinopathy, multiple evanescent white dot syndrome, acute idiopathic blind spot enlargement syndrome.

Evaluation

- Complete ophthalmic history, neurologic examination, and eye examination with attention to color vision, Amsler grid, contrast sensitivity, pupils, motility, and ophthalmoscopy.
- Check visual fields.
- If patient does not carry the diagnosis of MS, then obtain an MRI of the head and orbits to evaluate for periventricular white matter demyelinating lesions or plaques (best predictor of future development of MS).
- **Lab tests:** unnecessary if typical case of optic neuritis. When atypical features exist: antinuclear antibody (ANA), angiotensin converting enzyme (ACE), Venereal Disease Research Laboratory (VDRL) test, fluorescent treponemal antibody absorption (FTA-ABS) test, ESR; consider *Bartonella henselae* if optic nerve swollen and exposure to kittens.
- Check blood pressure.
- Consider lumbar puncture to rule out intracranial processes.
- Neuro-ophthalmology consultation.

Management

- If MRI is positive, consider systemic steroids (methylprednisolone 250 mg IV q6h for 3 days, followed by prednisone 1 mg/kg/day for 11 days and rapid taper 20 mg/day on day 12 and 10 mg/day on days 13-15). The Optic Neuritis Treatment Trial (ONTT) showed that this regimen led to visual recovery 2 weeks faster than other treatments; however, no difference in final visual acuity, and a decreased incidence of MS over the ensuing 2 years but no difference after 3 years. *Note:* do not use oral steroids alone, because this led to an increased risk of recurrent optic neuritis (ONTT conclusion).

Management—cont'd

- Check PPD, blood glucose, and chest radiographs before starting systemic steroids.
- Add H_2-blocker (ranitidine [Zantac] 150 mg po bid) or proton pump inhibitor when giving systemic steroids.
- The CHAMPS study group showed that patients receiving weekly intramuscular interferon β-1a (Avonex) following steroid therapy for a first episode of optic neuritis associated with at least two lesions on MRI greater than 3 mm had a reduction in onset of clinical MS over 3 years and improvement or less worsening of MRI lesions.

Prognosis

Good; visual acuity improves over months; final acuity depends on severity of initial visual loss; 70% of patients will recover 20/20 vision; permanent subtle color vision and contrast sensitivity deficits are common; after recovery, patient may have blurred vision with increased body temperature or exercise (Uhthoff's symptom). Approximately 30% will have another attack in either eye, and 30-50% of patients with isolated optic neuritis will develop MS over 5-10 years.

Anterior Ischemic Optic Neuropathy

Definition

Ischemic infarction of anterior optic nerve due to occlusion of posterior ciliary circulation just behind lamina cribrosa; two types.

Arteritic

Giant cell arteritis ([GCA] temporal arteritis).

Nonarteritic or Idiopathic

Associated with hypertension (40%) and diabetes mellitus (20%); arteriosclerotic changes are seen in optic disc vessels.

Epidemiology

Arteritic   Usually seen in patients >55 years old (mostly over 70), fellow eye involved in 75% of cases within 2 weeks without treatment; associated with polymyalgia rheumatica.

Nonarteritic or idiopathic   Usually seen in younger patients; fellow eye involved in 25-40% of cases; associated with hypertension and diabetes mellitus.

Symptoms

Acute visual loss (arteritic > nonarteritic) and dyschromatopsia.

Arteritic   May also have headache, fever, malaise, weight loss, scalp tenderness, jaw claudication, amaurosis fugax, diplopia, polymyalgia rheumatica symptoms (joint pain), and eye pain.

Signs

Sudden, unilateral, painless decreased visual acuity and color vision, positive RAPD, altitudinal visual field defect (usually inferior and large), swollen optic disc (pallor or atrophy after 6-8 weeks), fellow nerve often crowded with a small or absent cup, fellow nerve may be pale from prior episode (pseudo Foster-Kennedy syndrome; more common than true Foster-Kennedy, which is a rare syndrome due to frontal lobe tumor causing ipsilateral optic atrophy and contralateral disc swelling secondary to increased intracranial pressure).

Arteritic   May also have swollen, tender, temporal artery, cotton-wool spots, branch or central retinal artery occlusion, ophthalmic artery occlusion, anterior segment ischemia, cranial nerve palsy (especially cranial nerve VI); optic disc cupping is seen late.

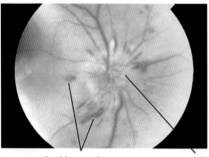 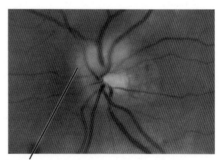

retinal hemorrhages   disc edema

Figure 11-3 • Anterior ischemic optic neuropathy with disc edema and flame hemorrhages.

Figure 11-4 • Anterior ischemic optic neuropathy with disc edema.

Differential Diagnosis

Malignant hypertension, diabetes mellitus, retinal vascular occlusion, compressive lesion, collagen vascular disease, syphilis, herpes zoster; also migraine, postoperative, massive blood loss, normal (low) tension glaucoma.

Evaluation

• Complete ophthalmic history and eye examination with attention to color vision, Amsler grid, pupils, and ophthalmoscopy.
• Check visual fields.

- **Lab tests:** STAT ESR (to rule out arteritic form; ESR > [age/2] in men and > [(age + 10)/2] in women is abnormal), CBC (low hematocrit, high platelets), fasting blood glucose, C reactive protein, VDRL, FTA-ABS, ANA.
- Check blood pressure.
- Arteritic: consider temporal artery biopsy (beware; can get false-negative results from skip lesions); will remain positive up to 2 weeks after starting corticosteroids.
- Consider fluorescein angiogram: choroidal nonperfusion in arteritic form.
- Medical consultation.

Management

ARTERITIC

- Systemic steroids (methylprednisolone 1 g IV qd in divided doses for 3 days, then prednisone 60-100 mg po qd with a slow taper; decrease by no more than 2.5-5.0 mg/wk) started before results of biopsy known to prevent ischemic optic neuropathy in fellow eye; follow ESR and symptoms carefully.
- Check PPD, blood glucose, and chest radiographs before starting systemic steroids.
- Add H_2-blocker (ranitidine [Zantac] 150 mg po bid) or proton pump inhibitor when giving systemic steroids.

NONARTERITIC OR IDIOPATHIC

- Consider daily aspirin.

Prognosis

Poor; visual loss is usually permanent.

Traumatic Optic Neuropathy

Definition

Damage to the optic nerve (intraocular, intraorbital, or intracranial) from direct or indirect trauma.

Etiology

Direct   Penetrating, surgical, bone fragment.

Indirect   Hematoma, head or facial injury to the ipsilateral frontal bone or maxilla (loss of consciousness is not necessary); usually involves intracanalicular portion of nerve.

Epidemiology

Occurs in 3% of patients with severe head trauma and 2.5% of patients with midface fractures.

Symptoms

Decreased vision, dyschromatopsia, pain from associated injuries.

Signs

Decreased visual acuity ranging from 20/20 to no light perception, positive RAPD, decreased color vision, visual field defect, optic nerve may appear normal acutely or show disc edema and hemorrhage, optic pallor develops later; may have other signs of ocular trauma.

optic nerve avulsion

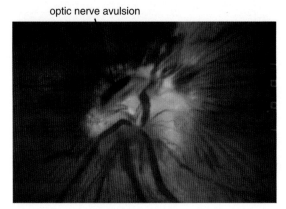

Figure 11-5 • Traumatic optic nerve avulsion.

Differential Diagnosis

Open globe, retinal detachment, Terson's syndrome, Purtscher's retinopathy, macular hole, vitreous hemorrhage.

Evaluation

- Check for associated life-threatening injuries.
- Complete ophthalmic history, neurologic examination, and eye examination with attention to mechanism of injury, color vision, pupils, motility, tonometry, anterior segment, and ophthalmoscopy.
- Orbital CT scan with thin coronal images through the canal to assess location of damage, mechanism of injury, and associated trauma.
- Check visual fields.
- Medical or neurology consultation may be required for associated injuries.

Management

- Consider megadose systemic steroids (methylprednisolone 30 mg/kg IV initial dose, then starting 2 hours later 15 mg/kg every 6 hours for 1-3 days); controversial because dosage, length of treatment, and efficacy are unproved.
- Consider surgical decompression if there is no improvement or there is radiographic evidence of optic canal fracture.

Prognosis

Usually poor, depends on extent of optic nerve damage; 20-35% improve spontaneously.

Other Optic Neuropathies

Definition

Variety of processes that cause unilateral or bilateral optic nerve damage and subsequent optic atrophy. Atrophy of axons with resultant disc pallor occurs 6-8 weeks after injury anterior to lateral geniculate nucleus.

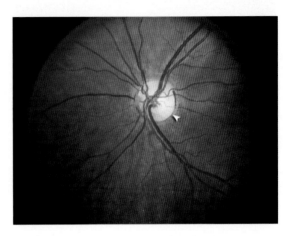

Figure 11-6 • Optic atrophy demonstrating pale nerve. The optic nerve pallor is most striking in the inferotemporal region of the disc *(arrowhead)*.

Etiology

Compressive

Meningioma, glioma, thyroid ophthalmopathy.

Hereditary

Behr's hereditary optic neuropathy (autosomal recessive [AR]) Occurs between 1 and 9 years of age; male predilection; moderate visual loss; no progression; associated with nystagmus in 50%, increased deep tendon reflexes, hypotonia, cerebellar ataxia, and mental retardation.

Kjer's hereditary optic neuropathy (autosomal dominant [AD]) Most common hereditary optic neuropathy; occurs between 4 and 8 years of age; mild, insidious loss of vision, tritanopic dyschromatopsia; slight progression; nystagmus rare, a wedge of pallor is seen on the temporal aspect of the disc. Recently mapped to chromosome 3q28, the *OPA1* gene, a mitochondrial dynamine-related GTPase.

Leber's hereditary optic neuropathy (mitochondrial DNA) Typically occurs in 10- to 30-year-old males (9:1); rapid, severe visual loss that starts unilaterally, but sequentially involves fellow eye usually within 1 year but can be within days to weeks; optic nerve hyperemia and swollen nerve fiber layer with small, peripapillary, telangiectatic blood vessels that do not leak on fluorescein angiography (optic nerve also does not stain); mitochondrial mutation—mothers transmit defect to all sons (50% affected) and all daughters are carriers (10% affected). Three common mutations in the mitochondrial genome at nucleotide positions 3460, 11,778, and 14,484 have been identified in these patients.

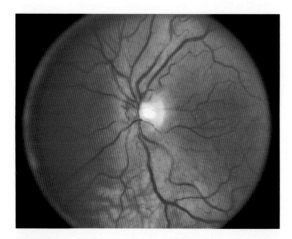

Figure 11-7 • Leber's hereditary optic neuropathy with optic nerve pallor.

Infiltrative

May be infectious or inflammatory from sarcoidosis, toxoplasmosis, toxocariasis, cytomegalovirus, and tuberculosis; or from malignancies including lymphoma, leukemia, carcinoma, plasmacytoma, and metastasis.

Toxic or Nutritional

Radiation, tobacco-related or alcohol-related amblyopia, ethambutol, isoniazid, chloramphenicol, streptomycin, arsenic, lead, methanol, digitalis, chloroquine, quinine, and various vitamin deficiencies including B_1 (thiamine), B_2 (riboflavin), B_6 (pyridoxine), B_{12} (cobalamin), and folic acid.

Symptoms

Decreased vision, dyschromatopsia, central scotoma.

Signs

Unilateral or bilateral decreased visual acuity ranging from 20/20 to 20/400, decreased color vision, and decreased contrast sensitivity; positive RAPD if optic nerve damage is asymmetric (if symmetric damage, RAPD may be absent); optic disc pallor, retinal nerve fiber layer defects, central or centrocecal visual field defects; abnormal visual evoked response; retrobulbar mass lesions may cause proptosis and motility deficits; opticociliary shunt vessels in meningioma or glioma.

Differential Diagnosis

As above; normal tension glaucoma.

Evaluation

- Complete ophthalmic history, neurologic examination, and eye examination with attention to color vision, pupils, motility, Hertel exophthalmometry, and ophthalmoscopy.
- Check visual fields.
- Head and orbital CT scan or MRI to rule out intracranial processes or mass lesion.
- Consider lab tests: CBC, vitamin B1, B2, B6, and B12 levels.
- Consider medical or oncology consultation.

Management

- **Compressive:** systemic steroids (prednisone 60-200 mg po qd) and surgical decompression for thyroid ophthalmopathy; consider surgical resection for some tumors.
- **Hereditary:** genetic counseling; no effective treatment. Molecular screening may add prognostic value.
- **Infiltrative:** leukemic optic nerve infiltration occurs in children and is an *ophthalmic emergency* that requires radiation therapy to salvage vision. Do not initiate steroids prior to oncology evaluation with bone marrow biopsy if leukemia is possible.
- **Toxic or nutritional:** discontinue offending toxic agent; consider vitamin B1 (thiamine 100 mg po bid), vitamin B12 (1 mg IM q month), folate (0.1 mg po qd), or multivitamin (qd) supplementation.

Prognosis

Poor; visual loss is permanent once atrophy has occurred.

Congenital Anomalies

Definition

Variety of developmental optic nerve anomalies.

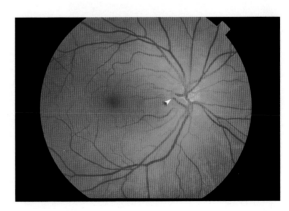

Figure 11-8 • Anomalous optic nerve. Note the atypical configuration of the vessels *(arrowhead)* as they emerge from the nerve head.

Aplasia

Very rare, no optic nerve or retinal vessels present.

Dysplasias

Coloboma

Spectrum of large, abnormal-appearing optic discs due to incomplete closure of the embryonic fissure; usually located inferonasally; associated with other ocular colobomata. May be associated with systemic defects including congenital heart defects, double aortic arch, transposition of the great vessels, coarctation of the aorta, and intracranial carotid anomalies.

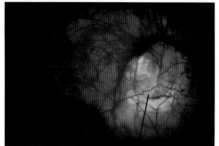

Figure 11-9 • Optic nerve coloboma demonstrating large abnormal disc that appears elongated inferiorly with irregular pattern of vessels.

optic nerve coloboma

Hypolasia

Small discs, "double ring" sign (peripapillary ring of pigmentary changes); unilateral cases usually idiopathic; bilateral cases associated with midline abnormalities, endocrine dysfunction, and maternal history of diabetes mellitus or drug use (dilantin, quinine, alcohol, LSD) during pregnancy.

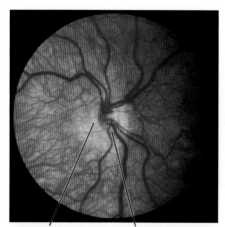

Figure 11-10 • Optic nerve hypoplasia demonstrating "double ring" sign or peripapillary ring of pigmentary changes.

"double ring" sign   optic nerve hypoplasia

Morning Glory Syndrome

Large, unilateral, excavated disc with central, white, glial tissue surrounded by elevated pigment ring; may represent a form of optic nerve coloboma; female predilection (2:1); usually severe visual loss; may develop a localized serous retinal detachment; associated with midline facial defects and forebrain anomalies. May be associated with the papillorenal syndrome, a *PAX2* gene mutation.

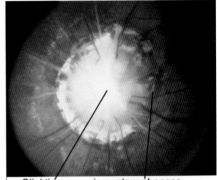

Figure 11-11 • Morning glory syndrome demonstrating characteristic appearance with central white glial tissue, surrounding pigmentary changes, and straightened spokelike vessels radiating from disc.

Glial tissue   pigmentary changes

Optic Nerve Drusen

Superficial or buried hyaline-like material in the substance of the nerve anterior to the lamina cribrosa; may calcify; 75% bilateral; may be hereditary (AD); associated with retinitis pigmentosa; may develop visual field defects usually inferonasal or arcuate scotomas (50%).

Pit

Depression in optic disc, 0.1-0.7 disc diameter, usually located temporally; appears gray-white; 85% unilateral; peripapillary retinal pigment epithelium changes in 95%; 40% develop localized serous retinal detachment in teardrop configuration extending from the pit into papillomacular retina; source of subretinal fluid (cerebrospinal fluid vs. liquefied vitreous) is controversial; retinal detachments often resolve spontaneously.

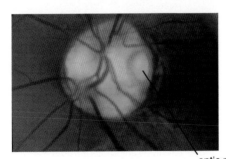
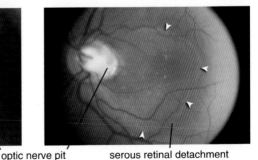

optic nerve pit   serous retinal detachment

Figure 11-12 • Optic nerve pit demonstrating round depression in neural rim at typical temporal location.

Figure 11-13 • Optic nerve pit with serous retinal detachment (arrowheads).

Septo-Optic Dysplasia (De Morsier)

Syndrome of optic disc hypoplasia, absence of septum pellucidum, agenesis of corpus callosum, and endocrine problems; may have see-saw nystagmus. Recently associated with mutations in the *HESX-1* gene.

Tilted Optic Disc

Displacement of one side of optic disc peripherally with oblique insertion of retinal vessels; associated with high myopia; can cause bitemporal visual field defects that do not respect midline.

Symptoms

Asymptomatic; may have decreased vision, metamorphopsia, scotomas, or visual field defects.

Signs

Normal or decreased visual acuity, abnormal appearing optic disc, variety of visual field defects, may have positive RAPD; calcified drusen appear on B-scan ultrasonogram and CT scan.

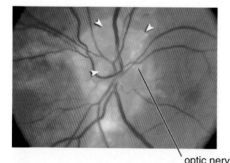
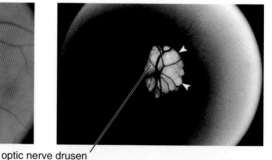

optic nerve drusen

Figure 11-14 • Optic nerve drusen *(arrowheads).* Multiple drusen are evident as elevated, chunky, refractile nodules.

Figure 11-15 • Optic nerve drusen demonstrating autofluorescence when fluorescein filters are in place through a fundus camera. The multiple drusen are quite evident as small, round bumps. This view is obtained without injecting any fluorescein dye.

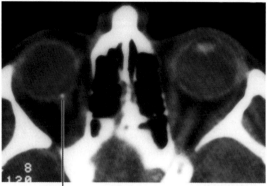

Figure 11-16 • Orbital CT of optic nerve drusen demonstrating calcification.

optic nerve drusen

Differential Diagnosis

See above; optic disc drusen may give appearance of papilledema (pseudopapilledema).

Evaluation

- Complete ophthalmic history and eye examination with attention to color vision, pupils, and ophthalmoscopy.
- Consider visual fields.
- **Fluorescein angiogram:** serous retinal detachment with early punctate fluorescence and late filling may be seen with optic pits; optic nerve drusen autofluoresce with only filter in place before any fluorescein administration.
- Consider B-scan ultrasonography to identify buried drusen.
- Head and orbital CT scan for dysplasias.
- Endocrine consultation for hypoplasia.

Management

- No treatment usually required.
- May require polycarbonate protective lenses if amblyopia or decreased visual acuity present.
- Laser photocoagulation to demarcate serous retinal detachments associated with optic pits (controversial); may also consider pars plana vitrectomy, peeling of posterior hyaloid, air-fluid exchange, and long-acting gas tamponade if laser fails (controversial).
- Treat any underlying endocrine abnormalities.

Prognosis

Stable; decreased vision from compression, choroidal neovascularization, or central retinal artery or vein occlusion can occur rarely with optic nerve drusen; basal encephalocele can occur in any of the dysplasias.

Optic Nerve Tumors

Definition

Variety of neoplasms (benign and malignant) that may affect optic nerve anywhere along its course.

Angioma (von Hippel Lesion)

Retinal capillary hemangioma (see Chapter 10); benign lesion that may involve the optic nerve; may be associated with intracranial (especially cerebellar) hemangiomas (von Hippel–Lindau syndrome) (see Figs. 10-118 and 10-131).

Astrocytic Hamartoma

Benign, yellow-white lesion seen in tuberous sclerosis and neurofibromatosis (see Chapter 10); may be smooth or have nodular, glistening, "mulberry-like" appearance; may be isolated, multiple, unilateral, or bilateral (see Figs. 10-124 and 10-125).

Combined Hamartoma of Retina and Retinal Pigment Epithelium

Rare, peripapillary tumor composed of retinal, retinal pigment epithelial, vascular, and glial tissue; may cause epiretinal membranes with macular traction or edema (see Chapter 10; Fig. 10-136).

Glioma

Two types.

Glioblastoma multiforme   Rare, malignant tumor seen in adults who develop rapid, painful visual loss in one eye with fellow eye involvement over the ensuing weeks; aggressive tumor with blindness in months and death within 6-9 months; may have central retinal artery or central retinal vein occlusion as tumor compromises blood supply; enlargement of optic canal present on CT scan; endocrine or neurologic deficits may appear if tumor invades other structures.

Juvenile pilocytic astrocytoma   Uncommon, benign, neural tumor seen in children; 90% occur in the first and second decades with peak between 2 and 6 years of age; causes gradual, unilateral, progressive, painless proptosis, decreased vision, positive RAPD, and optic disc edema; optic atrophy or strabismus may develop later; chiasmal involvement in 50% of cases; orbital CT scan shows fusiform enlargement of the optic nerve; histologically characterized by Rosenthal fibers, pilocytic astrocytes, and myxomatous differentiation; associated with neurofibromatosis type 1 in 25-50% of cases.

Melanocytoma

Benign, darkly pigmented tumor that lies over or adjacent to the optic disc, usually jet black with fuzzy borders; rarely increases in size; more common in blacks; malignant transformation is exceedingly rare.

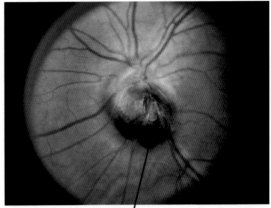

Figure 11-17 • Melanocytoma. This darkly pigmented tumor is obscuring most of the optic nerve head inferiorly.

melanocytoma

Meningioma

Rare, histologically benign tumor arising from optic nerve sheath arachnoid tissue or from adjacent meninges; usually seen in middle-aged females (3:1) in the third to fifth decades; signs include unilateral proptosis, painless decreased visual acuity and color vision, positive RAPD, opticociliary shunt vessels, and optic nerve edema or atrophy; may grow rapidly during pregnancy and involute after delivery; optic nerve pallor and opticociliary shunt vessels occur later; orbital CT scan demonstrates tubular enlargement of the optic nerve and hyperostosis; "railroad-track" sign seen on axial views and "double ring" appearance seen on coronal views; histologic features include whorl pattern and psammoma bodies (meningocytes that form whorls around hyalinized calcium salts).

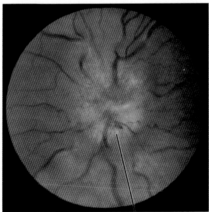

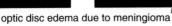
optic disc edema due to meningioma

Figure 11-18 • Meningioma producing optic disc edema.

Figure 11-19 • Fluorescein angiogram of same patient in Figure 11-18 demonstrating leakage of fluorescein from the optic disc.

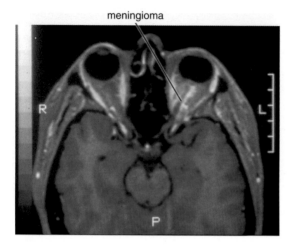

meningioma

Figure 11-20 • CT scan of same patient in Figure 11-18 demonstrating tubular enlargement of the optic nerve with "railroad track" sign.

Symptoms

Asymptomatic; may have decreased vision, dyschromatopsia, metamorphopsia, or pain.

Signs

Normal or decreased visual acuity and color vision, positive RAPD, proptosis, motility disturbances, increased intraocular pressure, optic nerve or peripapillary lesion, optic disc swelling or pallor, visual field defect; opticociliary shunt vessels in meningioma or glioma; angiomas may rarely cause vitreous or retinal hemorrhage.

Differential Diagnosis

See above.

Evaluation

- Complete ophthalmic history, neurologic examination, and eye examination with attention to color vision, pupils, tonometry, and ophthalmoscopy.
- Check visual fields.
- B-scan ultrasonography to evaluate course of optic nerve.
- Fluorescein angiogram to rule out retinal angiomas.
- Head and orbital CT scan or MRI (also to rule out intracranial lesions): optic nerve enlargement, railroad track sign (ringlike calcification of outer nerve), or bony erosion of optic canal.

Management

- Treatment depends on etiology and is controversial; younger patients with meningiomas or gliomas are treated more aggressively.
- May require treatment of increased intraocular pressure (see Primary Open-Angle Glaucoma section).

Management—cont'd

- Consider laser photocoagulation of angiomas (see Chapter 10).
- Treatment of malignant tumors with chemotherapy, radiation, or surgery should be performed by a tumor specialist.

Prognosis

Good for benign lesions, variable for meningiomas, and poor for malignant lesions.

Chiasmal Syndromes

Definition

Variety of optic chiasm disorders that cause visual field defects.

Epidemiology

Mass lesions in 95% of cases; most lesions are large, because chiasm is 10 mm above the sella turcica (microadenomas do not cause field defects); may occur acutely with pituitary apoplexy secondary to hemorrhage or necrosis.

Symptoms

Asymptomatic; patient may have headache, decreased vision, dyschromatopsia, visual field defects, diplopia, or vague visual complaints; systemically decreased libido, malaise, galactorrhea or inability to conceive may be present.

Signs

Normal or decreased visual acuity and color vision; may have positive RAPD, optic atrophy, visual field defect (junctional scotoma, bitemporal hemianopia, incongruous homonymous hemianopia), or signs of pituitary apoplexy (severe headache, ophthalmoplegia, and decreased visual acuity).

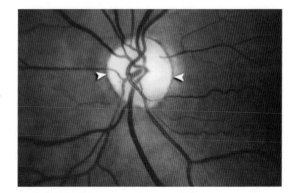

Figure 11-21 • Optic atrophy demonstrating "bow-tie" appearance of pallor in the horizontal meridian *(arrowheads).*

Differential Diagnosis

Pituitary tumor, pituitary apoplexy, meningioma, aneurysm, trauma, sarcoidosis, craniopharyngioma, chiasmal neuritis, glioma, ethambutol.

Evaluation

- Complete ophthalmic history, endocrine history, and eye examination with attention to visual acuity, color vision, pupils, and ophthalmoscopy.
- Check visual fields with attention to vertical midline.
- Head and orbital CT scan or MRI (*emergent* if pituitary apoplexy suspected).
- **Lab tests:** consider checking hormone levels.

Management

- Treatment depends on etiology.
- Pituitary lesions that require surgery, radiation therapy, bromocriptine, hormone replacement should be managed by a neurosurgeon or internist or both.
- Systemic steroids and surgical decompression for pituitary apoplexy.

Prognosis

Generally poor; depends on etiology.

▓ Congenital Glaucoma

Definition

Congenital: onset of glaucoma from birth to 3 months of age (infantile, 3 months to 3 years; juvenile, 3 to 35 years).

Epidemiology

Incidence of 1 in 10,000 births; three forms: approximately one third primary, one third secondary, one third associated with systemic syndromes or anomalies.

Primary   Seventy percent bilateral, 65% male, multifactorial inheritance, 40% at birth, 85% by 1 year of age. Mapped to chromosome 1p36 (*GLC3B* gene) and 2p22-p21 (*GLC3A* gene, *CYP1B1* gene). A mutation in the *CYP1B1* gene accounts for ~ 85% of congenital glaucoma.

Secondary   Inflammation, steroid induced, trauma, tumors.

Associated syndromes   Mesodermal dysgenesis syndromes, aniridia, lens-induced, persistent hyperplastic primary vitreous, nanophthalmos, rubella, nevus of Ota, Sturge-Weber syndrome, neurofibromatosis, Marfan's syndrome, Weill-Marchesani syndrome, Lowe's syndrome, mucopolysaccharidoses.

Mechanism

Primary Developmental abnormality of the angle (goniodysgenesis) with faulty cleavage and abnormal insertion of ciliary muscle. Associated with mutations in *CYP1B1* gene, a member of the cytochrome p450 gene family.

Symptoms

Epiphora, photophobia, blepharospasm.

Signs

Decreased visual acuity, myopia (primary or secondary to pressure induced change), amblyopia, increased intraocular pressure, corneal diameter >12 mm by 1 year of age, corneal edema, Haab's striae (breaks in Descemet's membrane horizontal or concentric to limbus), optic nerve cupping (may reverse with treatment), buphthalmos (enlarged eye).

Differential Diagnosis

Nasolacrimal duct obstruction, megalocornea, high myopia, proptosis, birth trauma, congenital hereditary endothelial dystrophy of the cornea, sclerocornea, metabolic diseases.

Evaluation

- Complete ophthalmic history and eye examination with attention to retinoscopy, tonometry, corneal diameter, gonioscopy, and ophthalmoscopy.
- Complete evaluation may require examination under anesthesia. *Note:* intraocular pressure affected by anesthetic agents (transiently increased by ketamine; decreased by inhalants).
- Check visual fields in older children.

Management

- Treatment is primarily surgical but depends on the type of glaucoma, intraocular pressure level and control, and amount and progression of optic nerve cupping and visual field defects (older children); should be performed by a glaucoma specialist; treatment options include:
- Medical (temporize before surgery): topical ß-blocker (timolol maleate [Timoptic] or betaxolol [Betoptic S] bid) or carbonic anhydrase inhibitor (dorzolamide [Trusopt] tid, brinzolamide [Azopt] tid or acetazolamide [Diamox] 15 mg/kg/d po), or both. Miotic agents may be associated with a paradoxical increase in intraocular pressure; brimonidine [Alphagan] may be associated with infant death.
- Surgical: goniotomy, trabeculotomy; also trabeculectomy, glaucoma drainage implant, cycloablation.
- Correct any refractive error (myopia).
- Patching or occlusion therapy for amblyopia (see Chapter 12).

Prognosis

Usually poor; best for primary congenital form and onset between 1 and 24 months of age.

Primary Open-Angle Glaucoma

Definition

Progressive, bilateral, optic neuropathy with open angles, typical pattern of nerve fiber bundle visual field loss, and increased intraocular pressure (IOP >21 mm Hg) not caused by another systemic or local disease (see Secondary Open-Angle Glaucoma section).

Epidemiology

Occurs in 0.5-2.1% of population >40 years old; risk increases with age; 60-70% of all forms of glaucoma; no sex predilection. Risk factors are increased intraocular pressure, increased cup:disc ratio, thinner central corneal thickness (less than ~550 μm by ultrasound or ~520 μm by optical pachymetry), race (blacks are 3-6 times more likely to develop primary open-angle glaucoma [POAG] than whites; POAG also occurs earlier, is six times more likely to cause blindness, and is the leading cause of blindness in blacks), increased age, and positive family history in first-degree relatives. Inconsistently associated factors include myopia, diabetes mellitus, hypertension, and cardiovascular disease. Mapped to chromosome 2qcen-q13 (*GLC1B* gene), 3q21-q24 (*GLC1C* gene), 8q23 (*GLC1D* gene), 10p14 (*GLC1E* gene, *OPTN* gene). A mutation in the *OPTN* gene accounts for ~ 17% of POAG.

Mechanism

Elevated Intraocular Pressure

Mechanical resistance to outflow (at juxtacanalicular meshwork), disturbance of trabecular meshwork collagen, trabecular meshwork endothelial cell dysfunction, basement membrane thickening, glycosaminoglycan deposition, narrowed intertrabecular spaces, collapse of Schlemm's canal. A subgroup of patients have been identified with mutations of the myocilin glycoprotein. This protein is also mutated in patients with autosomal dominant juvenile open-angle glaucoma (*GLC1A, TIGR* gene), which has been mapped to chromosome 1q21-q31.

Optic Nerve Damage (Various Theories)

Mechanical   Compression of optic nerve fibers against lamina cribrosa with interruption of axoplasmic flow.

Vascular   Poor optic nerve perfusion or disturbed blood flow autoregulation.

Other pathways leading to ganglion cell necrosis or apoptosis   Excitotoxicity (glutamate), neurotrophin starvation, autoimmunity, abnormal glial–neuronal interactions (TNF), defects in endogenous protective mechanisms (heat shock proteins).

Symptoms

Asymptomatic; may have decreased vision or constricted visual fields in late stages.

Signs

Normal or decreased visual acuity, increased intraocular pressure, cupping of optic nerve, retinal nerve fiber layer defects, visual field defects.

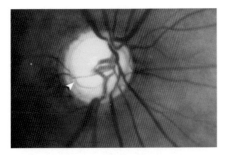

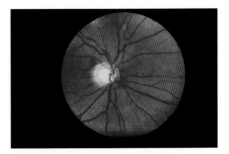

Figure 11-22 • Optic nerve cupping due to primary open-angle glaucoma. Note the extreme degree of disc excavation and course of the vessels at the poles and temporally as they travel up and over the rim giving a "bean pot" configuration *(arrowhead).*

Figure 11-23 • Physiologic cupping. Although the cup is large, there is a healthy rim of neural tissue 360 degrees.

Differential Diagnosis

Secondary open-angle glaucoma, normal tension glaucoma, ocular hypertension, optic neuropathy, physiologic cupping.

Evaluation

- Complete ophthalmic history and eye examination with attention to cornea, tonometry, anterior chamber, gonioscopy, iris, lens, and ophthalmoscopy.
- Check corneal pachymetry (IOP measurement may be artifactually high or low for thicker or thinner than average corneas, respectively).
- Check visual fields: visual field defects characteristic of glaucoma include paracentral scotomas (within central 10 degrees of fixation), arcuate (Bjerrum) scotomas (isolated, nasal step of Ronne, or Seidel [connected to blind spot]), and temporal wedge.
- Stereo optic nerve photos are useful for comparison at subsequent evaluations.
- **Optic nerve head analysis:** various methods including confocal scanning laser ophthalmoscopy (HRT, TopSS), optical coherence tomography, scanning laser polarimetry (Nerve Fiber Analyzer, GDx), and optic nerve blood flow measurement (color Doppler imaging and laser Doppler flowmetry).

Management

- Choice and order of treatment modality depend on many factors, including patient's age, intraocular pressure level and control, and amount and progression of optic nerve cupping and visual field defects. Treatment options include:
- **Observation:** intraocular pressure checks every 3-6 months, visual field examination every 6-12 months, gonioscopy and optic nerve evaluation yearly.
- **Medical:** topical β-blockers traditionally have been the first line of treatment; however, the newer topical prostaglandin analogues have become first-line drugs and have a better safety profile. If intraocular pressure is not controlled,

Continued

Management—cont'd

additional medications can be added. Follow-up (after intraocular pressure stabilization) at 3-4 weeks after changing treatment to evaluate efficacy. Treatment options include single or combinations of the following medications:

- Topical prostaglandin analogue (latanoprost [Xalatan], travopost [Travatan], or bimatoprost [Lumigan] qd; or unoprostone [Rescula] bid); increases uveoscleral outflow.
- Topical β-blocker (timolol maleate [Timoptic], betaxolol hydrochloride [Betoptic S] selective β_1-blocker, levobunolol hydrochloride [Betagan], metipranolol [OptiPranolol], carteolol hydrochloride [Ocupress] bid, or timolol gel [Timoptic XE] qd); decreases aqueous production; check for history of cardiac and pulmonary disease before prescribing.
- Topical α-adrenergic agonist (brimonidine tartrate [Alphagan-P] tid, apraclonidine hydrochloride [Iopidine] tid, or dipivefrin hydrochloride [Propine] bid); decreases aqueous production.
- Topical carbonic anhydrase inhibitor (dorzolamide hydrochloride [Trusopt], brinzolamide [Azopt] tid); decreases aqueous production.
- Topical cholinergic medication (pilocarpine [Ocusert] qid, carbachol tid, phospholine iodide bid); increases outflow through trabecular meshwork.
- Systemic carbonic anhydrase inhibitor (acetazolamide [Diamox], methazolamide [Neptazane] qd to qid); decreases aqueous production; rarely used due to systemic side effects.
- **Laser:** trabeculoplasty, sclerostomy, cyclophotocoagulation.
- Argon laser trabeculoplasty procedure parameters: 0.1 sec duration, 50 μ spot size, 600-1200 mW power, approximately 50 spot applications per 180 degrees, a contact lens is used to stabilize the eye and better focus the beam, spots are placed on the pigmented trabecular meshwork and the power setting is adjusted until a slight blanching of tissue is observed.
- Selective laser trabeculoplasty procedure parameters: 0.7-0.9 mJ power, time and spot size (400 μm) are fixed, approximately 50 confluent spot applications per 180 degrees, spots are placed to straddle the trabecular meshwork, and the power may need to be lowered (0.6 mJ) for heavily pigmented eyes.
- **Surgical:** trabeculectomy, glaucoma drainage implant, cycloablation.

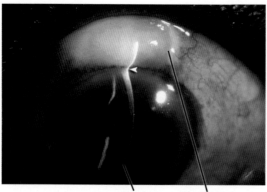

Figure 11-24 • Conjunctival filtering bleb following glaucoma surgery (trabeculectomy), demonstrating typical appearance of a well-functioning, thin, cystic, avascular bleb. Note the curve of the slit-beam at the inferior portion of the elevated bleb *(arrowhead)*.

slit-beam   filtering bleb

Prognosis

Usually good if intraocular pressure is controlled adequately; worse prognosis in blacks; visual loss is permanent.

Secondary Open-Angle Glaucoma

Definition

Open-angle glaucoma caused by a variety of local or systemic disorders.

Etiology

Pseudoexfoliation syndrome (see Chapter 8), pigment dispersion syndrome (see Chapter 7), uveitis, lens induced (see Chapter 8), intraocular tumors, trauma, and drugs; also elevated episcleral venous pressure (orbital mass, thyroid ophthalmopathy, arteriovenous fistulas, orbital varices, superior vena cava syndrome, Sturge-Weber syndrome, idiopathic), retinal disease (retinal detachment, retinitis pigmentosa, Stickler's syndrome), systemic disease (pituitary tumors, Cushing's syndrome, thyroid disease, renal disease), postoperative (laser and surgical procedures), and uveitis-glaucoma-hyphema syndrome (see Chapter 6).

Drug-Induced Secondary Glaucoma

Epidemiology

Steroid-related intraocular pressure elevation correlates with potency and duration of use; 30% of population develop increased intraocular pressure after 4-6 weeks of topical steroid use, intraocular pressure >30 mm Hg in 4%; 95% of patients with POAG are steroid responders; increased incidence of steroid response in patients with diabetes mellitus, high myopia, connective tissue disease, and family history of glaucoma.

Mechanism

Steroids   Unknown, possibly due to increased trabecular meshwork glycosaminoglycans.

Viscoelastic   Viscous substance injected during ophthalmic surgery obstructs trabecular meshwork, self-limited (1-2 days).

Alpha-chymotrypsin   Zonular debris blocks trabecular meshwork.

Symptoms

Asymptomatic; may have pain, photophobia, decreased vision.

Signs

Normal or decreased visual acuity, increased intraocular pressure; may have anterior chamber cells and flare.

Evaluation

• Complete ophthalmic history and eye examination with attention to cornea, tonometry, anterior chamber, gonioscopy, iris, lens, and ophthalmoscopy.

Management

• Treatment of increased intraocular pressure (see Primary Open-Angle Glaucoma section).
• Taper, change, or stop steroids.
• Consider releasing viscoelastic through paracentesis site on first postoperative day if intraocular pressure >30mm Hg and there is no vitreous in the anterior chamber.

Intraocular Tumor Secondary Glaucoma

Mechanism

Hemorrhage, angle neovascularization, direct tumor infiltration of the angle, or trabecular meshwork obstruction by tumor, inflammatory, or red blood cells.

Symptoms

Asymptomatic; may have decreased vision, pain, or systemic symptoms.

Signs

Normal or decreased visual acuity, increased intraocular pressure, iris mass, focal iris elevation, hyphema, hypopyon, anterior chamber cells and flare, pseudohypopyon, leukocoria, segmental cataract, invasion of angle, extrascleral extension, sentinel episcleral vessels.

Evaluation

• Complete ophthalmic history and eye examination with attention to cornea, tonometry, anterior chamber, gonioscopy, iris, lens, and ophthalmoscopy.
• B-scan ultrasonography if unable to visualize the fundus; consider ultrasound biomicroscopy to evaluate angle and ciliary body.
• Check visual fields
• Medical or oncology consultation for metastatic workup.

Management

• Treatment of increased intraocular pressure (see Primary Open-Angle Glaucoma section).
• Treatment for tumor with radiation, chemotherapy, or surgery should be performed by a tumor specialist.

Uveitic Secondary Glaucoma

Mechanism

Outflow obstruction due to inflammatory cells, trabeculitis, scarring of trabecular meshwork, or increased aqueous viscosity.

Symptoms

Asymptomatic; may have pain, photophobia, red eye, decreased vision.

Signs

Normal or decreased visual acuity, increased intraocular pressure (may be complicated by steroid response), ciliary injection, anterior chamber cells and flare, keratic precipitates, miotic pupil, peripheral anterior synechiae, posterior synechiae, iris heterochromia, iris atrophy, fine angle vessels, decreased corneal sensation, corneal edema, corneal scarring, ghost vessels, cataract; may have low intraocular pressure due to decreased aqueous production.

Evaluation

- Complete ophthalmic history and eye examination with attention to cornea, tonometry, anterior chamber, gonioscopy, iris, lens, and ophthalmoscopy.
- Check visual fields.
- Consider uveitis workup.

Management

- Treatment of increased intraocular pressure (see Primary Open-Angle Glaucoma section); do not use pilocarpine or prostaglandin analogue.
- Treat uveitis with topical cycloplegic agent (cyclopentolate 1% or scopolamine 0.25% tid) and topical steroid (prednisolone acetate 1%, rimexolone [Vexol], or fluorometholone [FML] qd to q1h depending on the amount of inflammation; beware of increased intraocular pressure with steroid use due to steroid response or recovery of ciliary body to normal aqueous production; consider tapering or changing steroid if steroid response exists); steroids are not effective in Fuchs' heterochromic iridocyclitis.

Traumatic Secondary Glaucoma

Mechanism

Angle recession   If more than two thirds of angle is involved, 10% of patients develop glaucoma from scarring of angle structures.

Chemical injury   Toxicity to angle structures from direct or indirect (prostaglandin, ischemia-mediated) damage.

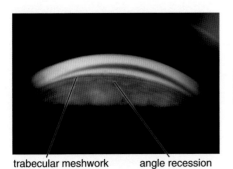

Figure 11-25 • Gonioscopy of angle recession demonstrating deepened angle with blue-gray face of ciliary body evident.

trabecular meshwork   angle recession

Hemorrhage   Red blood cells, ghost cells (degenerated red blood cells), or macrophages that have ingested red blood cells (hemolytic glaucoma) obstruct the trabecular meshwork; increased incidence in patients with sickle cell disease.

Siderosis or chalcosis   Toxicity to angle structures from iron or copper intraocular foreign body.

Symptoms

Asymptomatic; may have decreased vision, pain, red eye.

Signs

Normal or decreased visual acuity, increased intraocular pressure, anterior chamber cells and flare; may have other signs of trauma including red blood cells in anterior chamber or vitreous, angle recession, iridodialysis, cyclodialysis, sphincter tears, iridodonesis, phacodonesis, cataract, corneal blood staining, corneal scarring, scleral blanching or ischemia, intraocular foreign body, iris heterochromia, retinal tears, choroidal rupture.

Evaluation

• Complete ophthalmic history and eye examination with attention to cornea, tonometry, anterior chamber, gonioscopy, iris, lens, and ophthalmoscopy.
• Consider B-scan ultrasonography if unable to visualize the fundus.
• Consider orbital radiographs or head and orbital CT scan to rule out intraocular foreign body.
• Check visual fields.

Management

• Treatment of increased intraocular pressure (see Primary Open-Angle Glaucoma section).
• Laser trabeculoplasty is usually not effective.
• May require anterior chamber washout or pars plana vitrectomy for hemorrhage-related, uncontrolled elevation of intraocular pressure.

▊ Normal (Low) Tension Glaucoma

Definition

Similar optic nerve and visual field damage as in POAG, but with normal intraocular pressure (≤21 mm Hg).

Epidemiology

Higher prevalence of vasospastic disorders including migraine, Raynaud's phenomenon, ischemic vascular disease, autoimmune disease, and coagulopathies; also associated with history of poor perfusion of the optic nerve from hypotension, shock, myocardial infarction, or massive hemorrhage.

Symptoms

Asymptomatic; may have decreased vision or constricted visual fields in late stages.

Signs

Normal or decreased visual acuity, normal intraocular pressure (≤21 mm Hg), cupping of optic nerve, splinter hemorrhages at optic disc (more common than in POAG), peripapillary atrophy, nerve fiber layer defects, visual field defects.

Differential Diagnosis

POAG (undetected increased intraocular pressure or artifactually low intraocular pressure secondary to thin cornea [e.g., naturally occurring or after LASIK or PRK]), secondary glaucoma (steroid-induced, "burned out" pigmentary or postinflammatory glaucoma), intermittent angle-closure glaucoma, optic neuropathy, optic nerve anomalies, glaucomatocyclitic crisis (Posner-Schlossman syndrome).

Evaluation

- Complete ophthalmic history and eye examination with attention to cornea, tonometry, anterior chamber, gonioscopy, iris, lens, and ophthalmoscopy.
- Check visual fields.
- Check corneal pachymetry.
- Consider diurnal curve (e.g., intraocular pressure measurement q2h for 10-24 hours) and tonography.
- Consider evaluation for other causes of optic neuropathy; check color vision, lab tests (CBC, ESR, Venereal Disease Research Laboratory [VDRL] test, fluorescent treponemal antibody absorption [FTA-ABS] test, antinuclear antibody [ANA]), neuroimaging, or cardiovascular evaluation if age less than 60 years old, decreased visual acuity without apparent cause, visual field defect not typical of glaucoma, visual field and disc changes do not correlate, rapidly progressive, unilateral or markedly asymmetric, or nerve pallor greater than cupping.

Management

- Choice and order of topical glaucoma medications depend on many factors, including patient's age, intraocular pressure level and control, and amount and progression of optic nerve cupping and visual field defects. Treatment options are presented in the Primary Open-Angle Glaucoma section.
- Collaborative Normal Tension Glaucoma study conclusion: follow patients every 6 months with complete eye examination and visual fields. No treatment if stable unless other risk factors are present for progression (disc hemorrhage, history of migraine, or female); treatment goal is intraocular pressure reduction of 30% from baseline.

Prognosis

Worse than that for POAG.

C h a p t e r 12

VISUAL ACUITY, REFRACTIVE PROCEDURES, AND SUDDEN VISION LOSS

▐ Refractive Error

Definition

The state of an eye in which light rays are not properly focused on the retina and, therefore, images are blurred. As a result, uncorrected visual acuity is decreased. Visual acuity measures the ability to see an object at a certain distance. It is frequently recorded as a ratio comparing an individual's results with a standard. Snellen acuity (a measure of central acuity) is the most common method to test vision (Table 12-1). For children and illiterate adults, other tests may be used, including the "E" game, Landolt "C" chart, HOTV match test, and Allen card pictures.

Ametropia

Refers to a refractive error (e.g., myopia, hyperopia, or astigmatism).

Anisometropia

Refers to a difference in refractive error between the two eyes; usually 2D or more.

Astigmatism

The curvature of the cornea or, less commonly, the curvature of the lens varies in different meridians. If the cornea is steeper in the vertical meridian, it is referred to as "with-the-rule" astigmatism; if it is steeper in the horizontal meridian, it is called "against-the-rule" astigmatism. Astigmatism can also be designated regular or irregular. A cylindrical lens corrects regular astigmatism.

Table 12-1   Measures of Visual Acuity: Central Visual Acuity Notations

Distance Acuity Notations

Distance Snellen		Decimal	logMAR	Loss of Central Vision (%)
Feet	Meters			
20/10	6/3	2.00	−0.3	—
20/15	6/5	1.25	−0.1	—
20/20	6/6	1.00	0	—
20/25	6/7.5	0.80	0.10	5
20/30	6/10	0.63	0.20	10
20/40	6/12	0.50	0.30	15
20/50	6/15	0.40	0.40	25
20/60	6/20	0.32	0.50	35
20/70	6/22	0.29	0.55	40
20/80	6/24	0.25	0.60	45
20/100	6/30	0.20	0.70	50
20/125	6/38	0.16	0.80	60
20/150	6/50	0.125	0.90	70
20/200	6/60	0.10	1.00	80
20/300	6/90	—	—	85
20/400	6/120	—	—	90
20/800	6/240	—	—	95

Near Acuity Notations

Near Snellen		Jaeger Standard	American Point-Type	Distance Snellen	
Inches	Centimeters			Equivalent	Loss (%)
14/14	35/35	1	3	20/20	—
14/18	35/45	2	4	20/25	0
14/21	35/53	3	5	20/30	5
14/24	35/50	4	6	20/40	7
14/28	35/70	5	7	20/45	10
14/35	35/88	6	8	20/50	50
14/40	35/100	7	9	20/60	55
14/45	35/113	8	10	20/70	60
14/60	35/150	9	11	—	80
14/70	35/175	10	12	—	85
14/80	35/200	11	13	—	87
14/88	35/220	12	14	20/100	90
14/112	35/280	13	21	—	95
14/140	35/350	14	23	—	98

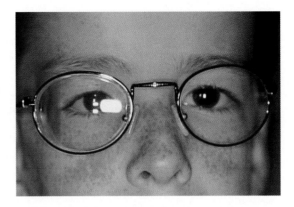

Figure 12-1 • Anisometropia with high myopia in the right eye (OD) (note minification from spectacle lens) and hyperopia in the left eye (OS) (note magnification from spectacle lens).

Emmetropia

No refractive error exists and thus no corrective lens is required to achieve good distance vision. In the emmetropic eye, parallel rays of light are brought to focus on the retina, and the far point is infinity, which is conjugate with the retina.

Hyperopia ("Farsightedness")

Light rays are focused behind the retina. A "plus" lens is used to correct this refractive error.

Myopia ("Nearsightedness")

Light rays from a distant object are focused in front of the retina and those from a near object are focused on the retina; therefore, distant objects are blurry and near objects are clear. A "minus" lens is used to correct this refractive error.

Presbyopia

Loss of accommodative response resulting from loss of lens elasticity or possible anatomic change in lens equator to ciliary body position. Average age of onset is 40 years old. A "plus" lens is used to correct this problem (bifocal "add").

Symptoms

Decreased vision when not wearing corrective lenses, distant objects are blurry and near objects are clear (myopia), distant and near objects are blurry (hyperopia), or near objects that are blurry become clearer when held further away (presbyopia).

Signs

Decreased visual acuity that improves with pinhole testing, glasses, or contact lenses.

Differential Diagnosis

Normal eye examination in presence of decreased vision: amblyopia, retrobulbar optic neuropathy, other optic neuropathies (toxic, nutritional), nonorganic (functional) visual loss, rod monochromatism, cone degeneration, retinitis pigmentosa sine pigmento, cortical blindness.

Evaluation

Complete ophthalmic history and eye examination with attention to pinhole acuity (corrects most low to moderate refractive errors to the 20/25 to 20/30 level), manifest (undilated) and cycloplegic (dilated) refraction, retinoscopy, pupils, keratometry, cornea, lens, and ophthalmoscopy.

Consider potential acuity meter testing, rigid contact lens overrefraction, and corneal topography (computerized videokeratography) if irregular astigmatism is suspected.

Management

- Glasses are the first line of treatment and can correct virtually all refractive errors with the exception of high or irregular astigmatism.
- Contact lenses (soft or rigid). Numerous styles of contact lenses are available to correct almost any refractive error.
- Consider refractive surgery (see below).

Prognosis

Good.

▉ Intraocular Refractive Procedures

May be used to correct moderate to high degrees of myopia and hyperopia.

Clear Lens Extraction

The noncataractous crystalline lens can be removed and replaced with an intraocular lens implant of appropriate power to correct the resulting aphakia. Disadvantage of this method is loss of accommodation. This procedure is controversial for myopia because of the risk of retinal detachment in pseudophakic eyes; hyperopic eyes with nanophthalmos may develop choroidal effusions.

Phakic Intraocular Lens

A lens implant is placed in the anterior chamber, posterior chamber, or fixed to the iris with the optic centered over the pupil. Prophylactic peripheral iridotomies are performed prior to surgery to prevent postoperative pupillary block, angle closure (see Chapter 11).

Symptoms

Postoperatively may have: photophobia, pain, decreased vision, glare, halos, and foreign body sensation.

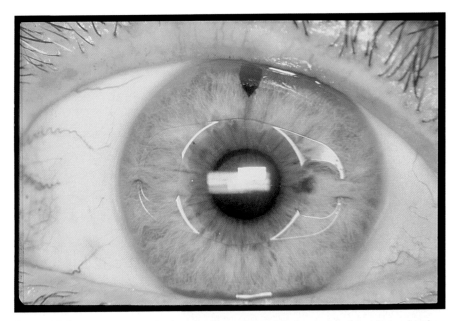

Figure 12-2 • Phakic intraocular lens demonstrating an iris-claw lens in the anterior chamber attached to the iris at the 3 o'clock and 9 o'clock positions. Note the peripheral iridectomy at the 12 o'clock position to prevent pupillary block.

Signs and Complications

Corneal edema (endothelial cell loss), cataract, glaucoma, pupillary block, iridocyclitis, and endophthalmitis; may have residual refractive error. Additional complications of clear lens extraction include posterior capsular opacification, cystoid macular edema, retinal detachment, suprachoroidal hemorrhage, choroidal effusion, retained lens material, and iris damage.

■ Corneal Refractive Procedures

Incisional

Radial Keratotomy (RK)

An incisional refractive surgical procedure for the correction of low to moderate myopia. Deep, radial, corneal incisions are created with a diamond knife to flatten the central cornea. Radial keratotomy can be combined with astigmatic keratotomy for compound myopia (myopia with astigmatism).

Astigmatic Keratotomy (AK)

An incisional refractive surgical procedure for the correction of astigmatism. Deep, midperipheral arcuate or straight incisions (parallel to the limbus) are made with a diamond knife on the steep corneal meridian, causing flattening of the cornea and reduced astigmatism.

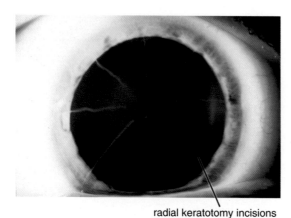

Figure 12-3 • Eight-incision radial keratotomy demonstrating near full-thickness corneal incisions at 90-95% depth.

radial keratotomy incisions

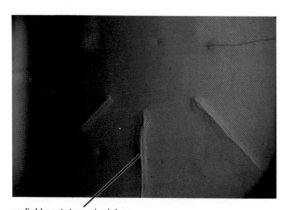

Figure 12-4 • Same patient as Figure 12-3 demonstrating the radial keratotomy incisions in retroillumination.

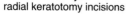
radial keratotomy incisions

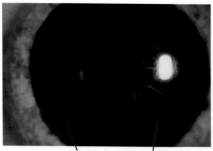

Figure 12-5 • Radial keratotomy demonstrating 16 irregular incisions with hypertrophic corneal scarring and varying optical zones centrally.

irregular radial incisions

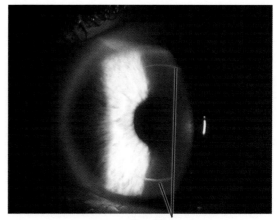

Figure 12-6 • Astigmatic keratotomy demonstrating a pair of 90% depth corneal incisions in the midperiphery of the vertical meridian.

astigmatic keratotomy

Automated Lamellar Keratoplasty (ALK)

A lamellar refractive surgical procedure to correct either myopia or hyperopia. A mechanical device (keratome) is used to cut a partial thickness flap in the cornea. For myopia, a second cut is made with the keratome in the corneal stromal bed. For hyperopia, one deep stromal cut is made to weaken the cornea. The corneal flap is then replaced.

Symptoms

Postoperatively may have: decreased vision (due to undercorrection, overcorrection, or irregular astigmatism), fluctuating vision, difficulty with night vision, halos, glare, star bursts, ghost images, double vision, and foreign body sensation.

Signs and Complications

Corneal scarring, infection, or perforation. May have residual refractive error. Additional complications of ALK include corneal ectasia, circular lamellar flap with or without haze, and epithelial ingrowth.

Excimer Laser

The excimer laser ablates corneal tissue to correct myopia (central ablation), hyperopia (peripheral ablation), regular astigmatism (cylindrical ablation), or irregular astigmatism (custom or wavefront ablation).

Laser in Situ Keratomileusis (LASIK)

A surgical procedure that employs a combination of automated lamellar keratoplasty and photorefractive keratectomy (PRK) techniques. A keratome is first used to cut a hinged partial thickness corneal flap that is then folded back. Laser energy is applied to the underlying stromal bed, and the flap is replaced. LASIK allows for faster visual recovery and minimal pain after surgery, but there is a higher risk of complications due to flap-related problems than with PRK.

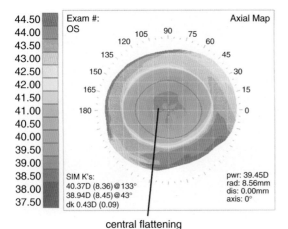

central flattening

Figure 12-7 • Post-LASIK corneal topography map for a myopic excimer laser ablation. Note the blue central flattening on the map created by the photoablation of corneal stroma.

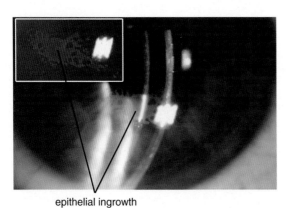

epithelial ingrowth

Figure 12-8 • Epithelial ingrowth after LASIK at the inferior corneal flap edge. The gray puddy-like pseudopods represent epithelium in the corneal flap interface. Inset shows transillumination of the epithelial ingrowth.

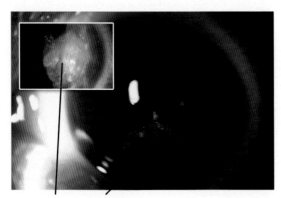

infectious keratitis

Figure 12-9 • Atypical mycobacterial keratitis after LASIK demonstrating the infectious keratitis in the corneal flap interface.

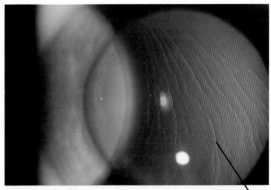

Figure 12-10 • Traumatic LASIK flap striae demonstrating vertically curved wrinkles in the flap.

flap wrinkles

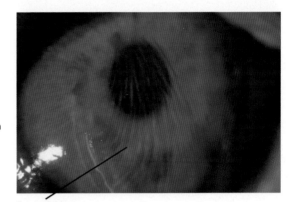

Figure 12-11 • Same patient as Figure 12-10 with traumatic LASIK flap striae demonstrating the curved striae that are enhanced with topical fluorescein and viewed with a blue light.

flap wrinkles

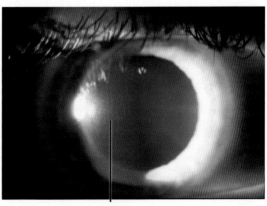

Figure 12-12 • Flap striae after LASIK demonstrating vertical folds with railroad track appearance.

flap striae

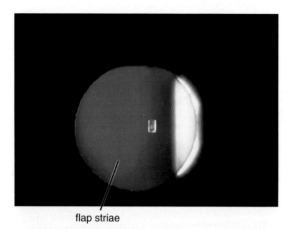

Figure 12-13 • Same patient as Figure 12-12 demonstrating flap striae as viewed with retroillumination.

flap striae

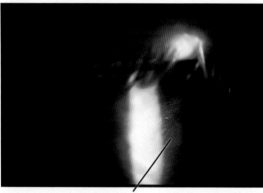

Figure 12-14 • Diffuse lamellar keratitis or "sands of the Sahara" after LASIK demonstrating characteristic appearance of white granular interface material distributed in a wavelike pattern.

diffuse lamellar keratitis

Laser-Assisted Subepithelial Keratectomy (LASEK)

A surgical procedure that employs a combination of PRK and LASIK techniques. A flap composed of only epithelium is created with topical alcohol, the epithelial flap is carefully retracted, laser energy is applied to the stromal bed, and the epithelial flap is replaced. This may combine the advantages of PRK and LASIK by decreasing the incidence of pain and haze associated with PRK and risk of flap complications associated with LASIK.

Photorefractive Keratectomy (PRK)

A surgical procedure that uses laser ablation after corneal epithelial removal. The final visual outcomes are good, but the visual recovery period is longer than with LASIK. Patients may experience initial pain due to the epithelial defect, and decreased vision due to corneal haze.

Symptoms

Postoperatively may have: decreased vision (due to undercorrection, overcorrection, or irregular astigmatism), fluctuating vision, difficulty with night vision, halos, glare, star bursts, ghost images, double vision, and foreign body sensation.

Signs and Complications

Corneal scarring, infection, or ectasia, decentration (apparent on corneal topography), or dry eyes; may have residual refractive error. Additional complications include evidence of a circular lamellar flap with or without haze (lost flap), flap striae, epithelial ingrowth, and diffuse lamellar keratitis (DLK, "sands of the Sahara"; LASIK).

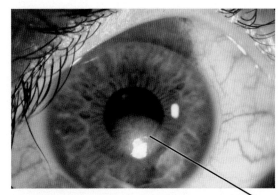

Figure 12-15 • Photorefractive keratectomy demonstrating moderate central corneal haze 6 months after a treatment for high myopia.

corneal haze

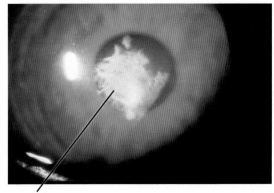

Figure 12-16 • Dense (4+) central haze and scarring after photorefractive keratectomy in a corneal graft. The edge of the graft is visible as a fine white line at the right edge of the picture extending from the 1 o'clock to 5 o'clock positions.

corneal haze

Implants

Intracorneal Inlays

This procedure combines a partial thickness corneal flap with a thin, contact lens–like, intrastromal implant that is placed in the central optical zone. The thickness and shape of the implant alter the corneal curvature to correct all refractive errors without removing corneal tissue.

Intrastromal Corneal Ring Segments (ICRS, Intacs)

Ring segments are placed into peripheral corneal channels outside the visual axis to correct low to moderate myopia by flattening the cornea without cutting or removing tissue from the central optical zone.

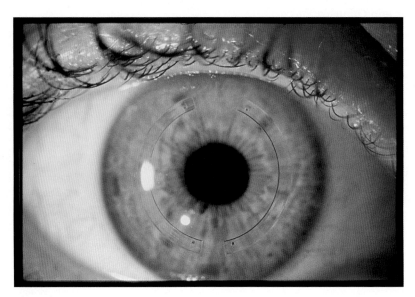

Figure 12-17 • Intacs (intracorneal rings) demonstrating two intracorneal ring segments well positioned in the cornea.

Symptoms

Postoperatively may have: decreased vision (due to undercorrection, overcorrection, or irregular astigmatism), fluctuating vision, difficulty with night vision, halos, glare, and foreign body sensation.

Signs and Complications

Implant extrusion, implant decentration, infection, stromal deposits (intrastromal corneal ring segments), flap wrinkling (intracorneal inlays), epithelial ingrowth (intracorneal inlays); may have residual refractive error.

Thermokeratoplasty

Thermal energy is applied to the peripheral cornea to achieve central corneal steepening in order to treat low to moderate hyperopia.

Conductive Thermokeratoplasty (CK)

Radiofrequency energy is directly delivered to the peripheral cornea through a probe in a ring pattern outside the visual axis.

Laser Thermokeratoplasty (LTK)

A noncontact, holmium:yttrium-aluminum-garnet (Ho:YAG) laser is used to apply thermal burns in a ring pattern outside the visual axis.

Symptoms

Postoperatively may have: pain, foreign body sensation, decreased vision (irregular astigmatism, regression), glare, and halos.

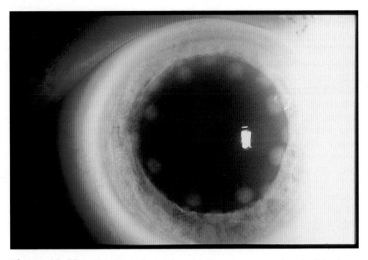

Figure 12-18 • This laser thermokeratoplasty treatment is a double ring, staggered pattern of eight spots each, and is visible as opaque white spots in the cornea overlying the pupillary border.

Signs and Complications

Corneal scarring in area of application; may have residual refractive error.

Evaluation and Management of Corneal Refractive Procedure Complications

Evaluation

- Complete ophthalmic history and eye examination with attention to pinhole acuity, manifest and cycloplegic refractions, pupil size, keratometry, cornea, lens, and ophthalmoscopy.
- Corneal topography (computerized videokeratography).
- Consider rigid contact lens overrefraction.

Management

- No treatment recommended unless patient is symptomatic and vision is decreased. Choice of treatment depends on type of refractive surgery performed.
- **Undercorrection or overcorrection:** modification of topical medication regimen, spectacles or contact lens, consider retreatment after corneal stabilization and failure of conservative management. Specific treatment must be tailored on an individual basis and is beyond the scope of this book, but should be performed by a cornea or refractive specialist.

Continued

Management—cont'd

- **Infectious keratitis:** culture (lift corneal flap), topical antiinfective agents (see Chapter 5); may require flap amputation.
- **Epithelial ingrowth:** lift corneal flap and scrape undersurface of flap and stromal bed; consider suturing flap.
- **Diffuse lamellar keratitis:** frequent topical steroids (q1h initially); may require lifting flap and irrigating stromal bed to remove inflammatory debris (grades 3 and 4 DLK); consider short pulse of oral steroids.
- **Flap striae:** lift flap, refloat, and stretch; may require removing epithelium and suturing flap; consider heating flap with warm spatula. On postoperative day 1, striae often can be removed with massage or stretching at the slit lamp.
- **Decentration or irregular astigmatism:** contact lens trial; retreatment with custom or wavefront ablation.
- **Halo, glare, and star bursts:** consider topical miotic agent (pilocarpine 0.5-1% qd to bid) or brimonidine (Alphagan-P 0.15% bid), polarized sunglasses, or enlarging treatment zone.
- **Dry eye:** topical artificial tears (see Appendix) up to q1h; consider punctual plugs; may require a bandage contact lens for corneal surface irregularities.

Prognosis

Usually good; depends on specific surgical technique and attempted correction.

Vertebrobasilar Artery Insufficiency

Definition

Impaired vertebrobasilar circulation produces neurologic deficits referable to the brain stem or occipital lobe.

Etiology

Hypertensive vascular disease, atheromatous occlusion, microembolization (heart), or changes in cardiac output.

Symptoms

Transient visual blurring (seconds to minutes), photopsias (flashes of light), diplopia, unilateral weakness, sensory loss, ataxia, nystagmus, dysarthria, hoarseness, dysphagia, hearing loss, and vertigo; history of drop attacks.

Signs

Small, paracentral, congruous, homonymous visual field defects.

Differential Diagnosis

Amaurosis fugax, migraine, papilledema, temporal arteritis.

Evaluation

- Complete ophthalmic history, neurologic examination and eye examination with attention to motility, pupils, and ophthalmoscopy.
- Check visual fields.
- **Lab tests:** complete blood count (CBC), erythrocyte sedimentation rate (ESR), and blood glucose (hypoglycemia).
- Check blood pressure.
- Head and orbital computed tomography (CT) or magnetic resonance imaging (MRI).
- Cervical spine radiographs (cervical spondylosis).
- Medical consultation for complete cardiovascular evaluation, including electrocardiogram, echocardiogram, duplex and Doppler scans of carotid and vertebral arteries.

Management

- No effective treatment.
- Aspirin (325 mg po qd).
- Medical or neurology consultation, because long-term anticoagulation may be required.

Prognosis

Usually poor.

■ Migraine

Definition

From the Greek *hemikranos* = half skull. A neurologic disorder caused by changes in intracranial vasomotor control. Often with headache, but not a necessary feature. Typically classified as classic, common, or complicated.

Classic Migraine (10-20%)

Well-defined prodrome or aura (10-40 minutes); usually visual or other fleeting neurologic signs including visual scintillations, dazzling zigzag lines (fortification phenomenon), photophobia or phonophobia, spreading scotomas, dizziness, and tinnitus followed by unilateral throbbing head pain, nausea, and sometimes emesis. Patients may have premonitory symptoms including hunger, thirst, elation, excessive energy, drowsiness, depression, and a feeling of impending doom. Strong family history.

Common Migraine (70-80%)

Poorly defined prodrome with mood fluctuations, fatigue, and gastrointestinal disturbances (anorexia, nausea, and emesis). Headache may occur without prodrome.

Complicated Migraine

Persistent neurologic deficits beyond headache including numbness or tingling, paralysis, aphasia, weakness that eventually resolve over minutes to hours; includes basilar artery migraine (mimics vertebrobasilar artery insufficiency), retinal migraine (monocular visual loss), ophthalmoplegic migraine (children, cranial nerve [CN] paresis [CN III > CN VI]), and cerebral migraine (motor or sensory defect).

Acephalgic Migraine

Visual aura without headache. Visual symptoms described as fortification phenomenon, scintillating scotoma, tunnel vision, double vision, amaurosis fugax, and altitudinal field loss; 25% have family history of migraine.

Epidemiology

Affects 15% of men and 25% of women; can occur at any age; family history of migraine 60%, or a history of motion sickness or cyclic vomiting as a child is common. In women, increased incidence during premenstrual tension and pregnancy.

Symptoms

Aura (see above), photophobia, headache, nausea, emesis.

Signs

None; may have visual field defect, cranial nerve palsy, or other neurologic deficits.

Differential Diagnosis

Serious: meningitis, subarachnoid hemorrhage, temporal arteritis, malignant hypertension, intracranial tumor, arteriovenous malformation, vertebrobasilar artery insufficiency, aneurysm, subdural hematoma, or cerebral ischemia.
Others: tension or cluster headaches, trigeminal neuralgia, temporomandibular joint syndrome, cervical spondylosis, herpes zoster ophthalmicus, sinus or dental pathology, uveitis, angle-closure glaucoma, after lumbar puncture, nonorganic, caffeine withdrawal, carbon monoxide inhalation, and nitrite exposure.

Evaluation

- Careful headache history (e.g., precipitating factors, location, frequency).
- Complete ophthalmic history, neurologic examination, and eye examination with attention to motility, pupils, tonometry, and ophthalmoscopy.
- Check visual fields.
- Check blood pressure and temperature.
- Consider lumbar puncture for suspected meningitis.
- Neuroimaging for complicated migraines or migraines with atypical features.
- Medical or neurology consultation.

Management

- Place patient in dark, low-noise surroundings; encourage rest.
- Aspirin (325-500 mg po qd) or nonsteroidal antiinflammatory drugs (ibuprofen 600 mg po qd).
- Patients who have more than three attacks per month:
- At first sign of aura give ergotamine (1-3 mg po 1 tablet at onset of headache, 1 more 15-20 minutes later); consider adding caffeine (caffeine 100 mg and ergotamine 1 mg [Cafergot] po 2 tablets at onset of headache, 1 more 30 minutes later).
- Consider sumatriptan (Imitrex IM) or oral narcotic medications (codeine, oxycodone prn) if headache severe.
- **Prophylaxis:** systemic β-blocker (propranolol 20-40 mg po bid to tid initially), tricyclic antidepressant (amitriptyline 25-75 mg po qd to bid initially), or calcium-channel blocker (nifedipine 10-40 mg po tid or verapamil 80 mg po tid); avoid precipitating agents (e.g., alcohol [especially red wine], foods, medications, stress).
- Treatment should be monitored by an internist or neurologist.

Prognosis

Good.

▨ Convergence Insufficiency

Definition

Decreased fusional convergence with near fixation and a remote near point of convergence.

Epidemiology

Typically occurs in teenagers and young adults, rare before 10 years of age; slight female predilection; usually idiopathic; common cause of asthenopia (eye strain); aggravated by anxiety, illness, or lack of sleep.

Symptoms

Eye strain (asthenopia), crossed diplopia, blurred vision, headaches, difficulty reading.

Signs

Inability to maintain fusion at near (patient closes one eye while reading to relieve visual fatigue), distant near point of convergence, reduced fusional convergence amplitudes; possible exophoria at near without exotropia (especially after prolonged reading).

Differential Diagnosis

Presbyopia, uncorrected refractive error (hyperopia), accommodative insufficiency.

Evaluation

• Complete ophthalmic history and eye examination with attention to manifest and cyclo-plegic refractions, motility (cover and alternate cover tests [exophoria at near]), near point of accommodation (normal is 5-10 cm, abnormal is 10-30 cm), and fusional convergence amplitudes (normal is 30-35 prism diopters, base-out causes diplopia; abnormal is <20PD).

Management

• Correct any refractive error (undercorrect hyperopes, fully correct myopes).
• **Orthoptic exercises:** training of fusional convergence with pencil push-ups. (Bring pencil in from arms length toward nose while focusing on eraser. When diplopia [break point] develops, the exercise is repeated. Each attempt is designed to bring the pencil closer without diplopia.) Alternatively, use base-out prisms (increase amount of prism diopters until blur point is reached, usually 4-6PD, then increase further until break point is reached); exercises are repeated 15 times, 5 times a day; can also use major amblyoscope (stereograms).
• When no improvement is noted with exercises, base-in prism reading glasses are helpful.
• Very rarely, muscle surgery with bimedial rectus muscle resection.

Prognosis

Usually good.

▊ Accommodative Excess

Definition

A clinical state of excessive accommodation (lens focusing) due to medications, uncorrected refractive errors, or ocular disease. Spasm of the near reflex is the triad of excess accommodation, excess convergence, and miosis.

Symptoms

Headache, brow ache, and variable blurring of distance vision, diplopia.

Signs

Abnormally close near point and miosis; relief of symptoms with cycloplegia.

Differential Diagnosis

Iridocyclitis, uncorrected refractive errors (usually hyperopes, but also astigmats and myopes), hyperglycemia (lens swells), use of anticholinesterase medications or sulfa-containing drugs.

Evaluation

- Complete ophthalmic history and eye examination with attention to manifest, cycloplegic, and postcycloplegic refractions, and pupils.

Management

- Stop offending medication if applicable.
- Correct any refractive error including prescribing a reading aid if esotropic at near.
- Consider cycloplegic agent (scopolamine 0.25% qd to qid) to break spasm (only occasionally needed).
- Instruct patient to focus intermittently at distance during periods of prolonged near work.

Prognosis

Good.

Functional Visual Loss (Malingering, Hysteria)

Definition

Visual abnormality not attributable to any organic disease process (nonphysiologic).

Malingering

Fabrication of existence or extent of disorder for secondary gain; usually involved in legal action or compensation claim.

Hysteria

Subconscious (not willful) expression of symptoms.

Symptoms

Decreased vision (monocular or binocular, usually very vague about quality of symptoms), diplopia, metamorphopsia, oscillopsia.

Signs

Decreased visual acuity (20/20 to no light perception), abnormal visual field (usually inconsistent or has characteristic pattern); may have voluntary nystagmus, gaze palsy, or blepharospasm; malingerer often uncooperative and combative, hysteric often indifferent but cooperative; otherwise normal examination (especially pupils, optokinetic nystagmus response, fundus).

Differential Diagnosis

Organic disease, especially amblyopia, early keratoconus, anterior basement membrane dystrophy, early cataracts, central serous retinopathy, early Stargardt's disease, retinitis pigmentosa sine pigmento, rod monochromatism, cone degeneration, retrobulbar optic neuropathy, other optic neuropathies (toxic, nutritional), and cortical blindness.

Evaluation

- Complete ophthalmic history and eye examination with attention to vision (distance and near, monocular and binocular, varying distance, fogging, red-green, prism dissociation, stereopsis, startle reflex, proprioception, signing name, mirror tracking, optokinetic nystagmus response), retinoscopy, motility, pupils, and ophthalmoscopy.
- Check visual fields (monocular and binocular); beware tunnel vision, spiraling fields, crossing isopters.
- Consider electroretinogram, visual evoked response, fluorescein angiogram, or neuroimaging in difficult cases or if unable to prove normal vision and visual field.

Management

- Reassurance.
- Usually not necessary to consult psychiatrist.

Prognosis

No improvement in up to 30%; may have coexistent organic disease in 20%.

▌ Transient Visual Loss (Amaurosis Fugax)

Definition

Unilateral or bilateral transient visual loss.

Etiology

Carotid disease, vertebrobasilar artery insufficiency, arrhythmias, cardiac valvular disease, coagulation disorders, vasospasm, migraine, orbital mass, anterior ischemic optic neuropathy, pseudopapilledema (optic nerve drusen), papilledema.

Symptoms

Brief (2-5 minutes), reversible dimming or loss of vision.

Signs

Asymptomatic; may have intravascular emboli in retinal vessels.

Evaluation

- Complete ophthalmic history, neurologic examination, and eye examination with attention to pupils and ophthalmoscopy.
- Check visual fields.
- Medical consultation for complete cardiovascular evaluation including electrocardiogram, echocardiogram, and carotid Doppler studies.

Management

- No treatment recommended.
- Treat underlying disease.

Prognosis

Depends on etiology; 1-year risk of cerebrovascular accident is 2%.

Amblyopia

Definition

Unilateral or bilateral loss of best corrected vision in an otherwise anatomically normal eye.

Epidemiology

Present in approximately 2% of general population.

Etiology

Strabismic

Most common form of amblyopia. Develops in a child with constant deviation of misaligned eye due to inhibition of visual input from deviated eye in order to prevent diplopia and visual confusion.

Anisometropic

Due to unequal, uncorrected refractive error between the two eyes which causes a constant defocusing of the image; usually requires high degree of myopic anisometropia (> –6D) but mild degrees of hyperopic or astigmatic anisometropia (1-2D).

Isoametropic

Bilateral amblyopia due to large, but equal, uncorrected refractive error; usually requires hyperopic refractive errors greater than 5D, myopic refractive errors greater than -10D, and astigmatic refractive errors greater than 3D.

Deprivation

Uncommon, usually caused by congenital or acquired media opacities such as cataracts, corneal opacities, or ptosis; often results in significant loss of vision.

Occlusion

Form of deprivation amblyopia resulting from excessive therapeutic patching during treatment of amblyopia.

Symptoms

Asymptomatic; may have decreased vision; may notice eye turn, droopy eyelid, or white pupil.

Signs

Decreased visual acuity (unilateral or bilateral), visual acuity often improves with neutral density filter; may have strabismus, nystagmus, ptosis, cataract, corneal opacity, small relative afferent pupillary defect.

Differential Diagnosis

Functional visual loss, optic neuropathy (e.g., toxic, nutritional, alcohol).

Evaluation

• Complete ophthalmic history and eye examination with attention to vision with neutral density filters (worsens in organic amblyopia) and single letters (improves acuity), cycloplegic refraction, retinoscopy, pupils, and ophthalmoscopy.

Management

• Correct any refractive error.
• Patching or occlusion therapy for children under 10 years old (full-time occlusion of preferred eye for no more than 1 week per year of age of child before reexamination) and continue until vision stabilizes. Discontinue if no improvement after 2-3 months of compliant, full-time patching. May require part-time occlusion to maintain visual level.
• Cycloplegic agent (usually atropine 0.5% or 1% qd) to blur image and improve compliance.
• Protective eyewear with polycarbonate lenses if significant amblyopia exists after 10 years of age to protect fellow eye.
• Consider surgery in cases of deprivation (e.g., cataract extraction) or strabismus.

Prognosis

Depends on extent and duration of amblyopia and age at which appropriate corrective therapy is initiated (the earlier the better, must be prior to 9 years of age); poor prognosis in deprivation amblyopia, good in strabismic amblyopia.

Cortical Blindness (Cortical Visual Impairment)

Definition

Rare syndrome of bilateral blindness due to widespread damage to occipital lobes.

Etiology

Cerebrovascular accident (bilateral occipital lobe infarction), rarely neoplasia.

Symptoms

Complete visual loss; rarely, denies blindness (Anton's syndrome).

Signs

Normal ocular examination (including pupillary response) except no light perception vision in both eyes; patient may demonstrate the Riddoch phenomenon (ability to perceive moving, but not static, objects) and "blind sight" (intact primitive mechanism that may allow navigation around objects).

Differential Diagnosis

Functional visual loss.

Evaluation

- Complete ophthalmic history, neurologic examination, and eye examination with attention to vision, pupils, and ophthalmoscopy.
- Head and orbital CT scan or MRI.
- Medical and neurology consultation.

Management

- No treatment recommended.
- Treat underlying condition.

Prognosis

Poor.

APPENDIX

Ophthalmic History and Examination

History

As with any medical encounter, the initial component of the evaluation begins with a thorough history. The components of the history are similar to a general medical history but are focused on the visual system.

- Chief complaint (CC)
- History of present illness (HPI)
- Past ocular history (POH)
- Eye medications
- Past medical and surgical histories (PMH/PSH)
- Systemic medications
- Allergies
- Family history (FH)
- Social history (SH)
- Review of systems (ROS)

Ocular Examination

The ocular examination is unique in medicine because most of the pathology is directly visible to the examiner; however, specialized equipment and instruments are necessary to perform a comprehensive examination. As with the general medical examination, there are multiple facets to the eye examination, and they should be performed systematically.

Vision

Visual acuity (VA)   Vision should be measured in one eye at a time and with correction if the patient wears glasses or contact lenses. Distance vision using a standard Snellen chart at 20 feet is the most common method and is denoted with VA, Va, or V and subscript of cc or sc (i.e., V_{cc} or V_{sc}) depending on whether the acuity is measured with (cc) or without (sc) correction, respectively. An occluder with pinholes (PH) can be used in an attempt to improve the vision and estimate the eye's best potential vision. If the vision improves with pinhole testing, an uncorrected refractive error or cataract is typically present. Vision that is worse

479

than 20/400 is recorded either as counting fingers (CF at the test distance; e.g., CF at 6 inches) if the patient can identify the number of fingers the examiner holds up; hand motion (HM) if the patient can identify the movement of the examiner's hand; light perception with projection (LP and the quadrants) if the patient can identify the direction from which a light is shined into the eye; light perception without projection (LP) if the patient can only determine when a bright light is shined into the eye and not the direction the light is coming from; or no light perception (NLP) if the patient cannot perceive light from even the brightest light source. Near vision is similarly measured (monocularly with or without correction) and is denoted with N. For infants, vision is commonly assessed by the ability to fix and follow (F&F) objects of interest or the presence of central steady maintained fixation (CSM).

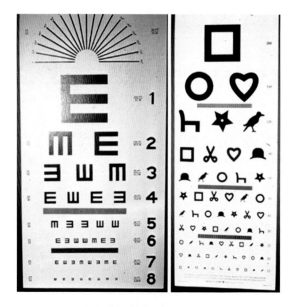

Figure 1 • Eye charts for nonverbal patients or patients who cannot read English letters. *Left,* Tumbling E chart. *Right,* Eye chart with pictures.

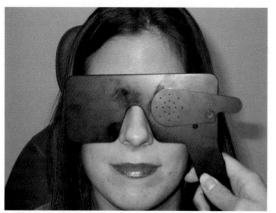

Figure 2 • Patient with pinhole occluder over her left eye.

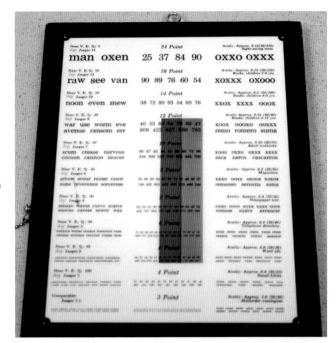

Figure 3 • Near vision chart.

Glasses Prescription

Refraction A subjective measurement of the refractive error performed with a phoropter or trial frame allows the patient to decide which lens is best. A manifest refraction is done before dilating the eyes and is denoted with M_R or M. A cycloplegic refraction is done after dilating the eyes with cycloplegic drops to prevent accommodation and is denoted with C_R or C.

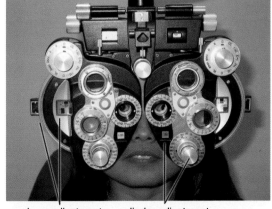

Figure 4 • Patient behind a phoropter undergoing manifest refraction.

sphere adjustment   cylinder adjustment

A cycloplegic refraction is particularly important when refracting children, hyperopes, and refractive surgery candidates, in whom a manifest refraction may not be accurate. The duochrome test is a useful method to check the refraction for overcorrection or undercorrection.

Retinoscopy   An objective measurement of the refractive error performed with a retinoscope; it is denoted with R.

Lensometer   An instrument that measures the power of spectacle lenses; the prescription the patient is wearing is denoted with W.

glasses placed here

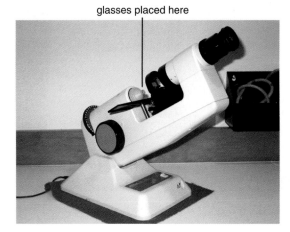

Figure 5 • A lensometer measures the power of spectacle lenses placed on the middle platform.

Other Specialized Tests

Potential acuity meter (PAM)   An instrument that measures the visual potential of the retina by projecting the eye chart onto the retina through any corneal and/or lens opacities. This test is most commonly used to assess visual potential before cataract surgery when there is coexisting retinal pathology.

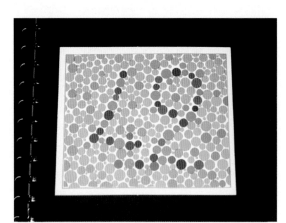

Figure 6 • Ishihara pseudoisochromatic chart with the number 42 evident.

Color vision   Color vision is tested monocularly, most commonly with Ishihara pseudoiso-chromatic or Hardy-Rand-Ritter plates. More extensive evaluation is done using Farnsworth tests. Gross macular function can be assessed by asking the patient to identify the color of a red eyedrop cap (any dilating drop bottle has a red cap). Red saturation (optic nerve function) can also be tested with the red cap by asking the patient whether the cap appears to be the same brightness of red when the eyes are alternately tested.

Stereopsis   Stereo vision must be tested binocularly and is commonly done with titmus or randot tests. The titmus test uses polarized images of a fly (patient is asked to grasp or touch the wings), animals (three rows of five cartoon animals each are pictured, and the patient is asked to touch the animal that is popping up), and circles (nine groups of four circles each are pictured, and the patient is asked to touch the circle that is popping up).

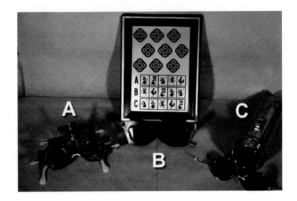

Figure 7 • Three specialized tests. *A,* Trial frame. *B,* Stereo vision tests with polarizing glasses. *C,* Worth 4 dot test.

Ocular Motility

The alignment of the eyes in primary gaze is observed, and the movement of the eyes is assessed as the patient looks in all directions of gaze by following an object that the examiner moves. Normal motility (extraocular movements) is often recorded as intact (EOMI) or full. If misalignment, gaze restriction, or nystagmus is present, then other tests are performed. Several methods are used to distinguish and measure ocular misalignment.

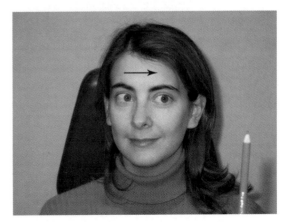

Figure 8 • Patient undergoing ocular motility testing. Note: Her eyes are following the pencil.

Cover Tests

The patient fixates on a target and an occluder is placed in front of the eye. Measurements are made for both distance and near with and without glasses.

Cover-uncover test   Distinguishes between a tropia and a phoria. One eye is covered and then uncovered. If the unoccluded eye moves when the cover is in place, a tropia is present. If the covered eye moves when the cover is removed, a phoria is present.

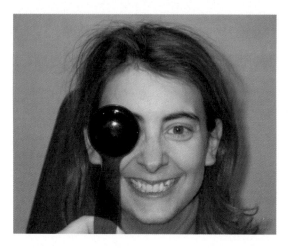

Figure 9 • Patient undergoing cover-uncover test to determine if she has a phoria or tropia.

Alternate cover test (prism and cover test)   Measures the total ocular deviation (tropia and phoria). The occluder is alternately placed in front of each eye until dissociation occurs, and then hand-held prisms are held in front of an eye until no movement occurs.

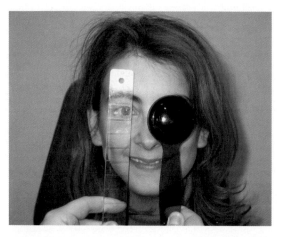

Figure 10 • Patient undergoing alternate cover test where the total ocular deviation is determined by holding prisms over the eye until no movement occurs.

Corneal Light Reflex Tests

Assesses ocular alignment by observing the relative position of the corneal light reflections from a light shined into the patient's eyes; can be used in patients who cannot cooperate for cover tests. The position of the corneal light reflexes is used to measure the ocular deviation.

Hirschberg's method   The deviation is estimated by the amount of decentration of the light reflex (1 mm of decentration corresponds to 7 degrees or 15 prism diopters). Thus light reflections at the pupillary margin (2 mm decentration), mid-iris (4 mm decentration), and limbus (6 mm decentration) correspond to deviations of approximately 15 degrees or 30 PD, 30 degrees or 45PD, and 45 degrees or 60PD, respectively.

Modified Krimsky's method   Prisms are placed in front of the fixating eye to center the light reflection in the deviated eye.

Forced Ductions

Under topical anesthesia the eye is grasped at the limbus with forceps and rotated into the deficient direction of gaze to determine whether a restrictive etiology exists. The forceps should be placed on the same side of the limbus in which the eye is being moved to avoid an inadvertent corneal abrasion should the forceps slip.

OKN Testing

OKN testing is used to assess patients with nystagmus and other eye movement disorders. A rotating drum (or strip) with alternating black and white lines is moved both horizontally and vertically in front of the patient and the resultant eye movements are observed.

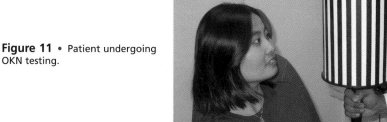

Figure 11 • Patient undergoing OKN testing.

Pupils

The size, shape, and reactivity of the pupils are assessed while the patient fixates on a distant target. Both the direct and consensual responses are observed. The swinging flashlight test is done to test for a relative afferent pupillary defect (see RAPD in Chapter 7), particularly if anisocoria or poor reaction to light is present. If the pupils react to light, then they will react to accommodation, so this does not need to be tested; however, if one or both pupils do not react to light, then the reaction to accommodation should be assessed because various conditions may cause light-near dissociation. The reactivity of each pupil is graded on a scale of 1+ (sluggish) to 4+ (brisk). Normal pupils should be equal, round, and briskly reactive to light. The most common abbreviation for denoting this pupillary response is "pupils equal round and reactive to light" or PERRL (or PERRLA if accommodation is also tested). A preferred method that provides more information is to note the size of the pupils before and after the light stimulus is applied (i.e., P 4 → 2 OU). If anisocoria is present, the pupils should be measured in both normal lighting conditions and dim conditions.

Visual Fields (VF)

Confrontation visual fields are evaluated monocularly with the patient looking into the examiner's opposite eye (used as a control) and being asked to identify the number of fingers presented or the movement of a finger in each quadrant. Normal fields are recorded as visual fields full to confrontation (VFFC or VF full).

Other specialized tests

Amsler Grid   A 10 cm × 10 cm grid composed of 5 mm squares can be used to test the central 10 degrees of the visual field. This test is more commonly used to assess central visual distortion in patients with age-related macular degeneration and other foveal pathology.

Tangent Screen   This is a manual test that is easily performed as the patient is seated 1 m in front of a 2 m × 2 m square black cloth over which the examiner presents test objects.

Goldmann Visual Field   This is a manually operated machine used to perform static and kinetic perimetry.

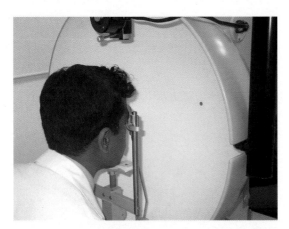

Figure 12 • Patient undergoing Goldmann visual field examination.

Humphrey Visual Field   This is a computerized static perimetry test with various programs to screen for and evaluate glaucomatous, neurologic, and lid-induced visual field defects.

External Examination

Orbit, eyelid, and lacrimal structures are evaluated for symmetry, position, and any abnormalities. Palpation and auscultation are performed when indicated.

Other specialized tests

Exophthalmometry This device measures the distance the corneal apex protrudes from the lateral orbital rim to assess for proptosis or enophthalmos.

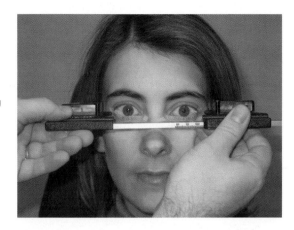

Figure 13 • Patient undergoing exophthalmometry test to measure for proptosis or enophthalmos.

Schirmer's Test Special strips of filter paper are placed over the lower eyelids to absorb tears and measure tear production to evaluate dry eyes (see Dry Eye Syndrome in Chapter 4).

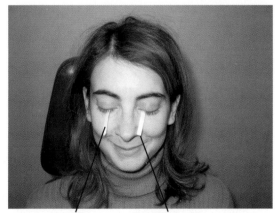

Figure 14 • Patient undergoing Schirmer's testing for dry eyes. This patient's tears have wet the strips, indicating that she does not have dry eyes.

tear line   Schirmer's strip

Jones' Dye Tests These tests are used to evaluate lacrimal drainage obstruction (see Nasolacrimal Duct Obstruction in Chapter 3).

Cranial Nerve Examination CN5 is examined to assess facial and corneal sensation, and CN7 is examined to assess facial movement including eyelid closure, when warranted.

Slit Lamp Examination (SLE)

This specialized biomicroscope allows detailed examination of the eye. The height, width, and angle of the light beam can all be controlled, and various filters can be changed to enhance visualization. A thin beam directed through the clear ocular media (cornea, anterior chamber, lens, and vitreous) acts as a scalpel of light illuminating a cross-sectional slice of optical tissue. This property of the slit-lamp allows precise localization of pathology. The technique of retroillumination (coaxial alignment of the light beam with the oculars) uses the red reflex from the retina to backlight the cornea and lens, making some abnormalities more easily visible. Furthermore, anterior segment lesions can be accurately measured by recording the height of the slit-beam from the millimeter scale on the control knob. Although the posterior segment can be evaluated with the aid of additional lenses, the SLE typically focuses on the anterior segment. Portable, hand-held, slit-lamp devices facilitate examination at the bedside. If a slit-lamp instrument is not available, a penlight examination can be done with a magnifying lens to briefly assess the anterior segment. Similarly, a direct ophthalmoscope or indirect ophthalmoscope and lens can be focused on the anterior segment structures for examination.

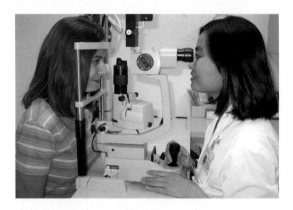

Figure 15 • Patient undergoing slit-lamp examination.

Components of the SLE

Lids, Lashes, and Lacrimal Glands (L/L/L)   The lids, lashes, puncta, and Meibomian gland orifices are inspected. The medial canthus or lid margin can be palpated to express discharge or secretions from the inferior punctum or Meibomian glands, respectively.

Conjunctiva and Sclera (C/S)   The patient is asked to look in the horizontal and vertical directions to observe the entire bulbar conjunctiva, and the lids are everted to observe the tarsal conjunctival surface. The caruncle and plica semilunaris are also inspected. The upper eyelid can be double everted to evaluate the superior fornix, and a moistened cotton-tipped applicator can be used to sweep the fornix to remove suspected foreign bodies.

Cornea (C)   All layers of the cornea are inspected. The tear film is evaluated for break-up time and height of the meniscus. The cobalt blue filter allows better visualization of corneal iron lines.

Anterior Chamber (AC)   The anterior chamber is evaluated for depth—graded on a scale from 1+ (shallow) to 4+ (deep)—and the presence of cells and flare (see Chapter 6). Normally, the AC is deep and quiet (D&Q).

Iris and Lens (I/L)   The iris and lens are inspected. The lens is better evaluated after pupillary dilation. If the eye is pseudophakic, the position and stability of the intraocular lens implant are noted, and the condition of the posterior capsule is assessed. The anterior vitreous (AV) can also be observed without the use of additional lenses. For aphakic eyes, the integrity of the anterior hyaloid face is evaluated, and any vitreous prolapse into the AC or strands to anterior structures is noted.

Special Techniques   *Dyes:* Fluorescein, rose bengal, and lissamine green can be used to evaluate the health and integrity of the conjunctival and corneal epithelium. The integrity of wounds is assessed with the Seidel test (see Laceration in Chapter 5).
Gonioscopy: A special mirrored lens placed on the cornea allows visualization of the angle structures.
Fundus contact and noncontact lenses: numerous lenses can be used to examine the retina and optic nerve. Although performed with a slit-lamp, these findings are recorded as part of the fundus examination (see below).

Tonometry (T)

Various instruments can be used to measure the intraocular pressure (IOP). Most commonly, IOP is measured as part of the SLE with the Goldmann applanation tonometer that is attached to the slit-lamp. Topical anesthetic drops and fluorescein drops (either individually or in a combination drop) are instilled into the eye, the tonometer head is illuminated with a broad beam and cobalt blue filter, the tip contacts the cornea, the dial is adjusted until the mirror-image semicircular mires slightly overlap so that their inner margins just touch each other, and the pressure measurement in mm Hg is obtained by multiplying the dial reading by 10 (i.e., "2" equals 20 mm Hg). If marked corneal astigmatism exists, to obtain an accurate reading the tonometer tip must be rotated so that the graduation marking corresponding to the flattest corneal meridian is aligned with the red mark on the tip holder. Central corneal thickness also affects pressure readings. It is important to record the time when the pressure is measured. If a slit-lamp is not available, portable hand-held devices such as the Tono-pen, Perkins, or Shiotz tonometers can be used. Estimating IOP by digital palpation (finger tension) is highly inaccurate.

Fundus Examination

The optic nerve and retina can be examined with or without pupillary dilation and with a variety of instruments and lenses. Direct ophthalmoscopy (DO) and indirect ophthalmoscopy (IO) are performed with a direct or indirect ophthalmoscope, respectively. The direct ophthalmoscope provides high magnification (15×) with a narrow field of view, whereas the indirect ophthalmoscope produces a wide-field of view at lower magnification (2-3×). The image obtained through the IO and slit-lamp fundus lenses are flipped and inverted, and this must be taken into account when drawing retinal diagrams. An easy way to correct for this image reversal is to turn the retinal diagram upside-down and then draw the pathology as it is seen through the lens; when the diagram is viewed right side up, the picture will be correct. A dilated fundus examination is often denoted as DFE, and the appearance of the disc, vessels, macula, and periphery are noted. A normal retinal examination is commonly abbreviated as d/v/m/p wnl. The dimensions and location of lesions are compared to the size of the disc; thus measurements are recorded as multiples of disc diameters (DD) or areas (DA).

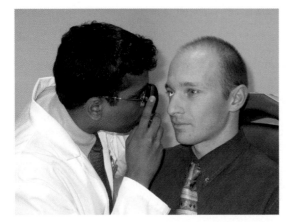

Figure 16 • Patient undergoing direct ophthalmoscopic examination.

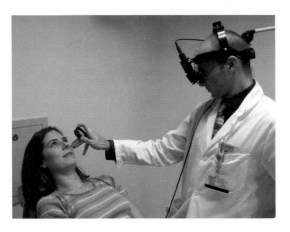

Figure 17 • Patient undergoing indirect ophthalmoscopic examination.

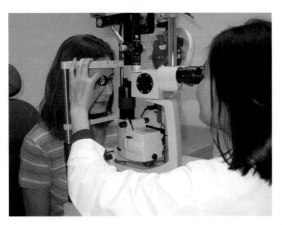

Figure 18 • Patient undergoing slit-lamp fundus examination with high magnification lens to evaluate the macula.

Components of the fundus examination

Disc   The optic nerve is inspected with particular attention paid to the cup-to-disc ratio (C/D), appearance of the neural rim (normally sharp and flat), and color (orange/yellow). The presence/absence of edema is also important.

Vessels   The retinal vessels are observed as they emerge from the optic cup and branch toward the periphery. Spontaneous venous pulsations can sometimes be seen at the nerve head. Any anomalous pattern or abnormality of the vasculature is recorded.

Macula   The macula, especially the fovea, is evaluated. Usually a bright light reflex is seen at the center of the fovea, especially in younger patients. In eyes with a suspected macular hole or cyst, the Watzke-Allen test can be performed by shining a thin vertical slit-beam over the center of the fovea and asking the patient if the light beam appears discontinuous or narrower in the middle (see Macular Hole, Chapter 10).

Peripheral Retina   The retinal periphery is most easily seen through a widely dilated pupil. The patient is asked to look in all directions of gaze so that the entire retina (360 degrees) can be viewed with indirect ophthalmoscopy. Visualization and differentiation of pathology near the ora serrata are aided with scleral depression.

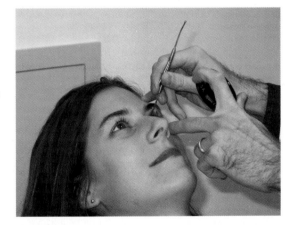

Figure 19 • Patient undergoing scleral depression in combination with binocular indirect ophthalmoscopic examination to evaluate the far peripheral retina.

Reference

Richard JM: *A manual for the beginning ophthalmology resident,* ed 3, San Francisco, 1980, American Academy of Ophthalmology.

AAO Suggested Routine Eye Examination Guidelines

Ages 0-2: screening during regular pediatric appointments.
Ages 3-5: screening every 1-2 years during regular primary care appointments.
Ages 6-19: schedule examinations as needed.
Ages 20-29: one examination.
Ages 30-39: two examinations.
Ages 40-65: examination every 2-4 years.
Ages 65 and over: examination every 1-2 years.

   (More frequent examinations may be recommended if any of the following risk factors exist: history of eye injury, diabetes, family history of eye problems, blacks older than 40 years of age.)

Common Ophthalmic Medications

Antiinfectives

Aminoglycosides

amikacin (Amikin) 10 mg/mL solution up to q1h
amikacin 25 mg/0.5 mL subconjunctival
amikacin 0.4 mg/0.1 mL intravitreal
amikacin 15 mg/kg/day IV in 2-3 divided doses
gentamicin (Genoptic, Gent-AK, Gentacidin, Garamycin) 0.3% qid
fortified tobramycin 13.6 mg/mL up to q1h
tobramycin (Tobrex, AK-Tob, Tobralcon, Tobrasol) 0.3% qid to q1h
neomycin–polymyxin B–gramicidin 0.025 (Neosporin, AK-Spore) qid to q1h
trimethoprim–polymyxin B–gramicidin 0.025 (Polytrim) qid to q1h

Fluoroquinolones

ciprofloxacin (Ciloxan) 0.3% solution or ointment qid to q1h
ciprofloxacin (Cipro) 500-750 mg PO bid
gatifloxacin (Zymar) 0.3% qid to q1h
levofloxacin (Quixin) 0.5% qid to q1h
levofloxacin (Levaquin) 500 mg PO qd
moxifloxacin (Vigamox) 0.5% tid to q1h
norfloxacin (Chibroxin, Noroxin) 0.3% qid to q1h
ofloxacin (Ocuflox) 0.3% qid to q1h
ofloxacin (Floxin) 200-400 mg PO q12h

Penicillins/Synthetic Penicillins

amoxicillin/clavulanate (Augmentin) 250 mg PO q8h or 500 mg PO bid
ampicillin 500 μg/0.1 mL intravitreal
ampicillin 50-150 mg/0.5 mL subconjunctival
ampicillin (Polycillin) 4-12 g/day IV in 4 divided doses
methicillin 200-300 mg/kg/day IV in 4 divided doses
penicillin G 12-24 million/units/day IV in 4 divided doses
ticarcillin (Ticar) 200-300 mg/kg/day IV in 3 divided doses

Cephalosporins

cefazolin 100 mg/0.5 mL subconjunctival
cefazolin 2.25 mg/0.1 mL intravitreal
cefazolin (Ancef) 50-100 mg/kg/day IV in 3-4 divided doses
cefotaxime (Claforan) 25 mg/kg IV q8-12h
ceftazidime 2.25 mg/0.1 mL intravitreal
ceftazidime 100 mg/0.5 mL subconjunctival
ceftazidime (Fortaz) 2 g IV q8h
ceftriaxone 100 mg/0.5 mL subconjunctival
ceftriaxone (Rocephin) 2 gm IV q12h
cephalexin (Keflex) 500 mg PO bid
fortified cefazolin 50-100 mg/mL up to q1h
fortified ceftazidime 50-100 mg/mL up to q1h

Macrolides

azithromycin (Zithromax) 250-600 mg PO Z-Pak
erythromycin (Ilotycin, AK-Mycin, Romycin) 0.5% qd to qid
erythromycin 0.5 mg/0.1 mL intravitreal
erythromycin 100 mg/0.5 mL subconjunctival

Peptides

bacitracin (AK-Tracin) qd to qid
fortified vancomycin 25-50 mg/mL up to q1h
neomycin–polymyxin B–bacitracin (AK-Spore, Neosporin, Ocutricin) qid to q2h
polymyxin B–bacitracin (Polysporin, AK-Poly Bac, Polycin B) qid to q4h
polymyxin B–oxytetracycline (Terak, Terramycin) qid to q4h
trimethoprim–polymyxin B–gramicidin 0.025 (Polytrim) qid to q1h

Sulfonamides

sulfacetamide sodium (AK-Sulf, Bleph-10, Cetamide, Ophthacet, Sodium Sulamyd, Sulf–10) 10% (Sodium Sulamyd, Vasosulf) 30% solution (AK-Sulf, Bleph-10, Cetamide, Sodium Sulamyd) 10% ointment, qid to q2h
trimethoprim/sulfamethoxazole (Bactrim) 1 double-strength tablet PO bid

Tetracyclines

doxycycline 100-200 mg PO qd (for blepharitis)
tetracycline 250-500 mg PO qd (for blepharitis)
tetracycline (Achromycin) 1% qid to q2h

Antibiotic/Steroid Combinations

gentamicin-prednisolone acetate 0.6% (Pred-G) solution or ointment qid to q2h
neomycin–polymyxin B–dexamethasone (AK-Trol, Maxitrol, Dexacidin, Dexasporin) qid to q2h
neomycin-dexamethasone 0.05% (NeoDecadron) qid to q2h
neomycin–polymyxin B–prednisolone acetate (Poly-Pred Liquifilm) qid to q2h
neomycin–polymyxin B–hydrocortisone (AK-Spore HC, Cortisporin) qid to q2h
oxytetracycline-hydrocortisone acetate (Terra-Cortril) qid
sulfacetamide sodium 10%–prednisolone acetate 0.2% (Blephamide) solution or ointment qid to q4h
sulfacetamide sodium 10%–fluorometholone 1% (FML-S) qid to q4h
sulfacetamide sodium 10%–prednisolone phosphate 0.25% (Isopto Cetapred, Vasocidin) qid to q4h
sulfacetamide sodium 10%–prednisolone phosphate 0.25% (Cetapred) ointment qid to q4h
sulfacetamide sodium 10%–prednisolone acetate 0.5% (Ak-Cide, Metimyd) solution or ointment qid to q4h
tobramycin 0.3%–dexamethasone 0.1% (Tobradex) solution or ointment qid to q2h

Antiamebic Agents

polyhexamethylene biguanide (PHBG, Baquacil) 0.02% up to q1h
propamidine isethionate (Brolene) 0.1% up to q1h

hexamidine (Desomedine) 0.1% up to q1h
paromomycin (Humatin) 10 mg/mL up to q1h

Antifungal Agents

amphotericin B 0.1-0.5% up to q1h
amphotericin B 0.25-1.0 mg/kg IV over 6 hours
amphotericin B 5 mg/0.1 mL intravitreal
clotrimazole 1% up to q1h
fluconazole (Diflucan) 800 mg PO loading dose, 400 mg/day maintenance
fluconazole (Diflucan) 0.2% up to q1h
flucytosine (Ancobon) 50-150 mg/kg/day IV in 4 divided doses
ketoconazole 1-2% up to q1h
ketoconazole (Nizoral) 200-400 mg PO qd to tid
miconazole 1% up to q1h
miconazole 25 μg/0.1 mL intravitreal
miconazole 30 mg/kg/day IV
natamycin (Natacyn) 5% up to q1h

Antiviral Agents

acyclovir (Zovirax) 200-800 mg; for herpes simplex virus: 200-400 mg PO bid to five times a day; for herpes zoster virus: 800 mg PO five times a day for 7 to 10 days
famciclovir (Famvir) 500 mg PO q8h
foscarnet (Foscavir) induction: 90-120 mg/kg IV bid for 14-21 days; maintenance: 90-120 mg/kg IV qd
ganciclovir (Cytovene) induction: 5 mg/kg IV bid for 14-21 days; maintenance: 5 mg/kg IV qd
idoxuridine (Herplex, Stoxil) 0.1% solution, 0.5% ointment qd to 5 times a day
trifluridine (Viroptic) 1% qd to 9 times a day
valacyclovir (Valtrex) 500 mg PO tid
vidarabine (Vira-A) 3% qd to 5 times a day

Miscellaneous Antibiotics

chloramphenicol (Chloroptic, AK-Chlor, Ocuchlor, Chloromycetin) 0.5% gtts, 1.0% ung qid to q4h
chlorhexidine 0.02% up to q1h
clindamycin (Cleocin) 50 mg/mL up to q1h
clindamycin (Cleocin) 15-50 mg/0.5 mL subconjunctival
clindamycin (Cleocin) 200 μg/0.1 mL intravitreal
clindamycin (Cleocin) 300 mg PO qid
clindamycin (Cleocin) 600-900 mg IV q8h
fortified vancomycin 50 mg/mL up to q1h
vancomycin 1 mg/0.1 mL intravitreal
vancomycin 25 mg/0.5 mL subconjunctival
vancomycin 1 gm IV q12h

Antiinflammatories

NSAIDs

celecoxib (Celebrex) 100 mg PO bid
diclofenac sodium (Voltaren) 0.1% qd to qid

diclofenac sodium (Voltaren) 75 mg PO bid
diflunisal (Dolobid) 250 mg PO bid
flurbiprofen sodium (Ocufen) 0.03% for prevention of intraoperative miosis
indomethacin (Indocin) 50 mg PO bid to tid
ketorolac tromethamine (Acular) 0.5% qd to qid
naproxen (Naprosyn) 250 mg PO bid
rofecoxib (Vioxx) 25 mg PO qd
suprofen (Profenal) 1% for prevention of intraoperative miosis

Immunomodulator

cyclosporine (Restasis) 0.05% bid for dry eye syndrome

Steroids

dexamethasone alcohol (Maxidex) 0.1% qd to q1h
dexamethasone sodium phosphate (Decadron, AK-Dex) 0.05-0.1% qd to q1h
fluorometholone acetate (Flarex, Eflone) 0.1% qd to q1h
fluorometholone alcohol (Fluor-Op, FML) 0.1% (FML Forte) 0.25% qd to q1h
fluorometholone alcohol (FML S.O.P.) 0.1% ointment qd to q1h
loteprednol etabonate (Lotemax) 0.5% (Alrex) 0.2% qd to q1h
medrysone (HMS) 1% qd to q1h
prednisolone acetate (Pred Mild) 0.12% (Econopred) 0.125% (AK-Tate, Pred Forte, Econopred Plus) 1% qd to q1h
prednisolone sodium phosphate (Inflamase Mild, AK-Pred) 0.125% (Inflamase Forte, AK-Pred) 1% qd to q1h
prednisone 60-100mg PO qd followed by taper; co-therapy (to prevent peptic ulcer disease) with famotidine (Pepcid), lansoprazole (Prevacid), omeprazole (Prilosec), or ranitidine (Zantac)
rimexolone (Vexol) 1% qd to q1h

Ocular Hypotensive (Glaucoma) Medications

α-Adrenergic Receptor Agonists (Purple Cap)

Mechanism of action: inhibit aqueous production, may enhance uveoscleral outflow
apraclonidine (Iopidine) 0.5% tid or 1.0% bid
brimonidine (Alphagan-P) 0.15% (Alphagan) 0.2% tid
Side effects: superior lid retraction, miosis, blanching of conjunctival vessels, dry mouth, dry nose, tachyphylaxis, lethargy, headache, allergic reactions

dipivefrin (Propine) 0.1% bid
epinephrine (Glaucon, Epifrin, Epitrate) 0.25%, 0.5%, 1%, 2% bid
Side effects: cystoid macular edema in aphakic eyes, hypertension, tachycardia, adrenochrome deposits in conjunctiva (epinephrine)

β-Blockers (Yellow or Blue Cap)

Mechanism of action: inhibit aqueous production by blocking β_2 receptors on nonpigmented ciliary epithelium
betaxolol (Betoptic S 0.25%, Betoptic 0.5%) bid
carteolol (Ocupress) 1.5%, 3% bid
levobetaxolol (Betaxon) 0.5% bid
levobunolol (Betagan) 0.25-0.5% qd or bid

metipranolol (OptiPranolol) 0.3% bid
timolol (Timoptic, Betimol) 0.25%, 0.5% bid
timolol gel (Timoptic-XE) 0.25%, 0.5% qd
Side effects: bradycardia, bronchospasm (contraindicated in asthmatics), hypotension, depression, lethargy, decreased libido, impotence

Cholinergic Agonists (Green Cap)

Mechanism of action: enhance trabecular outflow, may enhance uveoscleral outflow
carbachol (Isopto Carbachol, Miostat [intraocular 0.01%]) 0.75%, 1.5%, 2.25%, 3% tid
echothiophate (Phospholine iodide) 0.03%, 0.0625%, 0.125%, 0.25% bid
pilocarpine (Pilocar, Ocusert, Isopto Carpine, Pilopine HS gel) 0.5%, 1%, 2%, 3%, 4%, 6% qid (qhs for gel)
Side effects: miosis, induced myopia, accommodative spasm, brow ache, pupillary block, angle-closure

Carbonic Anhydrase Inhibitors (Orange Cap)

Mechanism of action: inhibit aqueous production
acetazolamide (Diamox; 125 to 250 mg tablets, 500 mg Sequels) up to 1 g PO qd in divided doses
brinzolamide (Azopt) 1% tid
dorzolamide (Trusopt) 2% tid (especially in dark irides)
dorzolamide 2% with timolol maleate 0.5% (Cosopt) bid
methazolamide (Neptazane) 25-50 mg PO bid to tid
Side effects: lethargy, depression, aplastic anemia, thrombocytopenia, agranulocytosis, Stevens-Johnson syndrome, paresthesias, renal stones, diarrhea, nausea (especially for oral medications), transient myopia, loss of libido, metallic taste. Remember that these agents are sulfonamide derivatives; beware in sulfa allergic patients.

Prostaglandin Analogues (Turquoise/Teal Cap)

Mechanism of action: enhance uveoscleral outflow
bimatoprost (Lumigan) 0.03% qd
latanoprost (Xalatan) 0.005% qd
travoprost (Travatan) 0.004% qd
unoprostone isopropyl (Rescula) 0.15% bid (docosanoid compound related to prostaglandin analogues)
Side effects: iris pigmentation, iritis, conjunctival hyperemia, cystoid macular edema, hypertrichosis, reactivation of HSV keratitis, flulike symptoms

Hyperosmotics

Mechanism of action: shrink vitreous by creating osmotic gradient
glycerin (Osmoglyn) 50% 8 oz PO
mannitol (Osmitrol) up to 2 g/kg IV of 20% solution over 30-60 minutes
isosorbide (Ismotic) up to 2 g/kg PO of 45% solution
Side effects: backache, headache, mental confusion, heart failure, ketoacidosis (glycerin in diabetic patients), nausea, emesis

Allergy Medications

azelastine hydrochloride (Optivar) 0.05% bid
cetirizine (Zyrtec) 5-10 mg PO qd

cromolyn sodium (Crolom, Opticrom) 4% qd to q4h
desloratadine (Clarinex) 5 mg PO qd
emedastine (Emadine) 0.05% qid
fexofenadine (Allegra) 60 mg PO bid; 180 mg PO qd
ketorolac tromethamine (Acular) 0.5% qid
ketotifen fumarate (Zaditor) 0.025% bid
levocabastine (Livostin) 0.05% qid
lodoxamide tromethamine (Alomide) 0.1% qd to qid
loratadine (Claritin) 10 mg PO qd
loteprednol etabonate (Alrex) 0.2% qid
naphazoline (Naphcon, Vasocon) qd to qid
naphazoline-antazoline (Vasocon A) qd to qid
naphazoline-pheniramine (Naphcon-A, Opcon-A, Ocuhist) qid
nedocromil sodium (Alocril) 2% bid
olopatadine hydrochloride (Patanol) 0.1% bid
pemirolast potassium (Alamast) 0.1% qid

Mydriatics/Cycloplegics

atropine sulfate (Atropisol, Isopto Atropine) 0.5%, 1%, 2% qd to qid
cyclopentolate (Cyclogyl) 0.5%, 1%, 2% qd to qid
eucatropine 5-10% qd to qid
homatropine (Isopto Homatropine) 2%, 5% qd to qid
hydroxyamphetamine hydrobromide 1%/tropicamide 0.25% (Paremyd) qd to qid (onset within
    15 minutes, recovery begins within 90 minutes)
phenylephrine (Neo-Synephrine, Mydfrin) 2.5%, 5%, 10% for pupillary dilation
scopolamine (Isopto Hyoscine) 0.25% qd to qid
tropicamide (Mydriacyl) 0.5%, 1% for pupillary dilation

Anesthetics

bupivacaine (Marcaine) 0.25-0.75% for peribulbar/retrobulbar injection
chloroprocaine (Nesacaine) 1-2% solution
cocaine 1-10% for topical anesthesia, pupil testing (Horner's syndrome)
fluorescein (Fluress [with benoxinate 0.4% anesthetic]) 0.25-2% for examination of conjunc-
    tiva, cornea, and intraocular pressure
lidocaine (Xylocaine) 0.5-4% for topical anesthesia (preservative-free for intracameral
    anesthesia)
mepivacaine (Carbocaine) 1-2% solution
proparacaine (Ophthaine) 0.5% for topical anesthesia
procaine (Novocain) 0.5-2% solution
tetracaine (Pontocaine) 0.5% for topical anesthesia

Miscellaneous

acetylcholine (Miochol; 1:100 [20 mg]) 0.5-2 mL intracameral for miosis during surgery
acetylcysteine (Mucomyst) 10-20% up to q4h
aminocaproic acid (Amicar) 50-100 mg/kg PO q4h up to 30 g/day
dapiprazole (Rev-Eyes) 0.5% for reversing pupillary dilation
edrophonium (Tensilon) 10 mg IV
hydroxyamphetamine (Paredrine) 1% for pupil testing (Horner's syndrome)
methacholine (Mecholyl) 2.5% for pupil testing (Adie's pupil)
sodium chloride (Adsorbonac, Muro 128) 2.5%, 5% solution or ointment qd to qid

Artificial Tear Gel Formulations

GenTeal gel   Moisture Eyes
Tears Again   Refresh PM
HypoTears   Tears Naturale
Lacrilube

Artificial Tear Solution Formulations

Tear Name	Preservative	Viscosity
Cellufresh	Free	Low
Refresh	Free	Low
Refresh Plus	Free	Low
Tears Naturale	Free	Low
GenTeal Mild	Free	Low
HyopTears PF	Free	Low
Moisture Eyes	Present	Low
GenTeal	Present	Low
Hypotears	Present	Low
Murine	Present	Low
Refresh Tears	Present	Low
Tears Naturale	Present	Low
Tears Naturale II	Present	Low
TheraTears	Present	Low
Bion Tears	Free	Medium
OcuCoat PF	Free	Medium
Refresh Endura	Free	Medium
Systane	Present	Medium
Aquasite PF	Free	High
Refresh Celluvisc	Free	High
Refresh Liquigel	Present	High
Murocel	Present	High
Aquasite	Present	High
Ocucoat	Present	High
Ultra Tears	Present	High

Color Codes for Topical Ocular Medication Caps

(Based on the American Academy of Ophthalmology recommendations to the FDA to aid patients in distinguishing among drops and thus minimize the chance of using an incorrect medication)

Class	Color
Antiinfectives	Tan
Antiinflammatories/steroids	Pink
Mydriatics/cycloplegics	Red
Nonsteroidal antiinflammatories	Gray
Miotics	Green
β-blockers	Yellow or blue
Adrenergic agonists	Purple
Carbonic anhydrase inhibitors	Orange
Prostaglandin analogues	Turquoise

List of Important Ocular Measurements

Volumes

Orbit = 30 mL
Globe = 6.5 mL
Vitreous = 4.5 mL
Anterior chamber = 250 µL
Conjunctival sac = 35 µL

Densities

Rods = 120 million
Cones = 6 million
Retinal ganglion cells = 1.2 million

Distances

Corneal thickness (central) = 0.5-0.6 mm
Anterior chamber depth = 3.0 mm

Diameter of

Cornea (horizontal) = 10 mm (infant), 11.5 mm (adult)
Lens = 9.5 mm
Capsular bag = 10.5 mm
Ciliary sulcus = 11.0 mm
Optic disc = 1.5 mm
Macula = 5 mm
Fovea = 1.5 mm
Foveal avascular zone (FAZ) = 0.5 mm
Foveola = 0.35 mm

Distance from limbus to

Ciliary body = 1 mm
Ora serrata = 7-8 mm
rectus muscle insertions:
    Medial = 5.5 mm
    Inferior = 6.5 mm
    Lateral = 6.9 mm
    Superior = 7.7 mm

Length of

Pars plicata = 2 mm
Pars plana = 4 mm
Optic nerve = 45-50 mm
Intraocular optic nerve = 0.7-1 mm
Intraorbital optic nerve = 25-30 mm
Intracanalicular optic nerve = 7-10 mm
Intracranial optic nerve = 10-12 mm

Length of orbital entrance

Width = 35 mm
Height = 40 mm

Extent of monocular visual field

Nasal = 60 degrees
Temporal = 100 degrees
Superior = 60 degrees
Inferior = 70 degrees

Miscellaneous

Visual field background illumination = 31.5 apostilb
Photopic maximum sensitivity = 555 nm
Scotopic maximum sensitivity = 507 nm
Fibers crossing in chiasm = 52% (nasal fibers)
Basal tear secretion = 2 µL/min

List of Eponyms

Adie's pupil: Tonic pupil that demonstrates cholinergic supersensitivity

Alexander's law: Jerk nystagmus, usually increases in amplitude with gaze in direction of the fast phase

Argyll Robertson pupil: Small, irregular pupils that do not react to light but do respond to accommodation; seen in syphilis

Arlt's line: Horizontal palpebral conjunctival scar in trachoma

Arlt's triangle: (Ehrlich-Türck line) base-down triangle of central keratic precipitates in uveitis

Bergmeister's papilla: Remnant of fetal glial tissue at optic disc

Berlin's edema: (Commotio retinae) whitening of retina in the posterior pole from disruption of photoreceptors after blunt trauma

Bielschowsky phenomenon: Downdrift of occluded eye as increasing neutral density filters are placed over fixating eye in dissociated vertical deviation (DVD)

Bitot's spot: White, foamy-appearing area of keratinizing squamous metaplasia of bulbar conjunctiva in vitamin A deficiency

Bonnet's sign: Hemorrhage at arteriovenous crossing in branch retinal vein occlusion

Boston's sign: Lid lag on downgaze in thyroid disease

Brushfield spots: White-gray spots on peripheral iris in Down's syndrome

Busacca nodules: Clumps of inflammatory cells on front surface of iris in granulomatous uveitis

Coats' ring: White granular corneal stromal opacity containing iron from previous metallic foreign body

Cogan's sign: Upper eyelid twitch when patient with ptosis refixates from downgaze to primary position; nonspecific finding seen in myasthenia gravis; also refers to venous engorgement over lateral rectus muscle in thyroid disease

Collier's sign: Bilateral eyelid retraction associated with midbrain lesions

Czarnecki's sign: Segmental pupillary constriction with eye movements due to aberrant regeneration of cranial nerve III

Dalen-Fuchs nodules: Small, deep, yellow retinal lesions composed of inflammatory cells seen histologically between retinal pigment epithelium and Bruch's membrane in sympathetic ophthalmia (also in sarcoidosis, Vogt-Koyanagi-Harada syndrome)

Dalrymple's sign: Widened palpebral fissure secondary to upper eyelid retraction in thyroid disease

Depression sign of Goldberg: Focal loss of nerve fiber layer after resolution of cotton-wool spot

Ehrlich-Türck line: (See Arlt's triangle)

Elschnig pearls: Cystic proliferation of residual lens epithelial cells on capsule after cataract extraction

Elschnig spot: Yellow patches (early) of retinal pigment epithelium overlying area of choroidal infarction in hypertension, eventually becomes hyperpigmented scar with halo

Enroth's sign: Eyelid edema in thyroid disease

Ferry's line: Corneal epithelial iron line at edge of filtering bleb

Fleischer's ring: Corneal epithelial iron ring at base of cone in keratoconus

Fischer-Khunt spot: (Senile scleral plaque) blue-gray area of hyalinized sclera anterior to horizontal rectus muscle insertions in elderly individuals

Fuchs' spots: Pigmented macular lesions (retinal pigment epithelial hyperplasia) in pathologic myopia

Globe's sign: Lid lag on upgaze in thyroid disease

Guiat's sign: Tortuosity of retinal veins in arteriosclerosis

Gunn's dots: Light reflections from internal limiting membrane around disc and macula

Gunn's sign: Arteriovenous nicking in hypertensive retinopathy

Haab's striae: Breaks in Descemet's membrane (horizontal or concentric with limbus) in congenital glaucoma (versus vertical tears associated with birth trauma)

Hassall-Henle bodies: Peripheral hyaline excrescences on Descemet's membrane due to normal aging

Henle's layer: Obliquely oriented cone fibers in fovea

Herbert's pits: Scarred limbal follicles in trachoma

Hering's law: Equal and simultaneous innervation to yoke muscles during conjugate eye movements

Hirschberg's sign: Pale round spots (Koplik spots) on conjunctiva and caruncle in measles

Hollenhorst plaque: Cholesterol embolus usually seen at vessel bifurcations, associated with amaurosis fugax and retinal artery occlusions

Horner-Trantas dots: Collections of eosinophils at limbus in vernal conjunctivitis

Hudson-Stahli line: Horizontal corneal epithelial iron line at inferior one third of cornea due to normal aging

Hutchinson's pupil: Fixed, dilated pupil in comatose patient due to uncal herniation and compression of cranial nerve III

Hutchinson's sign: Involvement of tip of nose in herpes zoster ophthalmicus (nasociliary nerve involvement)

Hutchinson's triad: Three signs of congenital syphilis—interstitial keratitis, notched teeth, and deafness

Kayes' dots: Subepithelial infiltrates seen in corneal allograft rejection

Kayser-Fleischer ring: Limbal copper deposition in Descemet's membrane seen in Wilson's disease

Khodadoust line: Corneal graft endothelial rejection line composed of inflammatory cells

Klein's tags: Yellow spots at base of macular hole

Koeppe nodules: Clumps of inflammatory cells at pupillary border in granulomatous uveitis

Krukenberg spindle: Bilateral, central, vertical corneal endothelial pigment deposits in pigment dispersion syndrome

Kunkmann-Wolffian bodies: small white peripheral iris spots that resemble Brushfield spots but occur in normal individuals

Kyreileis' plaques: White-yellow vascular plaques in toxoplasmosis

Lander's sign: Inferior preretinal nodules in sarcoidosis

Lisch nodules: Iris melanocytic hamartomas in neurofibromatosis

Loops of Axenfeld: Dark limbal spots representing scleral nerve loops

Mittendorf's dot: White spot (remnant of hyaloid artery) at posterior lens surface

Mizuo-Nakamura phenomenon: Loss of abnormal macular sheen with dark adaptation in Oguchi's disease

Morgagnian cataract: Hypermature cortical cataract in which liquified cortex allows nucleus to sink inferiorly

Munson's sign: Protrusion of lower lid with downgaze in keratoconus

Panum's area: Zone of single binocular vision around horopter

Parry's sign: Exophthalmos in thyroid disease

Paton's sign: Conjunctival microaneurysms in sickle cell disease

Paton's lines: Circumferential peripapillary retinal folds due to optic nerve edema

pseudo–von Graefe sign: Lid elevation on adduction or downgaze due to aberrant regeneration of cranial nerve III

Pulfrich phenomenon: Perception of stereopsis (elliptical motion of a pendulum) due to difference in nerve conduction times between eyes and cortex, seen in multiple sclerosis

Purkinje images: Reflected images from front and back surfaces of cornea and lens

Purkinje shift: Shift in peak spectral sensitivity from photopic (555 nm, cones) to scotopic (507 nm, rods) conditions

Riddoch phenomenon: Visual field anomaly in which a moving object can be seen whereas a static one cannot

Roth spots: Intraretinal hemorrhages with white center in subacute bacterial endocarditis, leukemia, severe anemia, collagen vascular diseases, diabetes mellitus, and multiple myeloma

Rizutti's sign: Triangle of light on iris from oblique penlight beam focused by cone in keratoconus

Salus' sign: Retinal vein angulation (90 degrees) at arteriovenous crossing in hypertension and arteriosclerosis

Sampaoelesi's line: Increased pigmentation anterior to Schwalbe's line in pseudoexfoliation syndrome

Sattler's veil: Superficial corneal edema (bedewing) caused by hypoxia (contact lens)

Scheie's line: Pigment on lens equator and posterior capsule in pigment dispersion syndrome

Schwalbe's line: Angle structure representing peripheral edge of Descemet's membrane

Schwalbe's ring: Posterior embryotoxon (anteriorly displaced Schwalbe's line)

Seidel test: Method of detecting wound leak by observing aqueous dilute concentrated fluorescein placed over the suspected leakage site

Shafer's sign: Anterior vitreous pigment cells (tobacco-dust) associated with retinal tear

Sherrington's law: Contraction of muscle causes relaxation of antagonist (reciprocal innervation)

Siegrist streak: Linear chain of hyperpigmented spots over sclerosed choroidal vessel in chronic hypertension or choroiditis

Soemmering's ring cataract: Residual peripheral cataractous lens material following capsular rupture and central lens resorption from trauma or surgery

Spiral of Tillaux: Imaginary line connecting insertions of rectus muscles

Stocker's line: Corneal epithelial iron line at edge of pterygium

Sugiura's sign: Perilimbal vitiligo associated with Vogt-Koyanagi-Harada syndrome

Tenon's capsule: Fascial covering of eye

Uhthoff's symptom: Decreased vision/diplopia secondary to increased body temperature (e.g., exercise or hot shower) seen after recovery in optic neuritis

van Trigt's sign: Venous pulsations on optic disc (normal finding)

Vogt's sign: White anterior lens opacities (glaukomflecken) caused by ischemia of lens epithelial cells from previous attacks of angle-closure

Vogt's striae: Deep stromal vertical stress lines at apex of cone in keratoconus

Von Graefe's sign: Lid lag on downgaze in thyroid disease

Vossius ring: Ring of iris pigment from pupillary ruff deposited onto anterior lens capsule after blunt trauma

Watzke-Allen sign: Patient with macular hole perceives break in light when a slit-beam is focused on the fovea

Wessely ring: Corneal stromal infiltrate of antigen-antibody complexes

White lines of Vogt: Sheathed or sclerosed vessels seen in lattice degeneration

Wieger's ligament: Attachment of hyaloid face to back of lens

Weiss ring: Ring of adherent peripapillary glial tissue on posterior vitreous surface after posterior vitreous detachment

Willebrandt's knee: Inferonasal optic nerve fibers that decussate in chiasm and loop into contralateral optic nerve before traveling back to optic tract

◼ Common Ophthalmic Abbreviations

(How To Read an Ophthalmology Chart)

AC	anterior chamber
AFX	air fluid exchange
AK	astigmatic keratotomy

ALT	argon laser trabeculoplasty
AMD	age-related macular degeneration
APD (RAPD)	(relative) afferent pupillary defect
ASC	anterior subcapsular cataract
AV	arteriovenous
BCVA (BSCVA)	best (spectacle) corrected visual acuity
BVO or BRVO	branch retinal vein occlusion
C or C_R	cycloplegic refraction
CB	ciliary body
C/D	cup/disc ratio
CE (ECCE, ICCE, PE)	cataract extraction (extracapsular, intracapsular, phacoemulsification)
C/F	cell/flare
CF	count fingers
CL (DCL, SCL, EWCL)	contact lens (disposable, soft, extended wear)
CME	cystoid macular edema
CNV/CNVM	choroidal neovascular membrane
CRA	chorioretinal atrophy
C/S	conjunctiva/sclera
CS	cortical spoking (cataract)
CSME	clinically significant macular edema
CVO or CRVO	central retinal vein occlusion
CWS	cotton-wool spot
D	diopter(s)
DD	disc diameter(s)
DFE (NDFE)	(non)dilated fundus examination
DME	diabetic macular edema
DR (BDR, NPDR, PDR)	diabetic retinopathy (background, nonproliferative, proliferative)
E (ET)	esophoria (esotropia)
EL	endolaser
EOG	electro-oculogram
EOM	extraocular muscles/movements
ERG	electroretinogram
ERM	epiretinal membrane
FA	fluorescein angiogram
FAZ	foveal avascular zone
FB	foreign body
FBS	foreign body sensation or fasting blood sugar
GA	geographic atrophy
H	Hertel exophthalmometry measurement or hemorrhage
HM	hand motion
HT	hypertropia
I/L	iris/lens
ILM	internal limiting membrane
IO	inferior oblique muscle
IOFB (IOMFB)	intraocular (metallic) foreign body
IOL (ACIOL, PCIOL)	intraocular lens (anterior chamber, posterior chamber)
IOP	intraocular pressure
IR	inferior rectus muscle
IRMA	intraretinal microvascular abnormalities

K	keratometry
KP	keratic precipitates
L/L/L	lids/lashes/lacrimal
LF	levator function
LP	light perception/projection
LR	lateral rectus muscle
M or M_R	manifest refraction
MA	macro/micro aneurysm
MCE	microcystic corneal edema
MP	membrane peel
MR	medial rectus muscle
MRD	margin to reflex distance
NLP	no light perception
NS (NSC)	nuclear sclerosis (nuclear sclerotic cataract)
NV (NVD, NVE, NVI)	neovascularization (of the disc, elsewhere [retina], iris)
NVG	neovascular glaucoma
OD	right eye
ON	optic nerve
OS	left eye
OU	both eyes
P	pupil(s)
PC	posterior chamber/capsule
PCO	posterior capsular opacification
PD	prism diopters/pupillary distance
PERRL(A)	pupils equal round reactive to light (& accommodation)
PF	palpebral fissure
PH	pinhole vision
PI	peripheral iridectomy/iridotomy
PK or PKP	penetrating keratoplasty
PPL	pars plana lensectomy
PPV	pars plana vitrectomy
PRP	panretinal photocoagulation
PRK	photorefractive keratectomy
PSC	posterior subcapsular cataract
PTK	phototherapeutic keratectomy
PVS	posterior vitreous separation
PVD	posterior vitreous detachment
R	retinoscopy
RD (RRD, TRD)	retinal detachment (rhegmatogenous, tractional)
RGP	rigid gas permeable contact lens
RK	radial keratotomy
RPE	retinal pigment epithelium
(R)PED	(retinal) pigment epithelial detachment
SB	scleral buckle
SLE	slit-lamp examination
SO	superior oblique muscle
SPK (SPE)	superficial punctate keratopathy (epitheliopathy)
SR	superior rectus muscle
SRF	subretinal fluid

SRNVM	subretinal neovascular membrane
SS	scleral spur
T (T_a, T_p, T_t)	tonometry (applanation, palpation, Tonopen)
TH	macular thickening/edema
TM	trabecular meshwork
V (VA, V_{cc}, V_{sc})	vision (visual acuity, with correction, without correction)
VH	vitreous hemorrhage
VF (GVF, HVF)	visual field (Goldmann, Humphrey)
W	wearing (refers to current glasses prescription)
X (XT)	exophoria (exotropia)

Common Spanish Phrases

Introduction

I am doctor . . .	Yo soy el doctor/la doctora . . .
Ophthalmologist	Oftalmólogo/oculista
I don't speak Spanish	No hablo español
I speak a little Spanish	Hablo un poco de español
Please	Por favor
Come in, enter	Pase(n), entre
Come here	Venga acá
Sit down (here)	Siéntese (aquí)

History

What is your name?	¿Cómo se llama usted?
Do you understand me?	¿Me comprende? *or* ¿Me entiende?
How are you?	¿Cómo está usted?
How old are you?	¿Cuántos años tiene usted?
Where do you live?	¿Dónde vive usted?
What is your telephone number?	¿Cuál es su número de teléfono?
Tell me	Dígame
Do you have?	¿Tiene usted? *or* ¿Tiene?
glasses	pejuelos/lentes/gafas
for distance	para ver de lejos
for reading	para leer
bifocals	bifocales
sunglasses	espejuelos obscuros/gafas de sol
contact lenses	lentes de contacto
prescription	receta/prescripción
insurance	seguro médico
allergies	alergias
Do you take?	¿Toma usted? *or* ¿Toma?
medications	medicinas
pills, tablets, capsules	pastillas/píldoras, tabletas, cápsulas
Do you use?	¿Usa usted? *or* ¿Usa?
drops	gotas
ointment	pomada
How much?	¿Cuánto?

Do you have problems?	¿Tiene problemas?
reading	al leer
with distance	al ver de lejos
with the cornea	con la cornea
with the retina	con la retina
Do you have?	¿Tiene usted? *or* ¿Tiene?
blurred vision	visión borrosa
diplopia	visión doble
excessive tearing	muchas lágrimas
How long?	¿Por cuánto tiempo?
How long ago?	¿Hace cuánto tiempo?
Does your eye hurt?	¿Le duele el ojo?
Never	Nunca
Once	Una vez
Many times	Muchas veces
What did you say?	¿Qué dijo? *or* ¿Cómo?
Please repeat	Repita, por favor
Again	Otra vez
Excuse me	Con permiso, dispénseme

Examination

Cover one eye	Tápese un ojo
Can you read this?	¿Puede leer ésto?
the letters/numbers	las letras/números
Better or worse?	¿Mejor o peor?
Which is better, one or two?	¿Cuál es mejor, uno o dos?
Put your chin here	Ponga la barbilla aquí
Put your forehead against the bar	Ponga la frente pegada a la barra
Look at the light	Mire la luz
Lie down	Acuéstese, boca arriba
Look up	Mire para arriba
Look down	Mire para abajo
Look to the right	Mire para la derecha
Look to the left	Mire para la izquierda

Diagnosis

You have . . .	Tiene . . .
normal eyes	ojos normales
myopia	miopía
hyperopia	hiperopía
presbyopia	presbiopía
strabismus	estrabismo
cataracts	cataratas
glaucoma	glaucoma
infection	infección
inflammation	inflamación
a retinal detachment	un desprendimiento de retina

Treatment

I'll be right back	Ahorita vengo *or* Regreso enseguida
I will put a patch/shield on the eye	Le voy a poner un parche/protector sobre el ojo
You need (do not need) . . .	Usted necesita (no necesita) . . .
an operation	una operación
new glasses	espejuelos nuevos
Don't worry	No se preocupe
Everything is OK (very good)	Toda está bien (muy bien)
I am giving you a prescription for drops/ointment	Le doy una prescripción para gotas/pomada
Take/put/use . . .	ome/ponga/use . . .
one drop bid/tid/qid	una gota dos/tres/cuatro veces al día
ointment at bedtime	omada por la noche antes de acostarse
in the right/left eye	en el ojo derecho/izquierdo
in both eyes	en los dos ojos
Do not bend over	No baje la cabeza
Do not strain	No haga fuerza
Do not touch/rub the eye	No se toque/frote el ojo
Do not get your eyes wet	No se moje los ojos
Do you understand the instructions?	¿Entiende las instrucciones?
I want to check your eye again tomorrow	Quiero examinarle el ojo otra vez mañana
I am giving you an appointment	le doy una cita
in one week	para dentro de una semana
in three months	para dentro de tres meses
Return when necessary	vuelva cuando lo necesite
Thank you	Gracias
Goodbye	Adiós

Suggested Readings

The following subspecialty textbooks provide more detailed information regarding conditions discussed in this book, as well as less common entities.

Arffa RC: *Grayson's diseases of the cornea,* ed 4, St Louis, 1998, Mosby.

Gass JDM: *Stereoscopic atlas of macular diseases,* ed 4, St Louis, 1997, Mosby.

Grant WM, Schuman JS: *Toxicology of the eye,* ed 4, Springfield, Ill, 1993, Charles C Thomas.

Kline LB, Bajandas F: *Neuro-ophthalmology review manual,* ed 5, Thorofare, NJ, 2001, SLACK.

Krachmer JH, Mannis MJ, Holland EJ: *Cornea,* St Louis, 1997, Mosby.

Mannis MJ, Macsai M, Huntley AC: *Eye and skin disease,* Philadelphia, 1996, Lippincott-Raven.

Miller NR: *Walsh & Hoyt's clinical neuro-ophthalmology,* ed 5, Baltimore, 1998, Williams & Wilkins.

Nelson LB, Calhoun JH, Harley RD: *Pediatric ophthalmology,* ed 4, Philadelphia, 1998, WB Saunders.

Nussenblatt RB, Whitcup SM, Palestine AG: *Uveitis: fundamentals and clinical practice,* ed 2, St Louis, 1996, Mosby.

Pepose JS, Holland GN, Wilhelmus KR: *Ocular infection and immunity,* St Louis, 1996, Mosby.

Ritch R, Shields MB, Krupin T: *The glaucomas,* ed 2, St Louis, 1996, Mosby.

Rootman J: *Diseases of the orbit,* ed 2, Philadelphia, 2002, JB Lippincott.

Ryan SJ: *Retina,* ed 3, St Louis, 2001, Mosby.

Shields JA, Shields CL: *Intraocular tumors: a text and atlas,* Philadelphia, 1992, WB Saunders.

Smolin G, Thoft RA: The cornea: scientific foundations and clinical practice, ed 3, Boston, 1994, Little, Brown.

Spencer WH: *Ophthalmic pathology: an atlas and textbook,* ed 4, Philadelphia, 1996, WB Saunders.

Tabbara JH, Mannis MJ, Holland EJ: *Infections of the eye,* ed 2, Boston, 1995, Little, Brown.

von Noorden GK: *Atlas of strabismus,* ed 4, St Louis, 1983, Mosby.

Walsh TJ: *Neuro-ophthalmology: clinical signs and symptoms,* ed 4, Philadelphia, 1997, Lea & Febiger.

Yanoff M, Fine BS: *Ocular pathology: a text and atlas,* ed 5, Philadelphia, 2002, JB Lippincott.

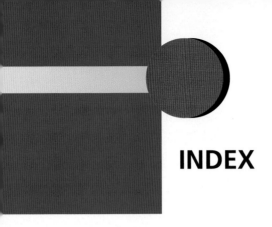

INDEX

Page numbers followed by *f, t,* and *b* indicate figures, tables, and boxed material, respectively.

Dear Friends,

Most people skip this page unless there's a chance they'll stumble across their own name. I hope you won't, because what I have to tell you is pretty amazing. About six years ago I felt the need to connect with other businesswomen. I'd recently moved my office out of my home and rented space in a commercial building, which is a bit unusual for a writer. I loved having my work life separate from home and family.

Even in my small hometown, it didn't take me long to meet other women who face the same struggles I do. After one luncheon date with Lillian Schauer, in which we both ended up in tears, I realized how often it's necessary to hide our emotions. I suggested we develop a support group for one another, and Lillian agreed. That was how my own Thursday Morning Breakfast Group was started.

For the past six years I've met with five incredible women—Betty, Lillian, Karla, Stephanie and Diana. We've been through a great deal together—weddings, births, celebrations, crises and death. A year and a half ago we lost our own Stephanie to ovarian cancer.

We continue to gather together to learn from one another, to share our challenges and seek advice, to talk about books we've read, our children, grandchildren.... You name it and we've talked about it. We talk, we listen, we laugh, we cry, but mostly we support and encourage one another. We are a bank president, an attorney and business owners, but more important we're women who share one of the strongest of female bonds: friendship.

So here's *Thursdays at Eight*, which is dedicated to each member of my Thursday Morning Breakfast Group (although I did not, of course, use actual events or real people in my story). Thank you for being a part of my life, for listening to my frustrations and helping me laugh at myself. I love you all.

Debbie Macomber

P.S. I enjoy hearing from my readers. Feel free to write me at P.O. Box 1458, Port Orchard, WA 98366, or visit my Web site at www.debbiemacomber.com.

DEBBIE MACOMBER
THURSDAYS
AT EIGHT

MIRA®

ISBN 0-7783-2380-3

THURSDAYS AT EIGHT

Copyright © 2001 by Debbie Macomber.

MIRA and the Star Colophon are trademarks used under license and registered in Australia, New Zealand, Philippines, United States Patent and Trademark Office and in other countries.

www.MIRABooks.com

Printed in U.S.A.

This story is dedicated to Lillian Schauer,
Diana Letson, Betty Roper and Karla Cain
The wonderful, wise and fascinating women
of my Thursday morning breakfast group.

For

Stephanie Cordall

March 13, 1948–November 12, 2000

We shall miss you, my friend

> "It's the good girls who keep the diaries; the bad
> girls never have the time."
>
> —Tallulah Bankhead

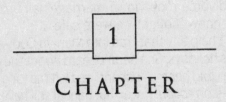

CHAPTER

CLARE CRAIG

January 1st

A promise to myself: this year is a new beginning for me. A fresh start, in more ways than one. I'm determined to put the divorce behind me. About time, too, since it's been final for over a year. Okay, thirteen months and six days to be exact, not that I'm counting...well, maybe I am, but that's going to stop as of *today*.

Michael has his new life and I have mine. I've heard that living well is the best revenge. Good, because that's what I intend to do. I'm going to live my life as a successful, happy (or at least, contented) single woman and mother. This is my vow. I will no longer expect another person to provide me with a sense of worth. I don't need a husband to make me feel complete. It's been a struggle to let go of the marriage, but holding on to all that pain and anger is getting me nowhere. I'm sick of the pettiness, sick of fighting and sick to death of the resentment, the bitterness. I just never thought anything like this could possibly happen to Michael and me.

I saw divorce mow down marriages all around us, but I somehow thought we were safe....

It didn't help any that I ran into Marilyn Cody over the Christmas holidays. She hadn't heard about the divorce, and when I told her my husband had left me for a twenty-year-old—*correction,* my ex-husband (I still have trouble remembering that)—I could see how shocked she was. Then, apparently thinking she was giving me good advice, Marilyn suggested I find myself a boy toy (or is it toy boy?) to get my confidence back. She was actually serious, as though going to bed with a man only a few years older than my own children would make me feel better. Marilyn is a good example of why I can't remain friends with the people Michael and I once associated with.

Losing Marilyn as a friend is no great loss, anyway. I read the pitying look in her eyes, and I didn't miss her innuendo that I could've kept my husband if I hadn't let myself go. It was all I could do not to get in her face and defend myself—as though *that* would prove anything. As a matter of fact, I happen to weigh within fifteen pounds of what I did at twenty-five, and damn it all, I take care of myself. If anyone's suffering from middle-age spread, it's Michael. The audacity of Marilyn to imply that Michael's affair is somehow *my* fault!

How the hell was I supposed to compete with a girl barely out of her teens? I couldn't. I didn't. Every time I think about the two of them together, I feel sick to my stomach.

The journal-writing class has helped. So did meeting Liz, Julia and Karen. They're my friends, and part of my new life. Forming a solid relationship with each of these women is one of the positive changes I've made. As the saying goes, "Out with the old and in with the new." I'm glad the four of us have decided to continue seeing each other, even though the class isn't being offered again. Thursdays for breakfast was an inspired idea.

Writing down my thoughts is the only way I got through the last six months. This should be a good time in my life. Instead, I've been forced to start over—not my choice and not my fault! Okay, fine. I can deal with it. I *am* dealing with it, each and every day. I hate it. I hate Michael, although I'm trying not to. The best I can say at this point is that I'm coping.

I will admit one thing. Michael's affair has taught me a lot about myself. I hadn't realized I could truly hate anyone. Now I know how deep my anger can cut...and I wish to hell I didn't.

My mistake—and I made a few—was in delaying the divorce as long as I did. Eternal optimist that I am, I clung to the belief that, given time, Michael would come to his senses. I was convinced that eventually he'd see how much he was hurting me and the boys. An affair with a twenty-year-old was sheer madness. Surely he'd wake up one morning and realize he'd destroyed his entire life—and for what? Good sex? I doubt she's *that* incredible in the sack.

In retrospect, I could kick myself for waiting so many months to see an attorney. I merely postponed the inevitable, because I was so sure he'd admit what he was doing and put an end to it. How I prayed, how I longed for the opportunity to save my marriage. If only Michael would come home again. If only he'd give us another chance. Little did I understand that his actions had utterly destroyed the foundation of our lives together. The minute he told me he'd fallen in love with Miranda (sure he had!), I should've hightailed it into a lawyer's office and set the divorce in motion. Doing that would have saved me a lot of grief.

At a particularly low point, when I was feeling absolutely desperate, I signed up for counseling. The irony didn't escape me, even then. *I* wasn't the one defiling our wedding vows, yet I was the one making appointments with a shrink!

Then, on a particular Thursday morning about a year and a half ago, I got up after another restless, miserable, lonely night. I remember leaning against the bathroom sink in such emotional pain I couldn't even stand upright. I looked at myself in the mirror and barely recognized my own face. Something *happened* in those moments. Nothing I can precisely identify, but the experience changed me. The victim disappeared and there I stood, straight and tall, glaring back at my reflection, determined to survive. Michael might want to kill our marriage, but he wouldn't kill *me* in the process. In retrospect, I realize that was when I'd reached my limit.

I got dressed and marched myself right down to Lillian Case's office. If there's anything to smile about regarding this ugly divorce, it's the misery Lillian put Michael through. Michael repeatedly claimed he wanted a friendly divorce, but as Lillian said, it was far too late for that.

The boys still aren't speaking to him. I'm not sure Mick ever will. Alex was always close to his father, and I know he misses Michael. We don't talk about him. I wish we could, but nothing I can say is going to take away the pain of having their father walk out the door. What Michael failed to understand was that in leaving me, he abandoned his children, too. He didn't just betray *me*. He broke faith with us all.

I probably should have figured out what was happening—that was what Marilyn seemed to insinuate. I *did* suspect something was wrong, but never, ever would I have guessed *this*. I thought maybe a midlife crisis or boredom with our marriage. Maybe that was how he felt; maybe it's why he did what he did. But he should've been honest with me about his feelings—not had an affair. Bad enough that my husband screwed another woman, but a friend's daughter?

I can only imagine what Carl would think if he were alive. It's all so crazy. Just a few years ago, Michael and I attended the party Kathy and Carl threw for Miranda's high-school graduation. Our top car salesman keels over from a heart attack and Michael, being a caring friend and business-owner, helps the grieving widow with the funeral arrangements and the insurance paperwork. Even crazier is the fact that I actually suggested it.

My one concern at the time was that Michael might be getting too close to the widow. Only it wasn't Kathy keeping my husband entertained all those nights. It was her twenty-year-old daughter. I don't think Kathy or I will ever get over the shock of it.

Michael still doesn't fully appreciate the consequences of what he's done. He sincerely believed that once we were divorced, everything would return to normal between him and his sons. Mick set him straight on that score. Alex, too. I know Michael hasn't stopped trying, but the boys won't be so easily won over. I've done my best to stay out of it. Nothing will ever change the fact that he's their father; how they choose to deal with him is up to them. I refuse to encourage either boy to forgive and forget, but I won't hold them back from a relationship with Michael, either. The choice is theirs.

Twenty-three years of marriage and I never looked at another man. Damn it all, I was a faithful, loving wife. I could have tolerated an affair if he'd given it up and returned to our marriage. But, no, he—

Okay, enough. I don't need to keep repeating the same gory details. As I said, this is a fresh start, the first day of a new year. I'm giving myself permission to move on, as my psycho-babbling counselor used to put it.

Part of moving on is belonging to the breakfast group—and continuing to write in my journal. Liz suggested we each pick a word for the year. A word. I haven't quite figured out why, let alone which word

would best suit me. We're all supposed to have our
words chosen before we meet next Thursday morning
at Mocha Moments.

I've toyed with the idea of *beginnings,* as in new beginnings, but I don't want to carry that theme around
with me for the next twelve months. At some point,
beginnings have to become middles and potential has
to be realized. I guess I'm afraid I won't be as successful as I want to be.

What I really need to do is discover who I am, now
that I'm single again. For twenty-three years my identity was linked to Michael. We were a team, comple-
menting each other's strengths and weaknesses. I was
always better with finances and Michael was the people person. He took a part-time job selling cars the first
year we were married in order to supplement our
budget, and quickly became the top salesman. His degree was in ecology and he had a day job at the town
planning office but made three times the money selling cars. Soon he was working full-time at the dealership and I was stretching every dollar he made, creating
a small nest-egg.

Then we had the chance to buy the Chevrolet dealership—the opportunity of a lifetime. We scraped together every penny we could. By the time the
paperwork was finished, we didn't have a cent between
us, but we were happy. That was when we—

I can't write about that, don't want to dwell on how
happy we were in those early years. Whenever I think
about it, I feel overwhelmed by the pain of loss and
regret. So much regret...

Word. I need a word. Not memories. I can't tie my new identity to the past and to who I was; I've got to look toward the future. So I need a word that fits who I am today, the woman I'm becoming. The woman I want to be.

Just a minute here. Just a damn minute! *Who I was, who I want to be.* Why do *I* have to change? There's nothing wrong with me! I wasn't the one who ripped the heart out of this family. I was a good wife, a good mother. I was faithful...

FAITHFUL.

That's it. My word. Not *beginnings*, not *discovery*, but *faithful.* From the moment I spoke my vows I was faithful to my husband, my marriage, my family. All these years I've been faithful to myself; I've never acted dishonestly and I've always put my family responsibilities above my own desires. I don't need to *find* myself. I found out who I am a long time ago and frankly I happen to like that person. I wasn't the one who changed; Michael did.

This feels good. The burden isn't on my shoulders to prove one damn thing. I'll remain faithful to *me.*

Happy New Year, Clare Craig. You're going to have a wonderful year. No financial worries, thanks to Lillian Case and a judge who's seen far too many men mess up their family's lives. Michael will be spending twenty very long years paying off my share of the dealership. Plus interest. I have the house, a new car every year, health insurance, the boys' college expenses and enough money to live comfortably.

I don't have anything to worry about. I can do whatever I want. I certainly don't have to work if I don't feel like it.

Hey! Maybe getting a job wouldn't be a bad idea. Maybe I should put my two decades of experience back into play. Didn't I recently hear that Murphy Motors was advertising for a general manager? With my experience, I could work any hours I chose. News of my taking that job would really get Michael. It's what he deserves. Turnabout is fair play (another of those handy sayings). Oh God, it's awful of me, but I love it.

This is what I've been waiting for. It's taken a long time to feel anything but horrendous, crushing pain. I'm smiling now, just thinking about the look on Michael's face when he learns I've been hired by his largest competitor.

Marilyn Cody was wrong, but then so was I. Living well isn't going to teach Michael a thing, is it? Knowing that he's lying awake at night, worrying about me sharing all his insider secrets with the Ford dealership—now, *that* will go a long way toward helping me find some satisfaction. And once I'm satisfied, I'll start to concentrate on living well.

* * *

"Mom, can we talk?"

Clare Craig glanced up from her desk to find her seventeen-year-old son standing in the doorway of the family room. They'd spent the morning taking down the Christmas decorations, as they always did on January sixth—Epiphany, Twelfth Night—and getting Mick ready to return to college. How like Michael he looked, she thought with a twinge of sorrow. Michael twenty-five years ago, athletic, handsome, fit. Her heart cramped at the memory.

"I'm not interrupting anything, am I?" Alex stepped inside, dressed in his soccer uniform. The holiday break was already over; school had begun earlier in the week. Mick had left that morning for college in San Francisco.

Clare capped the end of her fountain pen and set aside the checkbook and bills in order to give her younger son her full attention. "What can I do for you?"

Alex avoided her gaze. "We haven't been talking as much as we used to," he mumbled, walking slowly toward her desk.

"I've been busy." The Christmas tree had only come down that morning, but she realized he wasn't referring to the last few days; he meant over the past year.

"I know," he said with a shrug, his eyes darting around the room. "It's just that..."

"Is there something you wanted to tell me?"

He raised his head and their eyes briefly met. Reading her younger son had never been a problem for Clare.

"How about if we talk in the kitchen?" she suggested. "You thirsty?"

The hopeful look on his face convinced her to abandon paying the bills. She'd get back to all that later.

"Sure." He led the way through the large family room and into the kitchen.

Clare loved her expansive kitchen with its double ovens and large butcher-block island. Shining copper pots and kettles dangled from the rack above, the California sunlight reflected in their shine. Clare had designed the kitchen herself and spent countless hours reviewing every detail, every drawer placement, every cupboard. She'd taken pride in her home, in her skill as a cook and homemaker.

These days it was unusual for her to prepare a meal. Alex

had a part-time job at a computer store, and if he wasn't at school or work, he was with his friends or on the soccer field. Cooking for one person hardly seemed worth the effort, and more and more often she ordered out. Or didn't bother at all.

"I'll get us a Coke," Alex said, already reaching for the refrigerator handle. Clare automatically took two glasses from the cupboard.

Alex placed the cans on the round oak table. Many a night, unable to sleep, the two of them had sat here while Clare sobbed in pain and frustration. Alex had wept, too. It hadn't been easy for a teenage boy to expose his emotions like that. If Clare didn't already hate Michael for what he'd done to her self-esteem, then she'd hate him for the pain he'd brought into their children's lives.

"Mick and I had a long talk last night."

Clare had surmised as much. She'd heard them in Alex's bedroom sometime after midnight, deep in conversation. Their raised voices were followed by heated whispers. Whatever they were discussing was between them and she was determined to keep out of it. They needed to settle their own differences.

"He's upset with me."

"Mick is? What for?"

Alex shrugged. He seemed to do that a lot these days.

"Brother stuff?" It was what he generally said when he didn't want to give her a full explanation.

"Something like that." He waited a moment before pulling back the tab on his soda can and taking a long swallow, ignoring the glass she'd set in front of him.

"Does this have to do with Kellie?" Alex and the girl across the street had been dating for a couple of months.

Mick had dated her last summer and Clare wondered if the neighbor girl was causing a problem between her sons.

"Ah, Mom, we're just friends."

"If you and your brother had a falling-out, why don't you just tell me instead of expecting me to guess?"

He lowered his eyes. "Because I'm afraid you're going to react the same way Mick did."

"Oh? And how's that?"

Alex took another drink of his Coke. Clare recognized a delaying tactic when she saw one. "Alex?"

"All right," he said brusquely and sat up, his shoulders squared. "I've been talking to Dad."

Clare swallowed hard, but a small shocked sound still managed to escape. She felt as though she'd taken a punch to the solar plexus.

"Are you mad?" Alex asked, watching her anxiously.

"It shouldn't matter what I think."

"But it does! I don't want you to feel like I've betrayed you, too."

"I..."

"That's what Mick said I was doing. First Dad and now me. Mom, I swear to you, it isn't like that."

"Michael is your father," she said, her mind whirling as she struggled with her conflicting emotions. Alex would never intentionally do anything to hurt her. As much as possible, Clare had tried not to entangle her sons in this divorce. When Michael moved out of the family home and in with his under-age sweetheart, the two boys had rallied around her as if they could protect her from further pain. It didn't work, but she'd cherished them for their show of sympathy and support.

"He called... Dad did."

"When?" Now she was the one avoiding eye contact. She distracted herself by opening the can of Coke and pouring it carefully into her glass.

"Last week at Softline."

"He phoned you at work?" She shouldn't have been surprised; Michael was too much of a coward to risk having her answer the phone here at the house. Naturally he'd taken the low road.

"He invited me to dinner."

"And you're going?"

Clare felt her son's scrutiny. "I don't know yet. Mick doesn't think I should."

"But you want to, right?"

Alex stood and paced the area in front of the table. "That's the crazy part, Mom. I do and I don't. I haven't talked to Dad in over a year—well, other than to say I wasn't going to talk to him."

"He *is* your father," Clare said, to remind herself as much as her son.

"That's what Kellie said."

Sure Kellie said that, Clare mused darkly. She hadn't seen *her* mother betrayed and then dumped like last week's garbage. Kellie had two loving parents. She couldn't even imagine what divorce did to a person's soul or how it tore a family apart.

"I told Mick and I'm telling you. If my seeing Dad hurts you, then I won't do it."

Clare forced a smile but wasn't sure what to say.

"Kellie thinks I should be talking to Dad," he said, studying her closely, as though the neighbor girl's opinion would

influence her. Clare wasn't particularly interested in what
Kellie thought, but she knew how difficult the last two years
had been for Alex, knew how badly he missed Michael.

"Kellie's right," she said briskly. "You and your father
should be communicating."

"You don't mind?"

His obvious relief was painful to hear. She swallowed and
said, "Alex, you're my son, but you're also your father's."

"I can't forgive him for what he did."

"I know," Clare whispered. She sipped her Coke in order
to hide the trembling in her voice, although she was fairly certain Alex had noticed.

Her son glanced at his watch, did a startled double-take
and bolted out of the chair. "I'm late for soccer practice."

"Go on," she said, waving toward the door.

"Dad said he might start coming to my games," Alex
said, the words rushed as he hurried to the back door.

"Alex—"

"Sorry, Mom, gotta go."

Oh, great! Now she had to worry about running into her ex
at their son's soccer games. And what about his girlfriend—
was she going, too? If Alex chose to have a relationship with
his father, that was one thing, but Clare couldn't, *wouldn't*, be
anywhere in Michael's vicinity when he was with Miranda.

The anger inside her remained deep and real, and Clare
didn't trust herself to control it. But under no circumstances
would she embarrass her teenage son, and if that meant not attending the games, then so be it. Almost immediately, the resentment sprang up, as strong as the day Michael had left her.
He'd already taken so much! How dared he steal the pleasure
she derived from watching Alex play soccer? How dared he!

For a long time she sat mulling over her conversation with Alex. She knew how relieved he was to have this out in the open. Alex had been on edge for a while now, and she'd attributed his tension to the upcoming SATs. But it wasn't the tests that were bothering him, or his relationship with his girlfriend or even his part-time job. It was Michael. Clare was positive of that.

Once again her ex-husband had gone behind her back.

January 15th

I got the job! There was never any doubt I'd be hired. Dan Murphy nearly leaped across the desk when he realized what he had. He gave me everything I wanted, including the part-time hours I requested. He'll go ahead and hire a full-time manager and I'll be more of a consultant.

Damn, it feels good. I've never experienced this kind of spiteful satisfaction before—and I do recognize it for what it is. Until these last two years, I had no idea I could be so vindictive. I don't like this part of me, but I can't seem to help myself.

> "The teeth are smiling, but is the heart?"
> —Congolese proverb

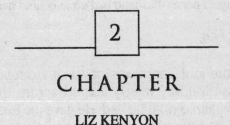

CHAPTER 2

LIZ KENYON

January 1st

For the first time in my fifty-seven years I spent New Year's Eve alone. I ordered in Chinese, ate my chicken hot-sauce noodles in front of the television and watched a 1940s movie starring Douglas Fairbanks, Jr. They sure don't make films like that anymore. Then at midnight, I brought in the New Year sipping champagne all by myself. I was in bed a few minutes after twelve, my thoughts full of Steve.

After six years the memories aren't as painful as they were in the beginning. What continues to haunt me are the last minutes of my husband's life. I wonder what went through his mind when he realized the huge semi had crossed the yellow line and was headed straight toward him. I wonder obsessively if his last thoughts were of the children or me, or if in those split seconds there'd been time to feel anything but panic and fear. I keep imagining his absolute terror when he knew he was about to be hit. Witnesses said he'd done everything possible to avoid the collision. At the last second, he must have faced the gut-wrenching horror of knowing there was nothing he could do. I've lived through my husband's final minutes a thousand times. The sound of the impact—crunching metal and shattering glass—the screeching tires, his scream.

I thank God he died instantly.

As I lay in bed, I remembered our last morning together, as clearly as if it had happened yesterday instead of six years ago. April twentieth was an ordinary day, like so many others. We both got up and dressed for work. He helped me fasten my necklace and took the opportunity to slip his hand beneath my sweater. While I made breakfast, Steve shaved. We sat across from one another and chatted about the morning news, then he kissed me goodbye as I left for the hospital. I remember he said he had a staff meeting that afternoon and might be late for dinner.

An hour later my high-school sweetheart and husband of thirty-one years was dead. My life hasn't been the same since; it'll never be the same again. I'm still trying to accept the fact that Steve won't come bursting through the front door wearing his sexy grin. Even now, I sleep on the far right side of the bed. Steve's half remains undisturbed.

The last three months have been hard. I knew when

Amy phoned to tell me Jack had been transferred to Tulsa that being separated from my daughter and grandchildren was going to be difficult. What I didn't realize was *how* difficult. Spending time with Andrew and Annie was what kept me sane after losing Steve. I miss them so much! And then, as if my daughter and her family moving to another state wasn't bad enough, Brian had to go and move out on his own. My son always did display impeccable timing.

He got a great job offer and I don't begrudge his taking it for a minute. And yet I have to admit I wish it hadn't happened quite so soon. It was hard to let him go and keep a smile on my face. I'm glad he's happy, though, and adjusting to life in Orange County. At the same time, I'm sorry he's living so far from Willow Grove. A couple of hours doesn't sound like much, but I know my son and he's far more interested in his social life than in visiting his widowed mother. That's the way it should be, I suppose, only I can't help feeling abandoned. First Amy, Jack and the grandkids, then Brian—and all at once I'm alone. Really alone.

I understand why I went to bed with thoughts of Steve. All my distractions have moved away. Even with the champagne, I couldn't sleep. After an hour I gave up trying. I sat in the dark with an afghan wrapped around my legs and contemplated my future. During the holidays I put on a brave front, acting as though I'm okay about being alone. I didn't want the kids to know how wretched I was feeling. Brian was here for Christmas, but he has friends he wanted to see and there's a new girl in his life.

I wonder if that son of mine is ever going to settle down. I guess he's one step closer now, living on his own; at least that's what I tell myself. Amy and I talked, but she phoned me and I know that with a single income and a large mortgage, they're on a tight budget, so the conversation was short. Normally I would've called back but it sounded so hectic there with the kids opening their gifts and all the craziness of Christmas morning. I put phoning off until later and then just didn't.

As for New Year's Eve, spending it alone was my choice. Sean Jamison casually suggested we get together for dinner. The problem with this doctor is that outside of his work, everything's casual with him. I'm not going to make the mistake of getting involved with a man who has a reputation as a womanizer (although I readily admit his interest flatters my ego). Besides, I'm older than he is. Not by much, six years, maybe seven, just enough to make me a little uncomfortable...not that I'd seriously consider dating him, anyway. My major complaint, in addition to the age difference, is that he's the exact opposite of Steve, who was genuine and unassuming. The good doctor is stuck on himself.

Still, he's obviously an interesting man. I wouldn't mind talking to him on a strictly-friends basis. Nothing romantic or sexual. Just conversation, maybe over coffee or a drink. After all, everyone can use another friend.

Speaking of friends, when Clare, Julia, Karen and I met after our last journal-writing class, we decided to continue the friendship by meeting for breakfast every Thursday. I came up with the suggestion that we should each take a word for the year. A word to live by, to help us focus our thoughts. A word to reflect what's happening in our lives and what we want to do and be. I'm not sure where that idea came from, probably some article I read, but it struck a chord with me.

Karen loved the idea, but then Karen's young and enthusiastic about everything. That's what makes her so much fun and why she fits in so nicely with the rest of us. We each bring something individual to the group, and yet we connect....

Last night, I started thinking about my word, considering various possibilitie. I still hadn't found the *right* word. It's like trying on dresses at Nordstrom's for a special occasion. I only need one and I want it to be perfect. It has to fit properly, look wonderful and feel great. My thoughts went around and around—Steve, my job, Amy and Brian. My word for the year—*love? Change?* Something else? Strangely, unexpectedly, I found myself remembering Lauren. Lauren. My baby daughter, whom I never had a chance to know. The baby I held in my arms so briefly. Born too soon, she died during the first week of her life, nearly thirty-six years ago. Every year on the date of her birth, Steve would bring me a bouquet of daisies, to let me know he hadn't forgotten her or the pain we endured as young parents, losing our first child. I'm really not sure why I started thinking about Lauren just then.

. Determined to dwell on the present and not the past, I turned my attention to searching out a suitable word for the year. It took a while but I found one that feels right for me. As I sat in the shadows, unable to sleep, listening to the grandfather clock tick away the minutes, my word came to me.

TIME.

I'm fifty-seven. In three years I'll be sixty. *Sixty*. I don't feel close to sixty and I don't think I act it. Still, it's the truth, whether I choose to face it or not. There always seemed to be so much time to do all the things I'd planned. For instance, I always thought that someday I'd climb a mountain. I don't know exactly why, just because it sounded like such a huge accomplishment, I guess. Now I know I won't be doing any mountain-climbing, especially at this stage of my life. It all comes down to choices, I guess. Besides, I've got other mountains to climb these days.

At one point, when we were in our twenties, Steve and I wrote a list of all the exciting things we were going to do and the exotic vacations we planned to take. The years slipped away and we were caught up with raising our family and living our lives. Those dreams and plans got pushed into an indefinite future. We assumed there'd always be time. Someday or next year, or the year after that. This is a mistake I don't intend to repeat and why the word *time* is appropriate for me. I want to be aware of every moment of my life. And I want to choose the right plans and dreams to fulfill in the years that are left to me. As soon as I settled on my word, I was instantly tired and fell promptly asleep.

Because I didn't go to sleep until after two, I slept late. I didn't make breakfast until past noon. I had the television on for company, but football's never interested me. That was Steve's game, though, and I found it oddly comforting to keep the channel on the Rose Bowl. For a few hours I could pretend that my husband was with me. The house didn't feel quite as big or as empty.

The house...that's something else I have to consider. I should make a decision about continuing to live here. I don't need three thousand square feet, but this was the home Steve and I bought together, where we raised our family. With the way real-estate prices have escalated, I'm sitting on a lot of money that could well be invested elsewhere.

It's silly to hold on to this place. The house was perfect when Andrew and Annie came to spend the weekend. Two rambunctious grandchildren need all the space they can get. It didn't bother me then or when Brian lived at home. We needed a big house in order to stay out of each other's hair, but for just me... Actually it's the thought of getting it ready to sell—sorting through all the stuff that's tucked in every nook and cranny, then packing up fifty-seven years of accumulated junk—that's giving me pause.

After Steve died, my friends advised me to delay any major decisions for twelve months. That's good advice to remember now. What I'm experiencing is a second loss. The loss of my children. I'm the only Kenyon left in Willow Grove.

I'm not entirely alone, however. My friends are here—those I've known all my married life, although it seems we've drifted apart since Steve died. My new friends live here, too—the women I met in the journal-writing class. I'm grateful to Sandy O'Dell for recommending I enroll. It was exactly what I needed, and I've learned a lot about myself through the process of writing down my thoughts every day. I wish now that I'd kept a diary when I was younger. Perhaps then I'd have found it easier to understand and express my own feelings.

Our teacher, Suzanne Morrissey, was an English professor assigned to the class at the last minute. Unfortunately, she didn't have any idea where to start, although she gave it a good try. Mostly, she had us read and critique literary journals, which was interesting but not all that useful. Still, I suppose keeping a journal isn't really something that can be taught. It's something you do.

What came out as I wrote in my journal was this deep sense of loss and abandonment I've felt since Steve's death. I'd assumed that after six years I'd dealt with all that, but coupled with Amy and Jack's move to the mid-West, followed by Brian's moving out...well, it's too much.

Amazing, isn't it, that I can cope with one crisis after another in my job at the hospital yet feel so defeated by the events in my own life?

Clare and I have been spending quite a bit of time together. That's probably natural, her being recently divorced and me a widow. Clare's situation is similar to mine a few years back when I realized, to my dismay, that my friends came in couples. Most of them are matched sets. Like me, Clare has come to recognize that she lost not only her husband but the framework of her social world, which crumpled right along with the marriage. Although her circumstances are different from mine, the outcome has been the same. The dinners, card-playing, even something as uncomplicated as a night at the movies—it all seems to be done in pairs.

Within a few months of Steve's death, I found myself drifting away from the very people I'd once considered our dearest friends. We have so little in common anymore that I couldn't see the point.

It was awkward, too. People didn't know what to say after the accident. In fact, I didn't want anyone to say anything. What I needed was someone to listen. Few of my friends understood that.

Clare's had a hard time adjusting to the divorce. Losing the people she once considered her friends is a bitter pill after everything she's been through with Michael. Maybe she should have taken it up with the attorney: custody of the friends. Who gets to stay friends with whom?

Really, it's odd that Clare and I should have bonded at all. We're very different kinds of people; in our previous lives, we probably wouldn't have felt the slightest interest in knowing each other. Right now, Clare's angry and bitter and struggling not to be. I still have my share of anger, too, yet I'm more accepting of the events that led me to this point (but then, my husband didn't leave me for another woman). I enjoy Julia and Karen, too, but it's Clare I identify with most. Perhaps it's the loneliness. That's something we both understand. Something people can't truly appreciate until they've experienced it themselves.

Time. This should be the best time of my life. I have a fabulous career. When I started out at Willow Grove

Memorial, I never dreamed that one day I'd end up as the hospital administrator. My children have grown into responsible adults. I had a wonderful marriage and I've got lots of memories to sustain me. Yes, this *should* be a good time, and it will be—once I learn how to live contentedly by myself.

* * *

Liz stared at the phone on her desk, dreading its ring. Her Monday had begun badly, and already she could see that this first week of the new year was going to be a repeat of December, with many of the same problems she'd faced then. The hospital was no closer to a new contract with the nurses' union, and the state health inspectors were scheduled for Wednesday afternoon. In addition, she'd had several hot flashes and been downing Chai tea with soy milk all morning. This was not a good start to the year, she thought gloomily.

She got up and removed her jacket, placing it on a hanger. Then she unfastened the top button of her white silk blouse and rolled the long sleeves past her elbows. Picking up a piece of paper from the desk, she fanned her flushed face and paused to look out the sixth-floor window to the parking lot below.

"I can see I've cornered you at a good moment." It was a deep male voice, one Liz immediately identified.

"Dr. Jamison," she said in a crisp, professional tone. He was rarely at Willow Grove Memorial. Most of his patients were admitted to Laurelhurst Children's Hospital, where he worked primarily with premature infants. Sean Jamison was an excellent pediatrician but he had a well-deserved reputation for being demanding, impatient and arrogant—an arrogance that found expression in his womanizing behaviour. Liz couldn't fault his medical skills, but when it came to dealing with staff, he could use a few lessons in emotional maturity.

"Come now," he said, his voice seductive, "we know each other well enough for you to call me Sean."

Liz stepped behind her desk and resumed her seat, motioning for him to sit down, too. "How can I help you?"

"This is more of a social visit." He claimed the closest chair and struck a casual pose, crossing his legs and balancing one ankle on the opposite knee. He relaxed, leaning back as if he was settling in for a long visit. "I stopped by to see how you're doing."

"I'm busy," she said quickly, thinking he might have time for chitchat but she didn't.

He ignored her lack of welcome. "How was your New Year's Eve?"

So that was it. He'd asked her out—well, sort of. What he'd done was propose that they get together, the invitation flavored with sexual innuendo, and she'd promptly refused. Although she'd been a widow for six years, Liz rarely dated. Opportunities were available, had she been interested. For the most part, she wasn't.

"I had a lovely night. What about you?" From Sean's reaction she'd realized it wasn't often a woman turned him down. Liz had certainly heard all the rumors about Dr. Jamison. He was tall, sandy-haired and craggy-faced, with an undeniable presence; comparisons to Harrison Ford were regularly made—by women from twenty to sixty. Sean possessed the ageless appeal of a man who was smart, handsome, wealthy and single. The hospital was full of gossip about him, and more than one of the female nurses had fallen under his spell. Divorced for ten years, Sean Jamison seemed to consider himself a prize to be caught. He never dated anyone for long and Liz disliked his arrogant approach in romance as much as she deplored his indifference to staff relations.

Liz and Steve had met in high school, and other than the normal ups and downs that were part of any long-standing relationship, they'd had a good, solid marriage. She wasn't interested in a fling, no matter how handsome or wealthy the man.

Sean's attention confused her, although she'd never allow him to see that. From what she understood, he generally went out with women several years younger than he was. While Liz kept fit and watched her diet, she wasn't a trim thirty-year-old. With loving humor, Steve had suggested that her hourglass figure had begun to show an hour and ten minutes. She still smiled whenever she thought of that.

"Stayed home New Year's, didn't you?"

"Yes," she admitted, and crossed her arms, letting him know she wasn't open to a discussion involving her private life, "but as I said, I had a perfectly lovely evening."

"All alone?"

"I happen to enjoy my own company." Standing, she braced both hands on the edge of her cherrywood desk. "I'm sorry to cut this short, but I have a meeting in ten minutes."

"I'm willing to give you another chance to go out with me."

"No, thanks."

He grinned, dismissing her rejection as though it was her loss, not his. Then he stood and turned away, ambling toward the door.

"Sean," she said, shocking herself just a little.

His smile firmly in place, he raised his eyebrows. "Change your mind?"

"As a matter of fact, no," she said, knowing that for some reason she didn't want this conversation to end the same way the others had.

"No?" He arched his eyebrows again, affecting a look of mild surprise.

"This is the second time you've stopped by my office to ask me out."

He didn't comment.

"I've turned you down both times," she reminded him. "And I'm wondering if you've asked yourself why."

"It's self-explanatory," he murmured. "You're afraid."

"It's more than that."

He shrugged carelessly, and she could practically read his response. *No big deal.* Plenty of women willing to take him up on his offer.

"It's your attitude."

For the first time in their lengthy association, Sean appeared to be at a loss for words.

"I'm not some bimbo you can schmooze into bed. This might come as news to you, but there's more to a relationship than what happens between a man and a woman in the bedroom."

He stared at her, as if daring her to continue. "I happen to think you're one of the finest pediatricians in this state," she went on. "I respect your diagnostic and medical skills, and I've seen the way you are with the children. My regard for your professional abilities is immense. But your manner with most people in this hospital leaves a lot to be desired, and frankly I'm not impressed."

"Is this the long version of why you're not interested in dating me?" he asked with barely disguised disdain.

"Actually...I'd like to get to know you."

His look implied that he wasn't sure he should believe her. "You have an odd way of saying so."

Despite his apparent indifference, she knew this couldn't be easy on his ego. "I suspect there's more to you than meets the eye."

"Great. Your place or mine?"

Liz wanted to groan out loud. He hadn't heard a word she'd said! "Neither." She held the door for him and added soberly, "When you're ready to see me as an intelligent, mature woman whose professional interests are compatible with yours, let me know." She leaned against the open door. "Otherwise you're wasting your time."

"I doubt that," he said as he stepped past and paused to touch his lips to her cheek. "Give me a call when *you're* ready for some excitement in your life."

Liz rolled her eyes. *Forget it, Doctor. I have enough excitement just dealing with all the staff complaints against you.*

Some people never learned.

"The thing that makes you exceptional, if you are at all, is inevitably that which must also make you lonely."

—Lorraine Hansberry

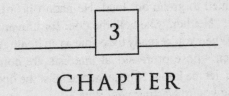

CHAPTER

KAREN CURTIS

January 1st

I woke at noon, nursed a tall, half-caff/decaff, double-sweet mocha latte for breakfast. Nichole phoned and wanted to hang out at the mall so we did. I ran into Jeff, who's working at Body and Spirit Gym, and we talked for a while. He's wasting his life teaching Tae-Bo classes to a bunch of overweight business executives who don't care about anything beyond their corporate image. I found it really hard to hold my tongue. Jeff is letting his talent go down the drain and it upsets me.

Jeff and I made a vow to one another in high-school

drama class that we wouldn't give up the dream. It was all I could do not to grab him by the shoulders and remind him. *It's too soon to throw away the future*, I wanted to tell him. Although I kept my mouth shut, I could see that Jeff was eager to make his escape. Hanging with me made him uncomfortable; it forced him to face what he's doing.

What bothers me most is knowing Jeff isn't the only one who's given up; Angie and Burt did, too. Last I heard, Sydney and Leslee had regular nine-to-five jobs. So did Brad. Out of the seven of us who made up the acting ensemble, there's only me left. I refuse to surrender to the mundane. I refuse to take second-best. I am an actor. Currently a starving one, but that's beside the point.

All right, I'll step down from my soapbox. God forbid, my biggest fear is about to become a reality. I'm beginning to sound like my mother, the Woman Who Always Knows Best. Now there's a thought to send me screaming into the night.

She and Dad insisted I get a college education. I disagreed, stood my ground, fought the good fight, but then—during a period of below-poverty-level existence—I caved. Hey! They might've won the battle, but the war's all mine. Since the day I was born, my domineering mother has attempted to run my life. From the moment I enrolled in college, she's demanded I be a teacher. A lifelong occupation, she said. A good job for a woman. Give me a break!

Well, I have that precious degree, but it's in history with a minor in education. I have no intention of using it, except where it'll aid my acting career. Fortunately

I've found a way in which to do that. Oddly enough, it also means my mother's kind of getting what she wants. But that's just a by-product. The important thing is I'm getting what *I* want.

You see, I'm a substitute teacher. Temporary and part-time. Due to the severe teacher shortage currently happening in southern California, anyone with a college degree—and it doesn't matter in what—can be hired as a substitute teacher. Isn't that incredible? I can have a degree in basket-weaving and qualify as a teacher for a whopping two-hundred-and-fifty bucks a day. Now, I don't mind telling you that's good money for part-time work. What's so fantastic is this: I can pick and choose the days I want to teach.

If I can fit subbing into my schedule, I spend two or three days a week in a classroom. Three at the most. That way, I still make enough money to support myself. On the days I don't work, I can audition for whatever's available.

Before the holiday break, my agent sent me out to audition for a TV commercial for a new kind of toilet brush. The district called first thing that morning and without fear of losing my job and without so much as a twinge of guilt, I said I had other plans. No problem; they simply went to the next name on the list. I headed out the door, knowing there'll be a job for me another day, if I want it. Sadly, I didn't get the commercial, but rejection's the name of the acting game.

As soon as school starts up after the holidays, I'll be ready to go back to substitute teaching. With so many days off, I have to admit I'm experiencing a bit of a cash-flow problem. Christmas didn't help, and neither did the cost of the one-day acting workshop last week. In fact, Jeff bought my latte for me today. But never mind, I'll survive. I always do, despite my mother's dire predictions.

I know I'm an embarrassment to her. She can't brag about me to all her society friends the way she does Victoria. My sister had the good judgment to marry an up-and-coming attorney who raised our family's social standing an entire notch. As far as I'm concerned, Roger is a twit, but no one's asking for my opinion. Good thing, too, because I'm not afraid to give it.

One positive aspect of Victoria's brilliant marriage is that Mom and Dad's attention is now focused on my sister and her first child instead of on me (although I do have to admit my nephew's a real cutie!). Basically Mom's been leaving me alone. Thank God.

I once heard a psychology professor say that the females in his class should take a good look at their mothers because in all likelihood we'll be just like them as we mature. Heaven help me—say it ain't so!

Mother means well. I can't fault her there. It's just that I'm such a bitter disappointment to her. Mom's so...so sterile. So predictable. There's no passion in her soul. I'm nothing like her, so I don't know how Professor Gordon could categorically state that in a few years I'll resemble her.

If anyone's like Mom, it's Victoria. To her, what people think and say is of ultimate importance. Social standing. Appearances. Money. None of that interests me. Well, maybe the money part, but only enough to get by.

Unless I earn it doing what I love, and that's acting. I guess I'm a woman who needs an audience. As a kid, my first word wasn't Mom or Dad but *look*.

When Mom heard I'd tried out for a role in a toilet-brush commercial, she freaked. The very thought of her daughter appearing on national television and admitting she cleaned toilets would have mortified her. However, I was thrilled with the part and devastated when I learned it'd gone to someone else. But that's all part of the business... And as Dad keeps saying, I've got a university degree to "fall back on."

Liz, Clare and Julia are three surprises that came out of me finishing my credits to get my degree. I love these guys and I'm thrilled we've decided to keep meeting, just the four of us. Me and three smart, professional women. I don't know what exactly I offer the group. My guess is comic relief.

The only reason I took that journal-writing class was because I needed an easy credit, and from the course description this was a simple way to raise my GPA. From the time I was a kid, I've kept a journal. There must be twenty spiral-bound notebooks tucked away in my bedroom closet, and they document my entire life. I signed up for the class, convinced I'd be bored out of my mind, and became friends with three of the most fascinating women I've ever met.

The English professor who taught the class was a real ditz. I knew more about keeping a journal than she did. But I didn't miss a single session, and that's only because of Liz and the others. They've kind of adopted me and I'm grateful. What I like is the perspective they give me, being older and all. Liz is the sort of person I wish my mother could be. Hey, if my mother wants to change me, then I should be granted the same privilege. If I'm a disappointment to her as a daughter, then she should know she's not my picture of the ideal parent, either.

Unlike Mom, Liz has been nothing but encouraging about my acting career. I know what the chances are of actually making it, but I can't allow unfavorable odds to dissuade me from trying. This is my dream. My life's ambition. If I don't go after it now, I never will. I honestly don't understand why my mother can't support my choices.

Enough already. This entire journal is turning out to be about my mother instead of me. I'd prefer not to deal with her today, or any day. Besides, Liz gave us an assignment.

I need a word before we meet next Thursday. We're all selecting a personal word. It's supposed to have special significance in our lives. Maybe I should use this as an acting exercise, do some free association.

Actually, I rather like that idea. Let's see. Acting. Goal. Audition. Wouldn't it be great to audition for a TV show like *Friends*? Friends. New friends. Liz, Clare and Julia. What I love about them is that they're so accepting of me. I love that they laugh at my jokes and make me feel a real part of the group. If only my mother were half as accepting...

That's it. I've got it! *Acceptance*. I want my parents to accept me for the person I am. I might not have turned out the way they envisioned, but I'm a good, decent, honest person. That should count for something. If my parents can welcome a twit like Roger into the family, they should be able to cope with a daughter who wants to act. And no, Mother, I don't think performing in a toilet-brush commercial is beneath me. I was emotionally wiped out for a week when someone else got the role.

ACCEPTANCE. *I've got to be me.* Ol' Blue Eyes really knew what he was talking about. Acceptance. I like it. My hope is that one day my mother will accept me for who I am and be just as proud of me as she is of Victoria.

*   *   *

Fresh from her first audition of the year, Karen excitedly wrote in her journal, sitting at her usual window table at Mocha Moments. The upscale coffee shop was bustling as customers moved in and out. She'd been the one to recommend the place to the breakfast group and felt good about the way they'd applauded her suggestion. Two summers ago she'd stood behind that counter, concocting lattes and serving up fiber-filled bran muffins. Despite being fired for repeated absences, she maintained a friendly relationship with the manager and often stopped by. She did almost all her journal-writing at this very table.

She was about to leave when Jeff slid into the chair across from her. "Whatssup?" he asked.

"Hey, Jeff." It was great to see him. One advantage of teaching those fitness classes was that he looked positively buff. His shoulders were muscular and his chest had filled out. He wore a winter tan so rich, it must have come out of a booth.

"Thought I'd find you in here," he said, flashing a smile. Oh, yeah, he was the California poster boy, all right, with his gorgeous white teeth, whiter than ever against the tan, and his sun-streaked blond hair.

"You were looking for me?" Her ego wasn't immune to having this hunk seek her out, especially here, where everyone knew her. They'd been together some in high school, but nothing serious. Her mother's generation called it dating, but all Karen and Jeff had really done was hang out together. They were part of the acting ensemble, and their commitment had been to that, which left little time for anything social.

"I've been thinking about what you said." Jeff leaned back in his chair and crossed his arms. "I'm impressed with your determination. You believe in yourself."

"Jeff, you've got as much talent as I do. You can make it, I know you can."

"Yeah, I know, but it takes more than talent."

Talent was cheap, Karen knew that; she ran into it everywhere. And as Jeff said, it wasn't enough. What made the difference was drive, determination and plain old-fashioned stubbornness.

A slim strawberry blonde with her hair tied back in a ponytail came into the coffee shop and walked up to the counter, where she placed her order. Jeff's attention drifted from Karen to the blonde. She wore navy-blue spandex and a matching sports bra, her face glistening with sweat. It was obvious that she'd recently been at the gym.

"You know her?" Karen asked.

"She's in one of my classes, along with her sugar daddy."

Karen stared. It couldn't be, could it? She'd once been at the mall with Clare, meeting for lunch, when a pert blond woman, younger than Karen, had emerged from Victoria's Secret. Clare had pointed her out. Could this be the woman

Clare's husband had dumped her for? Miranda Something? Nah. The world got smaller all the time, but it wasn't *that* small. "What's the name?" she asked.

"Miranda."

"No kidding! What about the sugar daddy?"

Jeff frowned as he mulled over the question. "I don't remember."

"It isn't Michael, is it?"

His eyes widened. "I think it might be. Yeah, I think it is. You know him?"

"Of him," she muttered, checking out the other woman. So this was Miranda. Clare had told her a bit of the story; Liz had told her more, and over the last few months, Karen had picked up a few of the nastier details.

"He dumped his family for her."

Jeff's attention went back to Miranda. "She's not bad-looking," he said thoughtfully.

"What's Michael like?"

Jeff frowned again. "You interested in him?"

"No." She wanted to clobber him for being so stupid. "He was married to a friend of mine. Tell me about him."

Jeff seemed to be at a loss. "I don't know." He shrugged. "Personality-wise he seems all right, but he's not much of an athlete. He had trouble keeping up with the class. Must've dropped out because I haven't seen him around lately."

"But you've seen Miranda?"

"Oh yeah, she's there."

"Really?" Karen's gaze narrowed as she studied the other woman more closely. "What do you think she sees in him?" she asked Jeff.

"The sugar daddy?" Jeff said. "What they all see. He's got money to burn."

Karen shook her head. "There's got to be more than that."

"Why do you care?"

"I don't. I told you, it's just that I know his ex-wife and I'm curious."

Jeff raised his eyebrows skeptically. "Miranda's okay, I guess. I don't know why she hooked up with this older guy, but as far as I'm concerned, to each his—or her—own. It's not exactly unusual, Karen. I see this sort of thing at the gym. The older men come in and hit on the younger women all the time. It's part of life in the fast lane."

"That doesn't bother you?"

"Me?" Jeff laughed. "Hey, I get more attention than I can handle. I'm happy to share the wealth."

"I wonder where *he* is this afternoon." Karen wondered aloud.

"Michael? Either she completely exhausted him and he's still too weak to get out of bed, or he's hard at work, keeping Miranda in the style to which she's become accustomed."

Karen doubted that. Clare's attorneys had taken her ex to the car wash. If Michael Craig was hard at work, the pennies weren't being spent on Miranda. Looking at the other woman, Karen felt a pang of something approaching pity. There had to be a real lack in this girl's life, or she wouldn't have hooked up with a man old enough to be her father.

* * *

January 16th

The first few times I filled in as a substitute were fun, but lately it's gotten to be like real work. Maybe it's because I've been with a group of junior-high kids all week. They wear me out fast. Makes me wonder if I was that energetic at their age.

Today I got smart. Instead of standing at the front of the class all day yelling at kids who have no intention of listening, I brought in a huge bag of mini-chocolate bars. That got their interest. Why did it take me so long to figure out that a little thing like bribery would tame the savage beasts? (Yes, I know I'm misquoting!)

Mom phoned. It's the first I've heard from her since Christmas. She wants to take me to lunch on Saturday. I agreed before I learned that Victoria was coming, too. Mom did that on purpose. She knows how I feel about Victoria. We don't get along. Why should we, seeing that we don't have a thing in common? Mom dotes on her precious Victoria. My entire childhood, I was treated like an outcast because I wasn't like my perfect-in-every-way older sister. Apparently, all that's changed since I started teaching. Now that I'm respectably employed (even if it's only part-time) Mom's free to brag about me to her friends, too.

As soon as I learned Victoria would be at lunch, I should've found an excuse to get out of it, especially when Mother told me we'd be going to the Yacht Club. But with my current cash-flow difficulties, I'm not above accepting a free lunch.

Jeff's been interesting lately. He seems to be fired up about acting again and asked if I'd recommend my agent. I was happy to pass on Gwen's phone number and apparently they're talking. I don't know if she'll take him on or not; that's not my decision. Jeff took me to dinner to thank me. There's a great Mexican place close to the gym. It was good to see him and talk shop, to recharge my own enthusiasm. Focus, that's what it's all about. No one else is going to do this for me.

I'm still bummed about not getting the toilet-brush commercial, but Gwen said the feedback from the director was positive. She's planning to send me for another audition with the same guy, although she warned me this next one involves a dog. She didn't say what kind, and asked if I liked puppies. Who doesn't? But let's not forget what W. C. Fields said about working with kids and dogs.... Anyway, the director liked me, but didn't think I was right for the role of fastidious housewife. I guess he must've taken a look at my apartment. Cleanliness and order aren't exactly my forte. If God had meant women to do housework, He wouldn't have created men first.

> "Parenthood: that state of being better chaperoned than you were before marriage."
>
> —Madeline Cox

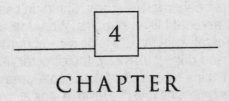

CHAPTER

JULIA MURCHISON

January 1st

This leather-bound journal is a Christmas gift from my husband and I've been waiting until today to make my first entry. My hope is that every morning I'll be filling the crisp, clean pages, writing out my thoughts, my concerns, my doubts, discovering who I am, one day at a time. That's something I learned in the journal class, along with a whole lot more. Taking that class was one of the best things I've done for myself in ages.

It's funny—here I am waxing poetic about this lovely journal that I've been waiting all week to start, and now that I have, I don't know what to write.

I'll begin with the kids, I guess. Adam and Zoe are

growing up before my very eyes. It seems like only yesterday that they were babies. Now they're both in their
teens, and before Peter and I know it, they'll be in college. It doesn't seem possible that Adam will be driving this year! He's champing at the bit to get behind
the wheel. He's ready, but I'm not sure Peter and I are.

Zoe at thirteen is turning into a real beauty. I look at
her, so innocent and lovely, and can hardly believe my
baby is already a young woman.

The Wool Station is a year old now. I've always loved
crafts, and opening my own small knit shop was a risky
venture. I thought about it for quite a while before making the commitment. Peter's encouragement was all I
really needed and he gave it to me. The store's been
wonderful for us both, bringing us together. And business has been good. The recent articles about all the
celebrities knitting these days certainly didn't hurt!
More and more women are looking for ways to express
themselves creatively; as well, knitting can calm and
relax you—as effectively as meditation, according to
one magazine I read.

Last year my shop brought in thirty-two percent
more than my projected gross income. (Peter's calculations, not mine. I'm hopeless with numbers.) At this
point, we're putting all the profit back into the business,
boosting the inventory at every opportunity. I'm not
making enough of a profit to draw a salary yet, but it
won't be long. A year, two at the most. I just wish I was
feeling better physically. Lately—ever since the flu bug
hit me before Thanksgiving—I've been under the
weather. I didn't bounce back nearly as fast as I thought

I would. Being thrust into the holiday season right afterward wasn't any help. I barely had a week to regroup when it was time for the big yarn sale. Then the shop was crazy all through December. Added to that were the usual Christmas obligations—buying gifts, wrapping them, sending cards, entertaining, etc. When I think about everything I've had to do, it's no wonder I haven't been feeling well.

Peter's mother flew in for Christmas Day. She had a meeting in the area and combined business with pleasure. I'm writing this with my teeth gritted. I don't enjoy dealing with my mother-in-law, who in my opinion never should have been a mother. She's cold and self-important and all she seems to care about is her career and her volunteer projects. Naturally, I'm grateful she had Peter, otherwise I wouldn't have my husband, but I swear the woman doesn't possess a single maternal instinct. Peter was left with a succession of nannies and baby-sitters most of his childhood while his mother climbed the corporate ladder and sat on one volunteer board after another. I don't disparage her commitment, just where it's been directed for the past forty years. It irks me no end that she can fly halfway across the United States for her causes, but practically ignores her only son and her grandchildren. Okay, enough. I've already written copious pages about my relationship with my mother-in-law.

Onto a far more pleasant subject, and that's the Thursday Morning Breakfast Club. We're each supposed to choose a word for the year. I've been giving it some thought, but my mind was made up almost from the minute Liz mentioned the idea. I wanted to wait to be sure this is truly *my* word. Experience tells me my first instinct is often the best. Still, I've taken this week between Christmas and New Years to mull it over, and I think I'm going to go with *GRATITUDE*.

I want to practice gratitude. I know that sounds hokey, but instead of concentrating on the negative, I want to look at the positive side of life. After that horrible flu, I'm grateful for my health, and yes, I can even find reasons to be grateful for my mother-in-law. (She must have done *something* right, considering how Peter turned out.)

I've decided to start every journal entry with five things for which I'm thankful. I'm calling it my *List of Blessings*. That way I can begin my day on a positive note.

I feel the breakfast club has become my own personal support group. Every Thursday at 8—what a treat! And to think that I never would have enrolled in the journal-writing class if not for Georgia. Leave it to my cousin to con me into something I didn't want to do, because *she* refused to go alone. Sure enough, I sign up for the class and three weeks later Georgia drops out. But I didn't feel abandoned since I'd met Liz and Clare and Karen by then and we'd bonded like super glue. I stayed in the class so I could be with them.

It began with the four of us meeting after class. We'd go to the Denny's restaurant near the college for coffee. Then when the session was over, Liz suggested we continue meeting. She's the one with all the good ideas. It made sense that we get together at the same time as the original class, but with teenagers at home it's difficult for me to take one night a week out of my already heavy schedule; doing that was hard enough while the course was in session. Trying to find a mutually agreeable time proved to be the biggest challenge. I suggested we meet for breakfast, and everyone leaped on that. Sometimes the obvious solution isn't immediately noticeable.

Georgia's sorry she dropped out of the class. I haven't invited her to join our breakfast group. Perhaps it's selfish of me to keep my newfound friends to myself, but I need this. I need them. The things we talk about, the things we share, are not always for Georgia's ears. She might be my best friend and my cousin, but I wouldn't want any part of the group's conversation to be repeated. Georgia, God love her, couldn't keep a secret if her life depended on it.

Peter and I didn't do anything all that exciting to bring in the New Year. The kids were with friends at church for an all-night youth program. We went out to dinner with the Bergmans. It's tradition now that we spend New Year's Eve together, but I wasn't really up to it this year. I would have preferred a night with just the two of us, but I didn't want to disappoint either Peter or our friends. We played cards and at the stroke of midnight, Peter opened a bottle of the best champagne we could afford and we toasted the New Year.

I didn't mean to get sidetracked. My word is *GRATITUDE,* and the first thing I'm going to do is write my

List of Blessings just so I'll remember to keep counting them. Then, seeing that the house is quiet for once,
I'm going to take a long nap.

COUNTING MY BLESSINGS
1. New beginnings.
2. My husband and his mother. God bless her!
3. Good friends like the Bergmans.
4. The sound of Adam's laughter and the sweet
   beauty of my daughter.
5. Sleeping for ten uninterrupted hours.

* * *

"Hi, Mom." Zoe walked into the kitchen not more than
ten minutes after Julia woke up from her afternoon snooze.
New Year's was always a lazy day around their house. Her
thirteen-year-old daughter fell into the seat across from her,
landing clumsily in the chair. Zoe laid her head on the
patchwork place mat and yawned. Her arms dangled loosely
at her sides.

"Did you have a good time last night?" Julia asked.

"Yeah," Zoe murmured with no real enthusiasm.

Julia knew that the church youth leaders had kept the kids
active with swimming and roller-skating, plus a number of
games that included basketball and volleyball. The night
ended with a huge breakfast at 5:00 a.m., and from there
everyone went home. Peter had picked up Adam and Zoe at
the church, and Julia had assumed they'd sleep for much of
the day. She was wrong.

"Did you and Dad have fun without us?" Zoe asked, as
though she expected Julia to announce that the evening had

been intolerably boring without their daughter to liven things up.

"We had a wonderful, romantic evening," she said, wanting Zoe to realize that she and Peter had a life beyond that of being parents.

Zoe frowned. Yawning again, she stood and made her way back to her bedroom.

"What was that all about?" Peter asked, coming in from the family room where the television was tuned to one of the interminable New Year's Day football games.

"Haven't a clue," Julia said, secretly amused.

"Come sit with me," Peter invited, holding out his hand.

A dozen objections ran through her mind. The kitchen was a mess and she was behind with the laundry, but she couldn't refuse him.

They snuggled up on the leather couch with Julia's head on his shoulder and his arm around her. It was peaceful; the only sound came from the television, the volume kept purposely low.

"I saw you writing in your new journal," he mentioned absently, his gaze on the TV.

"It's perfect," Julia said, cuddling close and expelling her breath in a long sigh.

Peter turned to study her. "What's wrong?"

"Nothing." He seemed to accept that, but Julia decided to confide in him about her gratitude plan. "Do I complain too much?" she asked, not certain she was going to like the answer. "The reason I ask is that I want to make an effort to be more appreciative."

"Really." Peter's gaze wandered back to the screen.

"I'm making a list."

"Good for you."

Julia doubted he'd even heard her. Still, she continued. "I want to work on me this year."

"That's nice, sweetheart."

Julia stifled a groan. "The kids are growing up and before long it'll be just the two of us."

"Hey, I'm in no rush," he joked.

"I'm not, either, but it's inevitable. Adam will get his driver's license this year and we'll be lucky to see either him or the car after that." Their son was a responsible boy and it would help Julia immeasurably not to be transporting him to and from track practice, which was an irony of its own. Driving him to the track so he could run.

"Zoe's going to be in high school soon," Peter added.

It seemed just the other day that their daughter was seven and missing two front teeth.

Peter slipped his hand inside Julia's blouse and cupped her breast. "I like the way we christened the New Year." His mouth nibbled at her neck with a series of kisses that grew in length and intensity. Julia straightened, and their lips met in a kiss they normally reserved for special nights.

"There *are* advantages to one's children growing up," Peter whispered, as his hands grew bolder with her breasts.

"Oh?"

"They seem to stay in their rooms a great deal more."

"That they do," Julia agreed, twining her arms around his neck and luxuriating in his kiss.

"Mom. Dad." Adam walked into the family room, his face clouded with sleep.

Peter quickly removed his hand and an embarrassed Julia tucked in her blouse.

Their son took one look at them and frowned darkly. "What's going on?"

"Ah...nothing," Julia mumbled, glancing away.

Adam wandered into the kitchen and made himself a cup of hot chocolate.

"I thought you two would be over the mushy stuff by now," he muttered disgustedly as he returned. "It's embarrassing to catch your parents in a lip lock."

"You just wait," Peter told his son. "When you're forty, you'll see things very differently."

Adam gave them an odd grimace, then carried his cup back toward his room. "I'm going online," he announced as he disappeared down the hallway.

"Where were we?" Peter asked and reached for Julia again.

"Advice is what we ask for when we already know
the answer but wish we didn't."

—Erica Jong

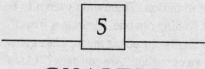

CHAPTER

CLARE CRAIG

"This is so nice," Liz Kenyon said, sliding into the booth
across from Clare in the Victorian Tea Room on Friday afternoon. Clare dredged up a smile, although the year wasn't
beginning well. Barely two weeks into January, and the issues
with Michael were once again staring her right in the face.

Clare was pleased—no, she was *relieved*— to see her
friend, even though they'd had breakfast with the others just
the day before. There were things she needed to talk about
that she wasn't comfortable saying in front of the whole
group. Liz was the person who'd understand. Who might
even have some practical advice or at least encouragement.

The restaurant was close to Willow Grove Memorial where
Liz worked as administrator, which made it convenient for
both of them.

A decisive woman, Liz picked up her menu, looked at it for no more than a minute, then set it aside.

Clare required much longer to make her selection, but only because she found it difficult to concentrate. Her head reeled, and making the simplest choice seemed beyond her at the moment. Spinach salad or a Monte Carlo sandwich? It wasn't a life-and-death decision but it took more effort than she was able to muster. There didn't seem to be a dish appropriate for spilling out one's heart to a friend.

When she finally closed her menu, Clare glanced up to see that Liz was watching her. "Are you okay?" Liz asked quietly.

With anyone else, Clare would have plastered on a phony smile and offered reassurances. She didn't think she could fool Liz. Nor did she want to.

Just as she was about to explain, the waitress arrived to take their orders, and looked to Liz first.

"I'll have the seafood sauté salad," Liz said and handed her the menu.

The woman nodded. "Good choice," she murmured.

She turned to Clare, but by then neither the spinach salad nor the sandwich sounded appetizing. "I'll have the same thing."

"Very good," the waitress said in the same approving tone she'd used earlier.

Liz waited until the woman was out of earshot. "I thought you didn't like seafood."

"I don't."

"Then why'd you order the seafood sauté salad?"

Clare wasn't aware of what she'd ordered; furthermore she didn't really care. She hadn't planned this lunch so she could eat. She needed support and advice, not food. "Oh, well," she muttered.

"Clare, what is it?" Liz studied her, staring hard. "Something to do with Michael, no doubt?"

Clare nodded and chewed at her lower lip. "Alex and Michael have been meeting behind my back," she said bluntly. "I knew they were talking—Alex admitted as much shortly after the first of the year. Then on Tuesday, Alex said he wouldn't be home for dinner because he was working late. It was a lie. I phoned the computer store and learned that Alex had left before five."

"You asked him about it?"

Clare nodded. "He'd gone to dinner with his father. He didn't mention Miranda, but I suspect she was there, too." The knot in her stomach tightened at the thought of her son dining with her ex-husband and his live-in lover. The pain never seemed to go away. Whenever Clare felt she was making progress, some new crisis would emerge. Some emotional stumbling block—like this one. She just hadn't expected it to involve her youngest son.

"It bothers you that Alex is seeing his father?" Liz asked.

"No." Well, she didn't really *like* it, but she was committed to her sons' right to communicate with their father. In any event, that part wasn't nearly as troubling as the lie. "I don't want to stand in the way of the boys having a relationship with Michael. Our differences don't have anything to do with Mick or Alex."

"Is that lip service or do you really mean it?" Liz had a way of cutting straight to the heart of the matter.

"I mean it—at least I think I do. Sometimes it's hard to know. I'm just so angry with Alex."

"Alex, not Michael?"

"Michael, too, because it seems to me that Alex is imitating his father's tactics. He didn't want to admit he was having dinner with Michael, so he did it without telling me."

"But he *did* tell you he'd been in contact with his dad."

That was true enough. "Alex said Michael had *phoned* him. Well, this is a lot more than a simple phone call. What I object to most is the secrecy. As if my not knowing was somehow supposed to protect me."

"What did Alex say when you confronted him?"

By the time her son had walked into the house, Clare had been so angry she'd barely been able to speak to him. To his credit, Alex didn't deny seeing Michael. He calmly told her where he'd gone, then he went to his room, leaving Clare to deal with impotent rage. She was convinced this was Michael's revenge for her taking the job at Murphy Motors.

"Alex lied to me, and I think Michael encouraged him."

"You don't know that."

"I know my ex," she snapped.

"Clare," Liz said softly. "I'm on your side, remember?"

"I know...I know. Part of me is relieved that the ice between Alex and Michael is broken. I mean, I realize how difficult our divorce has been on Alex. He was always so close to his father." She felt herself tense as she thought of the pain her ex-husband had inflicted on their family. Poor Alex had been put in an impossible position. He loved both his parents and yearned to please Michael as well as her. *That* she could understand, but not the lie. Surely he knew what his dishonesty would do to Clare when she found out.

It wasn't only his relationship with her that Michael had destroyed. Mick and Alex weren't getting along, and Michael was the source of that trouble, too. He'd managed to drive a wedge between the two brothers, and Clare feared that was about to happen between Alex and her, too.

"On his way out the door recently, Alex oh-so-casually said that Michael might be attending the soccer games. Now I find out he'll be there tomorrow afternoon."

"And you won't be there if your ex is?"

"Can you blame me?" She scowled. "At least Miranda's not coming. Alex told me that much, anyway."

"No, I don't blame you." Liz patted her arm. "It's perfectly understandable," she said. "I wouldn't go under those circumstances, either."

Clare instantly felt better. "What am I supposed to do now?"

"What do you mean?"

Michael had already taken so much from her, and Clare couldn't tolerate his stealing more. "I enjoy watching Alex play. I'm the one who drove him to and from soccer practice for the last twelve years. I'm the soccer mom who treated the team to ice cream and slumber parties. The other parents are my friends."

"And not Michael's?"

"No," she said so loudly that it attracted the attention of several people dining nearby. "No," she repeated, more softly this time. "It'll be awkward for everyone if Michael shows up. Not just me, but the other parents, too. His presence will be a distraction. Besides, I'm scheduled to work the concession stand."

"I see," Liz murmured with a darkening frown. "But I—"

The arrival of their meal interrupted whatever Liz was about to say. The waitress brought two huge Caesar salads piled high with sautéed shrimp, clams, scallops and an assortment of other seafood delicacies. Clare studied the salad for several minutes before she could produce enough enthusiasm to reach for her fork.

"Oh, Clare, you don't know what you're missing." Liz eagerly stabbed a fat shrimp.

Clare shook her head. "I'm not hungry," she said. Pushing aside a mound of seafood until she uncovered the lettuce, she managed a mouthful of that.

"Back to your dilemma," Liz said, looking thoughtful. "I think I have a solution."

Clare glanced up hopefully. "Tell me."

"You're going to contact Michael yourself."

"What?" The fork slipped from Clare's fingers and fell to the table. She retrieved it, glaring at her friend. "You must be joking."

"Not at all."

"I have no intention of *ever* speaking to Michael again."

Without a pause Liz sprinkled some pepper on her meal. "Don't you think that's a bit drastic?"

"There's no reason on this earth important enough for me to contact Michael Craig."

"What about your sons? Aren't Mick and Alex important enough?"

"Well, yes...but it's been over a year—"

"Does it matter how long it's been?"

"No, but..." Clare returned, growing frustrated. Liz made it sound like a foregone conclusion that she'd sort this out with her ex-husband in a calm and reasonable fashion—when reasonable was the last thing she felt. "Let me get this straight. You're suggesting I phone Michael and the two of us would decide which games each of us will attend."

"Correct." Liz beamed her an encouraging smile.

"Why do I have to be the one who calls him? Can't Michael understand this is awkward for me—for all the parents?"

"It's unlikely. Men don't think that far ahead."

Clare hesitated, doubting she could swallow another bite. The knot in her stomach had doubled in size. She'd come to Liz looking for suggestions and sympathy. Her friend had offered a little of both, but Clare didn't think she could follow her advice. "I—I can't do it," she admitted, her voice faltering.

"You can and you will."

"I don't think so...."

It'd been almost thirteen months since she'd heard Michael's voice. Clare wasn't sure she could trust herself not to respond to him in anger. Liz couldn't understand that, couldn't know. If her friends had any idea of the rage she still battled, it would frighten them. In fact, the intensity of her own anger terrified Clare.

"I'm not saying you should ask him to a picnic lunch."

Despite herself, Clare smiled.

"All you need to do is make a phone call. Suggest you split the games up. He attends half and you attend the other half. It'll save you both a lot of angst."

"Couldn't I write him instead?"

"Sure. Just as long as you communicate with him."

"I prefer that we not speak." Clare wondered why she hadn't thought of that sooner. A written explanation wouldn't leave room for any misunderstanding. She'd be clear, succinct and to the point. Michael believed in brevity—he was always quoting that line from *Hamlet* about "the soul of wit." Well, then he'd find her message very witty, indeed.

"Whatever's most comfortable for you," Liz said.

"I wouldn't even need to write a letter," Clare went on, feeling inspired. "I could take the schedule and underline the games he can attend and tell him to stay away from the ones I've selected." She wouldn't mention the dinner. That was between Alex and his father—but ultimately she blamed Michael. He'd lived a lie for several months before confessing to the affair, and apparently her son had learned that kind of deception.

"You could mail him the schedule," Liz agreed without much enthusiasm. "When's the next game?"

"Tomorrow." As she answered, Clare realized that even with overnight delivery service, Michael wouldn't get the schedule in time for the upcoming game. Okay, so she'd skip this game and make arrangements for someone to replace her at the concession stand. No big deal—only it was. It was a very big deal.

"Clare?"

Clare looked up.

"You didn't hear me, did you?"

"Hear what?" Her friend was right; she'd been so caught up in her own thoughts she hadn't heard a word in the last few minutes.

"I said your heart will tell you the best thing to do."

Now that was an interesting concept. If she'd listened to her heart, Michael would have died an agonizing death two years ago.

And she'd be making license plates in a federal pen.

> "You may be disappointed if you fail, but you are doomed if you don't try."
>
> —Beverly Sills

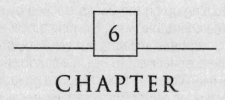

CHAPTER

LIZ KENYON

January 19th

Here it is Friday night, and I'm nestled in front of the television watching *Seinfeld* reruns and munching on popcorn while writing in my journal. I'm almost tempted to feel sorry for myself. Even Tinkerbell is showing signs of sympathy by sitting in my lap. Steve never did understand my affection for cats, but he liked Tinkerbell.

Work this week was dreadful. I hardly had a chance to deal with one crisis before I was hit with another. I don't even want to *think* about the nurses going out on strike. I didn't get home before seven once this entire week, so it's no wonder that all I want to do is hibernate in front of the TV tonight!

The weekend's already arrived, which means an entire week has vanished. It makes my word for the year, *time,* all the more significant. I'm feeling a sense of panic—a sense that if I don't do something *now,* the weeks and months will slip through my fingers. Spring will be here, and then autumn and I won't have accomplished any of what I've planned so carefully—travel, catching up on the books stacked by my bed, doing some charitable work, learning a new skill.

At the Soroptimist meeting last week, before everything at the hospital went to hell in a handbasket, Ruth Howe, the head librarian, talked about a program at the juvenile detention center. The librarians are taking turns reading the Harry Potter books over the loudspeaker system each night. There are only three librarians, and Ruth came to the meeting hoping to find more volunteers.

It seems she read about such a program in Grand Rapids, Michigan. She spoke of the difference this had made in the young people's lives. When she first proposed the idea here, the detention center told her there was little they could do to control noise. She was welcome to come in, but the staff couldn't guarantee that anyone would listen.

Ruth and the other librarians weren't dissuaded. As expected, their reception was lukewarm in the beginning, but they faithfully showed up every night, despite the hoots and hollers of protest. Apparently the disruptions didn't last long. According to Ruth, the reading period is the only hour of the day or night when the facility is absolutely quiet. For many of the teenagers, this is the first time in their lives anyone has ever read to them.

I knew right away that it was something I'd like to do. Ruth got a couple of volunteers at the meeting, and I was tempted to sign up right then, but I hesitated....

A while back, I read something smart. The exact wording escapes me now, but I remember the meaning: I need to stop and consider my options before volunteering for something. If I say yes, then I need to think about what I'm saying no to first. In other words, if I were a volunteer reader at the detention center tonight, what *wouldn't* I be doing? The answer is obvious—sitting in front of the TV watching reruns, writing in my journal and fighting Tinkerbell for the last of the popcorn.

Where would I rather be?

But after a work week like this, would I feel like trekking all the way to Charleston Street to read a chapter or two aloud. I don't know how good I'd be. Reading to my grandchildren is vastly different from trying to entertain adolescent felons. Still, it appeals to me and is something I'm going to consider.

I'm afraid this whole year will speed by, and I won't have achieved anything. I'm determined to make *some* kind of contribution to society.

When I volunteer for an activity, I'm going to do so wholeheartedly and with absolute commitment. That means I have to pick the right one....

> "If you think you can, you can. And if you think you can't, you're right."
>
> —Mary Kay Ash

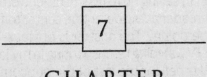

CHAPTER

CLARE CRAIG

At noon on Saturday, Clare checked her e-mail messages for the sixth time that day. It hadn't occurred to her until after her lunch with Liz that she could contact Michael without speaking to him *or* sending a letter. E-mail. She hardly ever used it herself, since she considered it a time-waster. But she remembered that Michael, who was enthralled with anything high-tech, did much of his correspondence by e-mail.

Her message had been short.

Michael:
Unless you want an
embarrassing scene, I suggest
you stay away from Alex's

soccer match this afternoon.
Next Tuesday's game is all
yours.
You will receive a schedule
of which games I'm attending.
You're free to attend the other half.
It's up to you.
Hugs and kisses.
Not!
Clare

It'd taken her most of an hour to write those few words. She hoped the small touch of humor would help.

By one o'clock, her stomach was so queasy she couldn't even manage a cup of tea. She hadn't asked him to e-mail her back but had assumed he would, if for no other reason than to confirm that he'd read her message. Clare needed his assurance that he'd do nothing to embarrass her in front of her friends. That was all she wanted; she should have known better than to expect cooperation from Michael.

At two, just an hour before she had to leave for the game, Clare found herself so agitated, she actually broke into a cold sweat. Her queasiness had developed into full-blown nausea. When she couldn't bear it another minute, she reached for the phone.

She hadn't called the dealership in a very long time, but the telephone number was still on her speed-dial. She punched the button.

"Craig Chevrolet," the receptionist answered in a light, pleasant voice. "How may I direct your call?"

"I'd like to speak to Hollie Hurst," Clare said. No reason to talk to Michael when his secretary knew his schedule.

"One minute, please."

She was put on hold while an easy-listening radio station played in the background. The receptionist was new. Clare hadn't recognized her voice and wondered briefly what had happened to Janet Harris. She wanted to think the young mother had quit in protest when she learned of the divorce, but that wasn't likely. Everyone at the dealership had stayed on. Being rational, she had to suppose it wasn't a question of personal loyalties. Michael, after all, signed the checks.

"Michael Craig."

"What happened to Hollie?" Clare demanded before she thought to slam down the receiver without identifying herself.

There was a short, shocked pause, followed by, "Clare?"

"I asked to speak to Hollie."

"She has the weekends off."

Clare should have remembered that. Recovering quickly, she lowered her voice. She hadn't expected him to pick up the phone, but she wasn't about to let him know the effect he'd had on her. "Well, hello, Michael."

"What's the matter, did the support check bounce?" He didn't bother to disguise his sarcasm.

Clare smiled. Thanks to Lillian, Michael was required to send her a hefty check each month. He had to be feeling the pinch.

"I guess you haven't read your e-mail?" she asked.

"Should I have?" He snorted. "I've been busy, you know. Making money I don't get to keep. You sent me an e-mail? What for?"

"I'd hoped to avoid this," she muttered.

He sighed as though bored with the conversation. "Instead of exchanging useless banter, get to the point, would you?"

"It's about Alex—"

"I have a right to see my son," Michael snarled, not giving her a chance to explain.

"Did I say otherwise?" she returned in like tones. "Whether Alex sees you or not is his decision. Not yours and certainly not mine."

"I agree," he said, but his voice still held an edge.

"See? We can agree on some things," she said with exaggerated sweetness.

"Is there a legitimate purpose for this call?"

"Yes." She made herself sound calm and businesslike. "I understand you're planning to attend Alex's soccer games."

Clare could feel Michael's tension through the phone line. "Do I need to call my attorney? Is that what you're saying?"

Clare laughed softly. "I can't believe you want to tangle with Lillian Case again."

"I'll do whatever is necessary if you try to keep me away from my son."

"Michael, really!" Her aggrieved tone was convincing, she thought. She was a better actress than she'd realized. Hell, Karen should take lessons from *her*.

"Do you enjoy this? Do you get some kind of sick thrill out of making my life miserable?"

Clare could almost see his face getting red. She could feel his anger—and she loved it. The exhilaration she experienced now made up for the months of strained, angry silence. Had she known the sense of triumph, of satisfaction, this would give her, she'd have phoned him much sooner.

"I didn't say anything about preventing you from seeing

his games, did I?" she asked, again maintaining a cool, even voice. "If you want to go to Alex's soccer matches, that's perfectly fine with me."

"You're damn straight I have a right to see Alex play!"

If he'd shut up long enough, he'd learn she had no objection to his being there. "Michael, listen," she said, trying to keep the smile out of her voice.

"No, *you* listen! If I need to have my attorney call yours, then so be it."

"Michael—"

"I'm warning you, Clare, I've had all I can take of your bullshit."

"I didn't phone to start an argument."

"The hell you didn't."

"No, really. All I wanted was to set up some sort of schedule. For Alex's sake." She waited for him to react.

"What do you mean?"

"Alex's soccer games. I was hoping we could be civilized about this. The last thing I want is to get the courts involved. Not again."

"I don't relish the idea myself."

She'd just bet he didn't. "You have to know how difficult it was for me to call you."

Silence.

"We haven't spoken in more than a year. I've put up with the situation, got on with my life. It isn't like I've made a pest of myself, is it?"

"Just say what you have to say."

"You want to attend Alex's soccer matches. So do I. He's my son, too. But I think it'd be best all the way around for us not to show up at the same time. That way Alex can concentrate on his game instead of what's happening off-field between his parents."

"All right," Michael said, sounding guarded.

"I tried to avoid this. If you'd read your e-mail, we could have solved everything without all this...unpleasantness."

"I assumed Alex told you I was planning to be there."

"Originally, all he said was that you might start coming to the games. Thursday night, he dropped the news—he said you were coming to *this* game. But that's not enough notice for me. Keith's mother asked me to help her at the concession stand and it would be irresponsible to cancel at the last minute. If you'd gotten back to me, I might have been able to find a replacement. I can't now."

"In other words, you don't want me there this afternoon."

"Exactly."

He hesitated. "All right, but I'm going to next Tuesday's game."

"And I won't," she said sweetly. "Now, was that so hard?"

"No," he admitted grudgingly.

"Goodbye, Michael," she said and replaced the receiver. Slumping in the chair, she buried her face in her hands. It shocked her to realize how badly she was trembling.

She'd talked to her ex-husband. During their conversation, she'd felt rage, exhilaration and a sense of bitter victory.

What she felt now was despair.

> "The worst part of success is to try finding someone
> who is happy for you."
>
> —Bette Midler

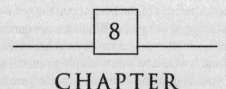

CHAPTER

KAREN CURTIS

This lunch was destined to be even worse than Karen had imagined. As she stood in the foyer of the yacht club restaurant, she saw her mother pull up to the valet attendant and step out of her Lexus. Catherine Curtis wore a pastel-blue linen dress with a huge wide-brimmed matching hat and white gloves. Victoria looked like her twin, only she had on a tailored blue suit with a white collar. Apparently, three-year-old Bryce was spending the day with his father. Karen was disappointed; she'd looked forward to seeing her nephew. It went without saying that her mother and sister weren't going to approve of her jean overalls from Old Navy.

"Hi, Mom," Karen said, standing when they entered the yacht club.

Her mother's expression spoke volumes. "Karen." She leaned forward and presented her cheek for Karen to kiss.

"You're early," was her sister's sole greeting.

"My car's on the fritz, so I took the bus." Actually, Karen had made a day of it, shopping in Willow Grove that morning, then catching the bus out to the marina. She'd read the current *Vanity Fair* during the forty-minute ride, which had been relaxing and enjoyable, calming her before the inevitable confrontation.

Her mother and Victoria exchanged glances.

"Don't worry," Karen said in a stage whisper. "No one saw me get off the bus. Certainly no one who'd connect me with the two of you."

"Shall we have the hostess seat us," her mother said, ignoring the comment.

"Yes, let's," her sister piped in with phony enthusiasm. The two headed in the direction of the restaurant, leaving Karen to trail behind. The temptation to slip away was almost overwhelming, but the consequences wouldn't be worth it. So, like an obedient child, she followed them.

The hostess directed them to a window table and handed them menus before she left. Karen sat across from her mother and sister and gazed out at the marina for several minutes. The water sparkled in the January sun, and boats of every size lined the long dock. Everything from the simplest sailboat to yachts with price tags that ran into the millions.

"What looks good to you?" Victoria asked Catherine. Karen observed, not for the first time, that Victoria rarely made a decision without consulting their mother.

"The crab and shrimp quesadillas, perhaps. With a small avocado salad."

"That's exactly what I was thinking," Victoria said, closing her menu. "What about you?" she asked Karen.

"I'll have the crab Louis."

"Excellent idea," Catherine said approvingly.

At least Karen had enough ordering savvy to please her mother.

Catherine set aside her menu and focused her attention on Victoria. "How's Roger?"

Karen frowned. She'd hoped all conversation regarding the twit would be over by now. They'd probably spent the entire drive out to the club admiring Roger and then discussing Karen—her lack of direction, her fanciful dreams, her multiple shortcomings.

Victoria smiled benignly at her mother. "Busy, as always."

Wishing now that she'd taken the time to change out of her jean overalls and into her new skirt, Karen leaned sideways, searching for the shopping bag. She'd purchased the skirt in a close-out sale, so the price was affordable. It would be the perfect thing to wear on the days she subbed for the school district; in fact, it was the most respectable thing she'd bought in years. She could hurry into the ladies' room and make a quick change. That way, she'd definitely gain a few points with her mother. Easy points.

Pretending to be enthralled by the witless conversation taking place, Karen edged the shopping bag closer with her foot. She reached for it without success, so she had no option but to lean down, peek under the table and grab it.

All at once her mother turned and glared at her accusingly. "What exactly are you doing?" she demanded.

Caught in the act, Karen flashed a brilliant smile. "What do you mean?"

"You're squirming around like a two-year-old in church."

"Oh," she said innocently. "I was getting my bag."

"Your bag? Whatever for?"

"I thought I'd change into my new skirt."

Her mother nearly leapt out of her seat, then regained control. Tight-lipped, she spoke in a slow, stiff voice. "This is neither the time nor the place for you to be changing your clothes."

"I intended to put it on in the ladies' room," Karen told her.

"At the Yacht Club? Karen, do I need explain that the facilities here are not dressing rooms?"

"Mom, don't get all worked up. I should've changed earlier. I meant to...." She hadn't, but then how could she know that her mother and sister would arrive looking like they expected to have lunch with the Queen of England?

"Please." Her mother was breathing hard. "Don't embarrass me any further."

"Embarrass you?" Karen asked in a puzzled voice. She'd had good intentions, and for her efforts she was rewarded with a hard, cutting look.

"Shall we order?" Victoria said, her voice slightly raised as the waitress approached the table.

Both her mother and sister ordered the shrimp and crab quesadillas, plus avocado salads as planned, and Karen asked for the crab Louis. As soon as the waitress left, the three went quiet.

Victoria was the first to speak, asking Catherine about her bridge club. It wasn't long before the two of them were involved in a meandering conversation about people who were of little or no interest to Karen.

She tried to comment once, but was cut off when their lunch arrived. The discussion continued with Karen feeling more and more out of place. It was just as bad as she'd feared. Worse.

Suddenly her mother turned her attention entirely on Karen. "You haven't contributed to the conversation once."

There was a very good reason for that; she couldn't get a word in edgewise. "What would you like to know?" she asked carefully.

Catherine raised her eyebrows. "You could tell me about school. I always knew you'd end up teaching. You're so good with children."

Karen felt gratified by the unexpected praise.

Victoria stared at her with more enthusiasm than necessary, obviously taking their mother's cue. "Mom's right," she announced. "You'd make a wonderful teacher. You're enjoying it, aren't you?"

"Well, *enjoying* isn't exactly the word I'd use. It's, um, a challenge."

"All children are a challenge," her mother said pointedly.

"How many days a week are you working?" Victoria asked.

"No more than three. Two's better, but that's pushing it financially. Teaching is exhausting and the little darlings couldn't care less, especially when they've got a substitute."

"Personally, I think teachers are grossly underpaid," Victoria said.

Her sympathy didn't go unappreciated, and Karen found herself warming to her sister. "Me, too. What I'm really hoping for is a part in a commercial. I'm trying out for another spot next week. The director liked me the last time and wants to see me again."

Her mother's eyes narrowed and she put down her fork.

"Naturally, I'd love a role in a weekly series," Karen added.

"But according to my agent I need a few credits first. She thinks I should get my feet wet doing commercials. Plus, the pay isn't bad, and there are residuals. Then she wants me to audition for a part in a situation comedy."

With great deliberateness, her mother smeared a dollop of sour cream on the quesadilla, and Karen saw that her hand shook as she did so.

"Even if you got a part in a commercial, you'd go back to substitute teaching, wouldn't you?" Catherine asked.

"Well, yes, I suppose, but teaching is only a means to an end for me. I—"

"I thought you were finally putting your college degree to good use. Your father and I paid a great deal of money for your education. You can't imagine how much it distressed us to hear that you're more interested in...in cleaning toilets than in making something worthwhile of your life."

"It wasn't exactly a housecleaning job," Karen muttered. "Not that there's—" She stopped abruptly, forcing herself to swallow the rest of her retort. "I deeply appreciate my education, Mom." Which was true, but only because it allowed her to support herself while trying out for acting roles.

"Are you seeing anyone?" Victoria asked, once again diverting the conversation to a different subject.

"Jeff and I went out the other night."

"Jeff Hansen?" her mother asked. "Isn't he the boy from your high-school drama group?"

"Yes, he's teaching aerobics classes at Body and Spirit Gymnasium, and wants to get back into acting. I hooked him up with my agent."

"Oh, dear," Catherine murmured. "I play bridge with

his mother.... She was so pleased when Jeff got a real job, and now this."

"Why do you think acting is such a horrible career?" Karen burst out. "Can you explain that to me once and for all?"

Her mother sighed as though the answer should be obvious. "You mean you don't know? Just look at the class of people who become professional actors! They're all involved with drugs and not a one of them stays married. These women get pregnant and most don't even bother to marry the child's father. They have babies by a bunch of different men. They take their clothes off for the whole world to see. They have absolutely no morals, Karen—and everyone knows the successful ones sleep with their casting directors. The unsuccessful ones are just unemployed."

"That's so unfair," Karen cried, not caring that she'd attracted attention to herself. "You're judging me by what's in the tabloids. There's more to being an actress than what those headlines scream and furthermore, you can't believe everything you read!" The only true thing her mother had said was that remark about unemployment, which Karen chose to ignore. "Besides," she added, "not all actors use drugs."

"I've read about those Hollywood parties with the drugs and sex and God knows what else. I don't want my daughter mixing with that kind of crowd."

"Mom, you don't know what you're talking about!"

"I do. They'll lure you in. Weird cults and casting couches..."

"I'm not doing drugs," Karen insisted. "I've never come across a cult, weird or otherwise. And I've never even *seen* a casting couch, let alone done anything on one."

"What about this director? He wants you to audition for another commercial?"

Karen sighed. "It's for a dog-food commercial. He told my agent he liked my style and—"

"I'll just bet he did," her mother said, lips pinched tight. "Exactly what are you going to have to do for that role?"

Enough was enough. As politely as possible, Karen placed the pink linen napkin on the table and picked up her purse. "I think it'd be best if I left." She kept her voice expressionless.

"Sit down right now!" her mother ordered. "I won't have you making a scene by leaving before we've finished our lunch."

Karen reached down for her shopping bag and held onto it with both hands. "If you're worried about creating a scene, then I suggest that the next time we meet, you refrain from insulting me."

"All I said was—"

"Thank you for lunch." Karen did her best to hide her anger—and disappointment. She should've known better. Whenever she saw her mother, they always played out some version of this encounter. The simple truth was that her family didn't respect her and had no confidence in her talent or, apparently, her judgment. And that hurt.

"Karen, wait," Victoria pleaded, rising to her feet.

Karen shook her head, fearing that if she stayed she'd end up saying something she'd regret.

> "What a wonderful life I've had! I only wish I'd realized it sooner."
>
> —Colette

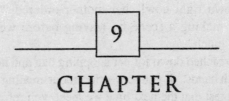

CHAPTER 9

JULIA MURCHISON

January 25th

List of Blessings
1. The security of order. Everything neatly in its place. Yarn arranged by color to form a rainbow effect in the store.
2. The welcome feel of my mattress after a long day on my feet.
3. Music and the way it nurtures me.
4. Zoe's snit fits when everything doesn't go exactly as she wants it to. Could this daughter of mine be taking after me? Never!

5. My customers, eager to create something lasting and beautiful.

I haven't been feeling well for weeks, and with my new-found determination to take care of myself physically, I've made an appointment to see Dr. Snyder, even though it means I'll have to leave the Thursday breakfast group early. The last time I saw Dr. Snyder was November when I had that dreadful flu bug and was flat on my back for an entire week.

I guess I haven't fully recovered from that virus. I assumed I'd feel better after the holidays, but I don't. In fact, I seem to be more tired now than ever. I can't seem to get enough sleep. Twice last week, I went to bed before Adam and Zoe did.

Peter, who almost never complains, mentioned it at breakfast this morning. But this is more than exhaustion. I'm constantly running to the bathroom. Could be I've developed a bladder infection. I certainly hope not.

My whole system is out of whack. Even my period is late. I'll be forty this year, but I didn't expect menopause to hit me this early. If it did, though, I wouldn't complain.

Reading this, it almost sounds like I'm pregnant. It's been so many years since I had the kids, I didn't put it together until just this minute. But that's impossible. I've been on the pill for years, and with the flu and the busyness of the season, Peter and I haven't been that active sexually.

After Zoe was born, Peter intended to have a vasectomy, but because we were both so young, the doctor advised us to hold off making that decision for a few years. We talked it over and agreed to wait. I went on the pill once I'd finished nursing, and all concern vanished from our minds. Five years later, Peter made an appointment for the vasectomy; I can't remember why he didn't go through with it. He'd gone in for his preliminary exam, but after discussing it with the specialist, he decided he wanted to think this through more carefully. So I continued taking the pill. Which is ninety-nine percent effective...

I'm *not* pregnant. I couldn't be. I'm methodical about my vitamins and my birth control pill. I don't miss. Ever. I refuse to think like this. A pregnancy now would be a disaster. I'm finished with the baby stage and couldn't imagine going back.

No need to borrow trouble when a baby simply isn't a possibility. Besides, I'd know if I was pregnant. I did with Adam and Zoe. Both times, within ten days of conception, I sensed the changes in my body. It felt as though everything inside me had welcomed this new life taking shape. There's no celebration happening now.

I'm ending this right here because I can't deal with what I'm thinking. *I am not pregnant.* I don't want to be pregnant and I refuse to torment myself with something that has only a one-percent chance of being true.

* * *

"I don't need a urine test," Julia insisted, meeting Dr. Lucy Snyder's unyielding gaze. "I already told you a pregnancy just isn't possible."

Dr. Snyder rolled the stool closer to the examination table where Julia sat, clutching the paper gown to her stomach, her bare feet dangling.

"The pelvic exam suggests otherwise," Doc Snyder said quietly.

"I *can't* be pregnant." Julia didn't know why she felt the need to argue when a pregnancy was now almost a certainty. The queasy feeling in the pit of her stomach had nothing to do with morning sickness and everything to do with her state of mind.

"With the pill, there's always that slight risk," the doctor murmured.

Julia adamantly shook her head.

"You say you never missed a pill? Not even once?"

"Not even once!" Julia cried, fighting back emotion so negative her voice actually shook.

Dr. Snyder read the chart. "What about when you had that flu virus?"

"I took my pills," Julia said.

"You kept them down?"

"Down? What do you mean down?" Julia asked.

"According to the chart, you suffered projectile vomiting for three days."

Julia's forehead broke into a sweat. "Yes... And I didn't eat solids for a full seven days." Her stomach hadn't tolerated anything other than weak tea and a few sips of chicken broth.

"I'd like you to have a urine test," the doctor said. "Just to be sure, one way or the other."

Numbness was spreading through Julia's arms and legs as she nodded. Dr. Snyder patted her shoulder and quietly slipped out of the room.

If she *was* pregnant, Julia could pinpoint the night it happened—after the tremendous success of her first yarn sale. She'd been incredibly happy. Adam and Zoe had spent the night

with her sister, and Julia and Peter had celebrated with a rare
evening out, followed by an incredible night of lovemaking.

After providing the nurse with the necessary sample,
Julia slowly dressed. Her fingers trembled as she fastened
the buttons of her blouse. She'd just finished when Dr. Snyder came into the cubicle with the results.

Their eyes met, and in that instant Julia knew the awful truth.
It was what she'd dreaded most. She was pregnant. Whatever
Dr. Snyder said after that was a complete blur. She walked out
of the office in a stupor and toward the parking garage.

The next thing Julia knew, she was at Benjamin Franklin
Elementary, the grade school where Peter had been prin-
cipal for the last four years.

"Mrs. Murchison, this is a pleasant surprise," the school
secretary said warmly.

For the life of her, Julia couldn't recall the older woman's
name, although she'd been working with Peter as long as
he'd been at Ben Franklin. Linda Dooley, she remembered.
It was Linda.

"Is Peter available?" Managing the question demanded
full concentration on Julia's part. Her head continued to
buzz, her mind skipping from one irrational thought to another. She'd left Dr. Snyder's not knowing where she was
driving or what she was going to say or do once she got there.
Obviously, she'd made a subconscious dedision that Peter,
her calm and reasonable husband, would supply the answers.

"You go on in." A look of concern came over Linda. "Is
everything all right, Mrs. Murchison?"

Julia shook her head. Nothing was right. Her entire life
was off-kilter. She didn't want this baby, didn't want to deal

with this pregnancy. Churchgoing, God-fearing woman that she was, her reaction would have shocked all who knew her.

"Julia?" Peter stood when he saw her. "What's wrong?" He left his desk and placed an arm around her shoulders, then gently guided her to a chair.

Julia sank down gratefully. Her legs had lost all feeling, and she felt on the verge of collapse.

Peter appeared to sense the gravity of the situation without her having to say a word. "What is it?" he asked. "Your mother?"

Julia shook her head again.

"Sweetheart, tell me."

Her eyes and throat burned with the need to cry, but she refused to allow it.

"You saw Dr. Snyder?" her husband prompted.

She nodded wildly. "The flu..." she managed, willing herself not to weep. Tears humiliated her. She wasn't like some women who used tears for effect. Nor did she look particularly fetching with red-rimmed eyes and a runny nose.

Peter's hands clasped hers. "It was more than the flu?"

Julia whispered, "Yes..."

"It isn't...cancer, is it?" Her husband had gone pale at the very word.

"No, you idiot!" she shouted, knowing even as she spoke how unreasonable she was being. "I'm pregnant!"

Peter stared at her blankly as though he hadn't heard or, like her, didn't *want* to hear.

"Don't look at me like this is a surprise or anything," Julia snapped. He was to blame, dammit! If he'd gone ahead with the vasectomy, they wouldn't be facing this situation now.

"Ah..." Peter straightened and buried his hands in his

pockets. "Were we planning on having a third child?" If this was an attempt at humor, she wasn't laughing.

"This is all your fault...."

His frown slowly evaporated into a soft, teasing smile. "You're joking, aren't you?"

"Do I look like I'm joking?"

"No..." He hesitated, confusion in his eyes. "You're really pregnant?"

Julia swore to herself that if he dared to smile, she'd slap the grin off his face.

"But how?" He shook his head as if he wanted to withdraw the question. "Not how, but when? I thought you were on the pill."

"I am on the pill."

"And you still got pregnant?"

"Yes...apparently I threw up the birth control pills when I had the flu a couple of months back."

"I see." His expression remained sober and concerned, but Julia knew her husband well enough to see that his reaction to the news in no way matched her own. Peter started to chuckle, but she cut him off abruptly.

"Don't laugh!" She wasn't kidding, either. A pregnancy wasn't a laughing matter. Not at this stage of her life. She was through with being a stay-at-home mother. She didn't regret any of it, but that phase was over now. There wasn't a single committee or volunteer job she hadn't done in the twelve years she'd been home with Adam and Zoe. She'd served as the Parent-Teacher Association president, been a Cub Scout leader for Adam, a Brownie leader for Zoe, an assistant soccer coach, Sunday School teacher, room mother and all the rest of it. She was still actively involved in her children's lives, but as teenagers they were less dependent, required less of her time. Finally, it was *her* turn, and she was unwilling and unable to go back and retrace her steps.

"You find this amusing, do you?" she yelled. "We have two teenage children, Peter. Can you imagine what a baby would do to our family?"

"Julia," her husband said, his eyes filled with sympathy. "A pregnancy isn't the end of the world."

"Oh sure, *you* can say that, but it isn't you who'll be getting up in the middle of the night! And what about Adam and Zoe? What about our friends? No one has a child at our age."

"It happens all the time."

"Not to us. Peter, you actually seem happy about this. I can't believe it!"

"I'm surprised, and obviously you are, too, but there are worse things. We'll adjust."

"You might, but I won't. I don't want this child." There, she'd said it, those dreadful words, but God help her, they were the truth.

Peter gazed at her as though he hadn't heard. "Give yourself time," he advised, as though all she needed was a few minutes to get over the shock.

"Time for what? Do you think that'll change my mind? Do you seriously believe that once I get used to the idea of being pregnant I'll feel differently?"

"Julia..."

"Why do you think our children's names start with A and Z? A boy, a girl. A to Z, and I was finished."

"Apparently not."

Julia jerked her purse strap over her shoulder and bounced out of the cushioned seat. "I can see that talking to you isn't any help at all."

"Julia..." Peter followed her outside his office and down the long empty corridor. "Listen, Julia. It's not so bad. Having another baby will be kind of exciting...."

Her husband didn't understand. Nor did her physician. As soon as she'd delivered the news—news Julia didn't want to hear—Dr. Snyder had distanced herself emotionally. Julia sensed it, felt it.

And Peter—sure, he'd been surprised, but he apparently shared none of her qualms. If anything, he seemed pleased. Thrilled, even. Excited.

Everything Julia wasn't.

> "Nobody has ever measured, even poets, how much
> the heart can hold."
>
> —Zelda Fitzgerald

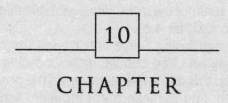

CHAPTER

LIZ KENYON

January 28th

I'm feeling depressed, and I'm not sure I want to an-
alyze the reasons. Perhaps it's just this time in my life.
I'm fifty-seven and alone. Never in a million years did
I think such a thing would happen.

Not to me.

The alarm wasn't set since it's Sunday, but I woke
at six anyway. After tossing for a half hour, I decided
I wasn't going to sleep any longer, no matter how
much I wanted to. So I got up and showered. When
the mirror cleared, I stared at my reflection and what
I saw made me feel like weeping.

When did those crow's feet appear? I don't remember noticing them before. It isn't only my eyes, either; there are lines at my mouth and neck that I swear weren't there a week ago. I looked old and beaten, and I'm feeling every day of my fifty-seven years.

Until recently—until I started a journal, in fact—I hadn't given much thought to age. Fifty-seven is still young. This morning, studying my reflection, I was forced to confront the truth. Fifty-seven *isn't* that young.

All at once it hit me.

As though losing Steve and having the children move away isn't bad enough, now I'm facing yet another loss, this one as devastating as the others. My youth. Oh, I don't mean that I thought I was still in my twenties or anything so foolish—just that I saw my life (and, admittedly, my looks) continuing into the future unchanged. And I know now it isn't true. There are supposed to be compensations for these losses...of beauty, health and endless possibility. Compensations like grandchildren, wisdom, insight. But as far as I'm concerned the trade hasn't been a fair one. My grandchildren are far away, and I'm definitely lacking in wisdom. All I feel is the loss and none of what I'm supposed to have gained.

Oh dear, I'm sinking to a new low. Self-pity. No. I won't allow it. I *refuse* to feel sorry for myself. Action must be taken and quickly.

To complicate matters, I'm convinced that Sean Jamison is partly responsible for this unwelcome and unappreciated epiphany. Rumor has it he's dating the new physical therapist.

I couldn't care less.

Obviously that's a lie—I do care—otherwise I wouldn't be writing about it. Nor has it escaped my notice that the woman is twenty years his junior and nearly thirty years mine. Naturally Sean finds her attractive. What man wouldn't? She's young, pretty and probably defers to him. I, on the other hand, am older (though maybe not wiser) and I have wrinkles. No contest there. Not that I'm interested in competing for Sean.

Really, it doesn't even make sense that I care. He isn't seeking what you'd call a meaningful relationship. He's attracted to me; he's made that plain and I have to admit I'm flattered. Truth be known, I'm attracted to him, too. I wish I wasn't, because it's clear that this is destined to be a dead-end relationship—if a relationship at all. Sean just wants me to blindly fall into bed with him.

Unfortunately I can't do that and be comfortable with myself. There's only been one man in my life and after thirty-one years with Steve, I can't get involved with a man who's looking for a bout of casual sex. To me, it has to mean more than a few hours of pleasure. I can't change the woman I am, even for Sean Jamison.

I shouldn't feel this disappointed. To his credit, Sean has been forthright about what he wants, but I'd hoped for something different from him. I've always believed there was real depth to the man. Apparently I was wrong.

In an effort to boost my spirits, I phoned Amy after breakfast. My Sunday-morning chats with my daughter and grandchildren are often the highlight of the weekend for me.

As always, the conversation made me feel better. I

told her I'd decided to be a volunteer reader at the Juvenile Detention Center and Amy applauded my decision. Getting out and doing something positive for the community is bound to improve my frame of mind.

Amy asked about the breakfast group and I was able to give her an update on everyone. She hasn't met any of these women who've become my friends, but she likes to hear about them whenever we talk. I think Amy wishes she could be part of such a group.

After I'd chatted with Andrew and Annie, I thought about my Thursday-morning friends. They're more than that, of course; it's just a quick way to distinguish them from my other friends. We're each at a completely different point in our lives, and yet there are similarities, too. I see myself in Clare's anger and grief, in Karen's passion, in Julia's sense of domesticity and order. And do they see their future selves in me? I think they must. I also think these friendships have become the truest and deepest I have.

I'm so thankful I met Clare, Karen and Julia. I need my friends, and never more than now.

> "The only thing that seems eternal and natural in motherhood is ambivalence."
>
> —Jane Lazarre

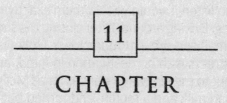

CHAPTER

JULIA MURCHISON

January 26th

List of Blessings
1. A clean kitchen.
2. A bathroom close to the bed.
3. Truth...whether I want to face it or not.
4. Dark clouds that match my mood.
5. My family.

Last night, I didn't come home until after ten. By that time Peter and the kids were worried sick. The minute I walked into the house, Adam flew into the kitchen and demanded to know where I'd been. He sounded like an outraged parent. Talk about role reversal. Zoe was next;

she burst into tears, stormed back into her room and slammed the door. Then Peter laid into me—only he didn't utter a word. He simply looked at me, and his expression said it all. He was furious with me for having worried them. He stomped out, leaving me alone in the kitchen.

I sat there for another hour. Had any of my family come in to listen, I would've told them exactly what I'd been doing. Driving around. After closing the shop, I left the strip mall and drove through town. I followed long, winding streets with no destination in mind, and then headed out to the highway. I went as far as McDonalds, where I had milk and a muffin, and turned back.

Peter was as upset as the children, but surely he of all people could understand why I did what I did. I couldn't look my children in the eye knowing I'm pregnant.

While I was driving around, I found myself at the cemetery for some oddball reason. My grandparents are buried there, but I barely remember them so I don't feel any deep connection. It probably had more to do with the way I was feeling. As if my life, the one I've been so careful to plan and nurture, is over. Corny symbolism, I know, but that's how depressed I felt.

Options are available to me. I'm well aware of what they are. I only wish I was the kind of woman who could walk into a clinic and be done with it, get rid of the burden. I never dreamed I'd even consider such a possibility. At first, the appeal of it was strong. No one need ever find out. Peter, of course. He wouldn't like it, would try to change my mind, but I know my husband and he wouldn't stop me. I thought about it, I really did. Even now, when I can be completely and totally honest, I can't make myself write the word.

An easy solution is what it sounds like, and for some women it might be the answer, but not me. I know myself too well. I hate that I'm pregnant, but I won't undo what's already been done.

Adam and Zoe realized something was wrong, but they seemed to think Peter and I had had a disagreement. I'm always home for them in the evenings. They're accustomed to having dinner on the table and me there to help with homework and to chat. Both of them were upset with me. Peter was, too. Later, when he'd cooled down, he asked if I'd eaten dinner and I told him yes. He said he'd ordered pizza for the kids. I went to bed and Peter came and asked if there was anything he could do. I told him no.

I thought of calling Georgia, but didn't. Much as I love her, I just don't know how to tell her about this. She's been married four times, twice to the same man, and she's childless. How could she understand what I'm feeling?

I could talk to the women in the breakfast group— except that I'm not ready. I'll tell them in a few weeks.

I wonder if the baby senses how much I don't want to be pregnant. Adam and Zoe were gifts; not this baby.

Is it wrong to hope I miscarry? The fact that I'm almost forty might mean the baby's at risk. There's a far higher chance of birth defects. Oh, God, I can't think about that now.

I feel so guilty and ashamed. Mostly I feel miserable.

* * *

Julia sat in her rocking chair, knitting by rote as her mind rapidly spun its thoughts. Thankfully, business had been slow all afternoon. The success of her shop was largely a result of the personal service she gave her customers, many of whom had become friends. Women—and a few men—visited her store; they trusted her advice and sought her opinion concerning their creative efforts.

Today, though, the quality of her service wasn't exactly what it should have been.

Preoccupied as she was, Julia found herself prone to mistakes. Irene Waldmann had certainly pointed that out. The older woman was a regular customer, and earlier that day Julia had made an error in calculating how much yarn she needed for her latest project. Mrs. Waldmann had noticed and complained at length. The woman's gruff personality made her hard to please, anyway, and she wasn't the type who would tolerate mistakes. Luckily, it'd been discovered early.

A car pulled into the parking space in front of her shop window and Julia glanced up to see Peter. They'd barely spoken that morning. Her husband and children had tiptoed around her as if they weren't sure what to expect.

As soon as they were out the door, Julia's stomach went queasy and the little coffee she'd managed to down was lost in a quick dash to the bathroom. This morning sickness was far worse than she'd experienced during the previous two pregnancies.

Maybe it was the baby's revenge for being unwanted.

When he walked into the store, Peter presented her with a bouquet of yellow daisies, her favorite flowers.

"To what do I owe this?" she asked, hating the edge in her voice but unable to hide it.

"I came to see how you're feeling."

She jerked on the yarn, pulling it unnecessarily hard. "Just great."

Peter took the empty rocker next to hers. If he'd tried to talk, forced her into a conversation, she might have been able to maintain her ugly mood. Instead he sat with her, gently matching his rocking motion to hers, the flowers in his lap, and said nothing. Not a word.

"This is God's big joke, you know," Julia whispered after a moment. "My word, I mean."

"Your word," he repeated. "What are you talking about?"

"My word for the year," she snapped, thinking it was obvious. He knew everyone in the breakfast club had chosen a word.

"Oh, you're talking about your friends from the journal-writing class. You told me what your word was, but I've forgotten."

Fearing she was about to break into tears, she just shook her head, not trusting herself to speak.

"Was it *surprise?*" he asked.

This was his idiotic attempt at humor, she assumed. Another time, she might have found him amusing, but not in her current mood.

"Gratitude," she managed.

"Gratitude," he said slowly.

"Funny, isn't it?"

He stopped rocking and placed his hand on her forearm. Julia continued knitting, afraid that if she stopped now she'd crumble completely.

"I'm sorry, honey," he said. "You're right, this is my fault."

"And mine... I should have— I don't know. Oh, Peter, I feel so awful, so guilty and ashamed."

"What did you do that's so terrible?" he asked, and rubbed his hand down her arm.

"I don't want this baby! I can't even think of it as a baby. Every child deserves to come into a loving home."

"I love the baby," he said.

He might have thought he was comforting her, but he wasn't. "Fine, you go ahead and love the baby. I don't. Maybe you should waltz on down to The Baby Emporium and stroll through the aisles and be happy. I'm not! And hearing you tell me how pleased you are isn't helping a damn bit." Her voice rose until she was close to yelling.

"Sorry," he said and raised both hands. "You're right. I won't say anything more."

"What are we going to do?" she wailed. "How will we cope?" She hoped he had some answers because she was completely out.

"I don't know," he answered.

"Neither do I."

They rocked a few more minutes while Julia knit, periodically tugging at the yarn, her fingers moving with confidence. She was working on a mohair sweater to display in the store. Maybe it should've been booties or a little blanket, she thought darkly, but even looking at the baby yarn was beyond her.

"Do you think we should tell the kids?" he asked.

Julia couldn't believe he'd pose such a question. "Absolutely not!"

He didn't respond for a long moment. "The only reason

I ask is because they were both so worried about you last night," he finally said. "You should have phoned."

"I know." She did feel bad about upsetting her family.

"Adam and Zoe are old enough to recognize when something's wrong. I think we should tell them. They have a right to know."

In other circumstances she would have agreed with him, but not now. "I don't think it's a good idea."

"Why not?"

"What if I miscarry? I could, you know. I'm going to be forty soon...and when you're older, the risk of a miscarriage is much higher."

"I realize that, but the baby might be perfectly okay, too. There's at least an equal chance of that."

"Still, this pregnancy isn't a sure thing, so we shouldn't say anything yet," she said, holding onto her one hope of escape. She wouldn't do anything to terminate the pregnancy, but if nature should take its course...

"I'm sorry you're so unhappy about all this," Peter murmured.

"I'm sorry, too," and Julia was, more than she cared to admit.

"Don't worry, sweetheart, everything will work out. Somehow or other."

"Somehow or other," Julia echoed. She wished she could feel differently about this baby. Her husband loved children. If it'd been his decision alone, they would have had a houseful of kids.

Peter glanced at his watch. "I'll head home and get dinner started."

Julia nodded.

"Don't worry, honey," he said, bending down to kiss her on the cheek.

A moment later, the door shut behind him. Julia tossed a ball of yarn at it.

Just as she was ready to close for the day, Georgia strolled in, sparking with her usual energy. They were cousins and best friends and about as opposite as any two women could be. In high school, Julia was the student-body president and class brain. Georgia was the flighty cheerleader with more beauty than common sense. She flitted in and out of marriage every few years, the way some people bought a new car. But despite their differences Georgia was the one person Julia knew she could trust.

"So. What's going on?" Georgia asked loudly, arms spread wide, bracelets clanking. Her cousin always made an entrance. It was her trademark. Everyone expected it of her.

"What—what do you mean?" Julia couldn't imagine how Georgia had heard her news.

"I haven't talked to you all week." Her cousin stood before her, hands now resting on her hips. "Must be *something* happening." Georgia's long blond hair was artfully arranged atop her head, with tendrils dangling down in all the right places. She was dressed in loose black clothes and heavy silver jewelry and looked stunning.

"I'm pregnant," Julia blurted out. She couldn't tell her mother, her sister or her own children, but felt no such compunction when it came to Georgia.

Georgia responded by sinking into the rocker recently vacated by Peter.

"Pregnant?" she repeated as though it was a foreign word whose meaning she wasn't quite sure of. "As in baby?"

Julia covered her face with both hands and burst into tears.

"Oh, Julia, you're not joking, are you?" Georgia got to her feet and grabbed her purse, spilling half the contents. Makeup, a hairbrush and loose change rolled across the table. "Damn, I need a cigarette."

"I thought you quit."

"I did, I'm down to five a day." She found what she was looking for, placed the low-tar low-nicotine cigarette between her lips and flicked her lighter. Stepping to the door, she took one deep puff, aiming a stream of smoke outside, then frowned at the cigarette. "I swear these things are giving me a hernia."

"It was an accident," Julia explained.

"All pregnancies are accidents," Georgia insisted. "What did Peter say?"

"He's thrilled."

"Naturally," she snorted and inhaled deeply on the cigarette. Leaning against the doorjamb, she waved her free hand toward the bouquet of daisies lying on the counter. "Peter?"

Julia nodded.

"I should've known."

Reaching for a tissue, Julia loudly blew her nose. "I haven't told anyone else—other than Peter."

"I was pregnant once," Georgia said.

"When?" They'd been close all these years, and this was the first she'd ever heard of it.

"Hell, I was just a kid."

"What did you do?"

"Not a damn thing. I lost the baby shortly after I married Ernie. I never would've married him otherwise."

Ernie was Georgia's first husband. The marriage lasted

all of two years, if that. Georgia had still been a teenager and Ernie was only a few years older.

"I always liked Ernie," she said with some regret. "But neither of us was cut out to be a parent."

Georgia rarely talked about her marriages, but Julia knew that Ernie had broken her heart. He'd managed a restaurant and apparently had something sweet going on the side with the pastry chef. The minute Georgia found out, the marriage was over. She'd married on the rebound—a mechanic, who had an affinity for the bottle. That marriage had turned into a love-hate relationship. When they were getting along, it was very good, and when they were on the outs, it was a free-for-all. They'd married and divorced twice before Georgia met her third and current husband. She and Maurice had been married a year and Julia hadn't seen him even once since the ceremony. She didn't know much about him, but Georgia appeared to be happy and that was all that mattered.

When she'd finished dabbing the moisture from her eyes, Julia glanced up and was stunned to see the tears trailing down Georgia's cheeks.

"Damn, I need a cigarette," she sniffled. She tended to punctuate her conversation with that remark.

"You have one in your hand."

"A real cigarette," Georgia said. "These aren't worth shit." Leave it to her cousin to make her smile. Julia started to laugh then, and soon Georgia was laughing, too. Without a pause, they were both weeping again, the border between laughter and tears invisible.

"Unbosom yourself," said Wimsey. "Trouble shared
is trouble halved."

—Dorothy Sayers

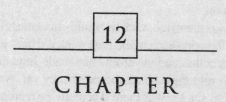

CHAPTER

THURSDAY MORNING BREAKFAST CLUB

Everyone had already arrived by the time Julia showed up
for the weekly breakfast meeting on the first Thursday of
February. Liz had ordered her usual coffee and croissant and
looked wonderful in her pinstriped power suit. Her dark hair
was stylishly short and utterly feminine. Julia knew her
friend's life was much easier now that the nurses' strike had
been averted. Liz's name had turned up in the local newspaper often in the past few weeks, and she'd played no small
role in the ultimate resolution.

Clare had her double-shot espresso and currant scone, and
sat next to Liz at the table for four. She looked less harried
now than she had when they'd first met, Julia noted; still,
the recent contact with her ex had thrown her, and her resentment and anger had quickly surfaced. She seemed to be

rebounding, though, and that was good for everyone involved—especially her sons. Julia didn't mean to be judgmental or critical; Clare had reason to feel the way she did. To Clare's credit, she'd made a gallant effort to get on with her life. She worked part-time and seemed less obsessive over the breakup of her marriage. Julia believed the group had been a good sounding board for her, and more than that, a real support.

Karen was there, too, with her multi-mix latte, a different flavor combination each week. Last week it'd been a coconut cream concoction and the aroma had made Julia nauseous. She hadn't told them about the pregnancy yet, wanting to delay it until she knew if there'd actually *be* a pregnancy.

Her three friends greeted her with welcoming smiles as she joined them. She ordered herbal tea and a blueberry muffin at the counter and carried them to the table where the others waited.

"Morning," she said, sitting next to Karen. "How's everyone this week?"

A chorus of "goods" followed. It was almost always like this. They started off slowly, each talking a little about the week that had passed, then gradually gaining momentum. Their lives were full of commitments, family obligations and stress. Outside of Thursdays, they rarely saw one another, but that had started to change. Liz and Clare got together occasionally; they seemed to have formed a close bond. And last Sunday afternoon, they'd all attended a movie.

Liz spread strawberry preserves across half her croissant as Karen animatedly described a recent audition for a dog food commercial. Apparently, the cocker spaniel had taken an instant dislike to her and growled every time she'd attempted to say her lines. Not surprisingly, she didn't get the part, but the way she told the story had them all laughing and offering sympathy.

"This director likes me, though," she concluded, "and Gwen, my agent, said she'd bring up my name the next time he's casting." She finished with a heavy theatrical sigh. "It seems my entire career rests on 'next time.' It really irritates me, too, because I love dogs and until the audition they've always loved me. You can bet I'll never own a cocker spaniel."

As they continued to talk about Karen's audition, Julia noticed that Liz had grown quiet. She wondered if her friend's lack of enthusiasm had anything to do with the recent troubles at the hospital. But the strike had been averted. Perhaps it was that doctor she'd mentioned a couple of times. Julia had caught on right away; Liz's offhand manner when she'd told the group about him had instantly signalled that there was more to the situation.

"Have you heard anything more from your doctor friend?" she asked.

Liz shook her head. It was obvious from the way she shifted in her chair and stared off into the distance that she didn't want to talk about Dr. Jamison.

"Is he bothering you?" Clare demanded. Her aggressiveness on Liz's behalf made Julia smile a little. Clare seemed ready to roll up her sleeves and do battle with Dr. Jamison.

"He's not exactly bothering me," Liz said, but Julia could tell she didn't like being put in the position of defending him.

Karen leaned across the table. "You're interested in him, aren't you? I thought you were when you first mentioned his name, and now I'm sure of it."

"I'm not," Liz insisted, but she didn't sound convincing.

"Who do you think you're kidding?" Clare said with a deep-throated laugh. "Somehow or other, the good doctor turns up in our conversation practically every week."

"Are you going to dinner with him? He asked you out again, didn't he?"

"As a matter of fact, he didn't and even if he did, the answer's the same. Really, I'm *not* interested."

"Yeah, right," Karen said good-naturedly. She propped her elbows on the table, clearly expecting Liz to supply more details.

Liz ignored her, paying careful attention to her croissant. "He hasn't stopped by the office in weeks, and from what I hear, he's seeing one of the physical therapists, which is perfectly fine with me."

"Is it?" Clare asked.

"Yes. I told you before I'm too old for him."

"Don't be ridiculous," Clare scoffed. "Besides, if he's as brilliant as you say, he'll soon figure out what he's missing."

"Valentine's Day is coming up," Karen said, raising her finely shaped eyebrows.

"Guys, I'm serious! I doubt I'd go out with him even if he did ask."

"You'll know when the time comes," Karen said confidently.

"Just be careful," Clare inserted. "Guard your heart." She dropped her voice on the last word, not meeting anyone's eyes.

"What about you, Clare?" Julia asked her. "How's the situation between Mick and Alex?"

A pained look came over Clare's face. "Mick isn't speaking to his brother yet, but I'm sure that eventually they'll settle this."

"You hate seeing your boys fighting about their father, don't you?"

Clare twisted her mouth. "Does anyone mind if we don't talk about Michael? I was just starting to get my appetite back."

They all grinned.

Clare relaxed, and Julia realized anew how hard her friend was struggling to keep the resentment out of her life.

"On a different subject, I'm thinking about selling the house once Alex graduates this summer," Clare said next. "I spent all week sorting through twenty years of junk, trying to decide what to do. I want to think positive, but it's damned difficult. When Michael and I built the house, it was with the intention of living there for the rest of our lives. That's why the master bedroom is on the main floor. We were looking to the future and didn't want to worry about climbing stairs when we hit our senior years."

"Then live there," Karen said. "No one's saying you have to move."

"No," Clare agreed, "but I'm not sure I can after Alex is gone. The house represents so much of what my marriage was to me, and now it's over. Everything I'd planned for the future is meaningless now."

"You'll make other plans," Julia assured her.

"I know," Clare said, sipping her espresso. "It just takes time."

"Have you talked to your mother lately?" Liz asked Karen.

Karen's reaction was immediate. She stiffened. "Not a word."

"What about your sister?" Clare asked.

Karen shook her head.

"I thought you said Victoria called you recently."

"She did," Karen admitted. "That's twice within the last month, which has to be something of a record. Generally I'm fortunate if I hear from her on my birthday."

"Any reason she's calling you more frequently?"

"None that I can figure out, except..."

"Yes?" Liz urged.

Again Karen shook her head. "I'm beginning to wonder if my sister's as happy as she leads everyone to believe."

"What makes you say that?"

"First, she hardly ever has people over. Second, I hardly ever see her and Roger together. Plus that last time she called, it sounded like she'd been crying."

"Did you ask her about it?"

"Sure I did," Karen replied, a bit indignantly. "She said she'd caught a bad cold." She rolled her eyes. "It wouldn't shock me, you know, if she's not Ms. Perfect, after all. But it *would* shock Mom."

"Maybe that's why she's calling you," Clare suggested.

"Maybe."

"What's her husband like?" Julia asked.

"He's a twit. He's a lot like my mother, only he's a man." Karen grimaced. "I can't imagine *anyone* marrying Roger."

"Your sister loves him," Liz reminded her.

"I know. In my humble opinion that means there's something wrong with her." Karen took a deep sip of her flavored drink; Julia thought it smelled like a cherry-vanilla combination. "Victoria and I were never close...."

"But she seems to be reaching out to you now," Julia said.

"Maybe she's hoping you'll reach back," Clare added.

Karen held the straw between her lips. "You think?"

Everyone nodded. There was silence for a minute or two.

"Have you heard anything from Jeff lately?" Liz asked suddenly.

"He's out of the picture. Looks like I'm going to be date-less on Valentine's Day. It won't be the first time and it probably won't be the last."

"What happened?"

She shrugged. "My agent decided not to take him on. He's got talent but no drive. He expected me to smooth the way for him, lead him by the hand. I've got enough trouble managing my own career. I can't baby-sit his. Once he figured that out, we had a parting of the ways. Trust me, it's no great loss."

"What about the guy you were telling us about a little while ago?" Clare asked.

"What guy?"

"George Somebody."

"I mentioned Glen?" She seemed surprised by this.

"I thought it was George," Clare said to Liz.

Liz smiled. "Apparently not."

"It's Glen."

"Tell us more," Liz said. "We're living vicariously through you."

Karen grinned and flipped a long strand of brown hair over her shoulder. "Sorry, there's nothing to tell. He's a high-school chemistry teacher. We met briefly in a parking lot across from the school where I was subbing. He's not my type."

"Damn," Liz muttered, and they all laughed.

"Just a minute," Clare said, turning to Julia. "What about you? Everyone else has been doing all the talking. How's your week been?"

Julia stared down at her hands. She hadn't planned to tell

her friends about the pregnancy until March, when she reached the twelve-week point, but she wanted to confide in them now, wanted it so much.

"Julia?" Liz asked, sounding concerned.

"What's wrong?" Clare asked with a gentleness Julia hadn't seen in her before. This show of compassion gave her a hint of what the other woman had been like before the divorce.

"You can tell us, whatever it is," Karen insisted.

"I don't know how," she whispered, fighting back the desperation that always seemed to hover.

"It's Peter, isn't it?" Clare cried, outraged and angry now. "He's found someone else."

"No." Julia shook her head, wanting to laugh because that idea was so incredibly ridiculous. "No," she said again, sighing deeply. "I'm pregnant."

The other three stared at her as if they weren't sure they should believe her.

"You're joking, right?" Karen said, looking from one to the other for a sign that she'd missed something earlier.

"I'm afraid not." If there was a joke, it'd been on her. "In case you haven't guessed, I'm not particularly pleased."

"Oh, Julia," Liz said, her eyes warm with sympathy.

"What are you going to do?" Clare asked next.

"Do," she repeated. "What *can* I do? I'll have this baby." *And resent it the rest of my life.* "I keep thinking this is God's sense of humor. Here I am trying to be so grateful, listing five blessings each and every morning—and now this? A pregnancy at age forty is one blessing I could've done without."

"Hey," Karen said, "we didn't talk about our word this week."

"Screw the word," Clare said fiercely. "We have more important things to deal with right now."

"What does Peter say?" Liz asked.

"Peter?" Julia said and laughed humorlessly, "is positively delighted."

"Figures," Clare groaned.

"He loves children...he's always wanted more. I was the one who insisted we stop at two." Her husband wasn't the only person who was thrilled with this news, either. Julia's mother had been overcome with excitement. "My own mother—" she threw back her head, eyes closed "—said the baby's a blessing in disguise."

"It's a mother thing," Liz said. "She's happy about adding another grandchild to her brag book."

"Have you told anyone else?" Karen asked.

"My mom and sister know, and my cousin Georgia."

"How'd they react?"

"Janice *laughed*. She said she couldn't help it. I'm the one who so carefully planned her life—always so organized and methodical—while Janice just kind of...improvises. And look at me now! Which is why she finds the situation hilarious." Julia exhaled softly. "When I told Georgia, she smoked an entire pack of cigarettes in thirty minutes. Then we sat and had a good cry together."

"That sounds like Georgia."

Julia reached nervously for her tea. Ever since learning of the pregnancy, Georgia had made a habit of visiting the shop every afternoon. Just yesterday, she'd brought Julia a bottle of vitamins that were large enough to choke a crocodile. With the vitamins had come a lengthy lecture on proper diet and the importance of exercise. It was Georgia's contention that Julia should get away from the shop more often; she insisted the two of them take up mall-walking. With that in mind, she'd purchased identical purple and hot-pink nylon running outfits. Julia declined, but Georgia had been relentless. Later, under pressure, Julia agreed to exercise, but only when she was feeling better.

"What about the kids?" Liz asked. "How did they react?"

"We haven't told them yet." Julia dreaded the thought. Her children were typical teenagers—meaning self-involved—and their entire world focused on their own needs. Peter had a blind spot when it came to his children; he sincerely believed they'd be just as delighted as he was. Julia doubted it.

"You have to adjust to it yourself first," Liz said and patted her hand.

"What about The Wool Station? Are you going to close it while you're on maternity leave?"

"I don't know," she said helplessly. So many questions remained unanswered. Peter was full of vague reassurances; he kept insisting they'd make it work.

Everyone was quiet for a while, as though they required a moment to absorb the news.

"If you need anything, you holler," Karen said. "I don't know much about babies, but I'll do what I can."

"I will, too," Clare assured her. "You have my complete support."

"And mine," Liz promised.

"Thank you," Julia whispered, grateful for these three dear friends. She had the feeling she was going to be calling upon them often in the months to come.

> "Life is under no obligation to give us what we expect."
>
> —Margaret Mitchell

CHAPTER

CLARE CRAIG

February 4th

I can't believe what happened yesterday. I saw Michael for the first time—outside a courtroom—since the divorce became final. Not by choice, mind you. Alex was in a soccer tournament in Fresno this weekend, and I assumed Michael wouldn't be there. My mistake. Michael's worked weekends for years and Fresno's a long drive. Needless to say, I took it for granted that he wouldn't show up.

Seeing my ex-husband was a shock. He's thinner now than when we were together, and what he wore—khakis and a Gap sweatshirt—reflected the change he's made in his life. If he's going to live with a twenty-year-old, I guess it's not surprising that he'd dress like one. As though he could fool anyone. It's pathetic.

What astonished me most was the pain I felt when I saw him. And not only pain but anger and resentment. I thought I was past this! It's disheartening to realize how far I have yet to go.

To be fair, I have to admit Michael didn't mingle with the other parents. He stood at the far end of the field, away from everyone else. In fact, he was there a good hour before I noticed him, which happened when Alex ran off the field to talk to him. Then, and only then, did I see that the stranger near the goalpost was Michael. From that point onward, the entire tournament was ruined for me.

Alex knew how upset I was and did his best to explain once we were alone. He told me he was surprised to see Michael at the Fresno game, too. I could tell he was pleased and didn't want to squelch his joy, but I was furious with Michael. He should have had the decency to let me know.

I've been depressed ever since last night. Alex isn't here right now; he's been gone a lot lately, busy with his job, soccer, school and friends. It wouldn't be appropriate to discuss my feelings with him, anyway. Usually when something like this comes up, I go to Liz. I suppose it's because she's older and she's been through the grief of losing her husband, but she always has a sensible perspective on things. I've been going to her a lot lately, relying on her too much, and I feel it's time I dealt with these problems on my own.

I spent last night wallowing in self-pity. I was exhausted after the long drive home, but I sat in the living room until the wee hours of the morning, thinking about all the times Michael and I attended the boys' games together. He missed some of the Saturday morning games, but for the most part we were there as a couple. I found myself crying again—all this heartache—and then I simply decided I couldn't let one man destroy me like this.

Easier said than done.

Sometimes I wonder if this pain will ever end. Michael's lost at least thirty pounds. So he's looking lean and craggy (very much his age, in my opinion). But he dresses in a style better suited to one of his sons. Miranda's obviously responsible for that. She's probably worn him to a frazzle with all her sexual demands. Good, maybe he'll die young and miserable. I've done my part to make sure he dies broke.

* * *

"Mom." Alex's raised voice rang over the telephone line. "I need a favor."

"What's up?" Clare had been busy working off her unhappiness over the soccer fiasco by scrubbing the shower stall in the master bedroom. She was determined to regain control of her emotions, and since it was Monday, didn't have the distraction of work. Her hours at Murphy Motors were Tuesdays and Thursdays.

"I need to write a makeup test this afternoon."

"English or algebra?

"Algebra."

Because of the soccer tournament, Alex had missed two important tests. Algebra was her son's poorest subject, and he resembled his father there, far more than he did her.

"What about the English midterm?"

"Mrs. Ford was cool about that. She said I could write it any time this week."

"Not so with Mr. Lawrence?"

"No. In fact, he said if I didn't take the test this afternoon, he'll give me a zero. And if I get a zero, you can kiss my chances of getting into Berkeley goodbye."

"Did you study?"

"Of course I did. I'll ace it if—"

"If what?"

"Mom," he said, then hesitated. "You know I wouldn't ask if there was any other way."

"What?" Clare demanded, growing impatient. Intuition told her she wasn't going to like this. Alex was generally straightforward when he wanted something; there had to be a reason he was being so indirect.

"I told Dad I'd pick him up at the hospital, and now I can't."

Clare's anger was immediate. "You're asking *me* to chauffeur your father around?"

"Yes." Alex's voice sounded small. "I know you and Dad are divorced, but that doesn't mean you can't be civilized."

Clare gritted her teeth and waited for the anger to pass. "I'm civilized, Alex. Are you suggesting I'm not?"

"No, Mom, please... I don't want to get into this with you. I wouldn't have asked if it wasn't important."

"What about his...friend?" Clare asked. Surely Miranda could pick him up.

"She can't just take off from work, you know."

Clare hadn't realized nail technicians were on such tight schedules.

"Can't he get a taxi?" If there was a way out of this, Clare planned to find it.

"Yeah, I guess, only I told him I'd be there and you always said it's important for us to keep our commitments."

Hmm. Moral righteousness. He was bringing out the heavy artillery.

Something wasn't logical here. A thought occurred to her that hadn't earlier. "Why can't he drive himself?"

"Mom, I'm between classes and I don't have time to discuss this, but apparently Dad's having some tests done at the hospital. He's not supposed to drive."

"Oh." She paused. "What kind of tests?"

"I'm not...sure." It was his turn to pause. "Will you do it or not?" he asked more sharply.

She desperately wanted to tell Alex that Michael could find his own damn way home. But deep down, Clare knew that if she refused, Alex would skip the exam and take the zero in order to fulfill his obligation to his father.

"Will you?" he repeated.

"All right," she muttered with ill grace, angry for allowing herself to be maneuvered into something she didn't want to do.

Alex quickly gave her the necessary information, then said, "Thanks, Mom. I knew I could count on you."

The line was disconnected before she had a chance to respond.

Dreadful though the situation was, it did give her an opportunity to speak to Michael about the next soccer tournament, scheduled for March. Look on the bright side, Clare!

They'd agreed to alternate attending the games. This afternoon would be a perfect chance to sort out the details and make sure there wasn't a repeat of last weekend.

Clare suspected that Alex was secretly hoping his parents would reunite. What a joke. As far as she was concerned, Michael had proven himself completely untrustworthy. But according to the books she'd read and what she'd heard in her support group, this was a common fantasy for children of divorce—regardless of age.

It worried her a little that Alex felt this responsibility toward his father. He was only a kid; he shouldn't have to ferry Michael around or be involved with his problems. Yet Alex had accepted the burden as if it were his own.

As the time approached to leave for the hospital, Clare dressed in her best business suit. Staring at her reflection in the bedroom mirror, she stripped it off. Too formal, she decided. She was striving for a look of casual elegance.

No. That might give him the impression that she was living a life of leisure. Whatever she chose to wear had to convey how terribly happy she was, how terribly busy. Her goal was to make Michael believe she was extremely inconvenienced by having her day interrupted. At the same time, her graciousness and generosity in coming for him would clearly state that she was the bigger person, capable of putting bygones aside.

Best of all, Michael had no idea she was picking him up. According to Alex, it was impossible to get a message to him, letting him know the arrangements had changed. That being the case, Michael would be caught off guard when she arrived. Good—he could suffer the same shock Clare had last Saturday. Not only that, *she* was prepared, and her carefully contrived demeanor would remind him of what he'd thrown away. A mature, classy, compassionate and capable woman.

Yes. She had it all figured out.

Life's unpleasant surprises did come with compensations.

After emptying almost her entire closet, Clare finally chose a canary-yellow pantsuit. It suggested cheeriness and optimism; even better, Michael had always liked it on her. Whenever she wore it, he'd sing "You Are My Sunshine," and he'd— Enough of that! She planned to swing into the hospital like a...like a ray of sunshine. Cordial but not overly so. Michael would be in her debt, and she preferred that to owing *him* anything.

The hospital. Apparently Michael's current lifestyle had taken its toll on his health. Poor boy, he just couldn't keep pace with a youngster. She'd be sure to reveal exactly the right amount of sympathy, with just a hint of contempt.

On the drive to Willow Grove Memorial, she repeatedly played through the scenario in her mind, imagining Michael's reactions and rehearsing her own.

Michael was supposed to be waiting for her in the hospital foyer. All that was required of her, according to Alex, was to drive up to the front doors.

She tried that, but when Michael didn't show up, she circled the block a couple of times. When he still didn't appear, she parked the car in the first available slot, and strode purposefully toward the hospital entrance.

Her mood darkened.

Searching for Michael was *not* part of the deal. It ruined the way she'd envisioned their meeting, completely spoiling the little script she'd created. If he wasn't inside where she'd been told he'd be, Michael could damn well find his own ride home.

No sooner had she walked into the marble-floored foyer than she heard someone call her name.

"Clare," Liz said, hurrying toward her. "What are you doing here?"

This was embarrassing. Being seen by her friend wasn't part of the deal, either. "Ah..." A lie would be convenient, but unaccustomed to prevarication, she couldn't think of one fast enough.

"Everything's all right, isn't it?" Liz pressed.

"Oh, sure..." She sighed. "I'm here to pick up Michael."

Liz's eyes widened, but she said nothing.

Reluctantly Clare explained Alex's predicament and hers, ending with Michael's non-appearance at the appointed place. "I guess I'll wait a few more minutes," she said.

Liz's expression was sympathetic. "Are you sure you're up to this?"

Clare's answer was a shrug. "I'm about to find out, aren't I?"

"Yes, you are." She glanced past Clare's shoulder. "Is that him over there?"

It was, and he looked dreadful. Pale and gaunt. Seeing him close-up, she realized he'd lost more weight than she'd noticed on Saturday; he was downright thin.

He stopped abruptly when he saw her.

"Where's Alex?" he asked, gazing around.

"Taking an algebra midterm," she replied stiffly, staggered by the differences she saw in him. She nodded toward Liz. "This is my friend Liz Kenyon, the hospital administrator."

Michael inclined his head, acknowledging the introduction with a brief smile. "Do you mind if we leave now?"

"I'll see you Thursday," Clare said, turning toward the doors.

"Okay." As Clare began to walk away, Liz squeezed her hand.

Outside the hospital, Michael paused. "Where's the car?"

"In the east parking lot." She pointed.

He nodded and started walking in that direction.

Clare followed more slowly behind him. She should have pursued her question about the tests. Alex probably knew *something* and she should've insisted he tell her. In her eagerness to wear the perfect outfit, to show him how completely she'd recovered from their divorce, she hadn't given it much thought. Whatever the tests were for, they must've been hellish.

Neither spoke as they walked toward the parking lot. By the time they reached the car, Michael's breathing was labored. She pretended not to notice.

Once inside the vehicle, Michael closed his eyes and leaned against the headrest. He'd broken into a sweat. She struggled not to react with pity or fear. Struggled not to react as a wife would.

Clare started the engine and backed out of the space.

"I appreciate this, Clare," he said, his voice barely audible.

"I won't pretend it was convenient," she said, keeping her voice cool, refusing to allow herself to feel anything, and hating it that she did. "I wouldn't be here if it wasn't for Alex."

"I know."

She waited until they'd merged with the flow of traffic before she broached the subject of their son and the remaining soccer matches.

"I thought we'd agreed to split up Alex's games," she said

in as reasonable a tone as she could manage. "If you wanted
to attend the tournament, you should've let me know."

Michael didn't answer, and when she turned to look at
him, he was staring out the side window.

So he intended to give her the silent treatment. Okay,
fine. But she wasn't conceding defeat. She—

"I'm sorry."

Again she had to strain to hear him. In an odd way, she was
almost disappointed by his apology. It sabotaged her anger.

"Sorry?" The least he could do was explain himself.

"Stop the car." His voice was harsh. Urgent. He pointed
to a side street and added. "Hurry...please."

"Stop the car?" she repeated. Even as she said the words,
she switched to the outside lane and pulled off the main
street, onto the road he'd indicated. The second she eased to
a stop at the curb, the passenger door flew open. Michael half
fell out of the car, bent over and vomited on the sidewalk.

Clare remembered Julia's horrible case of flu last November. That must be what Michael had, although even
worse. Doubled over, he heaved until there was nothing left.

When he'd finished, he leaned weakly against the side of
the SUV.

Without a word, Clare opened the back and found a bottle
of spring water and uncapped it. Next, she gave him a tissue
from her purse, which he used to wipe his mouth. She handed
him the water bottle.

Michael took it from her, rinsed his mouth, then used
what remained to wash off the sidewalk.

He climbed back into the car, more ashen than before.

"That must've been one hell of a test you had," she said.
"Or do you have the flu?" Clare didn't *want* to feel sympa-

thy for him, but despite everything, she did. It was impossible not to be affected by someone's pain. Even if that person had ripped apart her life. Even if she'd sworn to harden her heart against him.

"I wasn't at the hospital for tests," he said after a moment. "And I don't have the flu."

Clare glanced in his direction and waited for him to explain, her hand on the ignition key.

"I'm undergoing chemotherapy."

Chemotherapy? Michael?

"You have cancer?" Clare whispered.

> "The way I see it, if you want the rainbow, you gotta put up with the rain."
>
> —Dolly Parton

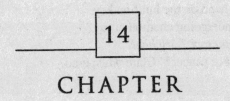

CHAPTER

LIZ KENYON

February 8th

I'm worried about Clare and Julia. Our meeting today troubled me.

Clare is my main concern. It didn't take me long to discover why Michael Craig was at the hospital on Monday, and it wasn't for any tests, the way Clare assumed. One look at her ex-husband told me he wasn't a well man. I wonder if Clare knows the seriousness of his condition, but unfortunately that isn't a question I can ask her.

My first reaction was that her son had practically blackmailed her into picking Michael up. I wondered if Alex did this on purpose so Clare would discover the truth on her own. It's a possibility, but not one I mentioned. In fact, as I learned later, she's not sure how much her boys know.

I suspected she was going to need to talk all of this over with someone, and I was right. After work on Monday, I got some Chinese takeout and drove to her house. It took her almost five minutes to answer the door, and she looked pale and shaken and very glad to see me.

We talked for several hours while we ate Szechwan chicken and shrimp egg fu yung, then drank black tea in front of her fireplace. Apparently Michael's still living with Miranda. It couldn't have been easy for Clare to drive him to the house he's sharing with another woman. I don't know what they said to each other, she and Michael. Doesn't matter, though. My main purpose is to help a friend.

Clare's a strong woman. She doesn't credit herself nearly enough. She's been through a great deal and unfortunately, there's more to come. However, by the end of the evening, I felt confident that Clare was handling this news as well as could be expected.

Then at the breakfast this morning, she looked like she hadn't slept all night. She seemed especially quiet, too, and Karen's attempts to draw her out were unsuccessful.

Clare isn't the only one experiencing problems. Julia seems completely drained. This pregnancy hasn't been easy on her physically or, of course, emotionally. She, too, was withdrawn and uncommunicative.

That left Karen and me. Karen, forever the actress, seemed grateful for an audience and did most of the

talking. While I enjoy her, I'd hoped Clare and Julia
would be more forthcoming, but neither of them really
entered into the conversation. Without them con-
tributing, the group simply doesn't work.

I'm making the effort to see more of Clare and Julia.
After all, I'm the one with the free time to invest in our
friendships. I can certainly give them the benefit of my
affection and sympathy—if not my wisdom!

With that thought in mind, I've decided I want to
learn how to knit, and Julia's agreed to teach me. She
doesn't hold regular classes; she found it was too difficult to run the store and teach at the same time. (She
can't afford to hire anyone yet, although that's her
eventual goal.) Evenings are reserved for her family
and after spending all day at the store, she's ready to
go home by six.

I've always wanted to knit (and I'll be meeting one
of my goals for the year—a new skill!). I'll buy yarn to
make a sweater for Annie, and while I'm learning the
basics, I'll have an opportunity to visit with Julia. We've
arranged our lessons for two lunch hours a week; I'll
bring the sandwiches, since she won't accept pay-
ment. We'll knit—and we'll talk. About the baby, her
feelings, whatever she wants.

Julia's baby must be why Lauren's on my mind so
much these days. To carry a child for six months and
then lose her, born three months premature, nearly destroyed us. Steve and I were so young and afraid. I've
never forgotten her, although I rarely mention her
name. Born now, my Lauren might have lived. A doctor like Sean might have given her a chance at life.

He came to my office earlier in the week. I didn't see him, but I knew he'd been there. I was in a meeting with the nursing director, finalizing the details of the new contract. When I returned, a long-stemmed rose had been placed on my desk. It's been almost a month since Sean and I talked. I'm not even sure if he's still seeing the physical therapist.

I wish I could pinpoint what it is about this man that I find so attractive. And dammit, I have to admit that I do. I know he's younger and he's arrogant and he's impatient and demanding—and he's got an inflated opinion of his own charms. And yet...and yet I can't stop thinking about him.

He's as different from Steve as any man could be. Perhaps what attracts me is the challenge. But really, do I need that at this point in my life? I don't think so. Then why do I care?

I can't figure it out.

I have plenty of challenges to occupy me. My job, of course. And my volunteer work. Now that I'm reading to the kids at the detention center, I'm finding the experience immensely satisfying.

Anyway, I put Sean's rose in a vase and left it on my desk (right next to my copy of the second Harry Potter book). All week that rose has been there to remind me of him. It's the first thing I notice when I walk into the office each morning and the last thing I see at the end of the day. I should have tossed it immediately, and didn't.

I generally trust my own judgment about people and relationships. This time I have the distinct feeling I'm setting myself up for a major letdown.

It's not a comfortable sensation. Sean obviously feels the same way or he would have asked me out again and he hasn't.

I can't decide if I'm relieved or disappointed.

> "It goes without saying that you should never have more children than you have car windows."
>
> —Erma Bombeck

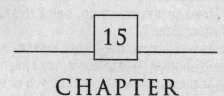

CHAPTER

JULIA MURCHISON

February 12th

List of Blessings
1. Hot baths and lavender soap and a matching cream that feels like silk on my skin. An early Valentine gift to myself.
2. A full night's rest—something I really appreciate now that I have difficulty sleeping.
3. Attics.
4. Heartburn medication.
5.

I was in for my monthly visit with Dr. Fisk, the OB-GYN who delivered both Adam and Zoe. We talked for almost fifteen minutes and probably would have spent more time discussing the pregnancy if she didn't have such a tight appointment schedule.

My attitude isn't good. I'm making an effort, but so far it hasn't really worked. My due date is September seventh. The ultrasound showed a healthy pregnancy; the fetus is developing normally. But I don't remember the nausea or the heartburn being this bad with either Adam or Zoe.

I might as well accept the fact that Peter and I are about to add another child to our family. I might as well assume that things will work out. I'm sick of worrying about how we're going to manage, sick of thinking about the complications a baby is adding to our lives. Babies are expensive, and our finances are already strained.

Peter has taken this pregnancy in stride—easy to do since he isn't the one who's pregnant. When the baby arrives, I'll let my good-natured husband worry about finding day care. I'll suggest he get up in the middle of the night to deal with the feeding and the constant needs of a newborn. Peter's conveniently forgotten how demanding an infant can be, but he'll remember soon enough.

The kids know something is up. We can't delay telling them much longer. Once again my husband has this rosy, unrealistic picture of how they're going to react. I hate to disillusion him, but I know exactly what Adam and Zoe will say, and it doesn't bear any resemblance to what he expects.

Saturday, while Peter had Adam and Zoe with him, gallivanting from one sporting event to the next, I went to the attic. I can't remember the last time I did that. What a mess. Obviously the kids have been up there.

I sought out anything we could use for this baby. As I recall, we gave the crib, high chair and other furniture to my sister, but Peter was sure we kept the bassinet. If so, I didn't find it. I looked everywhere, to no avail. There are no baby clothes to be found. Nothing. Zilch. Nada.

We'll have to start completely over. I simply don't know how we're going to afford all this. My shop's income has dropped—it's no wonder since I've had to close once or twice a week for doctor's appointments and all these tests Dr. Fisk considers necessary. Thank God Peter has excellent health benefits.

* * *

Nervous about confronting the children with news of her pregnancy, Julia took the chicken casserole from the oven and carried it to the table. She'd gone to extra trouble this evening, preparing a family favorite, accompanied by fresh green beans and hot rolls and followed by dessert.

Julia insisted on family meals, although Adam and Zoe were involved in a number of school activities that often ran late. Getting everyone to the dinner table at the same time was becoming more and more of a challenge.

"Dinner's ready," she called out when she'd finished. She stepped away from the table and waited for her husband and children to join her.

Peter was the first one in the kitchen. His eyes met hers, and Julia read the question in his gaze.

"Tonight?" he asked.

Julia nodded.

"How'd the doctor's appointment go?"

She shrugged. The appointment had been to discuss the ultrasound, and it had taken longer than she'd hoped. She was more than an hour late in opening the shop, which left her wondering how much business she'd lost. Or worse, how many people she'd irritated by not being there at the time posted. Between today and the two hours she was closed while she had the ultrasound on Monday, that was twice just this week.

"You're sure everything's all right?"

"Yeah." He knew the ultrasound revealed no problems; she'd mentioned it earlier. Peter had been relieved and so, of course, was she. This whole situation was hard enough without worrying about Down's Syndrome or spina bifida. Not that they'd know about *that* until she'd had the amniocentesis.

"Adam. Zoe," Peter yelled. "Dinner!"

As though he was doing his parents a favor, Adam slouched into the kitchen. He'd shaved his head recently, and after a growth spurt the past summer, was an inch under six feet. He was lanky and awkward and painfully conscious of his new height.

He pulled out his chair and fell into it. "I was on the computer," he said, as if that explained the delay.

"Where's your sister?" Julia set the milk carton on the table next to the salad and the green beans.

Adam raised his thin shoulders. "Her bedroom, last time I looked."

Peter walked to the hallway and shouted for Zoe again.

The thirteen-year-old arrived a minute later, full of high spirits. "Sorry," Zoe said, as she flew into the room. "I was on the phone with Ashley."

Ashley and Zoe were in constant communication. Julia's own best friend when she was thirteen had been Kathleen

O'Hara, who now lived in Seattle and worked as a journalist. Theirs had become merely a Christmas-card friendship, and she'd forgotten the intensity of relationships at that age. The two girls found it impossible to be separated for more than a few hours. All this would change, Julia realized, when boyfriends entered the picture; she hoped that wouldn't be for a few more years. As it stood now, Ashley and Zoe were at school together every day, then talked on the phone half the night, with e-mail to fill in any gaps. Weekends were spent at each other's houses.

"Shall we eat?" Peter suggested, sliding into his chair.

Julia sat down at the opposite end of the table.

Once they were all seated, they bowed their heads for a brief prayer. As soon as they'd finished, Peter reached for the spoon to serve himself some casserole. "Your mother and I would like to talk to you both after dinner," he said casually.

"Talk to us?" Zoe asked.

"About what?" Adam pressed.

"We'll wait until we've finished with dinner," Julia inserted, unwilling to disrupt this congenial time.

"Is it about me driving?" Adam was due to get his driver's license soon. Already he was pressuring Peter and Julia about purchasing an extra vehicle for him. Naturally, he assured them, he'd get a job to pay for the insurance, gas and maintenance.

Julia stabbed a green bean. She didn't have the heart to tell Adam that with the extra financial burden of a third child, there wouldn't be money for a car. They'd discussed buying a reliable used one, but that was completely out of the question now.

"I know what it is," Zoe burst out excitedly. She tossed her brother a superior look.

Adam scowled in her direction.

"We're taking a family vacation this year, aren't we?" Zoe said.

Julia and Peter exchanged glances.

Zoe's eyes brightened. "We're going to the Grand Canyon, right?"

"I'll drive," Adam offered.

"Do you mind if we put this discussion off until after dinner?" Julia said, wishing Peter hadn't announced their intention beforehand.

"I need forty dollars for gym class tomorrow," Adam announced, grabbing a second roll from the basket and slathering butter on it.

"Forty bucks?" Peter repeated, looking aghast.

"Children are expensive," Julia said pointedly. Peter didn't appear to recognize the sacrifice this new child was going to require, and she wasn't even thinking of the emotional implications, of which there were plenty.

"Speaking of money, I need new reeds for my clarinet," Zoe added.

School. Music lessons. Sports. Scouts. Church. All required commitments of money and time. Both Adam and Zoe were active teenagers, and a new baby wasn't going to change that. Last week alone, there'd been some meeting or other involving one of the kids every night for five evenings straight.

Julia couldn't imagine what they'd do next year when they had an infant at home. An infant who was on a feeding, eating and sleeping schedule. It wasn't as though she could drag a baby to these functions and expect anything to get done.

Peter wouldn't always be available to baby-sit either. He had work obligations of his own—PTA meetings, parent conferences and the like—that often took place in the evenings.

"*Are* we taking a vacation this year?" Adam asked.

"No." Julia corrected him before this line of questioning got out of hand and led to yet another disappointment.

Both children stared at her.

"Just tell us what it is then," Zoe pleaded.

"Yeah," Adam agreed. "Why don't you tell us?" He heaped another helping of the casserole onto his plate. During the last six months, their son's appetite had increased tenfold. Peter had joked recently that he was going to have to take on a second job just to afford groceries. A joke Julia now recalled with some bitterness.

"Maybe we should just tell them and be done with it," Peter said, looking at Julia.

"It's not fair to make us guess," Zoe said, her eagerness to hear this news spilling over.

"Gotta get back to the computer. I have a ton of English homework," Adam said, implying that he'd be working on it the instant dinner was finished. He'd be at the computer, all right, but it was doubtful he'd be tackling his English project. Julia was well aware that her son was hooked on "Age of Empires."

"I don't object, if your mother doesn't," Peter said.

Both children turned to Julia. "Tell us, Mom." "Come on, Mom."

Actually, she'd hoped Peter would be the one to make the announcement. Realizing she couldn't postpone it any longer, she set her fork down and placed her hands in her lap. She put on a brave smile. "Your father and I have some good news." She was determined to put a positive slant on this despite her own less-than-enthusiastic attitude.

"I *told* you it was good news," Adam shouted, exchanging a high-five with his sister.

"We're headed for the Grand Canyon," Zoe said. "Mom just said no 'cause she wanted it to be a surprise."

"I'm not sure a baby is what either of you have in mind." Peter threw out the words a bit desperately.

"Yellowstone Park." Adam's eyes flashed with enthusiasm. "I could help with the driving. We could be there in eighteen hours. We'd stay at the National Park, wouldn't we?"

"*Baby?*" The excitement vanished from Zoe's face as she took in her father's words. "What's this about a *baby?*"

Julia wished her husband had led into the subject with a little more finesse. Doing her best to appear pleased, she leaned forward and looked both her children in the eye. "You heard that right."

"A baby?" Adam shared a puzzled frown with his sister.

"Your mother's pregnant," Peter said. Julia preferred him to do the talking, since he was so damn thrilled about this baby. From Adam and Zoe's horrified expressions, he seemed to be the only one in the family who was. "Your baby brother or sister is due in September."

Both children turned their heads and stared at Julia as though they found this impossible to believe.

"I didn't know women as old as Mom could have babies," Adam said.

"This may come as a shock, but your mother isn't old," Peter told him, doing nothing to hide his amusement.

"I'll be forty this year," she murmured, in case Peter had forgotten the significance of that.

"You're honestly having a baby?" Zoe asked, her head cocked to one side. "You mean, we aren't going on a family vacation?"

"Not this year," Julia said. *And probably not for the next five. Or more.*

"Where will a baby sleep?" Adam asked, as if that thought had just occurred to him.

Julia understood her son's reasoning. Adam was concerned about being forced to share his room.

"We won't know that until the baby's born," Peter answered. "If it's a boy, then eventually he'll be with you. A girl will move in with Zoe at some point."

The ultrasound hadn't revealed the sex; at the moment Julia didn't care. She was merely grateful that the baby was okay—and that there was only one. She'd read that twins were more frequent with older mothers.

"Wouldn't it be better to move into a bigger house?" Zoe asked, looking from one parent to the other.

"We can't afford to do that," Julia said, pushing her dinner around the plate with her fork. Her appetite hadn't been good for several weeks, and this discussion wasn't helping.

"You mean if the baby's a girl, she'll be in the same bedroom as me?" Zoe's outrage echoed in each word. "I have the smallest bedroom already! Make Adam change rooms with me, then."

"Adam. Zoe." Peter entered the fray, his voice full of authority. "There's no need to argue about this now. After the baby's born, he or she will be with your mother and me for the first few months."

"Why can't you keep him with you all the time?"

"Don't you think you're both being a little selfish here?" Peter asked mildly.

Julia could tell he was disappointed by their children's reaction. Well, she'd done her best to warn him.

"No one my age has a baby brother or sister," Zoe said next, glancing at her brother for support. "This is...embarrassing."

"You might say we're a bit surprised ourselves," Peter countered. "It wasn't like your mother and I planned this."

"A baby now will change all our lives," Adam said and his insinuation was that any change couldn't possibly be for the better.

Which had been Julia's main concern from the first. "You're right. This pregnancy is going to alter the makeup of our family."

"Is that why Grandma's been phoning you so much?" Zoe suddenly asked.

Invariably, Zoe was on the line whenever Julia's mother called. Zoe made it abundantly plain each and every time that she resented having to end her conversations for something that wasn't related to her own small world.

Julia nodded. "My mother and sister both know."

"You told Grandma and Aunt Janice, but not us?" Adam scowled again.

"What am I going to tell my friends?" Zoe sounded near tears. "I can't *believe* you'd let something like this happen."

"Tell your friends you're about to become a big sister," Peter suggested.

"Oh, Daddy, how juvenile. This is so stupid."

Adam didn't say anything for a couple of minutes. Then he muttered, "This means you won't be able to afford a car for me, doesn't it?"

"We don't know that yet." Julia hurried to answer before Peter could say something too blunt and destroy their son's dream. "Maybe next year..."

"Are you closing the yarn shop?" Zoe asked.

"No." Of that Julia was certain. She'd come too far, sacrificed too much, to abandon everything now.

"Did you *want* more kids?" Adam asked her.

"No," Julia admitted.

Zoe stood and glared across the table at her and Peter. "Why'd you have to go and do this?" she wailed. "I don't want to share my room and furthermore, I refuse to baby-sit every afternoon after school. I know that's what you're thinking."

"Zoe, we haven't gotten that far. Your father and I are still dealing with this news ourselves. Don't worry, we won't ask you to baby-sit unless it's an emergency."

"What am I supposed to tell my friends?" she cried, tears glistening in her eyes.

"Tell them your parents are having a baby."

"At *your* age?"

"I'm not telling anyone," Adam announced. "They'll think it's a big joke."

"I hate you for doing this to us!" Zoe raced out of the kitchen. A few seconds later, her bedroom door slammed, the sound echoing throughout the house.

Wordlessly, Adam shoved his plate away. He left the table and marched down the hallway leading to his room. Seconds later, his door banged shut, too.

The kitchen was suddenly silent. Julia thought she was going to throw up. This had gone even more badly than she'd feared. She'd known the children would be surprised, and perhaps embarrassed, but she hadn't expected them to react this vehemently.

"Well," Peter said, leaning back in his chair. "What do you think?"

"Think?" Julia echoed as the knot in her gut tightened.

"It didn't go well, did it?"

"No, Peter," she said. "It didn't go well."

"Let me listen to me and not to them."

—Gertrude Stein

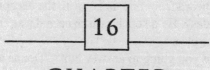

CHAPTER

LIZ KENYON

"He's here," Donna DeGooyer, the hospital social services director, said, peeking inside Liz's office on Thursday afternoon.

"Who?" Liz asked, playing dumb.

"You *know* who. I just saw Dr. Jamison down the hall and he's headed in this direction."

"Really?" Liz's pulse reacted immediately. For some unknown reason, she'd expected to hear from him yesterday—Valentine's Day. It was ridiculous to entertain any such notion. Men were not romantic beings. Steve's love for her was never in question, but he'd struggled with gift-giving and creating romantic interludes. Dr. Jamison had proven more than once that, except for his patients, he didn't spare a thought for any-

one other than himself. Or as Karen succinctly put it, "The
ego has landed." Even thinking he'd remember her on Valentine's Day was foolish. Embarrassing. And indeed he hadn't.
Yet he was on his way to her office that very minute.

"He's probably going to ask you out."

"Probably," Liz agreed, although she didn't think it was
probable at all. She'd spoken her mind to the good doctor
and hadn't heard from him since, with the exception of the
rose on her desk. He'd kept his distance and was, in fact, dating someone else.

"How are you going to answer him?" Donna asked.

Liz shrugged, trying to look cool and indifferent despite
her spinning head and sweating palms.

Donna glanced over her shoulder. "See ya," she said, and
with a naughty grin, she strolled calmly away.

No sooner had Donna left than Sean appeared, looking
better than any man had a right to. "Good—you're still
here," he murmured. "I thought you might be."

Liz glanced at the clock on her desk, surprised to see that
it was after six-thirty. "I was just finishing up some paperwork," she said.

"You sure you weren't waiting for me?" Only his light, teasing tone kept his remark from sounding arrogant. She bit back
the reply that sprang to her lips. Sean would believe what he
wanted to believe—which was, apparently, that she spent her
days longing to hear from him. Since it wasn't far from the
truth, she let it go. "Thank you for the rose," she said instead.

"What rose?" He leaned against the door frame and
crossed his arms.

"The one you left on my desk last week." He knew damn
well what she was talking about.

"Oh, the *rose*." He grinned that sexy, charming grin of his, and her heart began to race.

"You have plans for tonight?" he asked.

She hesitated—but not for long. "Um, no."

"How about a drink?"

"I thought you were dating...what's her name? The physical therapist."

He shrugged. "Not anymore. She's too manipulative."

It took her a moment to catch the pun, bad as it was. Then, despite herself, she smiled. A drink wouldn't hurt.

"Where?" she asked.

"The Seaside," he suggested.

"Sure." Liz was a little apprehensive, especially since it felt as though she'd just done something irrevocable and maybe dangerous: by agreeing, she'd acknowledged her attraction to him. And yet she couldn't have said no. For one thing, she was profoundly curious about *why* she found this man so attractive when he infuriated and annoyed her so much of the time.

Sean glanced at his watch. "Shall we meet there in fifteen minutes?"

"Fine."

He flashed her another easy smile, then turned and walked away.

Twelve minutes later, Liz was fortunate enough to find a spot in the parking lot outside the popular restaurant. She used another minute to refresh her makeup and dig around the bottom of her purse until she unearthed a miniature spray bottle of her favorite cologne.

"Here goes nothing," she said as she slid out of her car and locked it. At the very least, she'd have something to tell the breakfast group next Thursday.

They'd met that morning, and Clare had revealed that
Michael was undergoing cancer treatment. Clare vacillated between pity and wanting to remain indifferent. With
one breath she'd say it was Miranda's problem; with the
next, she'd worry frantically about his prognosis and the
chemo's side effects. Julia had finally told her children she
was pregnant, with predictable results, and Karen was still
upset about being disliked by the cocker spaniel, as if her
entire career hung in the balance. Liz had listened to them
all, but she'd left with the feeling that her own life lacked
meaning, and nothing to report.

The Seaside's bar was smoky and crowded. Valentine decorations—hearts and cupids—were still suspended from the
ceiling, and the usual classic jazz had been replaced by
schmaltzy love songs. Sean had yet to arrive, and she wished
now that she'd waited for him outside. If he stood her up, she
swore he'd never hear the end of it. A table became vacant
when the hostess led its occupants into the dining room. Moving quickly, Liz claimed the space.

A couple of minutes later, a harried waitress approached; Liz ordered a glass of Merlot and instantly at-
tacked the small bowl of peanuts, feeling she needed
something in her stomach.

Sean arrived before her wine did. He paid for her drink
and ordered an old-fashioned for himself. Neither seemed to
have anything to say, and Liz started to feel a bit desperate.

"I wish..."

"Well, what do you..."

Naturally, when she went to speak, he did, too. Sean
grinned and motioned for her to talk first. She nodded, fig-
uring they could make polite conversation, get involved in

hospital gossip or discuss books, politics, films, but what interested her most was Sean himself.

"Tell me about you."

He chuckled and reached for a handful of peanuts. "My favorite subject. What would you like to know?"

She imagined that he often spoke of his career, his success, but she was already aware of all that. "What would you like me to know?"

"All right." He took his time, munching on the peanuts, sipping his drink. "First, I don't usually work this hard to get a woman to go out with me."

She rolled her eyes. "Wrong path, take another."

He grinned. "All right. I've been divorced for ten years."

That was what he wanted her to know? It made her wonder if this was his way of saying there was no chance of a long-term relationship.

"Any children?" she asked while she sorted through her various unspoken questions.

"One. A daughter, Eileen. She lives in Seattle with her husband, who's a scientist for Boeing. They've got a three-year-old daughter named Emily."

"So you're a grandfather."

He looked away and nodded.

"Do you have pictures?"

He shook his head. "My daughter and I aren't particularly close."

"My daughter has two children," she told him to cover the awkwardness of his confession. He clearly had regrets, but this wasn't the time to ask him what had gone wrong, why he and Eileen were no longer in touch.

"How'd you get into hospital work?" he asked, obviously wanting to turn the subject away from himself.

Emboldened by the wine, Liz wagged her finger. "We were talking about you, remember?"

"All right." He seemed deep in thought for a few moments, then shrugged almost comically. "Not much else to say."

Liz didn't mean to laugh, but she did. "I can't believe that."

He laughed, too. "Well, not much more about my personal life," he said with uncharacteristic modesty. "And my professional qualifications you already know."

Liz nodded. She recognized that through this small crack in his ego she'd caught a glimpse of the real Sean Jamison. She had a feeling she'd like him.

But before she could learn more, he sidetracked the conversation, and Liz found she was talking about herself. He was curious about her volunteering at the detention center, which led them into a heated debate about the prison system, capital punishment and youth crime. Predictably, they disagreed vehemently on each topic.

"You are so closed-minded," she muttered.

"And you're just another bleeding heart."

"At least I *have* a heart," she countered.

Grinning, he checked his watch. "Do you have a stomach to go along with that generous heart of yours?"

"Yes..."

"How about dinner?"

By that time they'd had two drinks each and nothing to eat other than a small bowlful of salty peanuts.

"You're willing to continue this conversation?" she asked, certain he'd decided, as she had, that they shared little in common. Much as she respected his medical skills and was beginning to like him—his passion for debate, his intellect, even his humor—they were directly opposed on practically every subject.

"Sure. I'm always willing to argue. Aren't you?"

"If you feed me, I'm game." She needed to eat anyway, she told herself.

He leaned over and kissed her cheek, then stood. "I'll see about getting us a table."

The conversation over dinner didn't lack for stimulation. They argued every point, joked, teased and laughed. When they'd finished, Liz saw that the restaurant was closing for the night.

Sean looked at his watch. "It's 11:30—way past my bedtime. What about you?"

Liz groaned. "Mine, too. I need to be at the hospital early in the morning."

The bill had already been paid, so they got up to leave. Sean helped her on with her jacket and walked her to her car. "Just to be on the safe side, I'll follow you home."

"There's no need to do that."

"Don't argue with me, Elizabeth."

"I've spent the entire evening arguing with you," she reminded him sweetly, but actually she was touched by his protectiveness.

"You'll learn soon enough that I win most arguments."

"Yes, sir," she muttered sarcastically. "Although I'd say it was a draw."

He grinned at that but didn't respond.

Sean followed her home, as he'd promised, and when she pulled into the garage, he eased his vehicle behind hers, turning off the ignition.

Frowning, Liz climbed out of her car and met him. "Thanks again. I had ...an enjoyable evening."

"So did I."

She was gratified to hear him say it.

He reached for her and after the briefest of hesitations, she leaned into him and accepted his kiss. His mouth was warm and moist and firm, and she felt sensations she hadn't experienced in more than six years. She wound her arms around his neck and he held her tightly, his hands finding the small of her back and pressing their bodies close. He wanted her, and she was keenly aware of it.

"Invite me in," he whispered. Before she could respond, he kissed her a second time, then again—short, eager kisses that weakened her resolve. To put distance between them, she dropped her arms and stepped back.

"I'll turn an enjoyable evening into a pleasurable one for us both," he promised, his voice husky with desire.

Liz would be lying to herself if she didn't admit how tempted she was. She rested her forehead against his shoulder and waited for reason and sanity to return.

"Don't think," he pleaded. "Just feel." His lips, nibbling at her neck and earlobe, made for a persuasive argument.

"Sean," she said quickly before she had a change of heart. She lifted her head and placed her hands on either side of his jaw. "Your offer is tempting."

His eyes, clouded with passion, cleared and sharpened. "But?"

"If I was in my twenties, I'd probably do it."

"What has age got to do with anything?" he asked.

"Not so much age as common sense. I'm fifty-seven—" she made a point of reminding him that he was younger than she "—and I've acquired a bit more discretion. I find you stimulating and attractive and you're saying you feel the same way about me."

"Yes, God, yes." He kissed her suddenly in a deep, probing way that made her knees wobble.

When he released her, Liz closed her eyes in a determined effort to clear her head. "Now listen, because what I have to say is important."

He raised his head and their eyes met and held. "All right."

"It would be the easiest thing in the world to fall into bed with you. I'm part of the generation that said if it feels right, do it, and I—"

"Is this a lecture?" he asked, sounding bored.

"No, an explanation," she rushed to assure him. "I was married for thirty-one years, and in that time I learned that sex is more than pleasure. It's commitment and communication, shared dreams and lives. It's wonderful, but for me it has to mean something more than a...than a nightcap. I enjoyed myself tonight. I enjoyed being with you."

"In other words, thanks but no thanks. Some other time?"

She hesitated; it was more complicated than that, but she doubted he understood. "Sort of."

"I enjoyed your company, too, Liz, but I'm not interested in this touchy-feely philosophy you're pushing here. You don't want to go to bed with me? I can accept that. I don't like it, but the decision is yours."

She kissed his jaw to tell him she appreciated his listening.

"Tell you what I'll do," he said, heaving a ragged sigh. "I'll wait until you're ready and then you can give me a call."

"What?" He'd confused her.

"I don't ask a woman twice, Liz."

She glared at him, furious he'd turn this into a battle of wills. He hadn't heard a word she'd said. "You'll have a very long wait, Sean."

He chuckled, evidently amused. "I doubt that," he said with maddening confidence. "You'll come around soon enough and when you do, I'll be ready, willing and able."

> "Expecting life to treat you well because you are a good person is like expecting an angry bull not to charge because you are a vegetarian."
>
> —Shari R. Barr

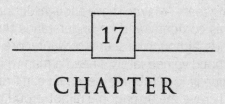

CHAPTER

KAREN CURTIS

February 23rd

Glen Trnavski, the high-school chemistry teacher I met in the parking lot a few weeks ago, called me after school yesterday. I guess he knew I needed some emotional support after eight-plus hours with fifth-graders. Despite what my mother thinks, I was never cut out to be a teacher. However, one bonus has been working with Peter Murchison, Julia's husband. I really like him and he's wonderful with the children.

Glen is actually kind of like Peter. Quiet, calm, a good sense of humor. He's different from the guys I know through drama—like Jeff. But quiet as he is, he's one of the most comfortable men I've ever met and when I analyzed why, I discovered it's because he *listens.* Not only does he listen, he seems to appreciate what I have to say. One thing I particularly like about him is his laugh—it comes from deep in his chest. He's *NOT* my type, though. Too even-tempered. Not bland, I don't mean that, but predictable. There's no fire in his belly, no all-consuming zeal.... Maybe I have enough for both of us?

I like his company and he understands that we're only friends, although he seems to want more. With all the rejection I've had lately, I need a man who's obviously falling in love with me—even if I can't return his feelings. I crave the attention. I'm not proud to admit it, but unfortunately it's true.

Speaking of rejection... I tried out for another commercial on Monday. This one was for hair spray and I should hear soon. I think I did well. I might not fit the role of meticulous housewife, but I can play an airhead to a tee. I've got real hopes this time. My agent said I should know what's up by the end of next week at the latest.

I haven't heard from my mother. That doesn't bother me, and I consider it a gift that she's decided to stay out of my life. Who needs the constant criticism? I'm always falling short of her expectations. Why can't she just accept me for who I am? Isn't that what every child needs? Love and acceptance. Mother wants me to do what *she* considers acceptable, so she can brag about me to her friends—and *then* she'll love me. That's completely backward! And it isn't fair and... Obviously this is still a big issue with me, otherwise I wouldn't continue to write about it. And I wouldn't have chosen "acceptance" as my word for the year. (Well, also I'd like to be accepted for an acting job! Positive thinking or what?)

Getting back to Glen. We're going to a movie tomorrow night. I probably shouldn't have agreed. I hate to string him along, but he did ask and it isn't like I've got hordes of men clamoring at my door. More's the pity. I love movies, and I don't mean to complain, but I find Glen...unexciting. Comfortable but unexciting.

I see as I review this journal entry that I've stayed away from the subject of my sister. She's been creeping into my Thursday morning conversations lately. Liz noticed. Nothing escapes her. Julia said she did, too.

When I asked them what they were talking about, Liz said I've spent my entire life competing with Victoria for my mother's attention. Well, duh! I knew that. Although Liz did say something that made me think. It annoyed me, too. She suggested I dress outrageously, (according to whom?) in order to provoke my mother. To get negative attention, in other words. I disagree. I don't do *anything* to get a reaction out of my mother. I dress the way I dress, which is stylish and unique (in my humble opinion, anyway). Because that's who I am. I'm me and nobody else.

Now that was profound!

Anyway, I hate to tell my friends they're wrong. My relationship with my mother has practically nothing to do with my older sister. Yes, I'm competitive with Victoria, but *she's* the one responsible for that.

She didn't have to be so perfect. She's always done everything according to form. The classic good girl. It was like she set me up to fail because there was no way

I was going to be prettier or smarter or more success-ful than she is. Enough said. The subject is closed and I'm going to bed.

* * *

By the time six o'clock arrived on Saturday night, Karen had serious doubts about her seven o'clock date with Glen Trnavski. She worried that she was using him to flatter her sagging ego, and worse, that he might read more into their date than he should. Friday night, she hadn't felt too con-cerned about this prospect, but in the light of day, her be-haviour didn't seem fair. She'd stressed the "just friends" stipulation, but still...

She'd halfway decided to phone and beg off when she got a call. If luck was with her, it would be Glen and he'd be the one canceling. That way, the problem would be solved with-out any action on her part.

"Hello," she said cheerfully.

No response.

"Hello," she said again, more loudly this time. "Is that you, Jeff?" she snapped. She hadn't heard from him since their spat and couldn't help wondering—and hoping....

Silence.

"You're really sick, you know that? If this is Jeff, then you already know what I think. If this is someone else, all I can say is *get a life*." With that, she banged down the receiver emphatically enough to make the person on the other end regret phoning.

Glen Trnavski arrived five minutes early with a bouquet of pink carnations.

Karen instantly felt guilty for wanting to cancel.

"How thoughtful," she said, holding the flowers to her

nose. Pink carnations might not be original, but it'd been a long time since any man had done anything so sweet and, yes, traditional. Karen was touched, although she reminded herself that this first date was supposed to be a non-date, more of an outing between two friends.

"Have you decided on a movie?" he asked, following her inside the studio apartment.

"You're letting me choose?" Other guys she dated generally decided in advance what movie they'd see. Or it was a decision they made together. "There's a new Julia Roberts film I wouldn't mind going to," she suggested. A "chick flick." Most guys were more interested in high adventure, blood and guts, gasoline explosions.

"Fine with me." He was so agreeable; she liked that and she didn't. This was not a man who was likely to argue anything to the wall. Or generate any fireworks.

After setting the carnations inside an empty mayonnaise bottle, one she'd saved for just such an occasion, Karen reached for her jacket and purse. Just as they were about to leave, the phone rang again.

"I'd better get that," she said hurrying across the room to pick up the receiver. She wasn't expecting to hear from her agent on a Saturday night, but she didn't want to miss anything important, either. Her cheap answering machine wasn't always reliable.

"Hello?"

Nothing.

Impatient, she slammed the receiver down and complained, "That happened earlier. I answer the phone and there's no one there. Well, there is, but they aren't speaking."

"Do you have any idea who it might be?"

"Not a clue." She certainly wasn't going to mention Jeff.

"What about caller ID?" Glen asked.

"Don't have it." She hated to admit she pinched her pennies to the point that she'd never enjoyed the luxury of caller ID. It was difficult enough paying her phone bill without all the extras. Her one extravagance was call waiting. Heaven forbid she miss a call from her agent because she was chatting with a friend. Of course, she could always punch star 69. She decided to try that now. Naturally, the number was unlisted and she groaned in frustration.

"If they call again, you simply won't be here," Glen said with such perfect logic she had no comeback. "They can leave a message—or not."

He was right, of course; there was no reason to worry about it. She turned on the machine, and with a lighter heart, grabbed a woolen cape she sometimes liked to wear. Glen took it from her and placed it around her shoulders. He was being traditional again, and she decided she rather liked it. This wasn't a gesture she was personally familiar with—except in old movies and period plays.

The movie was delightful, and they both laughed their way through it. Afterward they shared a gourmet veggie pizza and glasses of red wine at a popular Italian restaurant in the area. Despite her reservations about the wisdom of seeing Glen, Karen enjoyed herself and their time together. Her one disappointment was that she was home by eleven. When she invited him in for coffee, Glen politely declined.

As she entered her apartment, she couldn't help wondering if *she'd* passed muster. The first thing she noticed was the flashing light of her answering machine. In replaying the tape, she discovered there were no less than six hang-ups. *One* she could understand, even two, but six?

Whoever had called earlier and said nothing had obviously continued phoning. Karen was tempted to unplug the phone and be done with it.

She turned on the television for company, then stripped out of her jeans and vest. She'd just pulled on her pajamas when the phone rang again. Karen stared at it, certain that her caller was the jokester. The best thing to do was let the answering machine pick up, she told herself. However, seconds before the machine kicked in, Karen impulsively grabbed the receiver. She wasn't sure why, hadn't even known she was going to do it. One second she was staring at the phone, willing it to stop ringing, and the next she had the receiver in her hand.

"Hello," she yelled, furious with herself as much as the anonymous fruitcake on the other end.

Silence.

Karen was about to slam down the receiver and unplug her phone when she heard a soft, unrecognizable female voice say her name.

"Hello," Karen tried again. "Who is this?

"It's me."

Karen strained to make out the voice, but couldn't. "Who?" she demanded.

"It's Victoria."

"What's the matter with you?" Karen asked aggressively. "Are you the one who's been calling and hanging up? Why? You scared me, dammit!"

"I...I can't talk any louder, Roger might hear me."

Roger the twit, her brother-in-law. "You don't want him to know you're on the phone?"

"No..."

Karen thought she heard a soft intake of breath that might have been a sob. "What's wrong?" she asked more gently.

No response.

"Victoria? Are you still there?" The line hadn't been disconnected, but there was no further sound.

"I'm here," Victoria finally whispered.

Karen guessed her sister was in some kind of trouble, otherwise she wouldn't be phoning her, especially this late. And all those hangups... A sense of urgency filled Karen. The kind that required action. Something was terribly wrong. "I'm coming for you and Bryce."

"No." Her sister's response was sharp and immediate.

"Tell me what happened."

Victoria hesitated, sobbed once, then spoke again, her voice so low Karen had to concentrate in order to make out the words. "Roger and I had an argument."

Karen couldn't understand why her sister was calling her. What did Victoria need her to do? Sympathize? Give advice? That seemed unlikely, but just as she was about to ask, Victoria explained. "You were always so brave..." she said in a quavering voice. "You never let people get away with anything. I—I've always admired that. I...wanted to talk to you, tell you..." The words trailed off.

"Is everything all right between you and Roger now?" Karen asked.

Again the hesitation. "No."

"Are you sure you don't want me to come and get you?"

"I'm sure."

"Is there anything I can do to help you?" Karen asked, sitting down on the sofa and folding her legs beneath her. "Do you want to get away, talk, whatever?" She couldn't remember the last time she'd talked to her sister—*really* talked. Years ago, she guessed. Long before Karen had graduated from high school. Victoria was two years older, and Karen had looked up to her sister. Their real troubles had started when Victoria was away at college and Karen had gotten involved in the school acting ensemble.

"I don't think there's anything anyone can do," Victoria whispered.

Her sister was sobbing quietly and trying not to let Karen know. Karen's heart went out to her. "Did I ever tell you I think Roger's a total twit?"

Victoria responded with a hiccuping sound that was half laugh and half sob. "No, but I guessed. And...he knows."

"Good." Karen was glad to hear it.

"Oh, Sis, sometimes I think..." She didn't finish.

"Think what?" Karen probed.

"Nothing," Victoria said after a moment.

"Do you want to tell me about the argument?"

"It...it isn't important. The reasons never are."

"Victoria, listen. People don't always agree. We fought enough as kids, didn't we? It doesn't mean we don't love each other. We all say and do things we regret." Karen wasn't taking sides, nor did she want to put herself in the middle of a disagreement between her sister and brother-in-law. What she wanted to do was present a mature option, and give them both some breathing room. "Why don't you hop in the car and come on over here with Bryce? We can sit up all night and have a gabfest the way we did when we were kids."

"I can't."

"Sure you can. If you prefer, I could drive over to your place."

"No...no, that wouldn't work."

Karen's hand tightened around the receiver as a horrifying thought occurred to her. "Is there a reason you don't want me to see you?"

A soft sob, then, "Yes."

A chill ran down her spine. "The son of a bitch hit you, didn't he?"

"We're all in this alone."

—Lily Tomlin

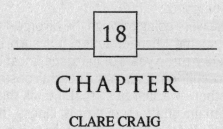

CHAPTER

CLARE CRAIG

March 9th

Most of my day was spent with Michael. Not *with* him as in the same room or even the same vicinity. But I thought about him constantly. He was back in the hospital for his second bout of chemotherapy and Alex was scheduled to pick him up at the same time as before.

Apparently Miranda can't be bothered. Her excuse is that she's building her customer base and can't be dragged away from the nail clinic without missing appointments. I can't stand the way Michael defends her!

Alex knows better than to discuss the little darling with me, although I doubt he would, anyway. He finds the subject of Michael's live-in lover as distasteful as I do.

I know it's hard for Alex to see his father this ill. It

is for me, too. I can sympathize with my son; Michael's his father, after all. My own reaction is harder to understand. Why should I care so much? But I do, especially since Michael's condition appears to be fairly serious. He's avoided my questions so far, but from what I've been able to learn, it's some form of liver cancer. Alex doesn't know any more details than I do, but this can't be good.

While we were going through the divorce, I thought I'd enjoy seeing Michael suffer, but surprisingly I don't. Twenty-three years of marriage, most of them good, two children plus a successful business we built together—we shared all that. I think this is why I can't remain unaffected by his illness. If ever I needed proof of the thin line between love and hate, here it is. The line's so thin, in fact, that sometimes it's transparent.

Michael's chemotherapy, and apparently he's being given one of the more aggressive drug combinations, takes nearly all day. He's at the hospital for almost eight hours and so weak he can barely walk when he's finished. For four consecutive days he receives the drug cocktail, then he doesn't get it again for three weeks. I don't know how many treatments he'll require, but Alex mentioned four sessions. Four months of this seems like a very long time.

Twice now, because of Alex's schedule at school and my part-time hours, I've been the one to chauffeur Michael home from the hospital. My friends in the Thursday morning group fear I shouldn't be doing this. As they pointed out, Michael does have other options that don't need to involve me. I understand their concerns and yet I still find myself volunteering.

I'm confused about my feelings for Michael right now. Love, hate. Compassion, anger. It's all there.

And apparently I'm not the only one who's confused. Michael doesn't know what to think about me, either. We talk more, but never about *her* or the divorce. The ride between the hospital and his place takes about thirty minutes, depending on traffic. So I guess it's only natural that we talk. After all, we spent more than two decades talking to each other.

The first time, our conversation was stilted and un-comfortable. More recently Michael described the side effects of chemotherapy. The weakness and nausea, the continuing weight loss, the depression. He's losing his hair but that seems too insignificant to mention. (Al-though it probably bothers his girlfriend.)

I was forced to stop the second time I drove him, too. I pulled off to the side of the road and just as before, Michael stumbled out of the car and immediately vom-ited. Then he did the oddest thing. He reached down and touched his vomit. *Touched* it. I had to know why. Michael would never do anything like that under nor-mal circumstances.

After he'd rinsed his mouth, he explained. It's the fire, he said. It feels as though his entire body is burn-ing from the inside out. The reason he touched the vomit was to see if it was boiling. That's the way it felt coming up from his stomach and through his throat. Like molten lava.

I gave him a few minutes to regroup and breathe in

the fresh air. He leaned against the bumper, too weak to stand upright.

I had to help him back into the car and I know he found it embarrassing. Once he was settled and we were on our way again, he casually asked about Mick. Apparently our oldest son remains unwilling to speak to his father. He knows about the cancer; I told him myself. But Mick is as stubborn and unforgiving as I am. It gives me no pleasure to write this.

Michael isn't the only one Mick isn't speaking to these days. I wonder if he knows that his sons are estranged from each other because of him. Alex and Mick haven't talked in weeks. It hurts me to see it, knowing how close they once were. The boys and I clung to one another all through the divorce, and now Mick can't forgive his brother for reconciling with their father. He was upset with me too when he learned I'd driven Michael home from the hospital. I guess I should count my blessings that he's still speaking to me. It's probably just as well that Mick's at college and not living at home right now, much as I hate to say that.

When we reached the place Michael's renting, he told me how much he regrets what's happening between him and his sons. Even though he sees Alex every week, Michael realizes their relationship will never be what it was. And Mick, of course, won't have anything to do with him.

Michael wanted me to know how much he loves them and how sorry he is, how he'd do anything to repair the damage. He looked sad and broken as he climbed out of the car and headed toward the small, dumpy rental house.

Not until he disappeared inside did I realize something important. When he talked about his remorse over everything that's happened, my name was missing.

> "See into life—don't just look at it."
>
> —Anne Baxter

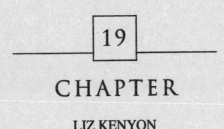

CHAPTER

LIZ KENYON

March 13th

Annie wrote me, and her sweet, precious letter was waiting when I arrived home from work. It thrilled me to hear from my granddaughter, but I felt restless and sad for the rest of the evening. Just a few months ago she lived here in Willow Grove and we had all the time in the world to be together. I miss our tea parties and baking muffins and snuggling up together in bed.

I read the letter twice, then wandered into the bedroom. The big fancy hats and white gloves we used for our tea parties are on the top shelf of my closet, gathering dust. What fun Annie and I had as we sipped tea—hers cooled with milk—from delicate china cups, the ones I inherited from Steve's mother. We'd nibble on cookies, having silly conversations with lots of laughter. It's a memory that brings tears to my eyes.

Amy and the kids and I chat every week, but it's not the same. I miss Annie and Andrew so much. They're my only grandchildren, an extension of my children, an extension of Steve and me and the wonderful years we shared.

My appetite was nil tonight, but I forced myself to eat dinner, although I didn't put any effort into cooking nor did I experience any pleasure when I sat down at the kitchen table to eat. When Steve was alive, our dinners were an occasion, always served in the dining room with good linen and china, usually accompanied by a glass of wine. I took pride in cooking. Now dinner is simply a necessity, a chore.

As soon as I finished eating and feeling sorry for myself, I wrote Annie, holding Tinkerbell in my lap, making a rash promise. I told her I'd visit her this summer. The thought lightened my mood and then on a wild impulse, I made the decision to drive from California to Oklahoma. I hate flying. I detest being cramped in a narrow seat, breathing recycled air. Invariably I'm stuck with an inconsiderate jerk who rams the back of his seat into my nose. Why should I fly when I have the time and the desire to drive?

I can already hear Amy and Brian's objections. My children are going to remind me that it's not safe for a woman to drive a distance of that length alone. They'll want to know why I'd take the risk when air travel is so convenient. And I can almost guarantee they won't like my answer.

Over the years, Steve and I took a number of driving trips, with the kids and without them. We always enjoyed our time on the road. Like so much else in my marriage, I've missed that. Spending all those days in the car is far from a hardship when you're with a person you love, a person you know so well. It's a distinct pleasure and definitely my favorite way to travel. However, it's just not a possibility now; there's no one like that in my life. But I can still enjoy my vacation. With three weeks due me, I can drive leisurely, stop when I feel like it, tour where I want to and still spend plenty of time with Amy and the kids.

I don't intend to be stupid about it, but if something dreadful happens, an accident of some kind, then so be it. I refuse to live the rest of my life in fear. I enjoy driving, I miss my grandchildren and I'm heading for Tulsa.

Only I won't mention my plans to the family. Not yet. No need to stir up their concerns this early. Besides, it won't matter; I've made up my mind. First thing tomorrow morning, I'll book the time off. I feel better already, just knowing I'll be with Annie and Andrew this summer.

Karen phoned just before I got ready for bed. She asked several questions about reporting spousal abuse. It didn't take me long to figure out who she was talking about, although she didn't actually mention her sister by name.

Karen is outraged and rightly so. She wants *the son-of-a-bitch* arrested. Although I don't know why she phoned *me* to ask these questions. I guess it's because I'm older and supposed to be wiser. And maybe she figures that I know about domestic crime because I work in a hospital. I told her that, to the best of my knowledge, a third party can't file charges. I explained that whoever was abused had to be the one to do it.

It was fairly easy to decipher what went on, although she was careful not to break any confidences. Karen has rarely mentioned her brother-in-law and never by name. She calls him "the twit," which appears to be a fairly accurate characterization. Reading between the lines, I listened as she explained that this *son-of-a-bitch* took a heavy hand to his wife. Just when it looked as if Karen had convinced *the wife* to file a report with the police, the twit sobered up and apologized. *The wife* has apparently forgiven him.

Karen is furious, not only with "the twit," but with her sister. She's having a difficult time accepting Victoria's decision. Again and again she talked about the danger she felt *the wife* and her child were in and how the *son-of-a-bitch* couldn't be trusted. I told her there was nothing more she could do without the wife's cooperation.

She didn't like hearing that any more than I liked telling her.

I will say one thing. For months now I've heard Karen complain about her sad relationship with her family. Even her word for the year has more to do with her family than with Karen herself—or so it seems to me.

At one breakfast meeting, she spoke of severing her relationship with her mother entirely. Each of us advised her not to do anything so rash, told her she'd regret it later. We all said family's too important to throw away like that. Karen took our words to heart, and I think she's glad she did. If ever her sister needed her love and support, it's now. From what Karen's said, *the wife* can't go to her parents. Karen might well be the only person Victoria can turn to.

* * *

It was nearly two and Liz still hadn't taken a lunch break. The way things were going, thirty minutes away from her office just wasn't feasible. Her one solution was to run down to the cafeteria and grab a sandwich to eat at her desk.

"You leaving?" Donna DeGooyer, the hospital social worker, looked stricken as she raced into Liz's office.

"What do you need?"

"Help and lots of it. I've got an adoptive couple coming to pick up a baby and an attorney who hasn't got the paperwork finalized and a young mother who's having second thoughts. The attorney and the birth mother are on their way to my office right now."

"I was just going to get a sandwich. Do you want to come with me?"

Donna did a double-take as she looked at her watch. "It's after two. Already? Go have lunch and I'll catch you later." Then she was gone as quickly as she'd arrived.

Taking her wallet with her, Liz headed for the basement where the hospital cafeteria was located. The food was cheap, and for institutional fare, she found it surprisingly good. The lunch crowd had thinned considerably and the room was nearly empty. She reached for a tray, sliding it along the steel rails as she studied the remaining choices.

This late in the afternoon the selections were narrowed down to only a few. As she picked up an egg salad sandwich and a small pastry, Sean Jamison stepped next to her and slid his tray alongside hers.

"Egg salad?" He sounded skeptical. "Hmm. And a danish. High fat, empty calories. I don't recommend it."

Ignoring him, Liz placed both items on her tray.

"You're a stubborn woman, aren't you?"

She didn't so much as glance in his direction. "If you haven't figured that out by now, you're a slow learner."

It'd been nearly a month since she'd last seen him. They'd parted on pleasant terms—sort of. He had said he'd wait for her to call him, and that wasn't going to happen. She liked Sean, enjoyed his company, but she wasn't interested in a casual affair, which was all he seemed to be seeking.

He helped himself to a sandwich—*and* a danish, Liz noted. What a hypocrite! She poured a cup of coffee and he did likewise.

"You eating here?" he asked as they moved toward the cashier.

Liz's original intention was to take lunch back to her office, but now she hesitated. "I was thinking of it."

"I was, too."

She paid for her meal, then chose a seat close to the window.

Sean paid for his lunch and positioned himself at the table directly across from hers. Liz glared at him. "Aren't you being a bit ridiculous?" she asked.

"Is that an invitation to join you?"

She sighed. "Don't be silly. You can sit here if you want."

He was out of his chair and at her table within seconds. She could tell by his cocky grin that he was pleased, as though her invitation—such as it was—had been a concession.

"It's good to see you," he said as he unwrapped the cellophane from his sandwich. "I'd hoped we'd get together before now. I don't mind telling you, it's been a long month. You're trying my patience, Liz. We both know what we want, so let's be mature about it."

Liz reached for the salt and pepper shakers and peeled back the bread to dump liberal doses on the egg salad. "Don't you ever give up?" she asked, not in the mood for verbal sparring.

"What?"

"You're wasting your time. I'm not calling you."

"Ah," he said with a beleaguered sigh, "so this is all a matter of pride."

"Come on," she scoffed, "you know better than that. I came away from our dinner date feeling good—until you wanted to turn me into one of your sexual conquests."

"Wrong. I happen to think you're an attractive woman and I believe we could enjoy each other in a mutually satisfying arrangement. What's so terrible about that?"

She was about to explain once again exactly what she objected to, but he cut her off.

"You're sexually repressed, aren't you?" he said. He seemed to be serious.

Laughing probably wasn't the most tactful response to his assessment, but Liz couldn't help herself. "You know what I've decided?" she asked, and then didn't give him a chance to answer. "I like you. I'm not sure why, because when it comes to male-female relationships, you're about as shallow as a man can get."

"Insults now?"

"No, the truth, and apparently there aren't enough people in this world brave enough to give it to you."

"Should I be grateful you're so willing to enlighten me?" He looked more entertained than insulted.

"Yes, but I doubt you will be. Frankly, I don't know who you've been dating for the last ten years, but the Hugh Hefner image lost its appeal a long time ago."

"Hugh Hefner?" he repeated as though that amused him. "Are you kidding?"

"I'm disappointed in you, Sean." This, too, was the truth. Her sincerity must have reached him because his grin slowly faded. "You see me as nothing more than a challenge," she said in a matter-of-fact tone.

He pushed his unfinished sandwich aside. "Hey, it's something we share because that's exactly how you see me. The only thing you're interested in is a ring on your finger. I went the marriage route once, remember, and all that got me was a whole lot of pain."

"I'm not asking you to marry me. I'm simply stating that I won't fall into bed with you without a committed relationship on both our parts."

"Sex isn't a four-letter word," he sputtered.

"But it is," she countered. "L-O-V-E."

"Been there, done that, not interested in doing it again."

Liz stared at him. She recalled that the only personal thing he'd told her was that he'd been married at one time. She hadn't realized the significance of that earlier.

"Was the marriage that bad?" she asked.

His face hardened. "Leave my ex out of this."

"All right." Apparently he'd carried the burden of his

failed marriage for the last ten years. Everything he said proved he'd never moved beyond the regrets and the pain.

"I don't need any more lectures from you or anyone else." He stood and emptied his tray, pastry, coffee and all, in the wastebasket on his way out of the room.

Liz knew it was unlikely she'd see him or hear from him again, unless it was work-related and unavoidable. Actually, that was for the best all around. They had nothing substantial in common, she decided, and a sadness settled over her.

She knew she had to relinquish the hopes she'd centered on Sean Jamison. Her natural tendency was to hang on, to keep hoping, but if she'd learned anything in the last six years, it was the danger that posed to her sanity and her heart. Sometimes you had to let people go—let your *feelings* for them go—in order to protect yourself.

She was back in her office when Donna returned, and from the relieved look on her face, Liz assumed that the adoption crisis had been resolved. Donna paused halfway inside the room. "You okay?"

"Of course I'm okay." Liz was surprised her friend could read her this readily.

"I just saw Dr. Jamison, and he's on another of his rampages. You two didn't happen to cross paths, did you?"

Liz nodded. "You could say so," she muttered. "We don't see eye to eye on certain subjects."

Donna sank down on the chair and crossed her legs. "I don't get it. As a physician he's brilliant and wonderful, and as a man he's a major jerk. The way he treats women is deplorable."

"I agree." And she did.

"The entry of a child into any situation changes the whole situation."

—Iris Murdoch

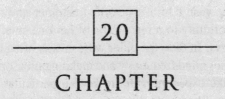

CHAPTER

JULIA MURCHISON

The Wool Station had been quiet all morning. Not an encouraging sign, Julia mused as she sat in her rocking chair and knitted a swatch to display the latest double-knit cotton yarn. She wanted this to sell, *needed* it to sell, seeing that she'd ordered it in fifteen different colors. The steel needles made a soft clicking that disrupted the silence. Her stomach had been queasy all morning, but she'd done her best to ignore it. Nor did she allow her mind to dwell on the battery of tests she'd recently undergone. The final results weren't in yet, and Julia wasn't sure she wanted to know. She'd had all the reality she could handle at the moment. If the baby did have Down's Syndrome or spina bifida or whatever, she'd deal with it when necessary and not before.

Some days the denial tactic helped, and she could pretend everything was okay. On other days, that was impossible. Her stomach rebelled. The morning sickness wasn't as bad as it had been when she first discovered she was pregnant. But it was bad enough.

A Mercedes pulled into the parking space in front of the store and Julia recognized Irene Waldmann. Great. Mrs. Waldmann wasn't Julia's favorite customer and she took every opportunity to remind Julia of her one small mathematical error. In fact, the older woman was often difficult, changing her mind frequently and making unreasonable demands—like expecting Julia to keep a particular wool in stock when it had been discontinued by the manufacturer. The root of the problem, in Julia's opinion, was that Mrs. Waldmann didn't really know what she wanted herself. Clearly wealthy, if her clothes and vehicle were any indication, she drifted from one project to another.

"Hello." Julia greeted her with a smile.

Mrs Waldmann ignored the greeting and headed for the rack where Julia kept the pattern books.

"Is there anything I can help you find?" she asked.

"Not just yet."

Finishing her row, Julia stood—and the room started to spin. She gripped the chair in an effort to steady herself. A moment later, her head cleared and then almost immediately her stomach heaved. The sensation was unmistakable.

"You'll have to excuse me for a moment," Julia said, rushing to the back of the store. She made it to the small rest room just in time. The little breakfast she'd managed to eat was soon gone.

Mrs. Waldmann's eyes were wide when Julia reappeared.

Until recently she'd kept the news of her pregnancy from her customers. But instances such as this needed explaining.

"You'll have to forgive me," she said, faltering slightly. "I'm—I'm pregnant."

Mrs. Waldmann stared back at her in open curiosity. "Pregnant? At your age?"

"It looks that way." How comforting to be reminded that she was past her prime. Her instinct had been to explain that this pregnancy wasn't intentional, that she and her husband were as surprised as everyone else. But she held her ground, refusing to defend herself or her situation. It was private— no one's business but theirs.

"Well," the other woman said, spinning the pattern rack. "That settles that."

"I beg your pardon?"

"I was just wondering what I should knit next." She twirled the rack until she found the infant section and reached for a pattern.

Julia was confused. "I'm sorry, did I miss something?"

"Apparently so," the older woman said dryly. "I've decided to knit a baby blanket for this new child of yours."

"For me?"

"Do you have a hearing problem?"

"N-no, I mean, b-but why..." Julia knew she was stuttering; she couldn't help it.

"I imagine this is a case of the cobbler's children without any shoes. I take it this pregnancy is unexpected?"

"Well, yes but—"

"Have you knit anything for your baby?"

"No, not yet, but—" She had every intention of doing so.

The problem was finding the time between her family and her commitment to The Wool Station's customers.

"Just as I thought," Mrs. Waldmann said, with—could it be?—a hint of humor. "You can use a blanket, can't you?"

"You'd do that for me?" Julia asked, taken aback by the generosity of the offer. Especially from a customer she'd often considered a burden.

"Boy or girl?" Mrs. Waldmann asked gruffly.

"We chose not to know," Julia answered.

Mrs. Waldmann nodded approvingly. "Good for you. There are too few surprises left in this life."

At the moment, Julia would happily live with fewer. The last four months hadn't been easy. Adam and Zoe's attitudes toward her pregnancy hadn't improved. The only people who seemed happy about it were her husband and her mother. All right, her sister and Georgia, too. George seemed to think the baby was destined to be "special."

"What do you think of this?" Mrs. Waldmann handed her a complicated pattern.

"This is an heirloom piece," Julia commented, wondering if the other woman realized the work involved in such a blanket.

"My thought exactly."

"But—"

"Shall I do it in ecru or would you prefer a soft yellow?"

"Ah..."

"Don't suggest that sickening lime color. I never could stand that."

"The yellow sounds very nice." Julia couldn't quite hide her astonishment. Mrs. Waldmann—of all people—knitting her a baby blanket!

"Good, that's what I would have chosen myself. There's something so...warm about yellow, don't you think? So uplifting."

"Yes," Julia agreed. Turning over the pattern, she read the amount of yarn required, then counted out the skeins, selecting the lemony yellow fingering weight.

Mrs. Waldmann concentrated on the pattern, her brow furrowed. Never having seen anything the other woman had completed, Julia worried that his project might be beyond her capabilities, but she dared not suggest it.

"You don't need to do this," she felt obliged to tell Mrs. Waldmann a second time.

"Didn't anyone ever warn you not to look a gift horse in the mouth?" Mrs. Waldmann asked her briskly.

"Yes, but really this is too much."

"Don't you tell me what is and isn't too much. I want to do this and I will."

"It's so nice of you."

"Oh, hardly. I know I'm not the easiest woman in the world to deal with. But you've always been patient with me and I appreciate it."

"I appreciate the business," Julia told her in turn, and it was true, especially on days like this. She needed to take in two hundred dollars a day just to meet her rent and utilities. The morning was half-gone and this was her first sale. Some days were like that.

Mrs. Waldmann wrote the check, tore it out and gave it to Julia. She hesitated as though she was about to say something, then evidently changed her mind. Julia handed her the bag.

"Thank you again," she said.

Mrs. Waldmann nodded. "I'll see you in a few weeks."

"I'll look forward to it."

At dinner that evening, Julia mentioned Mrs. Waldmann and what she'd done. It was a way of bringing the baby into the conversation in a casual manner; she thought this kind of comment might help the children adjust.

"Why would she do something like that?" Adam asked, sounding more annoyed than pleased.

"Some people like babies," Zoe answered, in a tone that suggested she wasn't one of them.

"What did you say her name was again?" Peter asked, frowning as he propped his elbows on the table, dangling his fork above his dinner plate.

"Irene Waldmann."

"Waldmann, Waldmann," he repeated thoughtfully. "The name rings a bell."

Julia noticed that as soon as she mentioned the baby both Adam and Zoe had grown sullen and unpleasant. She'd hoped that in time they'd be more accepting, more generous of heart.

She glanced at her family. She hated to bring discord to the table, but she couldn't ignore their attitude.

"I understand that this isn't easy," she said to her children. No further explanation was needed; both Adam and Zoe knew she was talking about the baby.

"How could you do this?" Zoe demanded, once again. "Nothing will ever be the same."

"We can't afford a car now." Adam glared at her, resentment in every word.

"Or a vacation," Zoe chimed in, close to tears.

"Stop it!" Peter banged his fist on the table. "Just listen to you," he said. "Just listen! You're only thinking about yourselves."

Rarely had Julia seen her amiable, easy-going husband display such anger and disgust.

"No one said it was our duty to provide you with a vehicle just because you're turning sixteen. Nor is there anything written about a parent's obligation to take children on expensive vacations. Your mother and I know you're disappointed about missing out on those things, but guess what, life is filled with disappointment. I'm ashamed of your selfishness. You think a little embarrassment in front of your friends, or having to share your bedroom with a younger brother or sister, is some major tragedy. Get a little perspective!"

Both children stared openmouthed at their father.

"Your mother and I have tried to be patient, to give you time to accept our news. But you know something? This baby is entitled to as much love and welcome as you received when you came into our family."

Silence followed. Then Zoe sniffled and bowed her head. "Can I be excused?"

"You're finished with your dinner?" Most of her meal remained untouched.

Zoe nodded.

"All right."

"Me, too," Adam muttered.

Frowning, Peter waved him off and the children hastily left the table.

Julia could tell by the belligerent way they stalked out of the room that nothing had changed.

Her husband shook his head. "I don't think I've ever been more disappointed in my children."

"Give them a chance," Julia urged, feeling guilty about her own ambivalence and resentment. Peter was right. This child deserved the same love as Adam and Zoe. Unfortunately the kids weren't the only ones who needed to hear it. Julia had to remind herself, as well.

* * *

List of Blessings
1. Irene Waldmann
2. Salt and how desperately I miss it
3. Comfortable shoes
4.
5.

March 21st

Adam and Zoe are barely speaking to Peter and me. The last few days have been a real strain. Peter suggested we just let them have their little temper tantrum and not react to it. Eventually they'll come around. I only hope he's right. I knew they were upset with us; I hadn't realized it was to this extent.

Peter came to the shop after school this afternoon. He had a copy of a newspaper article from the early 1990s. It was about a Manchester high-school graduate by the name of William Waldmann who'd been killed in Desert Storm. He was the only child of Irene and Brad Waldmann.

The other night at dinner, when I mentioned Irene's

name, Peter had said it sounded familiar. So he looked
it up on the school Internet and found the article.

My heart aches for Mrs. Waldmann. Her only son. I
can't imagine what it would be like to lose a child. The
grief would be unbearable. Knowing this helps me understand why she was so willing to knit a baby blanket
for me. There are no grandchildren in her future.

Georgia stopped by the store this morning on her
way home from work. Her job at the gallery has the
craziest hours; they spent all night setting up for a
major exhibit that's opening today. She filled in for me
while I ran to Dr. Fisk's for my appointment. Thankfully
I was in and out in forty minutes, which is something
of a record. I hate leaving the shop, but there's no help
for it. Nor was I comfortable closing for even an hour;
I've done that too many times already. If there's one
thing customers demand, it's consistency. If I say my
store's open from 10 to 5, then I'd better be open during those hours.

Georgia brought me a new maternity top. I looked
at it and wanted to weep. She was only trying to be
kind, but I hate the thought of growing into *that*.

Liz came for her knitting lesson at lunchtime.

She says the tension at the hospital is getting to her,
and she finds that knitting helps relax her at night.
We've done some squares, just to practice different
stitches, and today she bought yarn to make a sweater
for her granddaughter. We cast on and began, following a simple pattern I selected for her

I wasn't fooled. She comes more to check up on me

than because of any real desire start knitting. I know she and the others are worried about me. The last few weeks I haven't said much at breakfast. I won't for a while yet. I told Liz that, and the reasons for it, and she understood. I'm trying my hardest to make the best of this situation. I'm disappointed in my children, but no more than I am in myself.

"Only friends will tell you the truths you need to
hear to make...your life bearable."
—Francine du Plessix Gray

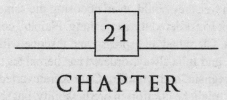

CHAPTER

THURSDAY MORNING BREAKFAST CLUB

Karen arrived at Mocha Moments early, and ordered her
current favorite latte, a caramel and mocha combination that
tasted like a liquid candy bar with twice as many calories.
Luckily, Karen didn't need to worry about her weight. A lot
of her friends were fanatical about every morsel they put in
their mouths. Not Karen; she ate what she wanted and when
she wanted. A good metabolism was just the luck of the
draw, she supposed.

She carried her drink to the table and slid into a chair,
planning to talk to her friends about Victoria. She had great
news, too, about getting the hair spray commercial, and she
was eager to let everyone know. Still, it was her sister's
dilemma that preoccupied her most. She was grateful Victoria had reached out to *her,* even if she'd now begun to back

off. Karen wanted to help her older sister, but deciding how
to do that was giving her a major headache.

Liz entered the coffee shop and walked up to the counter
to order her breakfast. Liz was almost always the first to arrive, but today Karen had come early.

The majority of people were creatures of habit, she mused,
and the four of them were no exception. They sat at the same
table whenever they could, even choosing the same chairs.
Every week Liz ordered the same thing. Plain ol' coffee and
a croissant. Clare had an espresso and a scone with black-
berry jelly, and Julia always ordered tea, herbal tea now that
she was pregnant, and a muffin. Only Karen varied her orders; there might be comfort in predictability, but she found
more reassurance in being different.

She wished again that her mother was more like Liz. Karen
got on far better with her father, but her mother had dominated
him for years. She used to wonder if there'd been a mix-up at
the hospital and she was actually someone else's daughter. Or
if she'd been adopted—a favorite childhood fantasy of hers.

"Good morning," Liz said, sitting down gracefully. "You're
bright and early this morning." She wore a dark red suit with
a double-breasted jacket and straight skirt. The matching high
heels were fabulous. So few women wore heels anymore, and
Liz, already tall, didn't need the height. They made her look
more powerful, yet strikingly feminine.

"Morning," Karen returned with a smile.

Clare and Julia were only minutes behind Liz. Soon all
four were at the table, each with her signature breakfast.

"Karen was here when I arrived," Liz said, and the other
two women turned to her. This was obviously Liz's way of
letting them know there was something on Karen's mind.

"Is it your sister?" Clare asked. At their previous week's breakfast, Karen had finally told them about Victoria's situation.

"Yeah," she said. "Guys, I want to throttle her. Her husband punches her in the face. First she won't let me call the police, and now...now she's acting like it was all a big mistake."

"She wants to put the whole thing behind her, right?" Liz asked, frowning thoughtfully.

"Yes, but it's more than that. She's embarrassed she even phoned me."

"This isn't the first time Roger's hit her, is it?" The question came from Clare.

Karen couldn't be sure, but she guessed this was a pattern between Victoria and her husband. Abuse, followed by apologies and promises. Roger was a bully who took out his frustrations on his wife. Six years earlier, when Victoria had started dating Roger, there'd been an incident that Karen had never forgotten. It'd happened at a family function—Thanksgiving dinner, if she remembered correctly. A command performance.

Victoria had brought Roger to meet the family, and all through dinner her mother had fussed over him, ingratiating herself in a way that made Karen cringe. The entire meal had been a disaster. Her mother had set out her best china and silver in an effort to impress Victoria's wealthy beau. She'd chatted endlessly, casually dropping names as if their family was part of the social circle that frequented the elite clubs and shops of Beverly Hills.

As the miserable meal progressed, Karen had watched Roger drink glass after glass of wine. She noticed that at every opportunity he criticized Victoria until her sister had dissolved into tears and run from the table.

Karen's first inclination was to go after her and advise her to dump the creep. He might come from a wealthy family and work at an established law firm, but that didn't excuse bad manners or classless behavior. Before she could move, their mother had apologized for Victoria's rudeness.

Karen had been furious. To her parents' dismay, she'd stalked out of the room. The ensuing argument with her mother had resulted in Karen's leaving in a huff. She'd threatened never to return, although of course she did. But her already difficult relationship with her mother grew even more strained.

Within a week of that infamous Thanksgiving, Victoria and Roger were engaged. Their wedding had been a gala event, with her mother using the opportunity to do some major sucking up. From the moment Victoria married Roger, Catherine Curtis had placed her eldest daughter on a pedestal. Karen thought wryly that her mother never complained about *Victoria* not using her college degree; in fact, she'd encouraged her to stay home and be the kind of wife "a man of Roger's standing" required.

"I think Roger might have hit her before," Karen said, although she had no actual evidence. "I do know he's been abusing her emotionally for years."

"You weren't able to convince her to file a police report?" Julia asked, shaking her head as though she found it difficult to comprehend how any woman would endure such treatment from her husband.

"Not for lack of trying," Karen informed her friends. She'd done everything but make the call herself. Victoria had seemed so small and broken when they'd first talked. Karen was forced to wait until Monday morning, after Roger had left for the office, before Victoria would let her visit.

The bruises on her cheek and upper arms were dark and ugly. Karen was enraged, but didn't dare show it. She talked to her sister about contacting the authorities, calling her doctor, visiting a women's crisis center—taking some kind of action—but Victoria wavered and then later refused to discuss it.

"It was all her fault, right?" Clare said. "That's what she told you, isn't it?"

Karen nodded. "That's exactly what Victoria said. If she'd had Bryce in bed when Roger returned from his client dinner, everything would've been okay. Can you *believe* it?"

"I'm afraid that sort of confused thinking is typical of abused women."

"I just can't understand why this is happening to my sister," Karen said.

"It's not uncommon," Liz told her. "And the women's reactions are more complex than many people understand. It's easy for us to say she should leave him, but she may be feeling shame, fear, desperation, even a sense of aloneness."

"In a way, things are even worse now," Karen murmured.

"Worse?" Julia repeated. "Has he hit her again?"

"I almost wish he had. It might help Victoria see the light."

Liz pulled the corner off her croissant and slowly shook her head. "My guess is the bastard's turned into a regular Prince Charming."

Karen stared at the older woman. "How'd you know?"

Liz answered with a sad smile. "I've seen it far too often. And I've heard of quite a few similar cases."

"He's so sorry," Karen said in a syrupy sweet voice, imitating her sister. According to Victoria, Roger was sick with remorse the minute he saw her bruises. He'd begged her forgiveness, apparently close to tears, and seeing how sorry he was, Victoria agreed. "It'll never happen again," Karen reported, "or so Victoria claims."

"Until next time," Clare added, her deep voice weighted with sarcasm.

"What can I do?" The frustration and anger were consuming her. Any excitement she felt over getting a role in a commercial paled against what she'd learned about her sister. Victoria was all she could think about. This was her *sister*, and although they had their differences, Karen couldn't tolerate the thought of anyone mistreating her.

"You can't talk to your parents?" Julia asked.

"No. I wish I could, but...I can't." Karen had considered that herself, and after careful thought, recognized that it would only cause more problems within the family. In Victoria's current state of mind, she might deny the entire incident and then hate Karen for breaking her confidence. The same went for contacting social services. Roger would be furious and Karen was convinced he'd take it out on Victoria.

"You could suggest Victoria get some counseling," Liz advised.

"I've already tried that—she said no. Besides, it wouldn't do any good. Roger's the one who needs therapy."

"Your sister could use some help herself," Clare said, not mincing words. "She's letting her husband beat her and then making excuses for him."

"True." But Karen hated to admit it.

"Talking out my feelings with a counselor after Michael left helped me tremendously," Clare told her.

"Speaking of Michael, how is he?" Karen asked, anxious now to change the subject.

"He's finished with the second round of chemotherapy,"

Clare said. She pulled her scone apart, turning it into a pile of crumbs. "I haven't seen him in several days, but Alex calls him every afternoon."

"Does that bother you?" Julia asked. "Because it would me."

Clare shook her head, but Karen didn't know if that was an answer to Julia's question or if she simply didn't have one.

"I always thought I wanted to see him suffer...." she finally said.

"And now that he is, you're finding it difficult to watch," Liz murmured.

Clare nodded.

"Is the...girlfriend around?" Karen wondered whether Michael was getting any support, emotional or otherwise, from Miranda Armstrong.

Shrugging, Clare reached for her espresso. "I wouldn't know. She must be, because he's still at the house."

Michael had moved into a rental place with Miranda Armstrong and if he was still living at the same address, presumably it was with her. Karen thought that was a reasonable assumption.

"How's Mick dealing with this?" she asked.

Clare's sigh said it all. "Not well. He isn't speaking to his father. He's angry with Alex and infuriated with me. He said we're the most screwed-up family he's ever known and wants nothing to do with us."

"He doesn't mean it," Karen rushed to assure her friend. "I'm always saying stuff like that to my parents. Oh, I mean it at the time, but I regret it later."

"When was the last time you talked to Mick?" Liz asked.

"Sunday afternoon."

"Give him a week," Julia suggested.

"Two weeks," Karen said, "then call him yourself. That's what my father usually does. He has his little speech down pat. I can almost recite it along with him, but by the time he phones I'm always glad he does, so I listen and pretend to take his advice." It was all part of her family's particular routine; every family had its own version. Actually, she was grateful her father stepped in when he did, breaking the stalemate between her and her mother.

"Little speech?" Clare was smiling, which pleased Karen.

"Yeah. First Dad says he can't understand why my mother and I can't get along. Then he goes on to remind me of the importance of family. He finishes up by telling me how much he loves his girls. When we're done, I feel better and apparently so does my mother."

Karen didn't mention that she never spoke to her mother during these conversations. Vernon Curtis was the peacemaker in the family.

"How's life treating you?" Julia asked, looking at Liz.

"No complaints," she responded.

"Have you run into Dr. Jamison lately?" Clare wanted to know.

For all her bitterness over her failed marriage, Clare was something of a romantic, Karen thought.

"No," Liz said abruptly.

"He's been at the hospital, though, hasn't he?"

"I wouldn't know." She focused her gaze across the room, refusing to meet their eyes. "Sean and I have agreed to disagree."

"Is that regret I'm seeing in you?" Julia asked softly.

Liz considered her question for a long moment. "Perhaps.

But it's been six years since Steve was killed. In that time, I've learned I don't need a man in my life. If and when I decide to become involved, it'll be with a man who appreciates and respects me."

"You might not *need* a man," Karen said, leaning closer, "but that's not the same as wanting one."

"Besides, you had your kids around for most of those six years," Clare added, "and now you're alone."

"She's right," Julia said emphatically. "With your son and daughter moving out of the area, this is the first time you've had to deal with certain issues—like being alone and what you want to do with your future. There are no distractions around you now, and it makes a difference."

Liz would make a great poker player, Karen decided. Her face was unreadable. "Maybe I'll get serious about dating," she said, but Karen couldn't tell if she meant it or not.

"*You* need to start dating, too," Julia said, staring at Clare.

At the shocked look that descended on Clare's face, they all burst into laughter.

"You're joking, right?" Clare shook her head as though the idea was ludicrous.

"No, I'm not," Julia insisted. "In fact, I have an uncle I want you to meet."

Clare's mouth opened and then closed, but no sound came out. Finally, she asked, "Who?"

"My uncle Leslie. He's gorgeous and fun and visiting the family. We're having him to dinner Saturday night, and I want you to join us."

"Me?" Clare pressed her palm to her chest. "What about Liz—she doesn't have all the baggage I do. Anyway, I'm not ready. I—"

"This is totally nonthreatening," Julia broke in. "My uncle's only going to be in town for a couple of weeks. He's divorced, too. He understands."

"I don't know..."

"You're going," Liz stated in no uncertain terms.

"Why me?" Clare challenged. "*You* should be the one."

Karen caught the glance Liz and Julia exchanged. It told her what she'd already suspected. Julia had originally gone to Liz, but she'd refused and suggested Clare instead.

"You'll come, won't you?" Julia pleaded.

"I..." Clare looked uncertain and then seemed to arrive at a decision. "Yes, I think I will."

Liz positively beamed.

"Are you sure you're up to this?" Clare asked Julia. "Entertaining and all?"

"Of course I am."

"The pregnancy's going okay?"

She nodded, but Karen noted a small hesitation. "I haven't been sick all week."

"Has the baby moved yet?" Clare asked.

"She's moving all the time."

"She?"

"I don't know, but I like to think I'm having a girl."

"I have a name for her," Karen said. "You should call her Thursday."

"Thursday?"

"Sure, why not? You could name her after us."

"Sorry," Julia said, instantly nixing the idea. "I'm far too traditional for something like that. Besides 'Thursday's child is full of woe'—don't you remember the old rhyme?"

"Before we get sidetracked," Liz said, "I believe Karen has something else she wants to tell us."

All eyes turned to Karen.

Karen blinked and stared back at her friend.

"Don't you have some good news about a recent audition?"

Karen shrugged, pretending to make light of her success, then joyfully threw her arms in the air. "I got the role!"

> "It is not easy to find happiness in ourselves, and it is not possible to find it elsewhere."
>
> —Agnes Repplier

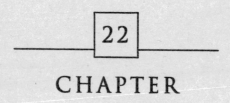

CHAPTER

CLARE CRAIG

April 7th

I can't believe I actually agreed to this dinner party. It's insane! The last time I went out with a man other than Michael was nearly twenty-six years ago. The minute Julia suggested the idea I should have refused. I have no idea what made me agree. How could I have done such a thing without thinking it through more carefully?

I'm not ready to date again. But if I phone now, just hours before I'm supposed to show up, I'd be putting Julia on the spot. To be honest, I'm not as worried about that as I am about what she'd tell the others in our group. Then everyone would know what a coward I am.

Okay, the decision is made. I'm going.

No, I'm not. I can't. I wouldn't know what to say. Idle chitchat with a stranger has never been my forte, even if this stranger is the nicest man in the world (according to Julia, anyway, who also says we'll have lots in common). The truth is, I don't know why I'm afraid. As Julia pointed out, this is totally nonthreatening. Having dinner with the uncle of a good friend. Really, what's so scary about that?

I think what terrifies me is the idea of any man in my life other than Michael. I didn't realize how insecure I am.

I refuse to believe that after all these years as a competent businesswoman, I'm letting a dinner date do this to me. I guess it isn't insecurity as much as the fear of making myself vulnerable again. I don't *want* to put myself at risk, especially when I know how crippling the pain of rejection can be.

Liz reminded the group that she doesn't need a man in her life. I agree with her. I don't need a man, either. I'm a smart, attractive woman, dammit! I'll admit my personal life has been a disaster recently. I'm coming back, though, slowly but surely, from the edge of insanity. I'm recovering from the grief of Michael's betrayal. Getting over the anger.

This evening, I'll go to Julia's with a brave smile and zero expectations. I have something to prove to myself. *I am healing.* I'm almost whole again. Oh sure, I take a few steps backward every now and then. For instance, my job with Murphy Motors—in some ways, that was a mistake. The main reason I wanted the job was to get back at Michael. I wanted him to spend his nights worrying about what I was doing, but my ploy lost its effectiveness when I learned he had other, more important things keeping him awake.

* * *

"Clare," Julia said, reaching for her hand when Clare arrived, giving her fingers a brief squeeze. "You look wonderful."

She should, Clare mused, seeing the time and effort that had gone into her appearance. She'd chosen a velvet cocktail suit in deep green, with a silk camisole, after trying on every party outfit she owned. Thankfully, Alex wasn't home and hadn't been around to see her agonizing over this dinner party—or to scoff at her primping. She was afraid he'd disapprove, which was the last thing she needed right now. In any event, he'd taken off that morning and she hadn't seen him all day. That wasn't unusual. She'd left him a note saying she'd gone out for the evening. Hey, she could be just as mysterious as Alex!

"Come and meet my uncle Leslie." Julia led her into the family room, where Peter sat talking to a distinguished-looking older man. Each held a glass of wine and glanced in Clare's direction.

Leslie and Peter stood as she entered.

"Clare, this is my uncle, Leslie Carter."

She stepped forward, her hand outstretched. "I'm delighted to meet you." Then smiling at Peter, she added, "And it's good to see you again, Peter."

"You, too." He headed into the open-plan kitchen, where an empty wineglass was waiting. "Can I pour you some wine?"

"Please." The dining-room table was set for four. Julia had mentioned earlier that the children were out with friends.

They all sat down on the two comfortable sofas in the family room. Julia placed a dish of baked artichoke dip and crackers on the coffee table in front of Clare.

"I understand you're visiting the area," Clare said, helping herself to a cracker and dip. Leslie Carter was a handsome man, just as Julia had promised. He had clear blue eyes, and was beautifully tanned. He'd gone almost completely bald, but it was extremely attractive on him—sexy in a Sean Connery way, Clare thought. In contrast to her, he'd dressed casually in a white polo shirt, crisp slacks and deck shoes. She guessed he was somewhere in his late fifties, perhaps early sixties. Julia hadn't said.

"I retired a few years ago," Leslie explained.

"He's a whiz with finances. In fact, he's been giving Peter and me lots of tax tips and he's got some good financial advice about the store."

Clare smiled.

"He's traveling around the world in his sailboat," Peter said enthusiastically.

"So far I haven't gone any farther than the West Coast of the United States," Leslie corrected.

"But you're going to Hawaii from here, right?"

"That's the plan."

"Alone?" Clare asked, thinking such a venture must surely be unwise.

"No. I have a small crew accompanying me."

"You must love sailing," Clare said.

"I do, but it's a recent passion."

"Uncle Leslie didn't even own a sailboat until three years ago," Julia told her.

"It was something I always thought about doing, but delayed. Then the excuses seemed to run out." Leslie leaned forward and reached for a cracker. "Once I got started, I wondered what took me so long."

"You say you retired a little while ago?"

"Yes, I was a management consultant for a number of companies in the Pacific Northwest."

Julia stood and headed into the kitchen. "Is there anything I can do to help?" Clare asked.

"Not a thing," Julia assured her. "Go ahead and visit while I put the finishing touches on the salad."

"Let me help," Peter said, as if on cue.

All at once Clare and Leslie were alone. She nervously twirled the stem of the wineglass between her hands while her mind raced with possible conversational gambits.

"I understand you were recently divorced," Leslie said.

"Actually, it's been a while. A little more than a year, I believe." She knew exactly how long it'd been, practically down to the hour. "You're divorced, too?"

He nodded. "Five years now. It was an adjustment at first. I was prepared to grow old with Barbara, but she... It seems we grew in different directions. She wanted a new life that didn't include me."

"So did my ex," Clare said with a short, humorless laugh. "Only Michael found a younger woman who made his new life a little more exciting." She gave a small shrug. "Why stick with apple pan dowdy when there's cheesecake available?"

"Barbara's new friend is named Troy. They're living together."

"Children?"

He shook his head. "I suppose I should be grateful for that, but I'm not. My life felt damn empty for a long time following the divorce. How about you?"

"Two sons. Mick's almost twenty and Alex is seventeen. I don't know what I would've done without them."

Leslie nodded. Clare sensed that the failure of his marriage had damaged this man, and that he was still recovering, just as she was.

"The salad's ready," Julia said, entering the room again.

"In case you weren't aware of it, my niece is an excellent cook," Leslie informed her as he got to this feet.

This was Clare's first opportunity to sample Julia's cooking. If the artichoke dip was anything to go by, she was in for a treat. The salad was impressive—a rich mixture of greens topped with slices of fresh pear, crumbled bleu cheese and walnuts, served with a raspberry vinaigrette.

"Julia, you've outdone yourself," Leslie said after the first bite.

Clare agreed. "This is fabulous."

Julia beamed at their praise. "Thanks. If you want I'll bring the recipe to breakfast next week."

"I'd love a copy," Clare assured her, although she didn't know when she'd get a chance to prepare it. Alex and Mick were meat-and-potatoes eaters, the same as their father.

After the salad, Julia brought a baked salmon and a scalloped potato dish to the table. Both were beautifully presented and delicious. Clare had always suspected that her friend possessed finely tuned domestic talents, but she'd never guessed Julia was this accomplished. Dessert was a lemon torte.

Over coffee in the family room, they chatted about Leslie's upcoming trip to Hawaii. Julia got out her knitting and, for the first time that evening, Clare was aware of the bulge outlined by her dress. She wondered whether Julia had mentioned the pregnancy to Leslie, then realized that Peter probably had. Julia's husband and uncle seemed to get on well.

Clare found that Peter and Leslie were good company and entertaining conversationalists. Julia was quieter than usual but seemed content. She concentrated on her knitting and made only the occasional remark.

At nine-thirty, Clare decided it was time to head home.

"I should be leaving, too," Leslie said and stood with her.

"I had a wonderful evening," Clare told Julia and Peter, but the message wasn't for them alone. Despite all her anxiety, she'd actually enjoyed herself.

After another round of farewells and thank-yous, Leslie walked Clare to her car, which was parked behind his at the curb. The night was lovely and warm, the stars were out and the scent of blooming lemon trees filled the air.

"Thank you, Clare," he said as she unlocked her car—the newest Chevy Tahoe.

Clare knew what he meant. "Thank *you*."

He grinned; they understood each other. Not only had the evening been pleasant, it had given them hope for the future—not necessarily a future together, but with *someone*. Romance and male companionship weren't lost possibilities, Clare thought, as long as there were men like Leslie Carter.

"Enjoy your adventures," she said as she slid into the car. "I'd love to see you when you get back."

"Same here." Leslie closed the door for her, then walked to his own vehicle.

Clare drove home, feeling better about life than she had in...well, in years. Two years. She parked in the garage and was climbing out of the car when the door leading to the house was thrust open. Alex stood on the threshold.

"Where were you?" her son demanded.

"I had a dinner engagement," she answered calmly. Judging by his tone, he'd been worried. Maybe he'd be a bit more considerate about letting her know where *he* was from now on.

"You had a date?" Alex asked, his tone bordering on the belligerent.

"Hey, be reasonable! I didn't shrivel up and die after the divorce, you know."

Alex followed her into the house. "Who'd you go out with?"

"Who?" she repeated, frowning. "Why do you need to know that?" When he continued to glare at her, she asked, "Is my going out really so remarkable?"

"Yes."

Taken aback, she just looked at him.

"Where were you?" he asked again.

"Julia and Peter Murchison's house, if you must know."

"She's in your breakfast club, right?"

"Right." Clare went into her bedroom, kicked off her shoes and removed her earrings. Alex trailed behind her, then slumped onto the end of the bed.

"Did you have a good time?" he asked, obviously making an effort.

"Wonderful. Julia's uncle Leslie was in town and I met him." She went on to mention Leslie's sailing trip to Hawaii.

"That's cool." But Alex didn't sound overly impressed.

"Did anything happen while I was gone?" Something was troubling her son. Alex didn't generally follow her from room to room, nor did he grill her about where she'd been.

"Dad called," Alex said, his voice deceptively casual.

"And?" She didn't know what was coming but she tensed, anticipating bad news. With Michael she no longer knew what to expect.

"He wanted to talk to you."

"Me?" Now, that was a first.

"He...he—" Alex's voice faltered and he bit his lower lip. Clare turned around to face her son. "What's wrong?"

"Dad didn't want to ask me. Dammit, Mom, you should have been here! Dad needed you and you weren't here." Alex stood, his hands clenched at his sides.

"Why did your father need me?" she asked, ignoring the accusation in his voice.

"He needed someone to take him to the hospital—he didn't want to ask me."

"Did you drive him?"

"No... When I got there, he was so sick Mom, I didn't know what to do so I called 911. I thought he was going to die." Alex's voice broke. "You should have been there, Mom, you should have been there to help Dad. He needed you."

"It is never too late to be what you might have been."
—George Eliot

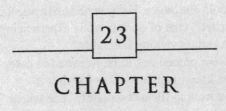

CHAPTER

LIZ KENYON

"Sharon Kelso is here," Liz's secretary announced over the intercom. "She's asked to speak to you and says it's important."

Liz sighed. Her afternoon was booked solid but her secretary certainly knew that. If the head of the nurses' union sought an impromptu meeting, then it went without saying something was up. In all likelihood, it meant trouble.

"Show her in," Liz said. She felt slightly sick to her stomach. Although a strike had been averted, relations between the hospital and the nursing staff remained tense.

Sharon Kelso was a large woman who presented herself as a no-nonsense professional. Liz liked and respected her. She considered her fair-minded but a tough negotiator.

Liz stood as Sharon marched purposefully into her office.

"Liz." The other woman inclined her head in greeting.

"Hello, Sharon, what can I do for you?" No need to delay this with idle conversation; they were both busy women.

"I'll need about ten minutes of your time."

"You have it," Liz told her and motioned to the chair. She waited until Sharon was seated before sitting down herself.

The head of the nurses' union paused to collect her thoughts before speaking. "I don't mean to be telling tales out of school," she began. Her pinched lips made it clear that she was upset. "One of our nurses is experiencing a problem with a certain visiting specialist."

There were procedures to be followed in cases like this and Sharon knew them as well as Liz did.

"Do you want to file a complaint?" Liz asked.

"That's an option we've considered," Sharon said.

"Can you tell me what this is about?"

"It involves recent corrective actions taken by Dr. Sean Jamison."

Liz should have known it had to do with Sean. She could barely keep from groaning aloud.

"At this point, the staff member involved and I prefer to handle the situation without the formality of filing a complaint," Sharon said. She appeared to be selecting her words carefully. "Once you hear what happened, you'll understand our hesitation. We don't feel it would serve a useful purpose to make an issue of this. There are extenuating circumstances."

There almost always were, but Liz didn't say so.

"Before I go any further, I want you to know my staff member accepts full responsibility for her part in this. However, I find Dr. Jamison's behavior offensive and unacceptable."

"Tell me what happened," Liz suggested.

The story that followed was short and to the point. "One of my staff made a small clerical error on one of the charts."

Liz knew there was no such thing as a small error, but didn't point that out.

"It was caught almost immediately, but when Dr Jamison learned about it, he blew a gasket. He insisted that the nurse in question not be assigned to any of his patients. Now, Liz, you and I both know that's an impossible request."

She nodded.

"He was rude, belligerent and unnecessarily harsh. We're not perfect. We can only do our best. No one deserves the kind of tongue-lashing Dr. Jamison gave her. It was humiliating and downright scathing, and furthermore he yelled at her in front of other people. I simply can't allow such unprofessional behavior to go unreported."

"I agree." Liz understood Sharon's dilemma. Knowing Sean, she could well imagine the scene. She was surprised she hadn't heard about it before now. Liz didn't blame him for his anger but took issue with the manner in which he'd expressed it. Under normal circumstances, Sharon wouldn't hesitate to file a formal complaint. The reason she didn't was understood; the nurse had been in the wrong and she didn't want documentation acknowledging her error.

"You'll talk to Dr. Jamison?" Sharon asked—less a question than a demand.

"I will," Liz promised, although it was the last thing she wanted. To this point, they'd managed to avoid each other. It wasn't difficult. Other than instances such as this, there was no reason for any contact.

"Thank you," Sharon said, rising. "We're pleased with our

new contract, and don't want anything to stand in the way of a long and healthy working relationship."

"I couldn't agree with you more," Liz returned, the knot in her stomach tightening.

Sharon left then, but Liz remained standing, considering how best to handle this situation. Sean might assume that her asking to speak to him was a convenient excuse to see him again. She shook her head in frustration; getting involved with him, however briefly, was a mistake.

She walked over to her desk and pushed the intercom button. "Cherie," she said, "leave a message for Dr. Jamison to stop by my office at his earliest convenience, would you?"

"Of course," Cherie returned, sounding delighted at the prospect. "I'll do it right away."

Sean didn't keep her waiting long. That very evening, just as Liz was shutting down her computer for the night, Sean appeared at her door. Cherie had long since gone home and Liz was there by herself. Sean often seemed to plan it that way.

"You wanted to talk to me?" He wore his usual cocky grin as he strolled casually into her office.

"This is a professional matter," Liz told him immediately. "Please sit down."

His face was carefully neutral as he claimed the chair across from her. "This has to do with the Tucker baby, doesn't it?"

"I wasn't given the full details."

"Was a formal complaint made? If so, I'm here to tell you the woman deserved everything I said. There's one thing I won't tolerate and that's—"

Liz held up her hand, stopping him. "A complaint wasn't filed."

He indicated no relief. "The woman deserved to have her wrist slapped. Her carelessness could have cost the Tucker baby his life. There are a lot of things I'm willing to put up with at this hospital, but sloppy record-keeping isn't one of them."

"No one's saying you were wrong about the nature of your criticism."

"Naturally, because I was right. Believe me, if I hadn't been, Sharon Kelso would have filed a complaint so fast, it'd make your head swim."

All of that was true, but Liz chose not to respond.

"What does she want?" Sean demanded. "An apology? Because I don't owe *anyone* an apology."

"Actually, no. The nurse in question is willing to accept responsibility for this error."

"Good, because that's what she needs to do."

"I believe," Liz said, "that Sharon came to me as a gesture of good faith. She wants to keep things low-key and nonconfrontational. She—"

"Like hell! She wants me reported as an unreasonable jerk." He shrugged. "I already know that, and so do you. When it comes to my patients I'm like a wounded bear."

"No one's faulting your skills or your commitment."

"Just my bedside manner?"

"No, I'd say it's your nurses' station tactics that are causing the problems."

His frown relaxed. "I'll admit I got damned angry." A grin began to emerge.

That was an understatement, Liz was sure.

He rubbed the back of his neck and expelled a slow sigh. "I probably did come down on her a little too hard," he was willing to admit, but with reluctance as if he, too, was making a concession to keep the peace. "I was afraid I was going to lose the Tucker boy. I hadn't slept in over thirty hours. I'll say something to her in the morning. That'll smooth things over."

"You were up for thirty hours? That's not good for you or your patients." Although she chastised him, she remembered doing the same thing herself once, years earlier, when her baby's life hung in the balance. Liz had been afraid to leave Lauren, afraid to fall asleep, afraid to even take her eyes off the baby. The staff had been gentle with her and Steve, but there'd been no physician by their side. No one to comfort her when her baby girl died.

How grateful the Tucker family must be to Sean. Liz found it difficult to think ill of a physician as dedicated to the well-being of his patients.

Sean glared at her. "Don't tell me how to do my job and I won't tell you how to do yours."

She remained calm. "You should learn how to deal with pressure—some method other than terrorizing staff. You need to find some kind of release."

"I know, but you won't cooperate. A week in bed with you would cure everything that ails me, and it'd probably do you good as well."

Liz gasped; she couldn't help it. She wasn't sure if she should be furious or just plain insulted. "I don't appreciate your making comments like that," she said in a stiff voice.

"Of course you don't. Why else would I make them?"

She stared at him and saw that he was smiling. Ten minutes with Sean Jamison and *she* was the one struggling to hold onto her temper.

"How do *you* relieve the stress of the job?" he asked, sounding genuinely interested.

"I...I do a number of things." Liz wasn't ready for his rapid switch from provocative to serious.

"Such as?"

"Most recently I took up knitting," she said, although she'd had to cancel her sessions with Julia this week.

"Knitting." His gaze was skeptical.

"One of the women in my breakfast group owns a yarn shop."

He grinned. "Ah, yes, this breakfast group of yours. Tell me, are the meetings just an excuse for men-bashing?"

Leave it to Sean to suggest such a thing. "Oh, hardly. The problem with you men is that you're so threatened by women getting together, you naturally assume it's all about you."

"Well, isn't it?"

"No," she said emphatically.

"All right," he said, sincere once again. "I agree with you, I need a way to release work pressure, but I don't know that knitting's my thing."

"Don't knock it until you've tried it," she joked.

He considered her words, then slowly nodded. "All right, I'll try it. Are you willing to teach me?"

This was more than a casual question, and Liz knew it. The last time they'd talked, Sean had made it clear that she'd have to come to him if their relationship was to advance. He'd riled her so much with his attitude and his arrogant tactics she'd vowed never to see him again. That hadn't stopped her from thinking about him, though. For weeks she'd pushed any thought of Sean Jamison to the farthest reaches of her mind. What irritated her was how often she'd been required to do so.

"It's a simple question," he teased, obviously well aware that it wasn't.

"Just you and me and a ball of yarn?" she asked, delaying a response while she weighed the risks.

"Sounds kinky, but I'm game if you are."

Liz groaned.

He knew she hated the sexual innuendoes and with a sheepish grin, raised both hands. "Just kidding."

She folded her arms across her chest. "You're serious about knitting?"

The teasing light left his eyes. "I promise to make an honest effort."

They both understood that he wasn't talking about knitting.

"What do you say, Liz?" His eyes continued to hold hers.

Her first inclination was to tell him to forget it; she didn't need the grief. Instead she found herself tempted. They'd gotten off to a bad start. He'd wanted one thing and she another. Finding a middle ground might not be possible, but if he was willing to try again, then she could do no less.

"All right," she agreed. "Don't make me sorry," she muttered as an afterthought.

He laughed, and the robust sound made her smile, too.

"Would I do that?" he asked.

> "You don't have to know how to sing. It's feeling as
> though you want to that makes the day worthwhile."
> —Coleman Cox

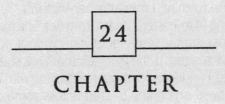

CHAPTER

KAREN CURTIS

April 19th

The breakfast group met this morning, and as usual we were all full of chatter and news. Julia and her husband bought a crib for the baby and set it up in their bedroom. Clare got a humorous card from Julia's uncle Leslie and showed it to everyone. She was a little giddy about it, and I found that rather endearing. Here she was, married all those years, and then she gets flustered over a silly card. Apparently the dinner party went well, although neither Julia nor Clare said much about it. We get sidetracked so easily.

The one who surprised us all is Liz who, just before we broke up, casually mentioned that she's seeing Dr.

Jamison again. You could have heard an egg crack when she dropped *that* news. Everyone went quiet. No one likes him, (well, not that we've actually met him, but we have a pretty clear picture). We're all wondering what a savvy, sophisticated businesswoman sees in a man who treats women like objects. On second thought, there must be more to the man. I sure hope so. I'd hate to think Liz is another Victoria.

Speaking of my sister, I heard from her. She mailed me one of those sappy, sentimental cards about how great it is to have a sister. If she truly felt that way, she'd listen to me. Hey, I understand about her staying with the twit, but the abuse isn't going to stop unless some changes are made. Victoria claims Roger loves her and is genuinely sorry. I'm sure he is and will continue to be—until the next time he slaps her around. Thinking about my sister and her marriage depresses me. So does the state of my own love life.

I haven't been out on a date for so long that I'm beginning to lose hope. I've been busy, but it isn't like there's someone in the wings just dying to ask me out, either. Glen Trnavski, maybe, although I haven't heard from him in a while. I've been substitute teaching at different schools lately, so I haven't had a chance to run into him. It's sort of pathetic that I'm even thinking about him, since we only went out once. He's a nerd, the kind of guy who dangles a slide rule from his belt loop, but a nice one and really very sweet. Doesn't matter—he hasn't called and neither has Jeff. Jeff and I will only argue, so it's just as well we're not in touch. Especially after our last conversation... Glen might be a little on the dull side, but at least he's focused. (Not on me, though. Ha! Ha!)

On a more positive note, the hair spray commercial airs for the first time next week. The filming took forever. I liked the director, but this ten-second spot isn't exactly *Gone With the Wind*. Unfortunately, the only part of me that shows is the back of my head. The camera shows me tossing my head as my perfectly shaped hair bounces about with every curl perfectly in place, thanks to "Beauty Hold." It's supposed to look like I'm playing tennis, but in reality I was hopping up and down on a trampoline. Needless to say, Mother's relieved no one will know it's me.

My rent is paid and I just got a check from the school district. I feel flush! It's only fitting that I celebrate my first national commercial. I haven't been to a movie in forever, but it's getting harder and harder to find someone who isn't one half of a couple to do things with. I never thought I'd have this kind of problem, but nearly everyone I know, male or female, is either married or has a significant other.

I could always ask Liz, but she works such long hours and besides, the little time she does have available is about to be taken up by the good doctor. Clare might be interested. She's fun, and I find myself liking her more and more.

* * *

"Do you want me to pick you up?" Karen asked. She'd followed her impulse and phoned Clare Craig, and to her delight Clare had immediately agreed. She seemed surprised that Karen had a Friday night free.

They took a few minutes to choose a film and decided on a comedy.

"Sure, pick me up," Clare said, "that way you can meet my son."

"Alex will be home?"

"He makes pit stops every weekend." Clare laughed. "I told him I should install a drive-through window so all I have to do is lean out and hand him money and food."

Karen laughed, too, and wished her mother had half the sense of humor the women in her Thursday morning break-fast group did. She and Catherine might have gotten along better if they'd found a reason to laugh together.

She finalized her arrangements with Clare and they ended the conversation.

Predictably, on Friday morning Karen got called in to substitute teach at Manchester High School. In the English department this time. She hesitated before taking the as-signment, but not for long. The money was too good to ignore and besides, Manchester High was where the elusive Glen taught chemistry.

High school was Karen's favorite age group. Somehow— maybe because of her own age—she found it easier to relate to the kids. She had three periods, then an hour's break before her two afternoon classes. The eleventh-graders were studying *Macbeth,* a play she knew fairly well, since she'd been in a college production, playing one of the witches. She gave the ninth-graders a creative-writing project. During her lunch break she ate in the teachers' lounge, thinking she might accidentally-on-purpose run into Glen.

She didn't, but when she asked about him, several of the other teachers sang his praises. Apparently he was popular with the staff. He might be popular with her, too, if he made more of an effort to seek her out. After school, Karen decided it would be all right to casually wander the halls until she located him. She found him in the chemistry lab with a handful of students clustered around him like groupies around a rock star.

Standing in the doorway, Karen was uncertain if she should interrupt. She cleared her throat. "Mr. Trnavski?" she said.

Glen glanced up and did a double-take. He was pleased to see her and made it obvious. "Karen, hi!"

"Hi," she said. "Um, I was subbing here and thought I'd stop by and say hello." She held up her right hand. "Hello."

"I was just finishing," he said, closing the text with a snap.

The students exchanged shocked glances, as though stunned that their teacher had a life outside of chemistry. "But..." one of them began.

"We'll go over this again on Monday," he said, dismissing them.

"But the test..."

"Has been postponed until Tuesday."

From the way they reacted, Karen knew the extra day to study had been an unexpected gift. The six students left, chattering away and patting each other on the back as if they'd just been granted parole.

He waited until they'd disappeared down the hall before he spoke. He might not have the sleek good looks that would attract Hollywood, she thought, watching him, but he wasn't bad on the eyes, either.

"You're looking fine," he said as the last student vacated the room.

His admiration was just what Karen's sagging ego needed. But if he was as interested in her as he seemed to be, she couldn't understand why he hadn't contacted her. "I haven't heard from you in a while."

Glen turned away and erased the blackboard. "As I recall, you said you wanted to be friends. Nothing more and nothing else."

"I said that?"

"Maybe not in so many words. But I got the message and decided not to waste either your time or mine." He brushed chalk dust from his palms.

"Oh." She did remember making some remark to that effect, but only because she hadn't really known what she wanted. Anyway, she'd said it months ago. Couldn't a girl change her mind? Glen was smart and funny, and the more she was around him, the more she liked him. "I've been known to make statements I later regret."

"Really?"

Karen nodded, hoping he'd take the hint and ask her out again.

He didn't.

Glancing at her watch, she decided to make a quick exit. No need to hang around, possibly waiting to be humiliated. The sole purpose for seeking him out was to let him know she was available, which she'd now done. She briefly considered asking him out, but figured he was too traditional to be comfortable with that. "Okay...see you later," she said breezily, then turned to leave.

"Can I phone you?" he called after her.

She turned back. "I'd be disappointed if you didn't."

"Do you have a date tonight?" he asked, following her into the hallway. He struck a casual pose, leaning against the door-jamb and crossing his arms. "Or would you like to go out?"

"Sorry," she said, "I already have plans."

"Another time, then?"

"I'd like that," she said, walking backward until she collided with the janitor, which totally ruined her exit.

Two hours later, Karen drove to the address Clare had given her and parked in front of the large, professionally landscaped house. It was the first time she'd been to any of the other women's homes, and she was impressed.

Alex answered the doorbell and stared at her.

"Hi, I'm Karen Curtis," she said, introducing herself. "Your mother's friend."

Alex was a tall seventeen-year-old, and although they'd never met, he seemed vaguely familiar.

"You came looking for Mr. Trnavski this afternoon, didn't you?" he asked as he held open the screen door.

"Is that Karen?" Clare's voice came from down a hallway.

"Yeah," Alex shouted over his shoulder.

If the outside of Clare's home was impressive, it paled in comparison to the inside. Every aspect of the house spoke of quality and craftsmanship. Karen thought about her parents' place, where her father's desire for comfort—comfortable armchairs, big TV—warred with her mother's often pretentious decorating ideas.

"Are you dating Mr. Trnavski?"

"We're friends."

"Man, I've never seen him get so flustered before."

Karen was thrilled to hear it.

"I see you've met my son," Clare said, entering the living room. She was trying to fasten an earring in place. She leaned her head to one side as she fiddled with the gold loop.

"Mom, this is Ms. Curtis from school."

"Yes, sweetheart, I know. Karen's in my breakfast group."

"Your breakfast group? I thought that was a bunch of old women like you."

Despite herself, Karen laughed. "I don't think you're earning points with your mother," she said.

Alex looked embarrassed. "You know what I mean."

His mother closed her eyes for a moment, as if to avoid the subject entirely. Then she resumed her struggle with the earring, finally succeeding.

"You're divorced, too?" Alex sat down on the sofa arm and gazed up at Karen.

"No. I've never been married."

"Not everyone in the group is divorced," Clare informed her son.

She didn't mention that she was, in fact, the only one of the four who was. Karen wondered why.

"Aren't you going to—" He stopped and frowned. "Isn't this Friday night?"

"Yes." Karen frowned, too. "Is that a problem?"

"Your divorce support group is tonight, isn't it, Mom?"

"Oh," Clare said. "That's what you mean. Well, it's an ongoing session and the people change."

"You're not going?"

"Not tonight. Karen and I are taking in a movie."

"Oh."

"I'll be just a moment longer," Clare told her, hurrying down the hallway.

Alex continued to stare at Karen.

"What's the matter?" she asked. "Didn't you realize teachers had a life outside the classroom?"

"It's not that," he said. "It's my mom."

Karen waited for him to finish.

"You don't understand. She's never missed a meeting of that group. She *needs* her group."

"Maybe she doesn't need it as much as you think."

Alex shook his head. "She needs it," he insisted.

"Then ask her."

"I will," Alex said, standing as his mother came back into the room. "What about the divorce support group? Don't you think you should go?"

Clare reached for her purse. "I decided not to."

"Well, I can see *that*. Why not?"

"Because, my dear son," Clare said and pressed her hand to the side of his face, "it's time to move on. I'm ready," she said, glancing at Karen. "How about you?"

"Ready," she echoed and smiled to herself.

"You don't get to choose how you're going to die.
Or when. You can only decide how you're going
to live. Now."

—Joan Baez

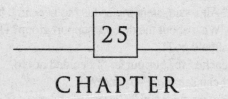

CHAPTER

CLARE CRAIG

Clare turned off the vacuum and heard the phone in the background as the Hoover moaned to a stop. Lunging for the cordless she had no idea if this was the first ring or the fifth.

"Hello," she said, slightly breathless. Although she could well afford a cleaning service, she preferred to do her own housework. She joked that it helped her work out her aggressions, which was true; she also felt that she could better maintain the kind of control she wanted over her environment.

Her greeting was met by a short hesitation. "Clare, it's Michael."

She knew he'd been released from the hospital a few days earlier; after Alex's 911 call, he'd been admitted a second time—and now he was home, in the tender, well-manicured hands of Miranda.

"Alex is at school," she reminded him in case he'd forgotten.

"Actually, I wanted to talk to you."

In the beginning she'd dreamed about the day Michael would need her, reach out to her, want her back in his life. During the two years since he'd moved out, it hadn't happened. But Clare had learned valuable lessons about herself. Each day she grew stronger, more confident and self-assured. They'd always been a team, the two of them, but she'd learned to fly solo.

"I'd like to invite you to lunch," Michael shocked her by asking.

"Lunch?" She nearly choked on the word.

"It's my way of thanking you for your kindness while I underwent chemo."

Clare sank onto the edge of the coffee table. He was telling her this was simply to let her know that he appreciated her help; she shouldn't put any stock in the invitation. He didn't want her back any more than she wanted *him* back, she told herself fiercely.

"No thanks are necessary." And they weren't. Her reasons were too complex to analyze. Suffice it to say she'd done it for him *and* for her. Because of their shared past and because of their children.

"I insist. I'd like to take you to Mama Lena's."

Her favorite Italian restaurant, no less. When they were first married and lived paycheck to paycheck, it was a special indulgence to dine at Mama Lena's. Every birthday and anniversary found them enjoying ravioli and eggplant Parmesan. The breadsticks and cheese, the antipasto, a glass of red wine—followed by espresso and tiramisu for dessert. The memories scrolled through her mind like silent movies.

"I...don't think that's a good idea," she said, fighting the urge to agree.

Michael paused. "Another restaurant then. You name it, any place you want."

"I know you appreciated my help, Michael, but I don't believe our having lunch is the right thing to do. Not at this point in our lives."

"I need to talk to you," he said after another long pause.

"Talk to me now."

"I can't," he told her with what sounded like regret. "All I'm asking is that you meet me. Any place you want, any time."

"All right," she said, curiosity getting the better of her. "Meet me at Mocha Moments at three o'clock tomorrow afternoon."

She felt comfortable there, safe. Michael wouldn't tell her what this was about over the phone, but she wasn't meeting him at Mama Lena's, where he could evoke memories of happier times, when life was sweet and all her illusions had yet to be shattered.

Clare didn't mention the phone call, not to Alex and not to Karen who called that evening to tell her excitedly about Alex's chemistry teacher asking her out to dinner. If Clare was tempted to discuss Michael's call with anyone, it would have been Liz. Instead, she kept the information to herself, wondering what it meant, and what the hell was so important that Michael had sought her out.

Perhaps she was reading more into this than she should. Since their relationship was fairly amicable now, Michael might simply want to discuss their sons. Maybe he wanted her advice about reconciling with Mick....

Then again, this might have to do with Alex's upcoming high-school graduation. Should they both attend and pretend to be a happy family for the sake of their sons? No. She couldn't see that happening, and there was Mick to consider. Naturally Michael was free to attend, but Mick wouldn't want his father sitting anywhere near him.

Another thought occurred to her as she sat with a cup of strong coffee the following day, waiting for her ex-husband to show up. Perhaps this was connected to his cancer treatment.

Precisely at three, Michael walked into Mocha Moments. He was even thinner than the last time she'd seen him but not so horribly pale. Some of the color had returned to his cheeks. He paused just inside the door and smiled when he saw her.

"Hello, Clare," he said, making his way to the table.

"Hello, Michael." She inclined her head toward him, choosing not to study him too closely for fear he might mis-interpret her interest. He glanced over his shoulder at the counter and the printed menu above the cash register. "I take it they don't have a waitress here."

"Everyone sees to his or her own."

"You want a refill?" he asked, and shoved his hand in his pocket, removing his money clip.

When she shook her head, he stepped toward the counter, returning a few minutes later with a latte. Pulling out a chair, he sat down across from her.

"How are you?" she asked. Now that he was close, she realized he didn't look as good as she'd first assumed. The whites of his eyes had a yellowish tinge and while there was color in his face, his cheeks were still gaunt.

"I'm better now, thanks," he answered and sipped from his latte.

"The cancer?"

He didn't respond right away. "I didn't come here to exchange news."

"Fine, then get to the point and be done with it," she snapped, feeling a little hurt, a little insulted.

"Actually, I have a favor to ask of you."

He had a funny way of leading up to it, she thought, considering he'd just antagonized her. *She* wasn't the one who'd asked for this meeting; her being here was a favor to him.

"I don't have any right to ask this," Michael went on, his voice lower now. He stared down at his latte as if he'd find the solution to his troubles in the frothy milk.

"Ask me what?" she demanded, trying to temper the defensiveness she heard in her own voice.

"I wouldn't, if it wasn't for our sons."

"What is it?" she asked. Enough with this preamble!

"I want you to come back and work at the dealership," he said, his eyes boring holes in her.

"No—no way." She didn't need to think it over, didn't need to hear the reasons. Her answer was instantaneous.

Michael raised his hand. "Let me explain."

"I've already got a job." She'd set out to be an irritant to him by taking the part-time job at Murphy Motors. She regretted it; apparently Michael had lost business and now he was afraid.

"Give Murphy two weeks' notice."

"Michael, I can't... Listen, I made a mistake. I should never have taken that job, and—"

"Hear me out," Michael interrupted.

She laughed, and shook her head. It was as though they were still married. He hadn't bothered to listen to her then, either.

"This doesn't have anything to do with Murphy Motors,"

he said impatiently. "The entire future of Craig Chevrolet hangs on your answer."

"Michael, please..." He was overreacting. Naturally, he didn't want her working for his biggest competitor and now he was trying to lure her back. What he didn't understand, hadn't bothered to hear, was that she regretted the whole stupid idea.

"I swear to you, this isn't personal. I need you to assume my role."

"And just where will you be?" If he told her he needed time to take Miranda on some exotic vacation, she'd tell him exactly what he could do with his job offer.

He wouldn't look at her.

"What exactly will you be doing while I'm taking over as general manager?" she repeated. Although her voice remained calm, she refused to answer his question until he answered hers.

"It's not what you think," he hastened to add.

"How do you know what I'm thinking?"

"Oh, Clare, you've forgotten I was married to you for twenty-three years." Although he was smiling, there was little humor in his words. "Fine, I'll tell you." He dragged a shaky breath through his lungs. "I've been selected for an experimental drug treatment. It means I won't be able to continue my duties at the dealership."

"This has to do with the cancer?"

Again he wouldn't meet her gaze.

"You know the car business better than anyone. Despite our differences over the past few years, I trust you."

She didn't know what to say. Earlier, he'd avoided the question of his health, sidestepping it with the pretense of getting on with their discussion.

"The dealership is heavily mortgaged now, and unless this transition is smooth, I could lose everything."

He was afraid of losses? Clare was stunned by his insensitivity. She'd had her life ripped apart, her security shredded, her heart broken. Now he was afraid that if he spent a few weeks away from the business, it might falter—so he'd come to her. Yes, any erosion of the dealership's finances would have an impact on her and the boys, but to ask her to step in like this! As though they were still a married couple, still a team... Well, they weren't and that was entirely his doing.

She wanted to tell him what she thought, but the words lodged in her throat, making it impossible to speak. Then Michael astonished her even more, by laughing.

"You find this *humorous?*"

"No." He shook his head. "Not at all. I'm just amused by your predictability. You're so mad right now, you can barely think."

"You've got it. Hire Miranda, Michael, because I'm not interested." She stood to leave, but his hand on her arm stopped her.

"Miranda left me." The pain behind those words was barely concealed.

Clare felt her knees buckle. For two years she'd wanted him to experience just a fraction of the emotional agony she'd endured when he walked out on her.

"Aren't you going to remind me that what goes around comes around?" he asked hoarsely.

"No," she whispered. Not when he'd so plainly learned that lesson on his own. What surprised her was his willingness to admit it, especially to her.

"Clare," he said, pleading with her now. "Sit down, please."

She reclaimed her seat, not that she had any choice, since her legs were about to go out from under her. "When did she leave?" Clare asked, wondering how long Michael had been on his own.

"A while ago now."

She nodded.

"Actually, she moved in with a friend soon after I learned about the cancer. She has...trouble dealing with sickness."

Clare found it interesting and rather sad that he'd continue to make excuses for Miranda.

"I should have told you sooner." His voice had grown soft, and he slouched forward, looking suddenly old.

"It isn't any of my business." She glanced away, finding it difficult to look at the pain in his eyes. Michael was alone and knew what it was like to come home to a cold, empty house. She studied him for any signs of regret and saw none. Even now, sick and abandoned by the woman he'd given up so much for, he revealed no contrition, despite what he'd done to Clare and their family. That hurt, and she silently chastised herself for seeking more than he could give.

"Aren't you going to gloat?" he asked, some of the old fire returning to his eyes.

"No," she whispered.

"Will you do it?" he asked again. "Will you take over for me when I go into the hospital?"

Clare couldn't meet his eyes. "Let me think about it."

"I'll make it worth your while," he promised. "The dealership belongs to the boys. I don't want to lose it. And, of course, there are your support payments...."

She nodded. She wasn't likely to forget those.

"How long will it take you to have an answer?" he asked.

Rushing her into a decision wasn't going to help. "I don't know," she said, hardly able to take it all in. "I—I need to think through my options."

"A day."

"Longer."

"A week then?"

Why was he rushing her like this? "I don't know," she said a second time, resenting the pressure. "If you're going to force me to answer right away, then the answer is no. I've made a new life without you, Michael, and I can't see the point of getting our personal and financial affairs all tangled up again."

"Think it over, Clare. This is important."

"To you, you mean."

"It's important to our children," he reminded her.

"I need time," she repeated.

"Dammit, Clare, I don't have time. Can't you see? Do I have to spell it out for you? I'm dying."

"Dying?" The word barely made it past the constriction in her throat.

"According to the specialists, I'll be lucky if this treatment buys me six more months. The cancer is spreading.... Look at me, Clare. Look at me," he insisted. "I don't have much longer. Now, are you going to help me or not?"

* * *

April 25th
2:34 a.m.

I can't sleep. Every time I close my eyes I see Michael sitting at the table at Mocha Moments, telling me he's dying.

Dying!

He seemed to accept it, as if it were a foregone conclusion. After the initial shock, I had a thousand questions. He answered the first few, but didn't want to go into detail. The cancer started out in his liver and has spread throughout his body. There's nothing to be done. No miracle drug, no clinic that can save him and no cure in sight. He doesn't want the boys to know and begged me to keep his secret.

Everything about this afternoon is so vivid in my mind. I keep going over it and over it, almost obsessively. Miranda left him—I never did learn exactly when she moved out. I'm sure Michael didn't want me to know.

That made me wonder if he delayed seeing the doctor because of her. And I wondered—if we'd still been together, if there'd never been an affair or the subsequent divorce—whether I would've detected something wrong before it was too late. If Michael had gotten medical treatment sooner, would that have made a difference?

I'll never know.

I've been walking around in a haze ever since. Michael asked me to assume the management of the dealership, but he made it clear that once he leaves, he won't be back. Mick's major is business, and Michael's hope is that our eldest son will eventually step into the role of manager and shared ownership with his younger brother. Until that happens, Michael needs me to run the business.

I remember, soon after I filed for divorce, pleading with God to let Michael suffer. My sense of outrage demanded it. I wanted him to know that betrayal can destroy you, wanted him to feel the bitterness corroding everything he once considered decent and fair. But even in my most desperate moments, I wouldn't have wished this on him.

Alex, the son of my heart, knew the minute he walked in tonight that something was drastically wrong. I kept my promise to Michael, but I don't know how long I'll be able to hold back the truth.

I'll do what Michael asked, give my notice at Murphy Motors and return to the dealership. With the two of us working together, the transition should be seamless.

Michael is dying and he's come to me for help. I'm willing to step in and do what I can, for my children's sake...and for his. I don't *want* to care, don't want to become emotionally involved. But I am, and even though we're divorced, that's not going to change.

> "The greater part of our happiness or misery depends
> on our dispositions and not on our circumstances."
> —Martha Washington

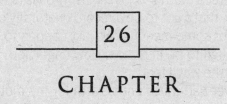

CHAPTER

JULIA MURCHISON

List of Blessings
1. My mother
2. Comfortable shoes
3. Consignment maternity clothes
4.
5.

May 13th—Mother's Day

The house is quiet and everyone's still asleep. I woke early, although this is the one day of the year I can sleep in without feeling guilty. The peacefulness was just too wonderful to ignore, so I'm sitting here in the family room, thinking over the events planned for today.

My mother's coming for brunch after church, and then she's going to my sister's for dinner. Janice wanted all of us to celebrate Mother's Day together, but I couldn't.

I wanted this day with my own husband and children—although that's not working out exactly as I'd hoped. Peter's mother is joining us. Two visits within a year. Now, that's got to be a record! Naturally she's in the area for some meeting. We just happen to be un-lucky enough to be here, too. How ungracious of me, but that's the way I feel.

I've never had much enthusiasm for my mother-in-law. She's so unlike my husband that it's difficult to see them as mother and son. She flew in from Seattle for a business meeting and insisted on staying in the hotel room her company arranged. I got the distinct impres-sion that visiting us is a burden. It's as though she'd like to forget she has a son and grandchildren. I sometimes find it difficult to hold my tongue with her. I have a won-derful, loving husband, but Peter owes his upbringing to a hodgepodge of daycare workers and nannies who provided him with the love and emotional support his mother was unable or unwilling to give her only child.

We invited Peter's mother to join us for church and then brunch afterward, but she declined, which didn't surprise me. Her excuse was that she didn't want to "intrude" on our time with my mother.

Peter is kind of defensive about his mother, so I said nothing, but I'm not looking forward to this af-ternoon. I only hope the children will behave themselves. This is probably wishful thinking on my part. Our kids are typical teenagers; the only people they care about are themselves.

* * *

"I am *not* playing the clarinet for Grandma," Zoe insisted as Julia added slices of cucumber to the salad, then placed it inside the refrigerator.

"Your father asked you to," Julia reminded her rebellious daughter.

"I hate it when he does that."

Julia understood her daughter's reluctance, but at the same time, she sided with Peter. He was proud of Zoe and wanted to impress his mother with her musical ability.

"When's Dad gonna get back?" Adam asked, slouching on the sofa, thumbing through the latest issue of *Car and Driver* magazine.

Julia read the digital readout on the microwave. "It's three-twenty. Give him another ten minutes."

"How come Grandma Murchison didn't want to sleep here?" Zoe asked, following Julia around the kitchen.

"Would you?" Adam demanded, his face hidden behind the magazine.

Zoe seemed to consider her brother's question. "Yeah, I would. If I only had a few hours to spend with my grandchildren, I'd make the most of every single one." She gave a slight shrug. "I mean, she doesn't get to see us very often."

"Grandma Murchison didn't come to see us this time, either," Adam told his sister.

"Yes, she did!"

Adam lowered the magazine. "Tell her, Mom."

"Tell me *what?*"

"I believe your grandmother flew in on a business-related matter," Julia confirmed, choosing her words carefully.

Zoe frowned. "What?"

"She's here for a finance meeting with some corporate bigwig," Adam said.

Peter's mother had seen her grandchildren maybe a dozen times in their entire lives. Adam was right; the only reason she was with them now was because her company had sent her.

"Apparently Grandma's real important," Adam continued, clearly in the know.

"That's what I hear," Julia muttered.

Zoe ran to the living-room window at the sound of the minivan pulling into the driveway. "Dad's back," she cried excitedly. Shoving her feet into an old pair of sandals, she raced out the front door.

Adam slowly set aside his magazine and stood, his shoulders hunched.

Julia removed the apron and brushed her hand down her blouse to remove any crumbs. She sighed deeply; other than a half-hour's respite when she first woke, all she'd done today was cook and clean.

Peter, ever thoughtful, had brought her a plant yesterday, but she'd been the one who'd organized two family meals to honor first her mother and now his. Everyone took for granted the effort and planning that went into each event. For brunch, she'd served a smoked salmon and asparagus frittata—admittedly wasted on her children—plus homemade rolls, muffins and fruit salad. Not to mention fresh-squeezed orange juice. Dinner was going to be a barbecue. At least

Peter would do that part, Julia thought grudgingly, although she'd marinated the chicken, made the salads and prepared dessert. She sighed again, feeling tired and out-of-sorts.

"We're back," Peter announced as he escorted his mother into the house.

"Brenda, welcome," Julia said, moving toward her. "It's so good to see you."

"Hello, Julia." The other woman leaned forward and pecked Julia's cheek. But her eyes didn't leave the small mound that identified the pregnancy.

"When is the baby due again?" she asked, eyebrows raised.

"September seventh," Adam said in a loud, clear voice. He sounded as though the date had been burned in his mind like a historical day.

"Adam's shot up about a foot since you last saw him," Julia said, sliding an arm around her son's shoulders.

"Hi, Grandma," he said with little warmth.

"Zoe, say hello to your grandmother," Peter instructed.

"Hi," Zoe mumbled, clasping her hands behind her back as if to say she had no intention of playing the clarinet on command.

"Please, come in," Julia said. This was all rather awkward, with the five of them standing in the entryway.

Brenda walked into the living room and sat down, choosing the most comfortable chair for herself.

"Iced tea, Mother?" Peter asked, evidently eager to please her.

"That would be nice." She patted her brow with a lacy cotton handkerchief. "The weather in southern California is considerably warmer than it is in Seattle this time of year," she murmured.

Peter hurried toward the kitchen. As soon as he'd left the room, Brenda turned to Julia.

"So, the new baby is due in September?"

Julia nodded and sat down, too. It was the first time since early morning that she'd had an opportunity to relax.

"Do you think a third child is wise at this stage of your life?" Brenda asked, her question as blunt as it was unwelcome.

"I beg your pardon?" What she *wanted* to do was scream "That's none of your business!" Brenda had no right whatsoever to comment on their personal lives and decisions. This was a woman who barely knew her grandkids' names, Julia thought angrily.

"The baby is a surprise," she managed to say calmly.

"This is a three-bedroom house, isn't it?" Brenda asked, looking around critically.

"Mom and Dad want us to share our rooms with the baby," Adam informed her. He ignored the furious glance Julia threw him.

"You can't do that to Adam and Zoe," Brenda said.

"For the first few months, the baby will be in our room," Julia told her.

"It'll ruin your marriage."

"Peter, I'd like a glass of tea, too," Julia said, in an effort to turn the conversation from the volatile subject of her pregnancy.

"Coming right up," he called back.

Julia wanted to wring her hands in despair when she realized that all her request had done was delay Peter's return.

"Zoe," Julia said, smiling grimly at her daughter. "Go get your clarinet."

The girl's eyes widened. "Mother, I *told* you I didn't want to play for Grandma."

"Please, Zoe," she whispered, desperately needing an ally.

The thirteen-year-old stamped out of the room, muttering as she went. Julia's feelings vacillated from embarrassment at her daughter's bad manners to relief at the coming distraction.

"Here we are," Peter said, returning with a tray of iced tea, clearly oblivious to the tension in the room. He served his mother first, then Julia, and took the third glass himself. The three of them sat in a small circle, with Adam standing next to his father.

"I thought we'd barbecue later, when it cools down a little," Julia said in an effort to fill the silence.

No one had anything to add to that.

"Do you like my purse?" his mother asked, holding up the briefcase-style leather bag. "I bought it specially for this trip."

"It's lovely," Julia said. *And obviously expensive...*

"It's my Mother's Day gift to myself." She turned to Peter. "Thank you, dear, for the flowers in my room."

Julia decided she should learn from her mother-in-law. Brenda wasn't waiting for her son or anyone else to go out and buy her what she truly wanted. Instead, she'd purchased it herself.

Julia had received a potted azalea from her husband. The kids had given her cards and gone in on a small basket of scented soap. She loved the significance of those gifts—but what she really longed for was a silk nightgown in a pale shade of ecru with a matching robe. The gown was on display at the local Nordstrom's, and Julia had been back to look at it three times. She wanted something beautiful, something to remind her that she was attractive and desirable even at five months pregnant. Unfortunately, the price tag was more than her shop pulled in during an entire day.

"Do I *have* to play?" Zoe bemoaned her sorry fate as she clumped back into the room, clarinet in hand.

"I'm sure Grandma would be happy to hear you perform," Peter told his daughter with a look that defied her to suggest otherwise.

"Do you know anything by Bob Dylan?" Brenda asked. "Maybe one of the early protest songs?"

Zoe glanced at her mother for the answer. Julia shook her head.

"Sorry, no."

"You choose then," Brenda said, with a resigned expression as if she had about as much interest in listening as Zoe did in playing.

The next ten minutes were taken up with Zoe's all-too-short performance.

"I'll have my driver's license this summer," Adam said as soon as his sister had finished playing and hurried back to her room.

Julia wished there was somewhere she could hide.

"Driving?" Brenda seemed astonished.

"I'll be sixteen next month," Adam boasted.

"And you're pregnant," Brenda said, turning to Julia.

Julia looked away.

"I certainly hope you can afford this child."

"Mother..." Peter murmured.

"Think about it," her mother-in-law pressed. "You're just making ends meet as it is. Julia's business is barely off the ground. What are you going to do with the baby while you're at work? Have either of you given that any thought?"

"My mother's retiring this year," Julia began.

"You expect your mother to step in and provide day care?" Brenda asked sharply. "That's completely unfair of you."

"My mom—"

"Mother," Peter said, more loudly this time.

"Far be it from *you* to offer any help," Julia cried, feeling trapped.

"Do you expect *me* to pay for your mistakes?"

Zoe came back to the living room, obviously drawn by the shouting. She and Adam stared wide-eyed, listening to the heated exchange between their mother and grandmother. Peter was trying to calm them down, without success.

Julia stood abruptly and glared at her mother-in-law, husband and children. "This might come as a shock to you all, but my baby is not a mistake."

"You mean to say you got pregnant on purpose?" Brenda demanded.

Julia stiffened. "No...no more than you did." She was instantly ashamed of her outburst. Brenda had chosen never to marry and had raised Peter entirely on her own. "My child is a surprise, but he or she is no mistake." Then, because the entire episode had distressed her so much, she left the room.

Peter followed her into the bedroom a moment later. "Honey..."

"All I want is a few minutes alone. I'm sorry if I upset your mother."

"No. I'm sorry *you're* upset." He sighed, and slowly exhaled. "Things got out of hand before I realized what was happening. I'm sorry, sweetheart." He sat on the edge of the bed. "What would you like me to do now?"

"I...don't know. Give me a while to rest and let our tempers cool, and I'll come back and apologize."

Peter rubbed the length of her arm. "Take as long as you need. And Julia?"

She glanced up at him, raising her head from the pillow.

"Don't apologize."

Exhausted and emotionally drained, Julia decided to rest her eyes and immediately fell asleep, waking two hours later. When she rejoined the others, it was as if nothing had happened. She found her mother-in-law with Adam and Zoe, arranging dinner dishes on the patio table. Brenda had rolled up her sleeves and donned one of Julia's favorite aprons.

"We were about to wake you," she said, setting a couple of salad bowls in the center of the table. "The potatoes are roasting in the oven. I hope that's okay."

"Thank you," Julia said faintly.

"You're up," Peter said, carrying a platter of barbecued chicken toward them.

"Just in time, too." She kissed his cheek, letting him know she felt much better. Because she'd been so exhausted, she'd allowed his mother's attitude to get the best of her, something she genuinely regretted.

"We wouldn't have eaten without you, Mom," Zoe assured her, slipping an arm around Julia's thickening waist. It was the first time in weeks that her daughter had made such a loving gesture. Julia felt tears gathering behind her eyelids; she blinked rapidly, determined not to let them fall. With pregnancy she'd become so emotional.

While Peter turned off the barbecue, the kids went to the kitchen to bring out the potatoes and collect drinks.

Julia approached her mother-in-law. "I'm sorry," she said in a low voice.

Brenda hesitated, then nodded and without looking at Julia, whispered, "Me, too. I have a bad habit of saying things I shouldn't—poking my nose in. You and Peter are wonderful parents. Everything I never was." Her mother-in-law busily rearranged serving dishes for a moment. "I realize this pregnancy is unplanned, but you're right, the baby's no mistake." She glanced toward Peter and her eyes softened. "I was never meant to be a mother, and when I discovered I was pregnant with Peter, I had doubts about my ability to raise a child. Over the years, I made my fair share of mistakes, but I've always loved my son and wouldn't exchange the experience of motherhood for anything in the world. You and Peter will be just fine." Having said that, Brenda did something completely and totally out of character.

She hugged Julia.

"Make no judgments where you have no compassion."
—Anne McCaffrey

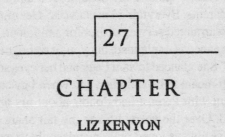

27

CHAPTER

LIZ KENYON

May 17th

Amy's belated Mother's Day gift arrived in the mail this afternoon. It was an eight-by-ten portrait of Andrew and Annie. My goodness, how my grandbabies have grown. I had to work hard not to break down and weep. I miss them all so desperately.

The gift certificate Brian sent me is on the kitchen counter. I haven't gotten down to Barnes and Noble to use it yet. At first I was disappointed that he'd mail me a generic present instead of coming up to spend the day with me. On second thought, it seemed a perfectly wonderful gift. Thoughtful, too. It's my son's way of saying he approves of me volunteering at the juvenile detention center. I think I may start reading the C. S. Lewis books next—once the last Harry Potter is finished. I'll have to see if that's okay with Ruth, although I'm sure it will be. I'll get a copy with the gift certificate—which is fitting because the Lewis stories were Brian's absolute favorite childhood reading. Okay, that settles it. I'll use my gift certificate to buy *The Lion, the Witch and the Wardrobe,* plus a book on knitting and, if there's any money left, the new Barbara Kingsolver. A satisfactory decision, if I do say so.

The kids called me Sunday morning, but if not for Sean, I would've spent Mother's Day alone. I've discovered something about him. All his provocative remarks about women are intended to get a rise out of me. It used to work, but lately I've been letting the ridiculous things he says just pass me by and that flusters him so much he doesn't know how to react.

Well, I'm on to his game. From now on I'll just pretend not to hear him. Maybe I should occasionally mutter a disparaging remark about men in the medical profession, just to rattle his cage, and see how he likes it.

He still makes cursory efforts to talk me into bed, but I'm not easily persuaded. He'd enjoy a weekend fling, or so he's let me know. The problem is, I'm confused. He can have his pick of women and he seems to want me.

We've gone out to dinner twice in the last week, and I cooked him a meal Sunday night. Afterward, I broke out the yarn and knitting needles and attempted to teach him to knit, which was hilarious because Tinkerbell thought the yarn was for her. I can't remember a time I've laughed more. I know why he chose not to be a surgeon! All his talk about agile fingers was simply that—talk. Sean was all thumbs. Somehow in the process of casting on stitches, he got the yarn completely twisted around his fingers. After fifteen minutes he gave up entirely and suggested we take in a movie. We saw the latest Mel Gibson film and shared a bag of popcorn. After the popcorn was gone, we held hands for the rest of the show.

He asked me not to tell anyone that all we've done is hold hands (and kissed once or twice—let's not forget that). But if word got out that we've spent all this time together and none of it in bed, it'd destroy his reputation. I had to roll my eyes but agreed to keep quiet.

I'm actually beginning to wonder if there's any truth to the rumors about him and all these women he supposedly dates.

* * *

The doorbell chimed and Liz set aside her journal. A check of the peephole revealed Sean standing on the other side. Liz was dismayed by the way her heart reacted at the sight of him. He'd come to mean so much to her, and that kind of feeling left you vulnerable. In a split second, she shook off her sense of fear. *Seize the moment*, she told herself.

"Surprised to see me?" he asked as she opened the door. When she merely smiled, he stepped into the house and leaned forward, kissing her briefly on the mouth, as though this was an accepted practice between them.

He had kissed her before, and both times the kisses had been full and passionate. This casual approach was welcome. But when he started to pull away, Liz stopped him, splayed her fingers through his hair and stepped closer to kiss him herself.

When she lifted her head, she found him staring down at her with an oddly puzzled look. Obviously he didn't know what to make of this sudden change in attitude.

"You must be really glad to see me," he whispered.

"I am," she assured him. He followed her into the kitchen. "Have you eaten?"

"I had something at the hospital earlier. Have you?"

"A while ago." It was after eight.

"Am I interrupting anything?"

"Nothing that can't be put off until later. What can I do for you?"

"Now that was a leading question if I ever heard one."

"Okay, bad choice of words."

"Have you got an hour or two?" he asked with a grin.

"Of course."

"Grab a sweater then."

Curious, she did as he asked, returning from her bedroom with a light sweater and her purse. He held out his hand and she took it.

"Tell me where we're going," she said as he led her outside to his Lexus and opened the passenger door.

"You'll find out in a few minutes."

A few minutes turned into twenty. He headed toward the freeway on-ramp, drove for several miles, then exited, ending up in a residential neighborhood that was unfamiliar to Liz.

She noticed that the houses were middle-class, with well-maintained yards. Sean eased to a stop in front of a corner house. Nothing distinguished it from any of the others.

"You're taking me to meet friends?" she asked. Then why didn't he say so?

"My very best friends," he said, climbing out of the car.

Liz looked around. "Do you mind telling me where we are?"

"Thirty-fifth and Jackson," he returned without a pause.

"All right, *why* are we here?"

"Ah," he said grinning broadly. "Now you're asking the right questions. My dear Liz, I'm about to show you what I do to release the tension in my life." He gestured to the house. "My alternative to knitting."

"You didn't mention anything about this earlier."

He grinned again. "I had my reasons."

"Does your tension relief have anything to do with Rolfing?" she asked, wondering if this place belonged to some kind of massage therapist.

"Rolfing," he echoed and laughed.

"Never mind."

He led her up the sidewalk and gently tapped on the door. Liz was certain no one could possibly hear his knock. Just when she was prepared to suggest there was no one home, the door opened. A large African-American woman stood there, wearing a stern look. As soon as she saw Sean, she broke into a wide smile, her face brightening with pleasure.

"Dr. Sean, aren't you a sight for sore eyes! Come in, come in."

Sean pressed his hand to the small of Liz's back and directed her into the large foyer. And Liz saw the babies. What would have been the living room was set up with six cribs and an equal number of rocking chairs. Each of the cribs held an infant, and most of them were crying.

"Who'd you bring with you?" the woman asked, eyeing Liz curiously.

"Clarissa, this is my friend Liz Kenyon. Liz, Clarissa Howard."

"Hey." The woman planted her fists on her ample hips. "I thought you said I was the only woman for you."

"Looks like you're going to have to share me," Sean joked.

Clarissa laughed boisterously, then faced Liz, her smile benevolent. "Any friend of Dr. Sean's is a friend of mine. Welcome to Little Lambs."

"These are all crack or heroin babies," he said. "Clarissa and her staff are here to love them through the worst of the withdrawals."

"Dr. Sean is our favorite physician," Clarissa told Liz, her gaze adoring. "The babies love him, too, isn't that right?"

Sean didn't answer. Instead he walked over to the farthest crib. "How's little Donovan doing tonight?"

"Not well, not well at all."

"Rough day?"

Clarissa nodded.

With a tenderness Liz had rarely seen in a man, Sean reached into the crib and lifted the emaciated infant and held him gently. "Only three weeks old," Sean whispered as he settled into the closest rocking chair. "Poor little tyke came into this world facing one hell of an uphill climb."

"Little Faye could do with being rocked," Clarissa said boldly, staring at Liz. "She's over there."

Liz knew an order when she heard one. Smiling, she found the crib marked with Faye's name. She gathered the baby in her arms and sat in a rocker. The baby gazed up at her, eyes wet with tears, lower lip quivering.

"Poor sweetheart," Liz whispered, gently brushing the curls from the baby's brow.

"Like Donovan, our Faye has a struggle ahead of her," Sean said.

Liz had seen a number of reports on crack and drug babies over the years. Women addicted to any illegal substance tended to neglect everything else in their lives. Their health in general was poor. Statistics showed that they ate junk food and skipped meals and had poor sleeping habits. They abused themselves in a multitude of ways. Studies had indicated that a large percentage of pregnant drug-users also smoked cigarettes and drank alcohol throughout the pregnancy. Consequently, the babies were born with low birth weights and often prematurely. Some had Fetal Alcohol Syndrome. Some, as Sean had said, suffered because they'd been born to drug-addicted mothers.

Liz had heard about Little Lambs when it was in the setup stages, but Willow Grove Memorial hadn't been part of the project. She'd never heard anything about Sean's involvement.

Clarissa took a third child and settled herself between Sean and Liz, humming quietly as she rocked, the baby cuddled in her loving arms.

Thirty minutes later, the room was quiet. Liz glanced over and realized that Sean's eyes were closed.

Clarissa's gaze followed hers. "He falls asleep nearly every time."

"Does he come often?" Liz asked.

"Quite a bit, but it's been a week or so since his last visit." The man was full of surprises.

"Dr. Sean's crazy about babies," Clarissa added. "I don't understand why he didn't have a houseful of his own."

Other than that one mention of his ex-wife and daughter, Liz knew almost nothing about Sean's life outside of medicine. Although he hadn't said so, Liz was under the impression that he hadn't told many people about his family.

"Do you love him?" Clarissa shocked her by asking next.

The question caught Liz unawares, and she wasn't sure how to answer. "I don't know."

"Someone should. He needs a woman, and you're the first one he's ever brought here."

That lifted Liz's spirits. "Have you known him long?"

Clarissa nodded. "He helped create Little Lambs and recommended me for the job. Far as I'm concerned, there's no better man than Dr. Sean. If he wanted me to walk over redhot coals, I'd do it for him, without asking why."

If Sean was aware of this conversation, he'd be gloating, Liz thought. He must love hearing Clarissa sing his praises. She leaned forward, wondering if she could detect a sassy grin on his face.

"He's out," Clarissa assured her. "It's amazing how rocking the babies calms *him* down."

Liz had to agree that was quite a switch. "He told me this is what he does to unwind."

Clarissa's chair made creaking sounds as she continued rocking, still humming softly.

"I tried to teach him to knit." Which, Liz had to admit, seemed a bit ridiculous now.

"Dr. Sean?" The other woman pinched her lips. "He doesn't need that; you don't either. Both of you just come see me and my babies."

"All right," Liz agreed.

A full hour passed before Sean woke. He yawned, looked in Liz's direction and asked, "You ready to go?"

"Whenever you are."

He replaced a sleeping Donovan in the crib, and within a few minutes they were preparing to leave.

Clarissa walked them to the door.

"It was a pleasure meeting you and your babies," Liz said.

The other woman nodded, then gripped Liz's elbow. "You find out."

"Find out?" Liz repeated.

"What we talked about earlier."

"Oh." Liz was sure her red face gave her away. She didn't dare look at Sean, certain he'd know they'd been discussing him. *Do you love him?* Clarissa had asked, and Liz figured she expected the answer to be *yes.* Clarissa was openly encouraging Liz to delve deeper into her feelings for Sean.

"What was that all about?" Sean asked as they strolled toward his car.

"Nothing important," she said dismissively.

Not until they were on the street, driving back to her house, did she chance a look in his direction. From what Clarissa had said, she was the first woman he'd ever brought to Little Lambs.

What she didn't understand was why. What did she actually mean to him? What did he *really* want from her?

"You're frowning," he said. They'd stopped at a traffic light before heading onto the ramp that led to the freeway. He reached over and squeezed her hand, his fingers lingering in hers.

"Just thinking." Liz smiled so he'd know she wasn't

upset, only perplexed by the complicated man she was beginning to know.

"Any thoughts you want to share with me?"

"One," she said, realizing even as she spoke that she was taking a risk. "I think there might be some hope for this relationship, after all."

Sean gave no outward response for a moment. Then he said, "That's what I've been trying to tell you. I don't know why you women don't listen to men more often."

Liz groaned and shook her head, but not before she saw him trying to suppress a laugh. She was smiling, too.

> "Life is the first gift, love is the second, and understanding the third."
>
> —Marge Piercy

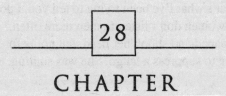

CHAPTER

KAREN CURTIS

"**Y**our father and I would like you to join us for lunch next Saturday," Catherine Curtis informed Karen in her most prim voice. She used the tone guaranteed to set Karen's teeth on edge every time.

Pressing the telephone receiver hard against her ear, Karen felt as if she'd received a summons to appear in court instead of an invitation from her mother. Whatever Catherine wanted was important enough to add the influence of her father's name.

Karen knew it wasn't her company they sought—or at least her mother didn't. Something was up, and she suspected she wasn't going to like it.

"You'll come?" her mother said.

"Don't go to any trouble, though," Karen warned. Lunch

for her generally consisted of a sandwich on the run or something she could pick up at a drive-through window.

For Catherine Curtis, on the other hand, every meal was an occasion. Karen didn't know anyone outside her parents' circle of friends who went to such effort for lunch. It was just *lunch,* for heaven's sake. Her mother had built her entire social life around a bridge club that met every Friday at one. The women were constantly in competition, trying to outdo each other with elaborate luncheon menus and fancy centerpieces.

"I'll see you on Saturday then."

"Any reason you and Dad want to talk to me?" Karen asked. Better to get a heads-up now than be blindsided later.

"Can't your father and I invite you to the house without a reason?" her mother asked with a light, tinkling laugh—a laugh that was so forced, Karen had to cringe.

"You always have a reason, Mother," she said grimly.

Catherine gave a beleaguered sigh but no other response.

"I was just there for Mother's Day." Being in close proximity to her mother twice within the same month was above and beyond the call of duty.

"You've already agreed to come," Catherine reminded her.

"Yes, and I will, but I want to know why."

"Because I asked it of you. Let's not get into this now. I'll look forward to seeing you at noon on Saturday."

"Yes, Mother," Karen muttered, banging down the telephone receiver. She'd allowed herself to be manipulated again. Would she never learn?

Saturday arrived far too soon, long before Karen was ready. She chose a dress her mother had bought her when Karen was still in high school. Sensible, demure—and a style completely wrong for her. Karen didn't know why she still held on to it.

By the time she arrived, her stomach was swarming with nerves. She knew from experience that her mother was likely to serve a five-course meal, and Karen didn't have the appetite to enjoy even one bite.

The first thing she noticed when she pulled into the circular driveway in front of her parents' home was that Victoria's car wasn't there. Always before, her sister had been included in these lunches. Not today, which led to immediate speculation that this conversation had something to do with her sister.

Before she could change her mind, Karen parked her ten-year-old Ford Tempo.

The front door opened and her mother stood in the entrance. Karen's engine was still hacking and coughing, although the ignition had been turned off. She was sorry her mother was there to hear it. Catherine had never approved of Karen's car, but to Karen it represented independence and integrity, since she'd purchased and paid for it herself.

She walked toward the door as the old Ford coughed one last time, as if to remind her how badly it needed servicing.

"Could you park your...vehicle over by the garage?" her mother called.

And out of the neighbors' sight, Karen added mentally. "Sorry, Mom, but I'm having trouble with the transmission. It'd be better if I left it someplace where I won't need to reverse."

Her mother started to speak, then seemed to change her mind, and turned away.

Karen followed her into the house. This wasn't the home she'd grown up in and she'd never felt as though she belonged here. Her father's chain of produce warehouses had prospered dramatically over the past ten years, and her parents were living off the fruit of his labors. She smiled at the pun.

Status had always been important to her mother, and the big home, fancy cars and children she could brag about to her friends were included in her requirements.

They were apparently having lunch in the kitchen. The kitchen, though, was the size of Karen's entire apartment. It was newly renovated with oak cabinets, a slate floor and lovely multi-paned windows—a nice traditional look, except that Catherine had added a few too many bits of "country" kitsch. The round oak table held a huge sunflower centerpiece, with sunflower-patterned place mats. Clearly a theme—no doubt based on a magazine article about decorating for summer. Karen glanced around expecting to find her father hiding behind the sunflower display. "Where's Dad?"

"He sends his apologies, but he was called into the office."

"On a Saturday?"

Her mother's sigh said it all. "I wasn't pleased," she said sternly. "You asked that I not go to any trouble, so I thought we'd have lunch in here."

"This is perfect." Karen clasped her hands to conceal any sign of nervousness. She'd hoped her father would be here. If Victoria wasn't around, her father could have served as a buffer.

Catherine opened the refrigerator and removed a sesame chicken and pasta salad. Bread, steaming from the oven, was already out and cooling.

"This is your favorite salad, isn't it?" Catherine asked.

Actually it was Victoria's, but now didn't seem the time to point that out.

"My all-time favorite," she lied. "How thoughtful of you to make it for me."

"Well, to be honest, I had Doris put it together."

Doris was the housekeeper who'd been with the family for a number of years.

"Oh." So much for thoughtfulness.

"You know I play bridge with the girls on Friday." Her mother's tone was defensive. "This salad needs to be made twenty-four hours in advance."

"I wasn't upset," Karen said, wishing they could have a normal conversation, one in which they weren't constantly offending each other.

"Shall we sit down?" Catherine said.

"Sure." Karen slid into her chair and unfolded her linen napkin. Catherine handed her the chicken salad; the warm bread followed.

Karen took her first bite, but it seemed to get stuck in the back of her throat. She knew it would be impossible to down another forkful until she learned what this was all about. "Where's Victoria?" she asked outright. She hadn't talked to her sister in some time and feared there'd been a repeat of the last incident. Karen felt her anger rise at the mere thought of that twit hitting her sister. Maybe she should change *twit* to *brute,* she mused darkly.

"Victoria?" her mother echoed. "Uh, what do you mean?"

"She's always here when we have our lunches."

Her mother paused for a moment. "I believe she's shopping—buying summer clothes for Bryce this afternoon."

"Oh." Karen never had a problem being articulate except when she was with her mother.

Catherine stabbed a shredded piece of chicken with her fork, eyes downcast.

Finally Karen couldn't stand it any longer. "Just tell me!"

Her mother's eyes widened. "Tell you what, dear?"

"Why you invited me here."

Her mother sighed. To Karen's surprise, she capitulated without any more of that conversational thrust and parry. "I'm concerned about Victoria," she said in a flat voice.

She knew. Thank God! Somehow, her mother had learned that Roger was beating Victoria. Relief swept through Karen. Surely her mother would step in now and help in ways that Karen couldn't.

"I'm worried about her, too," Karen blurted out, nearly weak with gratitude. "We need to do something, Mom."

"Yes, well..."

"Has she opened up to you? She called me a few months ago, absolutely desperate. I was deathly afraid of what Roger might do."

Her mother frowned. "Victoria phoned you?"

"I'm sure she would've called you and Dad, but she didn't want to alarm you."

"Oh, dear."

"How'd you find out? Did you see the bruises? She's gotten so good at hiding them, but it's more than the physical abuse, it's the horrible things Roger says to her. The worst part is that she believes them."

Her mother went pale and her hand crept to her throat.

Karen hesitated. "Are you all right?"

"I..."

A sick feeling came over her, and she realized she'd made a serious mistake in assuming that Victoria had confided in her parents. "You didn't know, did you?"

Ever proper, Catherine Curtis squared her shoulders. "I...don't know what to think. I have a hard time believing

Roger is the kind of man who'd do the things you're suggesting."

Horrified, Karen vaulted to her feet. Tears of anger and outrage stung her eyes. "You don't believe me? You think I'd make something like this up?"

"Sit down," her mother ordered, voice shaking.

"Do you think I'd fabricate this story out of some perverse jealousy?"

Her mother's hand trembled and when she spoke it was as if she'd forgotten Karen was in the room. "I've known for some weeks that things weren't…right between Victoria and Roger, but I didn't want to interfere." She shook her head. "I thought Victoria seemed depressed—that's what worried me. That's what I'd hoped to discuss with you."

Karen sank into her chair. "I saw what he did the last time. Well, the time she called me… Who knows what's happened since?"

"Roger hit her?"

Karen nodded.

"You say Victoria told you," her mother said, giving up all pretense of eating. Her hand continued to shake as she reached for her iced tea.

"Yes…"

"Did she tell you why she wasn't comfortable talking to me?"

"No," Karen answered. "I'm sure she just didn't want to upset you," she said again.

"Instead, she left that task to you."

"No…no, Mom, Victoria would never do that. I upset you all on my own. I mean, oh hell—you know what I mean!"

"Do I?"

The harder Karen tried, the worse it became. "Mom, listen to me, please. This is too important. We can't get all twisted up in our own egos. We have to help Victoria."

Catherine closed her eyes. "I agree. Tell me what you know."

Karen wasn't sure where to start. She felt tempted to mention that dreadful Thanksgiving dinner years earlier when Victoria had bolted from the table, but she didn't.

"Roger's a twit," she said instead. "And a brute."

"Is he...abusing Bryce?"

"No...not to my knowledge."

"You're absolutely certain about Victoria? Oh, of course you are. It's just that this is far worse than I imagined. Dear God, why couldn't she tell me?"

"I'm sure Victoria wanted to, but she doesn't know how."

Catherine's expression was stricken. "It's such a shock."

"I know it's hard to believe, Mom—it was for me, too. But I swear to you, it's the truth. I've seen the evidence."

Her mother looked away, as though just hearing the words brought her pain. "Why doesn't Victoria come to your father and me—surely she knows we'd do anything to help..." She let the rest fade.

"You said you were worried about her? That she seemed depressed?"

Caught up in her thoughts, her mother didn't immediately answer. "She's been so distant lately," Catherine finally said. "We were always close, Victoria and I, but lately she's made excuses to stay away. I felt something was wrong. I'd hoped you might know what was going on, and as it turns out you do."

Karen had no idea what to say next, what to suggest. She sipped at her iced tea while she waited for inspiration.

"I don't understand why Victoria didn't come to me," her

mother wailed. "I really don't." Karen had never seen her lose control to this extent. She realized Catherine was deeply hurt by Victoria's silence and probably felt a large measure of inadequacy.

"Listen, Mom, she's embarrassed and ashamed. Everyone assumes Victoria has the perfect marriage and she didn't want to disillusion any of us."

"But why would she allow this kind of treatment to continue?"

"Mom, the whys don't matter. We can sort all that out later. Right now, we both need to concentrate on how to help Victoria. She's at the point where she can't do it for herself."

Her mother stared down at her lunch plate. "She should have told me," she mumbled again. "She—"

"Yes Mom," Karen said impatiently. "But she couldn't."

"What are we going to do?"

"I don't know. Support and love her, first of all."

"Of course, that's understood."

"I wanted her to leave the jerk, but Victoria wouldn't hear of it. Nor will she involve the police. I talked until I was blue in the face and it didn't do one bit of good. She's afraid of hurting his career."

"If the law firm finds out about it, Roger could very likely lose his position," her mother said.

"That isn't Victoria's fault. He's the one hitting her."

"Oh, I agree. All I'm saying is that I can understand Victoria's hesitation. If Roger loses his job, the entire family will suffer. Plus, there's the humiliation of family and friends discovering she's married to a wife-beater."

"Of course," Karen muttered. "That's why she's kept it to herself."

"We must consider our options very carefully," her mother said. "Karen, let's give this some thought." She'd become the formidable matron once again, the woman whose strength of will wasn't easily defeated. Despite her flaws and pretensions, Catherine Curtis loved her daughters—*both* of them. Karen knew the truth of that, had in a sense always known it, but now she was overwhelmed by the insight. She suddenly understood that she was her mother's equal, in strength and determination, far more than Victoria.

She relaxed in her chair for the first time since she'd arrived. The burden of Victoria's life was lifted from her shoulders; she and her mother were allies, united in the quest to help her sister. She felt a hundred times better.

She shoved her plate and the sunflower centerpiece aside and leaned her elbows on the table. "Okay, Mom, let's get to work."

> "Learn the wisdom of compromise, for it is better to
> bend a little than to break."
>
> —Jane Wells

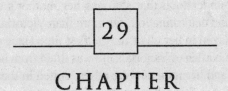

CHAPTER 29

CLARE CRAIG

The house was in chaos and that wasn't going to change any time soon. Mick was home for the summer. He'd arrived late the night before, his car loaded down with a year's accumulation of dorm room necessities.

Yawning, Clare ambled down the hallway to the kitchen, maneuvering around his half-size refrigerator with a microwave balanced on top. She paused to look inside the laundry room and gasped.

Rather than deal with what appeared to be an entire semester's worth of wash, she closed the door and continued into the kitchen. To her surprise the coffee was already made.

"Morning," Mick greeted her from the family room. All that was visible was his arm, which lay across the back of the sofa, and his head. His hair went in all directions and he was badly in need of a shave.

"How long have you been up?" she asked, reaching for a mug.

Mick merely shrugged.

"You haven't been to bed yet, have you?" Her son, like his father, was a night owl.

"I was too keyed up from the drive," Mick confessed. "I sat down in front of the television and then it was too much effort to move."

"Did you sleep at all?"

"Some," he muttered, but from the look of him, Clare doubted it.

She'd never understood why Mick always insisted on unloading the car the minute he arrived home. The boys were still hauling in one load after another when she'd gone to bed. She was relieved that Mick and Alex were back on speaking terms.

Her own relationship with Mick had also been strained, and Clare hoped that everything would resolve itself now that he was home. She hoped he'd make his peace with his father too. Her oldest son's anger toward Michael hadn't wavered. He refused to have anything to do with him, even though Alex and Clare saw Michael regularly.

"Do you feel like talking?" Clare carried her coffee into the other room and sat in the recliner across from Mick.

He stiffened. "Not if it's about Dad."

"All right." Her son was more intuitive than she'd realized.

"I'm glad school's out," he said. Mick was obviously searching for a topic of conversation.

"I'm not going to be around as much this summer," Clare

told him. To her relief, her taking over at the dealership had gone relatively well. Because she already knew the staff, the transition had been quick and smooth. Nevertheless, she worked far more than the normal forty hours a week.

"Alex told me you don't get home until eight o'clock," Mick said, frowning.

"Just some nights."

"I don't understand it. Why are you helping Dad? How *can* you, after what he did to you?"

"What he did to *us*," she corrected. That was what Mick was really saying. The pain their sons had endured was as great as her own.

"I can't forgive him."

"I'm not sure I've completely forgiven him, either," she said. Even now, Clare found it difficult to look past the agony Michael had brought into their lives.

"But you're helping him."

"I know."

"Why?" Mick cried. "Is it because of the cancer?"

It deeply pained her that neither boy was aware of the full truth regarding Michael's illness. She'd promised not to tell them Michael was dying, and, in fact, had only a few months to live; it was a promise she regretted now.

"What else could I do?" she asked, her voice low. "Michael came to me. The dealership was floundering, and someone needed to step in. Otherwise the business might fold entirely."

"Are you hoping Dad will come back?" Mick asked angrily.

Clare had given some thought to that question herself. A part of her *wanted* him to want her back, to plead with her to forgive him. The scenario had played in her mind a thousand times before and after the divorce, and in each version she'd rejected him. She didn't know what she would've done if Michael had actually attempted to reconcile.

"Are you, Mom?" Mick pressed.

She shook her head. "He doesn't want me anymore." That was the truth, painful though it was to admit.

Mick's face hardened. "Or Alex and me."

"That's not true," she insisted. "Your father loves you both."

Mick snorted. "Sure he does."

Clare wanted to argue, but stopped herself, hardly able to believe she'd turned into Michael's champion. As far as his father was concerned, Mick had already made up his mind.

"I'm glad Miranda left him," he added.

Clare hated the edge she heard in his voice and realized it was an echo of the anger she'd carried herself for all those months.

"I saw her, you know."

Clare glanced at him. "When?"

"Last Christmas, while I was home. She was with some guy."

"Someone her own age?"

Mick nodded. "She had her arm around his and was looking up at him with these big adoring eyes. I thought, you know, this was what Dad deserved. He cheated on you and now everything had come full circle and she was cheating on him."

"Poor Miranda."

"Poor Miranda?" Mick sounded incredulous. "You've got to be joking."

Clare avoided meeting his gaze. "It's taken a long time, but I finally understand what happened. Miranda lost her father without a minute's warning. One day he was alive, and the next day he was dead. That shook her whole world."

"And there was Dad, so helpful, taking care of every-thing," Mick said sarcastically.

Clare nodded, her throat tightening. "The poor girl got con-fused. In her pain and grief, she turned to Michael, somehow transferring the love she had for her dad to him. She was look-ing for another father figure more than she was a lover. In a way, I can understand that."

"Well, I can't." Mick's voice was stubborn, uncompro-mising.

"Michael offered her strength and comfort." Clare didn't condone the grief their actions had caused, but she wanted Mick to be a little more compassionate.

"That might excuse Miranda, but what about Dad?"

"I...I don't know. Perhaps there was something lacking in me." She'd gone over her own role in this fiasco again and again. "Miranda needed him and I...I didn't."

"All that tells me is you're strong and Dad's weak." Mick bolted off the sofa and stood in the middle of the family room, fists clenched at his sides. "We weren't going to talk about Dad, remember?"

"Right," she said, forcing a smile. She knew what her son was saying. It had been this way for more than two years now. Everything—every conversation, every argument, every thought—always went back to Michael.

"When I was in high school," Mick said, "Dad was around all the time and it was no big deal."

Even when he'd declared he *didn't* want to discuss Michael, Mick was the one bringing him into the conversation.

"Now Dad's gone, and I feel his absence far more than I ever did his presence."

How articulate Mick was. She stared at him with a re-newed sense of love and appreciation.

"I hope you'll go see him," she said.

Mick's response was immediate. "No way!"

"Oh, Mick, don't turn your back on him out of any sense of loyalty to me. Your father needs you."

Her son shook his head vehemently, his face unyielding. "What about all those times I needed him and he was playing daddy with Miranda? Don't push the issue, Mom."

The pain vibrated from him, and Clare could see that Michael had a lot of work ahead of him if he hoped to heal the broken relationship with his oldest son.

"What's everyone doing up?" Alex asked, wandering into the family room in his swimming shorts. He yawned and scratched his head.

"Mick never went to bed," Clare told him.

"Hey, why not?"

"I was watching reruns of *The Brady Bunch*."

"The Brady Bunch?" Alex repeated. "Why would you do that when there's all those stations? What about VH-1?"

Mick shrugged. "I don't know. I was in a groove."

Strangely, Clare understood. Her son wasn't interested in the entertainment value of a decades-old situation comedy. What he saw was a happy blended family. With the Bradys, problems all seemed trivial and the parents loved each other and everyone worked out their differences. This was the fantasy family, whose lives were far removed from his own.

* * *

June 10th

Michael phoned the dealership six times from the hospital this afternoon. The chemo's especially rough on him this go-round, and the doctors felt it was best if he stayed there for the week.

I was busy each and every time he phoned. I waited until I had a free minute before I called him back. He asked me to take over for him, but I've discovered that he wants to keep close tabs on everything I do. I know I was being unfair and unreasonable, but I let Michael have it.

I should apologize for that outburst. It must have been very hard for him to step down and let me assume the leadership. We're different people and our work methods don't necessarily agree. Nor do we handle staff in the same way.

I don't think Michael has quite realized what a financial mess the business was in. He'd obviously been putting work off for months, letting orders slide. I'm trying to get things in shape, but he has opinions on everything I do. Even from his hospital bed, Michael can't leave it alone. More than once I've been tempted to tell him exactly what he can do with this job.

I haven't, and I won't. I understand how difficult it was to turn the management over to me. He says he asked me to do this for the boys, and I know that's true. The dealership is their inheritance, but unfortunately they're not interested. Neither of them is willing to work here, even for the summer. Alex's job at Softline keeps him busy and Mick got a job as a lifeguard, which he loves. He's tanned and gorgeous and the girls are flocking to the house. Kellie is still dating Alex, but she's got her eye on Mick. A mother knows these things.

On a brighter note, I had an unexpected but welcome surprise. Leslie Carter phoned me from Hawaii. We chatted for nearly thirty minutes. He talked about the sailing trip and what he learned about himself and his limits. I found it really interesting; he's a perceptive man. I told him about working at the dealership. We only met that one time, but he's stayed in my mind and apparently I've stayed in his.

Both boys were home when Leslie phoned and were full of curiosity. It was all a little embarrassing. Mick had a lot of questions, and for a while there, I felt like I was being interrogated. Really, there's nothing to tell. Leslie is a wonderful man and I'm glad I met him. I don't have any idea if I'll be seeing him again.

I hope I do, though. I really would like to know him better.

"The dedicated life is the life worth living. You must give with your whole heart."

—Annie Dillard

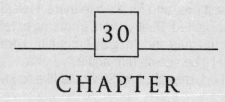

30

CHAPTER

Thursday Morning Breakfast Club

L<small>IZ</small>, by nature, was prompt and thus the first to arrive at Mocha Moments. She ordered her croissant and coffee, and secured the table by the window so she could watch for her friends.

These few quiet minutes helped her compose her thoughts. She needed to process the conversation she'd had with her son the night before. Brian, spurred on by his sister, was worried about her. Funny, her son had been perfectly content to call her once a month until he'd learned from Amy that their mother was dating again. Now he felt he should visit home and check out the situation.

Liz didn't know if she should be pleased by her children's concern or insulted by their lack of trust in her judgment.

Clare arrived soon afterward, looking harried. The last two Thursdays, she'd only stayed about ten minutes before rushing off to the dealership. Earlier in the week, Liz had left a message with Alex, but Clare hadn't called her back.

"Morning," Clare said, carrying her espresso and scone to the table. She was about to sit down but stopped in midaction. "I never did return your call, did I?"

"No."

"Damn, I'm sorry. It's just that I've been running around like a lunatic for the last couple of weeks." She sank into her seat.

"I noticed," Liz said, without chastisement.

"Hello, everyone." Julia pulled out her usual chair and joined them.

The maternity jumper seemed new and Liz was pleased to see some color in her cheeks. Julia dipped her tea bag in the white ceramic pot.

"How was your week?" she asked them both. Before they could answer, Karen appeared.

"Sorry I'm late." She greeted them with her cheerful smile as she bounced into her seat. The backpack went onto the floor next to her chair; this week's latte was plunked down on the table and some of it sloshed out of the cup.

Liz studied the frothy concoction Karen had bought and wondered what flavor combination she'd selected today.

"How is everyone?" Karen asked.

"I'm feeling great," Liz said and she meant it. She smiled widely; happiness seemed to radiate from her. Everyone at work had noticed. Her secretary, Donna De-Gooyer, people in the cafeteria—everyone—and they all knew the reason, too.

"So speaks a woman in love." Julia poured her brewed herbal tea into her mug.

"In love?" Karen raised her voice in excitement. "You're falling for that doctor friend of yours, aren't you?"

All three turned to stare at her.

Liz was uncomfortable with their scrutiny. She was surprised she'd been able to hide her feelings this long. "The operative word here is *friend*. Sean and I are just friends."

Clare eyed her skeptically. "Nothing more..."

"Nothing more," Liz quickly agreed, and she was serious. Sean wanted her in his bed, but he'd accepted her refusal with unexpected grace. As a result, their friendship had flourished, deepening beyond work talk and casual conversation. For the most part, he avoided any mention of his ex-wife and their divorce, but he'd divulged a few of the details. Liz felt certain she was one of the few people privileged with that information.

"Yeah, right," Karen muttered, not bothering to conceal her disbelief. "The way you feel about him is written all over you."

"Don't say that." Liz groaned aloud. "Brian's coming for a visit this weekend."

"To check out Sean?" Clare had two boys of her own and knew exactly what Brian was up to, Liz thought wryly.

"Well, he didn't admit it, but we both know why he's developed a sudden interest in visiting his mother," she replied.

"Amy sent him," Clare said, raising her eyebrows.

"That's my guess, anyway." Liz shook her head. "I never thought my children would react like this."

"React like what?" Julia peeled away the paper lining on her blueberry muffin, then looked at Liz, awaiting a response.

"Like my being attracted to another man is this huge shock." There, she'd come right out and said it. Liz was interested in Sean. Sure, they had their differences, but everything had changed the night he took her to Little Lambs.

He'd revealed an unprecedented trust in her and she, in turn, had shed her own prejudices.

"My dad died ten years ago," Julia continued, splaying her hand across her abdomen as the baby kicked. "And if my mom started dating after all this time, I'd wonder, too. It's only natural, don't you think?" She threw the question out to the group.

The other two agreed.

"I'll say one thing," Clare said, "you look happier than I've ever seen you. What was your word for the year again?"

"Time," Liz said. Funny Clare should ask, because she'd given a lot of consideration to her word lately. She'd chosen it because she was afraid life was passing her by and there were so many things she had yet to do, yet to experience. Falling in love wasn't something she'd anticipated. But it made every day, every hour, feel vivid and special—made her conscious of time in a new way.

"I suggest you don't waste any *time* making excuses, either," Karen said, half-humorously. "When Brian comes, just hold your head high."

"She's right," Julia said. "Brian might feel shocked, as I would, but be honest and ask for his support."

"What I can't get over is that my own children doubt my judgment."

"From some of the things you told us about him early on, *I* doubt your judgement," Clare muttered, then refuted her disapproval with a wide smile. "But if you see something redeeming in him, then it must be there."

"There is," Liz said with a soft sigh. She wouldn't be with Sean until the weekend, and already she was counting the days.

"Help me, please," Clare moaned. "My friend is falling in love and she can't think straight."

"Cut it out," Liz returned sternly, but was unable to keep back a smile. She *was* in love, and it felt absolutely wonderful.

"Love can have consequences," Julia said, placing her hands over the small mound that was her baby. "Before you ask, everything's developing nicely. I'm nearly seven months along now. I guess I spent so long trying to deny that I was pregnant, the weeks just slipped away."

"What about Adam and Zoe? Have they had an attitude adjustment yet?" Liz asked.

Julia shook her head. "Most of the time, they're still angry and upset with Peter and me, as though we purposely set out to destroy their self-involved little lives. That's one of the reasons we don't talk much about the baby around them."

"It's fairly obvious you're pregnant," Clare said. "It isn't like they can ignore it."

"Yes, they can," Julia insisted. "And they are. They don't understand that being parents to a newborn means more than having a package of disposable diapers on hand. This baby is going to cause a major lifestyle change, and *everyone's* been ignoring that fact, including me." Julia sounded near-frantic. "To complicate everything, Peter and I still don't know what we're going to do about day care."

"I thought you said Peter could get three months' paid leave after the baby's born, and that he'd bring him or her to you at the store for feedings."

"But that's only three months, and I don't even know how well it's going to work."

"You can't keep the baby at the store?"

"Not if I intend to give good customer service. I think

people would be tolerant for a little while, but not on an everyday basis. It is, after all, a retail store."

Liz agreed with her. "It's one thing with an infant," she said. "You might be able to manage. But when he or she begins to crawl..."

Julia nodded.

"I thought your mother was retiring," Karen inserted.

The worry in Julia's eyes diminished slightly, and Liz could see that her friend had pinned her hopes on her mother's help.

"Mom is retiring, but I can't expect her to leave one job and take on another, especially when it's this demanding. If she were to offer, then that'd be great. Peter and I would be thrilled. But she hasn't—and I can't ask her." Julia's voice faded with disappointment.

"What about Georgia?" Karen suggested.

"My cousin? You're joking, right? Georgia hasn't been around babies very much and doesn't know a thing about them. I love my cousin, but she'd hate me if I saddled her with this baby for more than an hour at a time. Besides, she already has a job."

"What about baby clothes and all the other paraphernalia you're going to need?" Liz asked.

Julia looked more distraught than ever. "Clothes are the least of my concerns. Between my sister and the women from church, I'll have more than enough clothes to see this baby through kindergarten."

"Day care is a big problem for a lot of women," Liz said, knowing how heavily the issue weighed on Julia's mind.

"I don't know what I'm going to do," she murmured again, eyes disconsolate. "I might have to close the shop. I'd hate that and it would make me resent my baby—which I don't want. But I don't want to throw away all my hard work, either." She shrugged helplessly. "The baby has to be my first priority."

"There don't seem to be any easy answers, do there?" Clare's voice revealed her sympathy.

"None—and the crazy part is, I'm actually looking forward to having this baby. After all the angst and doubt I had in the beginning, I didn't think that was possible. Now, if only my children would develop some tolerance..."

"Adam and Zoe will come around," Karen said. "Just be patient."

"Six months of substitute teaching, and the girl's an expert on child-rearing," Clare muttered under her breath.

"Hey," Karen countered. "I spend eight to ten hours a day, four days a week, dealing with teenagers. I know how they think."

Liz was surprised. "You must be substituting a lot more hours than you were before." Come to think of it, Karen hadn't mentioned an audition for some time now.

"I've been filling in at Manchester High School," she said.

"Isn't that where the chemistry teacher works?" Liz asked. "The one you hooked up with?"

"Yeah." Karen lowered her gaze.

Liz read the signs like a skilled scout. "You like this guy."

"I do," she admitted. "Glen is wonderful."

She was charmed by the way Karen's eyes brightened when she mentioned his name.

"Glen met my parents this weekend," she said with deceptive casualness.

"You took Glen to meet your *parents?*" Julia asked, unable to disguise her shock.

"Not exactly. Glen and I were rollerblading near the beach and we ran into my parents at the marina."

"Did mom and dad approve?" Clare asked, although the answer to that should be obvious.

"How could they not? Glen is smart and polite and traditional. Plus he's got a respectable occupation." She grinned. "He's everything my parents always wanted for me." After a brief pause, she added casually, "You know, I'm getting along much better with my mother these days."

"That's good news." Liz was sincere. Every week, it seemed, Karen had come with a long list of grievances against her mother. Liz recognized that this was a relationship between two stubborn people, neither of whom was willing to meet the other's expectations.

"How's your sister doing?" Clare asked next.

Karen didn't say anything right away, and it seemed to Liz that she struggled to answer. "Okay, I guess. She isn't speaking to me at the moment."

"Why not?"

If Clare had been able to stay for more than ten minutes the last couple of weeks, she'd know. Karen had told them about the lunch with her mother and how she'd inadvertently blurted out the truth about Victoria's marriage. Her mother had then confronted Victoria, and Karen's older sister had resented the intrusion.

Soon afterward, the two sisters had an angry exchange. In the end, Victoria had slammed the door in Karen's face, but not before she'd screamed that she wanted nothing more to do with her. Karen had felt horrible. She hadn't mentioned the episode since, but Liz knew the strained relationship continued to bother her.

"Here's what I wanted to tell you," Karen said, clearly eager to move on to another topic. "Guess what I've been teaching?"

"English?"

"No. Drumroll, please. Drama classes! And guys, I absolutely love it."

"Drama?" Liz repeated. "Karen, that's great!"

"Yeah, and with the year-round schedule, I can work all summer long, if I want."

Clare rolled her eyes. "I still can't get used to that. I'm just grateful only one of my boys was involved in it. Manchester High School didn't go year-round until after Mick graduated."

"Well, I'm just grateful they did," Karen said. "Otherwise I'd go back to being a starving artist. I've had work and I've had none and—"

"Work is better," Julia finished for her.

"Exactly!" Karen agreed.

"Get back to Glen meeting your parents," Clare insisted. "I want to hear about this. And I mean details, girl."

"Well..." Karen hesitated. She started to laugh. "You know what my mother said to Glen? That he was the first boy I'd dated who didn't have tattoos or a ponytail."

"She didn't!"

Karen nodded. "She did, but I think she was just so happy to meet someone she considered normal, she simply forgot herself."

Although Karen had made it obvious that she didn't want to discuss her sister, Liz was dissatisfied with their unresolved conversation about Victoria. She felt anxious about this woman, felt that her husband was a time bomb, waiting to explode. "Are you sure everything's all right with Victoria?"

"As far as I know," Karen said. "I tried to call her this week, but she hung up on me."

"Could it have been her husband who answered the phone?"

"No, it was Victoria, and as soon as she heard my voice she slammed down the receiver."

"How sad," Liz said sympathetically. "I'm sorry."

"I'm worried about her, naturally, but my fears are for Bryce, too," Karen said. "Every time Roger unleashes his anger on my sister, he's telling his son it's all right to hit someone smaller and weaker." She frowned darkly. "Mother said Victoria denied everything."

Liz had hoped that Karen's mother would be a catalyst in this situation. Realizing she had the love and support of her family might lend Victoria the courage to reach out for help.

"If she doesn't call you or your mother, who can she call?" Clare asked.

Karen lowered her gaze. "I don't know, but I refuse to give up. I'm stopping by her place this afternoon. She won't have any choice but to talk to me then."

"Good!"

"How did Alex's graduation go this weekend?" Liz asked Clare.

A moment's hesitation was followed by, "Good."

From the flat way she spoke, Liz knew something was wrong. So did the others, because everyone stopped to look at Clare.

"What?" Clare demanded.

"You'd better tell us what happened," Liz said. She hadn't noticed earlier that her friend was troubled, but she saw it now. Clare had looked tired and stressed ever since she'd started work at the dealership; today she also seemed distracted.

"Nothing's wrong."

"You might fool some of the people some of the time, but you can't fool us," Karen said, leaning forward, elbows on the tabletop. "Tell us what's going on."

A hint of a smile turned up Clare's mouth.

"We're waiting," Julia said, crossing her arms as though to say she'd sit there all day if necessary.

Clare exhaled noisily. "Michael insisted on attending the graduation."

Liz frowned. "He's been hospitalized all week."

"I know. Alex said he wanted him at the ceremony, if possible, and then Michael said he wasn't going to let his son down."

"How'd he get there?"

"Taxi." Clare drank the last of her espresso, but clung tightly to the small cup. "He wouldn't ask me because we'd had an argument."

"About the graduation?" Julia asked.

"No, the dealership. He's constantly checking up on me and it was driving me nuts. I talk to him nearly every day, but I haven't seen him since we had lunch together at the end of April." She paused and dragged in a deep breath. "Alex didn't say that Michael was going—he couldn't. He was afraid that Mick wouldn't show up if he learned his father planned to be there. He was probably right, too."

"How come you saw each other?" Julia asked.

"Assigned seating. Each family was allowed three tickets, and all three of ours were together."

"Oh, dear," Karen whispered.

"Michael looks dreadful, just dreadful. Mick was shocked... So was I. At first, he tried to pretend Michael wasn't there. I knew the medical procedure hadn't gone well, but I had no idea how badly he's doing. Later I glanced over and I could tell Mick was having a hard time seeing his father again, especially in this condition."

"How bad is he?" Liz asked, almost afraid of the answer.

"Bad. Really bad. He's down over fifty pounds now and...and his skin is this sickly yellow color." Clare pinched her lips together. "He's dying... He told me he was, but I don't think I actually believed it. I guess I couldn't bring myself to accept it."

"Now there's no denying it, is there?" Julia reached across the table and placed her hand on her friend's.

Liz placed her hand on top of Julia's and Karen set her own hand over all of theirs.

"I don't know how he endured the two-hour ceremony. He was so weak he could barely sit up."

"I wonder if Mick understood how ill his father is?"

Clare's eyes teared. "I think he knew more than I realized. Alex must have said something."

"It's so hard." Liz knew this from experience. Unlike her husband, her father had died a lingering death. "Even when you're prepared for a death, you're not really."

"Did they talk?" Karen asked.

"Not at first." Clare dug in her purse for a tissue. "It was as if they were invisible to each other. Then the graduates entered the auditorium and everyone stood as "Pomp and Circumstance" was played. Mick and I stood and...and Michael tried to."

"He fell?"

"No...Mick caught him and helped him back into his chair. The next thing I knew, they were both weeping and clinging to each other." Tears rolled down Clare's face. She half-sobbed, half-laughed as she said, "It was quite a display for the rest of the audience. Some of them were crying, too."

"Is Michael back in the hospital now?" Liz asked quietly.

Clare didn't answer immediately. "He's with us."

"With you?" Karen repeated.

"He can't go back to the rental house. At this point he's incapable of living on his own. So...he's living with the boys and me." She bit her lip hard, leaving tooth marks. "He's come home to die."

> "Time is a dressmaker specializing in alterations."
> —Faith Baldwin

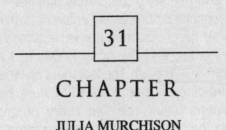

CHAPTER

JULIA MURCHISON

July 4th

List of Blessings
1. Sleeping in on a holiday.
2. America the Beautiful.
3. Fireworks.
4. Family barbecues, especially when Peter does the cooking.
5. Georgia, who helps me laugh at myself and at the curve life's thrown me.

I slept in late this morning, and while Peter and the kids are out picking up some last-minute supplies for the barbecue, I'm taking an hour for myself. After a long soak in the tub, I decided to write in my journal.

The last time I did that was a week ago. I can hardly believe seven days have passed. Usually I write every morning, but my body seems to require more sleep lately and when the alarm rings, I just can't drag myself out of bed. Peter feels that if I'm in need of extra sleep, I should take it. I do, but then the morning's one mad rush and my day's completely off-kilter.

This pregnancy is completely different from my previous two. At first I assumed it was because I'm fourteen years older, and my body knows it. I suspect there's more to it, though; the fact that I'm 40 explains some of the differences but not all of them. However, Dr. Fisk keeps telling me that every pregnancy is unique. Maybe this is just going to be a more difficult baby. That's certainly been the case so far!

At least my fears that there's something wrong with the baby have been calmed now that all the test results are in. I thank God we're going to have a healthy child. It was a real worry, although both Peter and I pretended not to be concerned, something we each did for the other's sake. I know how relieved I was with the good news and I could tell he was, too.

Today is going to be fun. Georgia and Maurice are coming over for a barbecue. The kids get a real kick out of my cousin, and she thinks they're fabulous. Georgia can be outrageous but these last few months I've been more grateful than ever for her friendship and emotional support.

Throughout this pregnancy, she's cried with me and laughed with me. When I was down in the dumps about being forty and wearing maternity clothes, she put on a smock and stuffed a pillow in her waistband just so I wouldn't feel foolish. You gotta love a cousin like that!

After the barbecue, we're all heading over to the pier to watch the fireworks. Adam and Zoe will probably meet up with their friends before then, and everyone will rendezvous back at the house at ten-thirty for banana splits, a family Fourth of July tradition.

Today, I refuse to worry. I refuse to give one minute's thought to the lack of day care arrangements for this unborn child. I refuse to feel upset about Adam and Zoe's selfishness. I will not, under any circumstances, weigh myself.

On the other hand, I will laugh and enjoy my family. I will eat whatever I want this afternoon and refuse to feel guilty for doing so. Also, I'm going to find an excuse to let others wait on me. I intend to sit with my feet up and enjoy the sunshine, appreciate my family and salute my country.

That's quite a manifesto for one day, but I plan to do everything within my power to make it happen.

* * *

"Don't *you* look comfortable." Georgia stood, hands on her hips in front of the lounge chair.

Shading her eyes, Julia glanced up. She smiled, revelling in the late-morning sunshine.

"I am in hog heaven." Julia rarely had an opportunity to indulge herself like this—to actually lie in the sun and do nothing. It was an interlude she cherished all the more for its brevity. Everything for the barbecue was in the refrigerator, including three different salads. For the first time in her married life, she was about to serve deli-made potato salad to her family.

Adam was sure to complain about that and he could go right ahead. If he wanted to peel potatoes for an hour, then more power to him!

"Where's Maurice?"

"He's smoking a cigar with Peter."

Julia swung her legs off the cushion. "Not in my house, they aren't."

"Hold up," Georgia said, giggling. "They're out front chatting with one of the neighbors."

"You should've said so earlier."

"And missed seeing you move so fast? That was an impressive feat."

"Especially in my condition." Julia rested her hands against her abdomen and admired Georgia's slim waist. Her cousin wore white slacks and a red, white and blue T-shirt with gold embroidered stars across the yoke. With her huge star-framed sunglasses and California beach tan, the effect was stunning.

"What do you mean, your condition? You've never looked better."

Julia rolled her eyes.

"None of that, either." Georgia wagged her finger at Julia. "It's true."

Every woman wants to believe she's beautiful while pregnant, Julia thought, but if ever there was a delusion, this was it. Her appearance was something Julia had avoided thinking about, along with day care, baby supplies...and just about everything else.

All her life, she'd been the organized one, the list-maker, the planner. This pregnancy had completely thrown her. She had two months to prepare everyone for the impact this baby would have on their lives. So far, all she'd done was buy a crib.

But she'd promised herself she wouldn't think about any of this today. Fortunately, Zoe provided a distraction.

"Mom, should I bring out the cheese dip?" she called from the house.

"Not yet," Julia called back.

"I'm hungry," Adam muttered, coming onto the patio and slumping into the chair next to Julia.

"So what else is new?" She twisted around. "All right, all right, you can bring out the goodies."

Adam rushed into the house to help his sister.

Georgia took the lounge chair he'd abandoned. "This is the life." She lay back with a long sigh and smiled into the sun.

"What's this?" Adam demanded, holding a plastic-coated nut-crusted cheese ball.

"What does it look like?"

"What happened to the one you always make?"

"I didn't make it this year."

"But—"

"Adam" Georgia inserted, "your mother's pregnant and she doesn't need to be standing on her feet all day cooking for the rest of us."

"Everything doesn't have to change because my mother was dumb enough to get pregnant," Adam exploded. "Nothing's the same anymore, and I hate it. She used to be a real person and now all she is...is pregnant." He pitched the cheese ball at the lawn and stormed back into the house.

"What got into him?" Georgia asked, frowning as she removed her sunglasses.

Julia shrugged. "He's sixteen, has his driver's license and doesn't have his own car the way most of his friends do."

"Now, just a minute here," Georgia drew herself to a sitting position. "Who said it was the parents' responsibility to provide their children with their own personal vehicles?" Her words echoed Peter's outburst of a few months ago. Correct though he was, his comments hadn't done a thing to change the kids' attitudes.

"It isn't that," Zoe said, walking onto the patio. "Adam's upset because he would've had a car if it wasn't for..." She angled her head toward Julia's abdomen.

"There was no guarantee of that," Julia argued. She'd heard all this countless times. "Can we talk about something else, please?"

"Like what?" Zoe asked.

"What about names for the baby?" Georgia suggested cheerfully. "Personally, I think babies should always be named after someone, like a favorite cousin," she said. "That would mean George or—"

"The baby's all anyone wants to talk about," Zoe cried. "It's the baby this and the baby that. If Mom's sick of Adam wanting his own car, then I can be sick of this baby." She raced back into the house and slammed the sliding glass door so hard it bounced and slid partway open again.

"My goodness, what's *with* those two?"

"The joys of sharing and family life," Julia said. But she wouldn't let either one of them ruin her stress-free, worry-free holiday. "I'm ignoring them both and suggest you do likewise."

Georgia didn't say anything for a moment. "Are you running a fever?" she finally asked. "Are you unwell?"

"Me? What makes you say that?"

Georgia hesitated. "Being able to ignore this stuff doesn't sound like you."

"Well, it is for today." Julia settled back in the lounger and closed her eyes. That was when she felt a sudden, inexplicable pain. She froze for a moment, then placed her hands on her stomach. It wasn't the onset of labor; that she would have recognized.

"Something's wrong." She choked out the words, holding her abdomen tightly, nearly blinded by pain.

"Julia, what is it?"

Julia heard her cousin but couldn't answer. Suddenly she felt liquid gush from between her legs. At first she assumed her water had broken, then she saw the blood and nearly fainted.

"Blood...oh my God, there's blood everywhere!" Georgia ran toward the house screaming, her voice filled with panic. "Call 911! Someone do something."

Peter was at her side almost immediately, his face pale. "Honey, it's all right. Help's on the way."

"What's happening?" Julia cried, clinging to his arms. "What's wrong?"

"I don't know... We need to get you to the hospital."

"It's the baby...the baby's in trouble." The panic was rising in Julia. She saw it reflected in the face of her cousin who stood next to her sobbing, hand over her mouth. Peter looked wild-eyed as he tried to comfort her. Zoe was off to one side, crying all by herself.

The next few minutes were a blur until Julia heard the sound of the emergency siren. The paramedics, directed by Adam, came through the gate into the backyard. Two young men lifted Julia from the lounger and placed her on a stretcher.

"Mom, Mom..." Zoe, weeping and nearly hysterical, grabbed her hand. "What's wrong? Tell me what's wrong."

"I don't know, honey, I don't know."

"Everything's going to be all right," Peter assured them both, but his words rang false.

The paramedics carried the stretcher toward the waiting ambulance. The blood continued to gush from between her legs. So much blood. Such intense pain and a fear so paralyzing Julia could barely think.

"I'll bring the children to the hospital."

Was that Georgia? Julia could no longer tell. Peter climbed into the ambulance with her. One of the paramedics wrapped a blood pressure cuff around her upper arm and shouted out a series of numbers to the driver. The siren blared.

"Everything will be fine in a few minutes," Peter told her, holding tightly on to her fingers.

She clutched his hand hard, but she could feel herself weakening. "Call Liz," she pleaded, certain she was about to pass out. As the hospital administrator, Liz could ensure that Peter and the children would be kept informed of her condition.

"Liz?"

"Kenyon," Julia whispered, fighting off unconsciousness. "Thursdays at eight."

"The breakfast group friend."

"Yes...yes." Her eyes remained closed. She felt light-headed, dizzy. Unreal. She had to make a determined effort to hold onto consciousness. Yet she felt almost euphoric and couldn't understand why.

The next time she opened her eyes, she realized she was at the hospital. There was a brilliant light suspended above her. Although it took a tremendous effort, she tried to lever herself up on one elbow to see who was in the room. An IV bottle hampered her progress. The nurse who stood beside her pressed a gentle hand to Julia's shoulder.

"Mrs. Murchison..."

"My husband, I want my husband."

"You'll see him soon, okay?"

Julia couldn't imagine where Peter would be. She needed him. She wanted him with her.

"What's happening to my baby?" she asked a moment later. It was difficult to think clearly with everyone about her moving in slow motion.

A sympathetic nurse clasped her hand. "We're doing everything we can to look after your health and that of your baby."

A man she couldn't see said something Julia didn't understand.

"Who are you?" she demanded. Julia hated it when people didn't identify themselves.

"Dr. Lowell. You're at Willow Grove Memorial Hospital. Your placenta has ripped away from the uterus. We've called in Dr. Fisk and as soon as she arrives we'll be taking the baby by Caesarian section."

"It's too early." She wasn't quite seven months pregnant.

"Don't you worry, we have one of the finest preemie doctors in the state."

"Dr. Jamison?" Julia asked, remembering what Liz had told her about Sean Jamison.

"Yes. He's already on his way."

Relief washed over her, and she relaxed. Liz had repeatedly lauded Sean Jamison's qualifications; she obviously held his medical skills in high regard. "Good."

"I'm going to give you something that'll make you feel sleepy now," the nurse told her.

"All right...but please tell my husband everything's going to be fine. Can you do that for me? He's very worried and I want him to know I'm okay."

"I'll tell him right away." The nurse patted her hand. "Everything *will* be fine."

"Thank you," she whispered, her voice thick and a bit slurred. Julia sincerely hoped the nurse knew what she was talking about.

> "The ultimate lesson all of us have to learn is un-
> conditional love, which includes not only others
> but ourselves as well."
>
> —Elizabeth Kubler-Ross

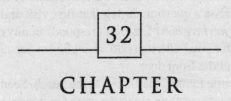

CHAPTER 32

LIZ KENYON

Sean had found a premium parking spot at the beach. Liz could hardly believe their good fortune. The sky was the purest shade of blue, and the sun, as always, shone bright along the California shoreline. A refreshing breeze blew off the water. A perfect fourth of July.

With his radio playing a Lovin' Spoonful ballad from the sixties, Sean eased his convertible into the empty parking slot. Liz could have driven around for hours and not located a single space within a mile of the beach.

"Hey, it's just clean livin'," Sean said with a chuckle when she said as much.

"Sure it is," she joked back, happier than she could remember being in a long while. They'd spent the morning at

Little Lambs. Sean had brought Clarissa a bouquet of red, white and blue carnations as a Fourth of July gift. They visited with each of the babies and Liz was delighted to see that little Faye showed some improvement. As they were about to leave, Clarissa had pulled her to one side.

"I see you have your answer," the other woman whispered.

Liz hadn't immediately made the connection. Then she recalled Clarissa's question during that first visit and understood. *Do you love him?* Liz didn't respond, merely nodded.

"Good for you," Clarissa said, chuckling to herself as she let them out the front door.

From Little Lambs, they drove to the beach. Sean waited until they were strolling along the crowded sidewalk before he broached the subject of her son's recent visit. "Are you going to tell me if I passed inspection or not?"

He tried to sound casual, but Liz knew he was concerned about the meeting with Brian.

"Feeling insecure, are you?"

"You haven't said a damn word," Sean muttered as they walked side by side, holding hands.

"That was intentional."

"Dammit, Liz, I was on my best behavior. I was as good as I can be. If your son found fault with me, then—"

"Brian thought you were fabulous," she interrupted. "He thinks you're the best thing since bottled water." Restraining her smile would have been impossible.

"He's a great kid."

"Of course you'd think so," she teased, "since he likes you."

"Yup." He grinned. "One thing's for sure, Brian's got terrific judgement."

"Would you stop?"

"Hey," Sean countered, "I'm just getting started. Naturally, once he's back, Brian will call Amy and tell her everything's copacetic. Then Amy will be reassured that you're seeing a real prince of a fellow, and all will be well."

Liz smiled at his enthusiasm. She didn't bother to add that neither of them needed a course set for this relationship. Not at this stage of their lives. For now Liz was content to have someone special to share the small everyday things. A companion, a friend, maybe—in time—a lover. Someone who loved and appreciated the woman she was. Someone who made her laugh. Someone who inspired her and encouraged her to take the occasional risk. Liz hoped for the opportunity to play that role in Sean's life as well.

"Will I meet your daughter one day?" she asked.

Liz saw the pleasure leave Sean's face. "Unfortunately that isn't likely," he said in a stiff voice.

"Why not?"

"First of all, Eileen lives in Seattle."

"She never visits?"

"No. Say, I could go for an ice cream bar. How about you?"

"Quit changing the subject. The only thing I want is more information about you."

Sean sat down on a nearby bench and leaned forward, bracing his elbows on his knees. "I don't want to talk about Eileen."

"I can see that, but why not?"

"If you must know," he snapped, "the subject of her mother invariably comes up and my ex-wife is off limits, even with you."

Liz sat on the bench beside him. She didn't remark that this wasn't always true; he'd mentioned Denise any number of times. But every mention was a glancing one, as though he couldn't bear to linger on her memory. "You must have loved her very much," Liz said quietly.

Sean turned away. "It's a beautiful day. Let's not spoil it with talk of a relationship that's been dead for years."

"Why don't you tell me what happened and get it over with?" she urged softly, her hand on his forearm.

"Happened?" he repeated. "Just what generally happens when a man's foolish enough to fall in love with a fickle woman. I don't mean to be rude, Liz, but I'm serious. I don't want to discuss Denise."

"Then we won't." She respected his wishes and wouldn't pressure him. She believed that eventually, as the trust between them grew, he'd tell her more. No point in forcing the issue.

Sean reached for her hand just as his beeper went off. Liz knew the sound all too well. Earlier he'd warned her that he was on call, and the beeper meant that her Fourth of July was about to be interrupted.

While he read the message on his pager, Liz's cell phone rang inside her purse. So few people had the number that she knew it must be important.

Liz felt around until she found her phone, and flipped it open on the third ring. "Hello."

"Is this Liz Kenyon?"

Peter Murchison introduced himself and explained the circumstances. "I'm leaving now," she told him, then snapped the phone closed and dumped it back in her purse.

Sean waited for her. "I've got to get to—"

"I know. The Murchison baby's mother is a good friend of mine. That was her husband. Julia asked if I'd come to the hospital."

"Let's go."

When they relinquished their parking space, there were a hundred vehicles all eager to claim the same spot. No sooner had Sean backed out than it was filled. Liz didn't spare even a thought for the leisurely day that had just disappeared.

As they headed toward the hospital, Liz reached for her cell phone again. She hit the "on" button and saw Sean giving her a puzzled look.

"Who are you calling?"

"The rest of the Thursday morning breakfast group."

"How likely is it that you'll reach them?"

"About a hundred percent," she assured him with total confidence.

"On a holiday?"

"Sean, I'll reach Karen and Clare because I won't give up until I do."

"Why? You aren't Julia's family."

"No, we're her *friends,* and this baby is important to us. We were there when she found out she was pregnant. We've watched her deal with family, friends, even her customers' reactions, and we're going to stand by her now."

"Must be a woman thing," he muttered. "If I needed emergency surgery, my golfing buddies wouldn't parade over to the hospital and sit there worrying about me."

"I would."

He turned to stare at her and nearly ran a red light.

"Sean!" she screamed as he entered the intersection.

Sean slammed on the brakes and Liz vaulted forward, the seat belt cutting into her shoulder. Her phone flew onto the dash.

"Dammit, Liz, you can't go saying things like that when I'm driving."

"Things like what?" He frowned at her and she couldn't imagine why.

"Never mind."

She shook her head and retrieved her phone to resume her calling.

By the time Liz and Sean arrived at the hospital, Julia had delivered a baby boy, weighing in at two pounds, ten ounces.

Sean went to assess Baby Murchison's situation while Liz made her way to the waiting area. The room was full of people who milled around, most of them pacing restlessly, talking in low, anxious voices. She recognized Julia's cousin Georgia from the journal-writing class and introduced herself to the others.

"I have a brother," Adam said beaming proudly as he repeatedly shook Liz's hand.

Was this really the same boy who'd given his parents nothing but grief from the moment he learned Julia was pregnant? Right now, he seemed pleased and excited. Liz hoped his enthusiasm lasted.

"Dad said we're going to name him Zachary Justin," Zoe said and impulsively hugged Liz. "Mom talks about you all the time," she whispered.

This was Zoe who did nothing but complain how embarrassed she was about the pregnancy?

"I think your mother's wonderful," Liz told her. "She's very proud of you and your brother."

Zoe's eyes filled with tears. "I think my mom's wonderful, too."

Clare arrived ten minutes after Liz, with Karen following a half hour later. The three of them stood in one corner, talking quietly while Peter, the kids, and Julia's family settled in another section of the room. Every now and again they'd exchange comments or questions.

At about four-thirty, Peter was summoned by a nurse, apparently for a conference with Sean. As he left, tension in the room increased perceptibly.

"Two pounds is terribly small," Clare murmured.

Liz didn't want to alarm the others, but the fact remained that poor Zachary faced a life-and-death struggle.

The room went quiet when Peter returned. "According to Dr. Jamison," he began, "Zachary's chances of survival are very good." He paused, then continued in a steady voice. "About ninety percent of infants born weighing less than three pounds survive."

"Ninety percent?" The odds sounded good to Liz, who felt a giddy sense of relief.

"Just a minute." Peter held up his hand and silenced the group. "Before we start celebrating, we need to recognize that there could still be problems."

Liz thought Peter Murchison looked as though he was close to collapsing from the strain.

"What else did the doctor say?" Adam pressed his father. It was the question they all wanted to ask.

"Dr. Jamison said there's no guarantee Zachary won't develop any number of other complications."

"Such as?" a woman asked fearfully. Liz knew her to be Julia's mother.

"Cerebral palsy."

Everyone grew quiet again.

"Apparently there's also a real fear that Zack could develop chronic respiratory problems."

"When will we know?"

"Not for some time." Peter's face was bleak.

"Oh, my." Georgia breathed hard and sat down. Her husband sat with her and reached for her hand.

"This is only the beginning," Peter said, as he slumped into a chair. "Of course, he might escape it all, but as of right now there's no way of telling."

"Will Zachary be transferred to Laurelhurst?" Liz asked. That was where Sean's babies were usually sent because the neonatal intensive care unit there offered the technology and expertise that would give little Zachary the best chance at life.

"Dr. Jamison is making the arrangements now," Peter said, tiredly rubbing the back of his neck.

"How's Julia?" Clare asked.

"Julia's resting... Naturally she's worried about Zachary." Clare nodded. "Is there anything I can do?"

"Yes," Georgia cried. "Pray."

"Zack might...die?" Adam asked, as though the information was just now beginning to sink in.

"Yes."

"I want to see him," Zoe pleaded. Her voice was shaky. "He's my baby brother."

"You can't now," Peter said as he wrapped his arms around his two older children. "I don't know yet what the policy is at Laurelhurst, but I'll do everything I can to make sure you get to see him."

Clare drove Liz to the children's hospital, where she waited for Sean until after dinnertime. When he stepped out of the neonatal center and found her, he seemed surprised.

"I thought you'd gone home."

"Hey, you can't get rid of me that easily."

Sean threw his arm around her shoulders. "I'm glad you waited."

"How's Zachary doing?"

He exhaled sharply. "About as well as can be expected. He's a little fighter—I'll give him that."

"That's good, isn't it?"

Sean nodded. "Yes, but statistically he's the wrong gender and the wrong race."

"I beg your pardon?" Liz knew premature girls fared better than boys, but she didn't know about race.

"We're not sure why, but black girls are the most likely survival candidates, followed by white girls and then black boys. White boys are at the bottom of that hierarchy."

"What are the chances he'll survive undamaged?" From what Peter had said earlier, the baby's odds of survival sounded good. It was everything else they needed to worry about. "Fifty-fifty?"

He shook his head.

"Less? More?" She wanted him to give her something to focus on, something to diminish her worry.

"I don't give estimates," Sean said. "Too often, I'm proved wrong."

> "The idea of strictly minding our own business is
> rubbish. Who could be so selfish?"
>
> —Myrtie Barker

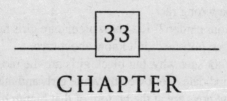

33

CHAPTER

KAREN CURTIS

August 1st

I spent the entire day on a shoot. This commercial has
the potential to get me a bit role on a sitcom, and I
should be thrilled. Normally I would be, but so much
is happening. I'm beginning to wonder if my head's
screwed on straight.

Glen's been on my mind a lot. I can't believe I'm falling
for a chemistry teacher. A brain, but he's so much fun and
so levelheaded and just all-around wonderful. Last week
he casually mentioned that the high school has an opening for a full-time drama teacher. That was all he said. He
didn't urge me to apply, didn't give me any of the details,
but he knew. He *had* to know.

The most fun I've had all year was the few days I filled in for the drama teacher. That includes *everything* else I've done, even the hair spray commercial that was shown nationally. Even the times Glen and I have gone out. I absolutely *loved* teaching that class.

I don't have the certification required for a full-time teaching position. Oh, there are ways around that, but I have to decide if this is something I really want to the exclusion of all else. I don't know. It was a point of pride with me, too. A teacher is what my mother always said I should be. I refuse to believe she knows me so well.

Last week, when Gwen called me to audition for a bit role in *Tom, Dick and Harriet,* a pilot for a situation comedy, I hesitated. Normally I would have leaped at the chance. I hemmed and hawed until my agent asked if I actually wanted this audition, because she had thirty other clients who'd die for the opportunity. I told her I wanted it, but I don't know if that's true anymore. I'm finally close to the goal I've been after for ten years—and I'm on the verge of saying no to it all. I wish to hell I could figure out what's wrong with me.

Perhaps it's all the worry about Victoria, who still isn't speaking to me. My sister's attitude has really got me down. I've tried to explain, but the minute she recognizes my voice, she hangs up the phone. I went to her house but she wouldn't answer the door. I sent her a letter, which she blatantly ignored. A week later I mailed her a schmaltzy card about the bond between sisters. I thought if anything would work on her, it would be that. Still, not a word. I wonder how long she intends to let this continue.

Fine! Whatever! If that's the way she wants to be, then it's her loss. I've done everything I can to repair our relationship.

Mom's having difficulties with her, too. My mother called me twice last week. Twice! Apparently, Victoria's embarrassed that Mom knows about Roger's explosive temper. It seems my sister had hoped we'd all blindly look the other way and pretend this is acceptable behavior. In your dreams, big sister—or maybe your worst nightmare.

It isn't just the falling-out with Victoria that's bothering me, or the job dilemma. The breakfast group is deeply involved with Julia and her baby. Little Zachary isn't responding as well as Dr. Jamison would like. It's tearing poor Julia apart. She's spending as much time as she can at the hospital. When she isn't with the baby, then Peter is. Julia's mother is retired now and thankfully, she's filling in at the shop. Georgia is there, too—she took vacation days to do this—and one of Julia's customers. An older woman whose name I don't remember.

Adam and Zoe finally came around. After months of claiming they wanted nothing to do with this baby, they're helping out at home and at Julia's shop, doing whatever they can. They've been incredibly helpful these last three weeks.

The situation is so intense. We all know it can go either way with Zachary. He might be all right; he might end up disabled. If he lives... Statistically, the odds for normal development aren't in his favor, and there's always that ten per cent who don't survive. Julia's in agony over it and blames herself, which makes no sense. We tell her repeatedly that she did everything she could, but she doesn't listen. She's going through this terrible guilt. If she'd eaten better, rested more, tried to do less... Everyone understands how she feels, although we know none of it is true.

Dr. Jamison has been wonderful. I remember when Liz first started seeing him and what a jerk we all thought he was. Our opinion of him has taken a one-hundred-and-eighty degree turn. He's been so kind to Julia and Peter, answering their questions, spending time with them. He hasn't minimized the dangers of Zachary's situation, and although it's painful, I know Julia wants the truth.

Last Thursday, we threw a baby shower for her. Clare gave Zachary Justin Murchison a silver baby spoon with his name engraved on it, plus three outfits. We all laughed because Zachary will probably be close to a year before he fits into them.

Liz knit him a cap and booties that look impossibly small and delicate, and she gave Julia a complete collection of Beatrix Potter stories. I found a store in L.A. close to the studio that sells clothes especially designed for preemies. My baby gift was the cutest little outfit that looks more like doll clothes. It was more than I could afford, but I don't care.

The baby shower lifted Julia's spirits. Mine, too, and everyone's. I never realized how strongly I'd feel about Julia's baby. My admiration for her grows all the time. In some ways, she's stronger than the rest of us put together. When she first discovered she was pregnant, I expected her to quietly terminate the pregnancy. I wanted to ask her why she didn't, especially when it became clear what an inconvenience the baby was going to be in all their lives. We would've understood and we certainly wouldn't have judged her. But she didn't do it.

Julia has taught me so much about inner strength and conviction. Even now, when the outcome with Zachary remains so uncertain, in my heart of hearts, I feel she did the right thing.

What with my own career, or lack thereof, my sister's problem and Julia's baby, I feel emotionally drained. This heat isn't helping, either. It's miserable, and just now that's the way my whole life feels.

* * *

Karen set aside her journal and took a sip from her glass of iced tea. She stretched out her legs as she tried to make herself comfortable on the patio chair—a cast-off she'd rescued from her parents' garage. At least this apartment had a balcony, tiny though it was. She sighed; her confusion seemed to be growing, until she felt as though she was walking in waist-deep mud. Every step forward was impeded.

Wiping away the sweat on her face, she got out of her chair, wincing as her bare thighs stuck to the vinyl cushion. She recalled summers as a child when she'd wait with her sister to hear the ice-cream truck come down the street. Then she'd race Victoria to see who could reach it first.

Her heart ached constantly over the estrangement between her and Victoria. In the past, weeks had often gone by, whole months during which they didn't speak, but that was different. It just meant they lived dissimilar lives, had dissimilar interests. It didn't mean they didn't care about each other. They were *sisters*.

"That does it," Karen muttered and without further thought, went inside to grab her wallet and car keys, then headed out. She made only one stop along the way.

Standing in front of her sister's door, she leaned on the doorbell.

Victoria appeared, looking frazzled and worn-out. She would've slammed the door shut if Karen hadn't put out her foot to prevent it.

"Remember when we were kids and we used to race to the ice-cream truck?" she asked.

"We're no longer children," Victoria muttered. Her hand was on the door, ready to close it.

"I usually won, didn't I?"

"Is there a point to this question?" Victoria feigned boredom.

Karen was tempted to remind her sister that *she* was the actress in the family. "Here," she said instead, and thrust out a chocolate-coated ice-cream bar with the wrapper peeled off. Unfortunately, in the late-afternoon heat, it'd already started to melt.

Victoria stared at it, as though she didn't know what to say.

"Go ahead, take it," Karen said.

"Do you seriously believe that offering me *ice cream* will wipe out what you did? You don't get it, do you?"

"No. Why don't you tell me?"

"No."

"I'm so sorry, Vicki. I never meant for any of this to upset you. I was only trying to help. I'm here now because I want us to talk this out."

The bar continued to melt and Karen caught the melting chocolate in the palm of her hand.

"Come inside and get rid of that before it leaves a mess on my porch," Victoria snapped. She opened the door wider so Karen could enter the house.

The foyer and living room were immaculate—even with a three-year-old underfoot all day. Karen's gaze fell on the coffee table and she was astonished to see that the magazines were not only in precise rows but stacked in alphabetical order.

"Throw that out." Victoria eyed the melting ice-cream bar and nodded toward the kitchen.

Karen discarded it in the sink and thought it was a real shame her sister hadn't eaten it. Victoria was thinner than she remembered. Too thin.

"Where's Bryce?" she asked. Normally her nephew would be leaping around her the minute she arrived.

"It's naptime."

Victoria didn't offer her anything to drink or suggest she sit down, so Karen stood with her back to the kitchen sink. A moment of stilted silence followed.

"How are you?" she asked. She searched Victoria's face and bare upper arms for bruises.

"None of your damn business."

Karen swallowed an angry retort, reminding herself that she hadn't come here to argue. "How's Bryce?"

Victoria shrugged.

"How many times can I say I'm sorry?"

"I thought I could trust you... I thought, I hoped, you'd be the one person in the world I could talk to."

"And then I blew it. Is that what you're saying?"

"How could you tell Mom? She's the last person I expected you to go to." Victoria's sense of betrayal seemed to overwhelm her; fears gathered in her eyes. "Do you hate me so much?" she cried.

"No, of course I don't hate you—"

Victoria didn't allow her to finish. "Now Mom's full of questions and Dad talked to Roger, and everything's a thousand times worse, all thanks to you."

"You don't actually think I could hate you?" Karen asked, close to tears herself. "You're my sister. The thought of anyone abusing you is more than I can bear."

"Sure, it is," Victoria taunted. "As I remember, you did your fair share of hitting me, too."

"We were just kids!"

Victoria turned her back. "Go away."

"No, I can't. I won't leave. Not until we've settled this."

Victoria shook her head. "Nothing you can say is going to make things right."

"You let your husband hit you."

Victoria whirled around so she was facing her once again. "He didn't mean it," she said heatedly.

Karen wanted to scream with frustration. How could her sister defend Roger? "Are you telling me it was an accident?"

Victoria refused to answer.

"You're furious with me because I said something to our mother. That was an accident, too, but you won't even give me a chance to explain."

"Roger loves me."

"I love you, too," Karen said. "You're my sister."

It looked for a moment as though Victoria was prepared to listen. Karen could actually see the indecision in her face—until they heard the sound of a car door slamming.

"Roger," Victoria whispered, and her eyes widened with panic.

A minute later, the door off the garage opened and Roger stepped into the kitchen. He hesitated when he saw Karen, and his lip curled with contempt.

"I didn't invite her," Victoria explained hurriedly.

"If you know what's good for you, you'll get out of my house," he threatened.

"Nice to see you, too," Karen muttered.

Roger set his briefcase on the kitchen table and Karen watched as the blood drained from Victoria's face.

"I want to talk to my sister," Karen insisted.

"She doesn't want to talk to you."

"Victoria can speak for herself, thank you," Karen said curtly, hands clenched at her sides. She wanted to hurt him the same way he'd hurt her sister.

"Fine, you tell her," Roger ordered his wife.

"It would be best if you left now," Victoria said, her voice low and pleading. "Please, just go."

Karen wanted to leave, but she was afraid of what would happen to Victoria if she did. She couldn't understand why her sister let Roger control her like this, why she let him belittle and abuse her.

"Shall I phone the police?" Roger asked no one in particular. He opened the refrigerator and took out a beer.

"Maybe you should," Karen said as calmly as her frantically beating heart would allow. "I'm sure they'd be interested in talking to me."

Roger slammed the beer down on the counter; at the violence of his action, Victoria cringed and leaped away. "Get the hell out of my house," he shouted.

"I'll go, but Victoria and Bryce are coming with me."

"No way."

"Victoria?" Karen stared at her sister, silently begging her to walk out the door and not look back.

Her sister wavered, and for a few seconds it seemed that she just might do it.

Hope surged within Karen and she smiled in encouragement.

"Fine, go," Roger stated calmly, as though bored by the whole scene. "But Bryce stays with me."

Any chance of her sister leaving was destroyed by those few words.

"I'll stay," she whispered.

Roger's smile stretched from ear to ear. "That's what I thought."

> "Courage is the price that life exacts for granting peace."
>
> —Amelia Earhart

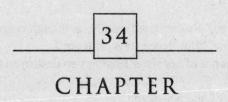

CHAPTER 34

CLARE CRAIG

When Leslie Carter unexpectedly walked into the Chevy dealership on a Friday evening early in August, Clare did a double-take. As general manager she had to oversee the sales staff and approve each deal. She was chatting on the phone with the head of the service department when she saw Leslie.

He had a luxurious tan from long days of sailing in the sun. He wore shorts and boat shoes and was so handsome it was difficult to take her eyes off him.

She watched as he approached the receptionist, who turned to shoot a glance in her direction. Clare swiftly ended the phone conversation, stepped away from her desk behind the glass wall and hurried into the showroom.

"Leslie, hi," she said, extending her hand. She felt a strong and immediate urge to hug him, but suppressed it, since this was only the second time she'd seen him. They'd talked occasionally over the intervening months and there'd been a couple of postcards, even some e-mail messages, especially after Zachary's birth. But she'd forgotten what he looked like. Absurd as it seemed, she'd forgotten he was this attractive, this downright good-looking.

Leslie stared at her extended hand, as though he was having the same thought—that this was too formal a greeting for someone who'd become a friend. He smiled warmly before clasping it between his own two hands.

"When did you get back?" she asked.

He peered at his watch. "About three hours ago."

He'd come almost directly to find her. His answer flustered and thrilled her.

"I thought I'd take you to dinner, if you're free."

"Let me find out." She already knew there was nothing scheduled for that evening, but glancing over her appointment calendar would give her a few minutes to gather her wits. With Michael living at the house now, she wasn't exactly free. But she didn't want to launch into a long explanation about her ex-husband or why he was living with her.

"Janet, would you get Mr. Carter a cup of coffee?" she asked as she disappeared into her glass office.

She made a pretense of looking in her book, then dialed the house. She couldn't very well announce that she had to check with her children before she agreed to a dinner date.

Alex answered on the second ring, his voice hushed.

"How's Dad?" she asked.

"He's sleeping."

"I'm going to be late, is that all right?"

Alex was silent. "How late?" he finally asked.

The boys took turns staying with Michael. He didn't want or need constant attention, but at this stage of his disease, no one was comfortable leaving him at the house alone. He was usually in a drugged state, and growing weaker day by day. Mick and Alex were with him during the days, and she often relieved them in the evenings.

"I'll be home before eight," Clare said. She and Alex reviewed the medication schedule for Michael, then she hung up.

Leslie was waiting for her. He stood when she returned to the showroom.

"When would you like to leave?" she asked.

"Is now too soon?"

"Now would be perfect."

Clare knew Leslie's arrival had stirred a lot of interest among the staff, but it didn't bother her. Her long hours had brought the dealership back to prosperity within a few months. With the staff's cooperation, she'd averted chaos and financial disaster. Her ideas had been welcomed and put into action, and all the employees had rallied around her. With some inventive, humorous television advertising, the dealership was reaching record sales.

True, the hours she'd put in were grueling. The reasons behind her renewed ambition, her drive, weren't entirely clear, even to her. Yes, the dealership was Mick and Alex's heritage, but there was more to it than that. Clare had something to prove to herself, and to Michael.

Living with her ex-husband wasn't easy; despite that, she felt the decision had been right. For Michael, for her and for their sons.

Clare didn't spend a lot of time alone with Michael. Because of her hours at work, she often didn't arrive home until he was asleep. But he remained in her thoughts—and in her heart. It had come as a revelation to discover she still loved him. Not the same way she had when they were married, of course. Now she loved him because of what they'd had, what they'd once been to each other. She loved him as the man who'd fathered her children.

"What's your favorite kind of food?" Leslie asked as he escorted her outside.

"Italian," she said automatically.

"Mine, too. Ever been to Mama Lena's?"

Clare nearly tripped over her own feet. "Yes." It had been Michael's and her favorite restaurant.

Some emotion must have been evident in her response because Leslie immediately said, "Someplace else?"

"Please," she whispered, not eager to explain.

"Luckily there's any number of good Italian restaurants close at hand. You choose."

Clare did, and before long they were sitting across from each other in an elegantly spare room, dipping warm bread into a small dish of flavored olive oil.

"I didn't know you were planning to get back this soon," Clare said, taking a leisurely sip from her glass of Chianti.

"I wasn't."

"Have you had a chance to check in with Julia and Peter yet?" she asked.

"I talked briefly to Peter earlier this afternoon," Leslie told her. "He was on his way to the hospital to relieve Julia, so we didn't get much of a chance to chat. He sounded pretty stressed so I didn't keep him long."

"I know." Liz gave her an almost daily update on the baby's progress.

"How is Zachary?"

Clare shook her head, unsure how to respond. "This is such an incredible baby. He wants to live so much. Julia and Peter are with him practically every minute. I talked to Julia the other day about his progress, and it's as though she's speaking in a foreign language. All these medical terms and procedures..."

"Little Zack's going to make it, isn't he?"

"We hope so. I gather that most of Zachary's problems have to do with his lungs. He isn't even supposed to be breathing air this soon, and it causes serious complications."

"Poor little boy."

"You can't imagine how small he is," Clare told Leslie. "Julia showed us a photograph at our baby shower, and he's barely as big as Peter's hand."

"Can they hold him?"

"They have." Clare wasn't sure how often. "Julia showed us another picture of Peter in a rocker with Zachary against his bare chest." Then feeling she should explain why Peter had removed his shirt, she added, "The baby needs Peter's body heat in order to keep warm. He can't regulate his own body temperature yet."

Leslie nodded.

"I pray every day that he survives." It was a prayer every member of the breakfast club shared.

From the subject of Zachary, they turned to talk of Leslie's adventure, sailing from California to Hawaii, and then the return flight home. The sailboat was berthed at Kauai while Leslie took a break from sea life. His crew of three had dispersed, two of them planning to stay in Hawaii, the other heading up to Alaska. He'd fulfilled his dream, achieved his goal and now had some decisions to make.

The meal was delicious; Clare had ordered a Caesar salad and her favorite eggplant dish. They lingered over a second glass of wine and then espresso. When they finished, Leslie drove her back to the dealership.

Precisely at eight, Clare arrived home, just as she'd promised. After dropping her purse on the kitchen counter, she ventured into the den, where they'd set up Michael's hospital bed.

"I'm back," she announced.

Mick sat at his father's bedside, the two of them watching television. Every time Clare saw Michael, she felt a sense of shock. He'd lost so much weight that he barely resembled the man she'd known. His skin held a yellowish tinge and his face was gaunt and drawn. The ravages of the cancer seemed more apparent every day.

"Who'd you go out to dinner with?" Mick asked. "Alex didn't say."

"A friend."

"Male or female?" Michael asked, turning his attention on her.

She hesitated, then decided there was no reason not to tell the truth. "Male."

Michael's eyes narrowed. "Anyone I know?"

She shook her head.

"I might," he insisted. "You can't say that until I have a name."

"Leslie Carter," she told him reluctantly. "He's Julia Murchison's uncle."

Michael frowned, and she could tell he was displeased. "Did you have a good time?" he asked.

"Yes." She wasn't going to lie, but she didn't intend to rub his face in it, either. This wasn't a revenge tactic. Her dinner with Leslie had been a pleasant outing and she refused to feel guilty about it.

Mick made a show of checking his watch. "I'm meeting a few friends later. Is it okay if I leave now?"

"Of course," Michael whispered. He closed his eyes, resting his head against the pillows.

When Mick left, Clare remained standing in the doorway. "Would you like a cup of tea?" she asked.

Michael nodded. "Please."

She made them each a cup and carried his into the room. Michael was out of bed, wearing his bathrobe and sitting in the nearby recliner. He rarely had much energy to move around anymore, especially toward nightfall.

"Can you stay for a few minutes?" he asked as she was about to leave.

Clare sat on the end of the bed. For a few moments, they both gazed at the television screen, as if a rerun of *Law and Order* was of utmost importance.

"I didn't know you were dating," Michael said in a casual tone.

Clare wasn't fooled. She opened her mouth to explain that Leslie was only a friend and that technically this was their first date, then changed her mind. She didn't owe Michael an explanation, nor did she feel at ease discussing this subject with him.

"When did you meet him?" he asked, again making his interest sound casual.

"Why?"

Michael still stared at the television. "No reason." He sipped his tea, then asked, "Do you intend to see him again?"

"Probably. Listen, Michael, I'm not comfortable talking about my social life with you."

"Sure," he said with an offhand shrug. "It's none of my business, right?"

"Right."

There was a pause during which they both watched the show. Then he murmured, "You might have waited."

"Waited," she cried, suddenly angry. "For what?" They'd been divorced for nearly two years, separated for three. He certainly hadn't waited to move in with Miranda.

He glared at her then. "I'm dying, Clare," he said in a low voice.

"Yes, I know. And I wish with all my heart that none of this—none of it—had happened. But you aren't my husband. *You* were the one who didn't want to be married to *me*, remember? Just because you live in my home now—"

"A house I bought and paid for," he shouted with more energy than she'd seen in weeks.

"Like hell," she tossed back. "I worked just as hard for this house as you did."

Michael clamped his mouth shut. "You can screw everything in pants for all I care, but I'd appreciate it if you'd—" He stopped abruptly and pressed his hand over his heart. His breathing came in deep, irregular gasps.

"Michael! Michael!"

He shook his head. His tea had fallen from the end table and spilled onto the carpet.

"Should I call for help?" Clare had already moved into the hallway, toward the phone. She didn't know what else to do.

"I'm all right... Just go."

Clare stood there in the doorway, irresolute. She couldn't tell if this attack was the result of their argument or a consequence of the disease. She started to leave, since that was what he seemed to want.

"No." He held out his hand to stop her.

She came slowly back into the room.

"I'm sorry—you're right," he said hoarsely. "Who you date is none of my damn business."

She nodded and turned away before he could see the tears in her eyes.

"It is best to learn as we go, not go as we have learned."

—Leslie Jeanne Sahler

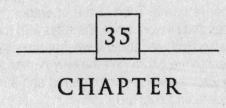

CHAPTER

JULIA MURCHISON

August 24th

The last time I wrote in my journal was the morning of Zachary's birth. It's hard to believe that was nearly two months ago. From the moment he was born, everything in our lives has been centered on him.

I'll be heading out to the hospital soon, since I try to get there by eight every morning. I'm writing this at the kitchen table, with a cup of tea at hand. (Yes, real tea once again!)

I used to worry about the shop. I'd get into a state if I had to close an hour early, certain I was losing a sale. In the last two months, I've barely given my fledgling business a thought.

Thankfully, my mother, Georgia and—to my ever-lasting surprise—Irene Waldmann are taking turns filling in for me. I realize this isn't a permanent solution, but all three claim they're enjoying themselves. It's one less thing to worry about. Mom's fully retired now and she loves to knit as much as I do. She came to me recently and suggested she continue working half-days after Zachary's home. Then in the afternoon, we can trade places and I'll work while she stays with the baby. I haven't talked to Peter about it yet, but the suggestion sounds ideal to me. Mom isn't the only person wanting to care for Zack—my sister volunteered and amazingly enough, Adam and Zoe, too.

My one concern is that Mom not feel any obligation, but she insists this is something she wants to do. She's alone and after working all these years, she'd miss the routine and the companionship, or so she says. When I asked her about traveling and doing the things she's always talked about, she said she still wants to do them, but for now it's more important to be a grandmother. When Adam and Zoe and Janice's children were born, she was too busy with her job to really enjoy them as much as she would've liked. Zachary's giving her a second chance and she's not about to lose it.

I can only say I'm grateful.

Adam and Zoe have been wonderful, and I'm grateful for that, too. Neither Peter nor I have given them much attention lately, and I realize our being at the hospital most of the time is hard on them.

Adam has shown a level of maturity I hadn't seen in him before. Maturity and a willingness to help in any way he can. Luckily, since he has his driver's license, he can take Zoe to her tennis lessons and run other necessary errands. He's chauffeured me to the hospital every afternoon, and we've had more time to talk one-on-one than we have in years. He's shared his goals with me and his plans for the future. I'm thrilled that he wants to go into teaching, like his father. He's a natural with kids, the same as Peter, and would be an asset to any classroom.

Zoe's been a great help all summer, too. She's taken it upon herself to cook dinners and take care of the laundry. I haven't had the time or inclination for housework; when I get home from the hospital, it's late, and I'm exhausted and emotionally drained. Without my having to ask her, Zoe took over. Dinner is waiting for me, and the house is clean. I still can't believe the way my children have pitched in—after all those months of complaining.

Peter, my wonderful, wonderful husband. I've never loved him more than I have in the last two months. Whenever I get discouraged about Zachary's condition, he finds a way to raise my spirits. He refuses to allow me to give up, or worry about the expense. I don't have any idea what the hospital and doctor bills will be or how much will be covered by our insurance. It's frightening to think about. Frankly, I don't care if we end up going bankrupt. I want my son to live and to grow up a normal and happy child.

Looking at him now, seeing the tubes and needles coming out of his tiny, emaciated body, my heart is so full of love it actually hurts.

When I see him struggle to draw each breath, it's hard

to remember how much I didn't want this baby. Now all my energy is focused on willing him to improve. He's not out of danger yet, but he's taken a turn for the better. If everything continues the way it is now, we might be able to bring him home close to his original due date in the first week of September.

I know why Liz fell in love with Dr. Jamison. His attitude toward women might be thirty years behind the times (although I suspect much of that's for show). But when it comes to dealing with preemies and their parents, he's a saint. What I like most about him is how deeply he cares. I've never had a physician as tender as he is, or as patient.

He and Liz are well-matched—in their intelligence, their sense of humor, their compassion. I know Liz delayed her vacation because of what's happening with me, although she denies it.

I've missed meeting the group for breakfast, but I didn't need to show up on Thursdays at eight to feel their support. At my lowest point, when I was sure we were going to lose Zachary, they threw a baby shower for me. I'm not likely to forget everything they've done. Their faith and love comforted me during my darkest hours.

Irene Waldmann came by the hospital one afternoon last week with the baby blanket she'd knit for Zachary. Peter was with him at the time so the two of us sat in the waiting area. Her gift meant a great deal to me—the blanket and helping out at the shop and all her concern for Zack and me. There was a time I thought of her as difficult. She's a bit prickly, but I should have seen past that. She mentioned the son she lost and tried not to let me see the tears in her eyes, but I did.

Peter and I decided to ask Irene to be Zachary's godmother. When I mentioned it to her, she grew extremely flustered and immediately left. But she visited again the next day.... Although she didn't come right out and say it, I think she's thrilled. Me, too.

Soon Peter and I will be making plans to bring Zachary home. I feel more confident than ever that our son will, indeed, be coming home.

* * *

Adam was waiting outside the hospital when Julia left at three-thirty that day. They ran into terrible traffic on the commute home, but she didn't mind; it gave them extra time to talk.

He dropped her off at the house and then went on to his part-time job at the neighborhood grocery, where he worked in customer service. When he got off at nine o'clock, he had instructions to come directly home for a celebration.

That afternoon, Zachary had weighed in at a whopping four pounds, and he was scheduled to be released within the week. Each and every one of those precious ounces had been reason enough to throw a party.

"Hi, Mom!" Zoe called out when Julia entered the house. "How's Zachary?"

"Fabulous." She hugged her daughter, then headed for her bedroom to change clothes. To her surprise, Zoe followed her and sat on the end of the bed while Julia shed her dress. She donned a pair of shorts and a tank top.

"I made spaghetti for dinner. I hope that's all right."

Zoe had developed her own sauce recipe that had quickly become a family favorite. "It's perfect."

"I added a can of sliced olives this time."

Julia had to think about that, then nodded. "Sounds good."

"I like cooking." Zoe drew up her legs and folded them beneath her.

Julia sat down next to her daughter. "Something on your mind?" It wasn't like Zoe to follow her around.

"I—I wanted to talk to you and Dad about Zachary, but it's been hard because either Dad was at the hospital or you were."

"I know." Julia hadn't seen as much of her daughter as she had Adam.

"I've...I've had these feelings and Aunt Janice said I should talk to you about them."

Julia took a deep breath, a little anxious about Zoe's concern and unable to guess what it might be.

"All right, let's talk."

Zoe was very quiet for a moment. "I'd better check on the sauce," she said abruptly. She hopped off the bed and dashed into the kitchen.

Although Julia was curious, she decided not to question her daughter. This had to come from Zoe voluntarily. She trailed after her into the kitchen.

Without being asked, Zoe poured her a glass of iced tea and set it out, with two cookies on a napkin—just as if she were serving her mother an after-school snack—which made Julia smile. Then, wooden spoon in hand, she lifted the lid to the simmering sauce and stirred.

"Do you remember when you told Adam and me you were pregnant?" Zoe asked conversationally.

Julia wasn't likely to forget. "I remember."

"I was really mad at you." She continued stirring the sauce, her back to Julia.

"You felt a baby would be an embarrassment to you in front of your friends." Julia spoke in a matter-of-fact voice, merely recounting Zoe's reaction, not judging it.

"I want you to know I don't think of Zachary as an embarrassment anymore," Zoe said in a rush. "I'm glad you had him. I'm proud of my little brother." She sniffled and rubbed her nose. "Mom, I'm sorry for all the things I said."

Julia left the table and Zoe turned, threw her arms around Julia's waist, and hid her face against her mother's shoulder.

"I was so afraid he wasn't going to live."

"That decision was in God's hands. It still is."

"I know..."

"There's something I have to tell you," Julia said, brushing the hair from her daughter's forehead. "When I first learned I was pregnant, I wasn't happy about it, either. I kept thinking of all the things our family would have to give up because of another baby."

"That's all I thought about, too," Zoe admitted, her eyes bright with tears. "I didn't once stop to think what Zachary would add to our family."

Julia was amazed at her daughter's insight. Zoe was right; Zachary had brought them all together again. As Adam and Zoe grew older, their family life had splintered, each member going in his or her own direction. They'd stopped functioning as a cohesive unit.

It was a process that had begun innocently enough as the children grew into their teens, and had escalated when Julia started her own business, since the focus of her energy and attention had gone into that. Even the things they'd once enjoyed as a family, like hiking and camping, had fallen by the wayside.

The kids had their own interests, which was completely natural. Equally natural, Peter and Julia appreciated having some time to themselves and the opportunity to see their friends. In the last couple of years, though, there'd been very few family occasions. She'd insisted on family dinners as much as possible, but too often they were rushed and per-functory, a source of tension more than pleasure.

Until now. Zachary had changed all that.

"Adam and I talked it over, and we both want to share our rooms with Zachary." She looked quickly at her mother. "Once he's old enough to sleep in his own crib, I mean."

Julia nodded. "He'll be in the bassinet in our room for a few months still."

"Adam thought Zachary should sleep in his room because he's a boy, but I convinced him it was only fair that he spend time with me, too."

Julia smiled despite the tears gathering in her eyes.

"Don't you agree?" Zoe leaned back to look at Julia.

"Of course I do," she said seriously. "Of course I do."

"Adam said once he leaves for college, Zachary can have his room full-time."

"That's considerate of you both."

"I'll watch him, too, Mom. After school and whenever you need me to. I know I said I wouldn't, but that was before he was born and I realized I was going to love him. He's my lit-tle brother, you know."

Julia hugged her close.

"And he's very special. No one thought he'd even live, did they? And...and now he's all right, isn't he? That's what Dad said." She gazed expectantly at her mother.

"Yes," Julia whispered. "Yes, he's fine. We've been very, very lucky."

"It's because he's a miracle baby," Zoe told her solemnly. "Our very own miracle baby."

"Vitality! That's the pursuit of life, isn't it?"
—Katharine Hepburn

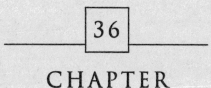

CHAPTER

LIZ KENYON

Liz had never purchased a vehicle of her own. Her car had been new six years ago; after Steve's death, she'd replaced the car destroyed in the accident with one identical to her husband's. She'd given her own car to Brian and driven the new one—for six years now. It had never occurred to her to purchase anything else. Never dawned on her that she might have distinct tastes and preferences.

Now she wanted a car of her own choice. She had the extras, the options and the color selected, but had yet to decide on make and model. The one person she could trust to guide her was Clare, who knew more about automobiles than Liz ever cared to learn.

They met at the dealership one hot August morning; Liz had stopped by on her way to work. Clare walked around the lot with her, pointing out the advantages of one style over another.

"So you're still determined to drive out to Oklahoma by yourself?" Clare said once she'd finished the tour.

Liz glanced away so Clare couldn't see her smile. She was astonished that a woman who managed an entire dealership, cared for her dying ex-husband, maintained a home and looked after two children, would ask such a question. "You seem skeptical. I *can* make the trip on my own, you know."

"You can do anything you put your mind to," Clare said, doing a quick about-face.

"Then why the concern?" They paused in front of a used two-year-old Seville in the very pearl-white color Liz preferred.

Clare shrugged off the question. "I was wondering if it's safe for you to be traveling alone, that's all."

"Why not? I'm not going to take any unnecessary risks. I have three weeks' vacation, so I've got the time for an extended trip. Besides, I happen to enjoy driving on the open road."

"What does your daughter think?"

"Same as you. She's afraid it's not safe. I haven't even pulled out of the driveway yet and already she's worrying."

"Well, maybe you should listen and just book a flight," Clare suggested.

"I could," Liz said as she strolled between the vehicles. She paused and looked back at the Seville. The sleek lines of the vehicle and the color were perfect, and the car had all the options she wanted; not only that, it was still under warranty. Liz sighed. She was definitely considering the Seville, but everything would be easier if she didn't have so many cars to choose from. The choices confused her, and every time she saw one she liked, it was more money than she wanted to spend or, if used, had too many miles to suit her.

"But you won't fly, will you?"

"Probably not," Liz agreed, walking back to the Cadillac Seville and looking inside the driver window.

"What does Sean have to say?"

So Clare was pulling her trump card, and far sooner than Liz had anticipated. "What does he say?" she repeated. "Actually, he hasn't said a thing."

Clare's gaze narrowed. "You haven't told him, have you?"

"Is there any reason I should?" Liz knew she sounded defensive, but she couldn't help it. To think Clare would suggest she submit her vacation plans to a man, any man, for approval! It was laughable.

"He isn't going to like it," Clare said, crossing her arms and exhaling slowly. "And you know it."

"Then he can take a number and stand in line like everyone else." She opened the Seville's door and slipped behind the wheel. Although the vehicle was two years old, it smelled of new leather. Liz adjusted the seat and placed her hands on the steering wheel.

"This is a beautiful car," she murmured. "And it's comfortable." She took a deep breath, relieved to have made a decision. "I'll take it."

Clare stared at her as though she hadn't heard. "Don't you want to test-drive it?"

"Not particularly."

"Liz, I can't let you pay sticker price. You're supposed to haggle with me."

"Why would I haggle?" Liz asked. "You're one of my best friends. If I can't trust you to be fair with me, then who can I trust? You're giving me a good trade-in value and this is a great price." She got out of the car. "Let me know what the total comes to and I'll write you a check." She headed toward her old car, which she'd left parked in front of the dealership.

"Where are you going?" Clare called after her.

"To work. I'm already late. Phone me when you've got the paperwork ready."

Clare hurried after her. "Think about what I said."

"Which part?"

"Just tell Sean, would you?"

Liz frowned. Naturally she'd tell Sean, but not until she was good and ready.

The office was buzzing with activity by the time Liz arrived. She breezed past Cherie, who was on the phone. Her secretary stuck out her arm with the day's mail. Liz took it from her without missing a stride.

When she entered her office, she was surprised to find Sean sitting behind her desk, his long legs outstretched, hands locked behind his head.

"About time you got here," he said, granting her one of his sexiest smiles.

"Is it, now? Have I kept you waiting long?"

"Yes, about six months, but we won't go into that."

Liz rolled her eyes; any reaction would only encourage him.

"I take it you have a reason for being here?" she asked, sorting through the mail as she stood beside her desk.

Cherie came into the room with a cup of coffee, which she handed to Liz. "Would you like a cup, as well, Dr. Jamison?" she asked hesitantly.

"Dr. Jamison is on his way out," Liz informed her secretary.

"Actually I'd love a cup," he murmured, but Cherie had already left.

Liz walked around to her chair. "Sean, I've got a million things to do and I can't do a one of them with you here."

"Hey, don't worry about my ego or anything," he muttered.

"You have a perfectly healthy ego."

"Aren't you going to ask me what I want?"

"Not on your life." Open-ended questions were his forte, and she'd learned the hard way to avoid them.

"A little birdie told me you're planning to drive to Oklahoma on your own."

"Clare?" The traitor! She'd never have believed her friend would go behind her back.

"Clare knows?"

"Who told you?" Liz demanded, in no mood for games.

"Your daughter phoned me."

"Amy?" Liz sputtered. "How *could* she?"

"And that isn't the only secret she revealed."

Liz could well imagine. "I apologize. Trust me, it won't happen again." She led him to the door and held it open for him. "Sean, please, I'm busy."

"Places to go and people to meet?" he said pointedly.

"Yes," she replied with equal emphasis. "Now get out of here."

"We're not through with this discussion."

They were as far as Liz was concerned. She playfully shoved him out the door and closed it. No sooner had she done so than the door opened again and Sean stuck his head inside.

He gave her a hangdog look and she laughed and leaned forward so they could kiss. And what a kiss it was. When they finished, Liz's knees were shaking and her head spinning.

"Dinner tonight?" he asked. "O'Shaunessey's?"

Liz needed a moment before responding. "Six o'clock?"

He nodded and was gone.

Smiling softly to herself, Liz tore into her day.

At five-forty-five, just as she was about to leave the office, Sean returned.

"I thought I was meeting you at O'Shaunessey's?" she said.

"You still can if you want," he told her, stepping toward her desk, "but I have something I want to discuss with you first."

"Fire away." She gestured toward the chair.

He remained standing. "I've been thinking about our conversation this morning."

Liz wrinkled her brow; she couldn't recall that anything of importance had been said.

"About you driving to Oklahoma by yourself," he quickly filled in.

Everyone was taking her to task about this, and she didn't like it. Before he could elaborate, she held up one hand. "Sean, don't even start."

"Too late. Liz," he said sternly, "it isn't going to happen. You aren't going alone."

Liz frowned at him.

"I'm coming with you."

Coming with her? "I beg your pardon? I don't remember inviting you."

"You don't have to. I've invited myself."

This took the notorious Jamison arrogance to a whole new level. "Sean!"

"Amy and I talked it over," he said, "and this seemed like the best solution. I haven't had a real vacation in ten years. If you want to drive, that's fine by me."

"You and *Amy* discussed this?"

He nodded, looking exceedingly pleased with himself. "I like her. She's a lot like her mother—smart, witty, beautiful."

"You've never met my daughter. How do you know what she looks like?"

"She sounds beautiful. Besides, how can she not be? She's your daughter."

All these months they'd been seeing each other and not once had Sean said she was beautiful. The compliment, although backhanded, robbed her of any witty reply.

"You know what else Amy suggested?" Apparently more relaxed now, he threw himself down in the chair. "She said she wished you'd marry me."

"She didn't!" If ever there was a blatant lie, this was it. Amy would *never* suggest such a thing.

"She did so," he said.

Liz stared at him, hardly knowing how to react. Then it dawned on her that he just might be serious. They'd never discussed making their relationship permanent. "Is this a proposal, Sean?"

The laughter faded from his eyes; her question appeared to catch him off-guard. He gazed at her a full minute, then muttered, "I don't know."

Neither did Liz.

"I hope you decide to let me take this trip with you," he said, standing now and heading toward the door. He seemed in a rush all of a sudden, as though he regretted introducing the subject of marriage.

Liz reached for her purse, locked up and followed him

out. "The truth is, I didn't really want to go alone, but there wasn't anyone I could ask to join me."

"I'm volunteering," he said, taking her hand and placing it in the crook of his elbow.

"Then I'd very much enjoy the pleasure of your company."

He looked as if he were about to kiss her, then hesitated. "How would you feel about a small side trip?"

"Side trip?" she repeated. "Sure. Where do you want to go?"

"Seattle."

"Seattle?"

Sean slapped the side of his head. "This room has developed an echo."

Laughing, she lightly punched his upper arm. "I'd love to visit Seattle. I hear it's beautiful."

"I think it's time you met my daughter." He shook his head. "Actually I think it's time I met her, as well. It's been nearly eight years since I saw her. A lot has changed."

Which meant he had yet to see his granddaughter. Liz could tell this trip was going to be one grand adventure.

They started slowly down the corridor. Everyone else who worked in the administrative offices had already left. "Did you mean what you said about me being beautiful?" she asked shamelessly, wanting to hear him say it again.

He shrugged. "You're not bad on the eyes."

"Well, thank you very much. You aren't either."

"I know."

Liz groaned aloud.

"Hey, are we going to share a hotel room on the drive?" He waggled his eyebrows outrageously.

"I think not."

"You are such a prude."

Liz enjoyed their banter, enjoyed these conversations in which they both gave as good as they got. "Perhaps I am, but you love me, anyway."

Sean chuckled. "Yes, I suppose I do."

> "People change and forget to tell each other."
>   —Lillian Hellman

CHAPTER

KAREN CURTIS

September 1st

I barely slept last night. Gwen had her secretary phone me Friday morning to ask for a meeting. When my agent calls, I'm there. Something inside me said she wanted to discuss my audition for the sitcom and I was right. The whole time I was driving into L.A.—and traffic was a bitch—I had this premonition that I'd gotten the role.

Any other time in the past four years I would've been *so* excited. But it wasn't excitement I felt. Instead, I experienced a crazy sort of letdown feeling. Get real! I mean, a television role is what I've wanted my entire life, what I've worked so hard to achieve, what I've sacrificed and struggled for.

By the time I found parking and made my way into

Gwen's office building, my stomach was full of knots. That was when it hit me. My head was telling me I should be jumping up and down for joy, and my body was telling me something completely different. It took me a while to connect with my feelings and realize that I didn't want the role.

I stopped in the rest room, washed my face with cold water and stared at myself in the mirror. I don't know what I expected to see because the face that stared back at me wasn't any different. Somehow, I felt it should be....

A weekly television show is the opportunity of a lifetime and worth thousands and thousands of dollars, in fees and residuals. I didn't understand what was happening to me or why I'd hesitate.

Then again, perhaps I did.

The last couple of weeks with the drama class at Willow Grove High School have been *fabulous*. I love the kids and I see so much of myself in them. Myself, ten years ago, that is. Creative, talented, passionate and totally in love with the idea of self-expression.

It's more than just teaching that I've enjoyed. Since I've been at the same school as Glen, we've eaten lunch together every day. I love being around him, love the way I feel, or more accurately the way he makes me feel. It's as if I'm the funniest, wittiest, most attractive woman in the world. No man has *ever* made me feel as special as he does.

I remember when we first met and how I wanted to

make sure he understood I was only interested in being his friend. No romance; I wanted fireworks. What I wanted—or thought I wanted—was a man just like me. Glen didn't seem passionate enough. Hard to believe I could have been that blind. Glen is so great. I really admire him. Not only is he brilliant, he's gentle and honorable and...I never thought I'd find this an attractive trait in a man, but he's humble. Yes, humble. We've gone out a couple of times since our movie date and both times I've been the one to suggest it. When I casually led up to the subject of getting together, he seemed genuinely surprised and pleased. Later, when I came right out and told him I'd welcome an invitation, it flustered him so much he asked me to chaperon one of the school dances with him. Then he decided that wasn't the kind of date I'd probably want and withdrew the invitation. It took me five minutes of teasing to make him believe I'd *love* to chaperon a dance with him. Any dance. Anywhere. Any day of the week. (Although I didn't mention that part.)

Well, to make a long story short, when I arrived at Gwen's office, her secretary ushered me into the inner sanctum where my agent awaited. All my worry was for naught. I didn't get the role. In fact, Gwen had viewed the audition tape herself and was disappointed in my performance. She suggested a series of classes for me. In other words I am no longer meeting her expectations. That was the reason she wanted to meet personally with me. I was being put on notice, so to speak.

I didn't sleep well on Friday, and now I'm afraid tonight's going to be an exact repeat.

* * *

The phone woke Karen out of a deep sleep. It took her a moment to realize the ringing wasn't actually part of her dream. Lying on her stomach, she stretched out her arm and groped blindly for the receiver. She opened her eyes just enough to glance at her clock radio and saw that it was just past 1:00 a.m. She hadn't even slept an hour and groaned at having her rest interrupted, especially when she'd had such a hard time falling asleep.

None of her friends would think twice about calling her any time, day or night. Okay, maybe not Glen, but then he was an exception to just about everything.

"This better be good," she muttered into the mouthpiece.

"Karen?" The timid voice was fragile and breathless.

"Victoria?" Instantly alert, Karen sat up, blinking rapidly. "Where are you?"

"Home—can you come and get me and Bryce?"

"Of course." Her response was automatic. Then it dawned on her that something must be terribly wrong if her sister was phoning her in the middle of the night, asking for a ride. "Are you all right?"

Victoria didn't answer.

"What happened? Tell me." Panic filled her throat.

"I might need you to take me to the hospital."

Karen was off the bed and pacing with the cordless phone in her hand. So this time Roger had gone too far. This time Victoria had had enough. She prayed her sister would press assault charges, prayed she'd leave him for good. "Where's Roger?"

"He's...asleep. Just hurry."

"I'll be there in fifteen minutes," she promised rashly.

Never in her life had Karen dressed faster. She pulled on sweats, then shoved her feet into tennis shoes without bothering to tie them. Not until she was in her car did she wonder why her sister hadn't simply left on her own. There was something Victoria hadn't told her.

Coming to a red light, Karen stopped and looked both ways; she didn't see any traffic in either direction. Unwilling to waste time waiting for the traffic signal to proceed through its cycle, she ran the light. Halfway through the intersection, she caught sight of a police car.

"Great, just great," she muttered. A heartbeat later, the patrol car was behind her, lights flashing.

Karen pulled over to the side of the deserted street and reached for her purse, extracting her driver's license even before the officer arrived.

As he approached her vehicle, Karen rolled down her window.

"Good evening," he said politely. "Did you happen to notice that the light at the intersection of Universal and Sixth was red?"

"Yes." She wasn't going to lie.

"So why the hurry?"

"My sister..." Karen started to explain, then realized this could be the most opportune event of her life. "Officer, listen, I realize I deserve a traffic ticket." She talked fast, hoping to get everything out without stopping to answer a lot of unnecessary questions. "I won't try to talk you out of giving it to me."

He raised his eyebrows. "This is a refreshing tactic."

"My sister just phoned me and...and I'm afraid her husband beat her again. She asked that I come and get her...."

Karen swallowed hard, knowing that if she involved the police she was going against her sister's wishes. Victoria wouldn't want her talking to the authorities. But she'd begged for help and this was the best way Karen knew to provide it.

"My brother-in-law is physically abusive," she continued, "and I don't know exactly what the situation is right now." Nor was she comfortable walking into circumstances that had the potential to be explosive. If Roger had no qualms about hitting his wife, he probably wouldn't hesitate to attack his sister-in-law. Especially a sister-in-law he considered an interfering bitch.

The young patrol officer asked her a few questions, returned to his vehicle for a moment and then walked back to her car. "The address you gave me is out of my area. A patrol car has been dispatched and will meet you there."

"Thank you." Karen was so grateful she felt like sobbing. "Can I leave now?"

He nodded, and gave her a written warning as well as a verbal one. She drove off immediately, careful to stay within the speed limit. She hoped she arrived at her sister's before the police did so she could explain to Victoria what she'd done and why. It'd taken tremendous courage for Victoria to call her, and Karen didn't want to destroy her fragile trust.

The outside lights were on when she turned into the driveway. As soon as she did, Victoria opened the front door. She held Bryce with her left arm, her right arm cradled against her side.

Karen leaped out of the car and hurried forward to help her sister and nephew.

"What happened to your arm?" Karen demanded.

"Daddy hit me real hard," Bryce sobbed, "then he pulled Mommy's arm."

So Roger had taken to hitting his son. Victoria had accepted the abuse for herself, but now that her husband had begun to hurt their child, she'd drawn the line.

"How bad is it?" Karen asked, wondering if she needed to get her sister to the hospital immediately.

"It doesn't matter. Let's go." Victoria's voice was edged with panic. "Please, it's all right."

"Mommy, Mommy?" Bryce started to cry louder.

"Everything will be fine, sweetheart." Victoria comforted him in soft tones. "Auntie Karen's here to take us to her house."

Karen ushered the two of them toward her car and was fastening Bryce's seat belt when she heard Roger's shout.

"What the hell do you think you're doing, bitch?"

"Go," Victoria cried.

"No." Karen turned to face her brother-in-law, who stood in the open doorway, his hands on his hips.

Swearing and clearly drunk, Roger stumbled down the steps and started toward his family. He was in a rage, his face red and twisted with anger. He stared at Karen, and then Victoria, who huddled protectively over her son in the back of Karen's vehicle.

"Stay out of this," he warned Karen.

"I wasn't going to say a word."

Her response apparently surprised him, because his gaze wavered from his wife and son to briefly clash with hers.

How dared he hurt her sister! How dared he strike a child! "You're a pitiful excuse for a man," she said contemptuously.

He swore again and lunged at her. Karen was quick on

her feet and managed to avoid his swing. Victoria screamed. Unfortunately, when Karen moved, she gave Roger access to his wife. Cursing, he reached inside the car and yanked on Victoria's arm.

Victoria let out a shrill cry of pain.

Hardly aware of what she was doing, Karen leaped onto Roger's back, pounding him with both fists. Everyone was shouting at once, Bryce was crying and Roger was bucking and heaving in an effort to throw Karen off.

Out of the corner of her eye, Karen saw the patrol car pull up to the curb and released her frantic hold on her brother-in-law. That gave him the slack he needed to strike out at her. She didn't see the punch coming until it was too late. He got her square in the jaw, hitting with enough force to knock her to the ground.

Almost immediately, the two police officers had Roger in a tight grasp. They dragged him away, toward their car. Roger's demeanor altered instantly.

"Officers," he said, sounding completely sober. "I'm glad you're here."

"Sure you are, Roger," Karen shouted back, although her jaw ached just from talking and she still felt so dizzy she thought she might faint.

While one officer spoke with him, the second approached Karen. "Can you tell me what's going on here?" he asked.

"My sister..." Karen pointed to Victoria, who climbed out of the car, holding Bryce against her left side.

"This is all my fault," Victoria sobbed.

"It *isn't* your fault!" Karen yelled, afraid that now, with the police involved, her sister would change her mind.

"I should never have called you," Victoria said.

Then they were talking at the same time, each one struggling to be heard over the other. Karen was trying to explain why the police were there, and Victoria kept insisting she was to blame. Roger was shouting, too.

"Who's married to whom here?" the older of the two officers asked.

It took several minutes to sort out the details. As she listened, Karen couldn't help thinking that her brother-in-law was the one who deserved a career on the stage. According to him, Karen was a meddlesome troublemaker intent on breaking up his marriage. He wanted to press charges against her for a malicious attack on his person. While it was true he'd struck out at her, he said, he'd only been defending himself. When he finished, he demanded that the police haul her away.

For one confused and crazy minute, that seemed about to happen. Then Victoria stepped forward.

"I...I phoned my sister..." she said in a small, hesitant voice.

"All right, all right," Roger said, staring at Victoria. "I'll be willing to drop the assault charges against your sister if you'll agree to put this...this incident behind us."

"You've got to be joking," Karen yelled.

Roger ignored her. "I'll admit I did get upset with my wife earlier and I probably overreacted." He turned to the officers, laughing as if it'd all been a misunderstanding that had gotten out of hand. He regretted his annoyance, he said; the last thing he wanted was to turn it into a federal case.

"I'm sorry, sweetheart," Roger said next, looking at Victoria again and sounding eminently reasonable. "I really do regret this. There's no need to get the police involved in a family matter, is there? You don't want this, and neither do I."

Victoria bit her lower lip, her eyes cast down. She actually seemed to be considering his words.

Karen didn't know what she'd say or do if her sister decided to go back to this bastard. She noticed that the neighbors' houses were now blazing with light. Great—an audience.

"I'm sorry, too," Victoria whispered.

Roger relaxed and glanced toward the police officers again. "A man works hard all week. Is it too much to ask that his wife have his dinner ready when he gets back from a Saturday golf game with clients?" He made a good-natured question out of it, but Karen heard the censure. In his view, this *was* all Victoria's fault.

"I'm sorry," Victoria repeated, her voice stronger and more confident now.

"I know you are," Roger said in cajoling tones. "Why don't we let these people go about their business and get back inside? Come on, sweetheart."

Karen thought she was going to be sick.

"I'm so sorry it's come to this," her sister continued. She turned to face the two police officers. "I'll be pressing abuse charges against my husband. I believe my shoulder's been dislocated. This isn't the first time he's hit me—doctor's records will confirm a number of recent visits in which I've been treated for so-called accidents."

Roger's anger exploded and he started toward his wife, fists clenched, but the police restrained him. Within minutes, he was in handcuffs and in the back of the patrol car.

Victoria sobbed and Karen gently placed both arms around her sister, offering what comfort she could. At the same time, she held tightly onto Bryce. He didn't understand what was happening or why. He clung to his mother and buried his face in her stomach, not wanting to look.

It was dawn before Victoria was released from the hospital emergency room, where her shoulder had been reset, and a police report filed. Not long after that, Karen brought their parents fully into the picture. Victoria, along with Bryce, moved back into the family home that day, and Vernon Curtis made immediate arrangements to collect their clothing and personal belongings. He also provided Victoria with an attorney whose name Karen recognised—Lillian Case. Their father had always been a practical man, Karen thought now, something his daughters had never valued enough.

At noon, an exhausted Karen prepared to return to her own apartment. She'd been a heroine in her family's eyes, and she basked in their love and approval. Before she left, Victoria hugged her and with tears in her eyes thanked her sister.

But the one with real courage had been Victoria. Roger was a formidable enemy, but his reign of terror had finally come to an end. Karen would relish sitting in the courtroom when her brother-in-law faced a judge.

She didn't wake until nearly six that afternoon. She sat up, stretched her arms luxuriously and reached for the telephone. Although she'd never called Glen, she knew his number by heart.

He sounded preoccupied when he answered.

"It's Karen."

"Karen...hello."

The joyful surprise in his voice warmed her from the inside out. "You doing anything important?" she asked.

"Not a thing."

"I thought I'd invite you to dinner."

"Sure. What night?"

"How about tonight?" she asked, smiling as she spoke. "It's a celebration."

"What time? And what are we celebrating?"

"A job."

"You got the part in that sitcom?" he asked.

"No, they turned me down flat." She felt such rightness about all of this. "Actually, it's a little premature to celebrate, but I'm fairly confident the position of drama teacher is still open."

"It was the last I heard," Glen assured her. "Are you applying?"

"I do believe I am."

Her announcement was met with a shocked silence. "Are you *sure* about this?"

"Yes," she told him. "I'm very sure."

All her life, Karen had known what she wanted; she hadn't known nearly as well what she *needed*. Only now was she beginning to understand the difference.

May the road rise up to meet you, may the wind always be at your back.

—Irish toast

CHAPTER

LIZ KENYON

September 7th

In a moment of weakness I allowed Sean to talk me into coming along on this driving vacation. Afterward, I had some reservations, but I have to admit, I'm enjoying his company. We left early this morning. I had our route all planned. The first night I thought we'd stay in Flagstaff. We could drive farther, but I wanted to have plenty of time for stops and sightseeing.

One day on the road, and all my careful calculations went down the drain. We're in Las Vegas. Sean's idea, naturally. I'd been here once before, years ago, with Steve. Has this town changed! We're staying at the New York, New York. As soon as we checked in, I went to the video poker machines and Sean headed for the blackjack tables. I didn't see him again until dinnertime. He got us tickets to see Lance Burton's magic show, and we didn't call it a night until after one. Tomorrow we hit the road again. I almost hate to leave.

September 13th

I meant to document every day of the trip, but by the time I get to bed, I'm too exhausted to write. Sean and I ended up spending two nights in Vegas. We'll probably stop there on the way back, too, if time allows. Naturally it depends on our route. I asked him about visiting his daughter, and as best I can determine, he hasn't made contact with her. It's hard to keep my opinions to myself, but on the subject of his ex-wife and daughter, I'm doing exactly that.

Those two nights in Vegas were a wonderful start to this vacation. It's like an amusement park for adults. I came away a hundred dollars richer and Sean isn't saying, which leads me to believe he lost at the blackjack tables. We sat and played slot machines for a couple of hours during our last night there, laughing and joking with each other. The mood was light, energetic, *fun*. It's very easy to love this man. Far too easy.

The third night, we stayed in Amarillo, Texas, which made for a long day on the road. I was anxious to get to Amy and Jack's, and Sean seemed to realize that, pushing ahead. We arrived in Tulsa by nightfall. Amy had dinner waiting for us. She'd also prepared *two* guest rooms, one of them the den with pull-out couch. Sean offered to take that—an offer I accepted.

Andrew and Annie were all over Sean, and he's just great with kids. Both my grandchildren think he's wonderful and so does Amy. In fact, the four of them are getting along famously.

Yesterday afternoon Jack took Sean to play golf, which both deemed a success.

Amy and Jack have adjusted well to the move. Jack got a big promotion with the shipping company and enjoys his job at corporate headquarters. Amy loves being an at-home mom and is grateful for the opportunity.

Our second day in Tulsa, Annie wanted to have a tea party the way we used to when she lived in California, so we did. Sean was invited, too. I wonder if he realizes what an honor that was.

September 17th

Sean phoned his daughter this afternoon. He'd been putting it off and I know it's been on his mind since before we left. Amy and I sat on the patio with the children while he used the phone in the den. He didn't come out for at least twenty minutes, and the instant I saw his smile I knew the conversation had gone well.

After talking to Eileen, he was eager to head for Seattle, which we'll do first thing tomorrow morning. I've so enjoyed this time with my daughter and her family, but it's been a week now and that's long enough. They need to return to their everyday work and school routines.

Sean never did tell me what caused the estrangement between him and his daughter. Nor has he mentioned what caused his divorce—other than "fickleness" on his wife's part. What does that mean?

An affair? It's not that I want to hear all the ugly details. It's a matter of trust. I want him to trust me enough to share his past, and I don't know if that's possible for him or not.

September 20th

We arrived in Seattle and the city is just as beautiful as I'd expected. I met Eileen, Sean's daughter, her husband, Ron, and their four-year-old daughter, Emily. The meeting was a bit strained at first.

Eileen looks a lot like Sean, but any resemblance stops there. She's quiet and soft-spoken and delicate. Her husband works for Boeing and is currently putting in a lot of overtime. He's not around much.

Wanting to give Sean as much time as possible with his daughter, I've gotten acquainted with Emily. She's a delightful child.

This evening, as we were driving back to the hotel, Sean finally told me about his divorce. His ex-wife had been involved in an affair with his former business partner—more or less what I'd suspected. As is often the case, Sean was the last to know. The divorce was messy, and because his daughter was in high school, Sean felt Eileen would be better off with her mother. The problem was that she wanted to live with Sean and he turned her down. Eileen was crushed by what she saw as his rejection and afterward refused to speak to him. Apparently his daughter's hurt and disappointment was fueled by her mother. Sean told me his ex has been married and divorced twice in the last ten years.

Sean admitted he'd played a role in the estrangement, though. When Eileen refused to answer his phone calls and letters, he gave up trying to communicate with her. He couldn't force her to let him into her life, or so he reasoned. He kept track of her from a distance, but rather than face continual rejection from the one person he truly loved, he buried himself in his work. It was during this period that he helped establish Little Lambs. Still, he sees now that he should have persisted in trying to stay in touch. He particularly regrets missing her wedding and the birth of his granddaughter.

After our talk, we walked along the Seattle waterfront to the hotel. I feel that the bond between us has grown. There's trust and commitment now. I'm happy, happier than I've been since Steve died.

While Sean was in his room changing for dinner, I stood on my balcony, which overlooks Puget Sound, and watched the sun set over the Olympic Mountains. This has been one of the best vacations of my life.

> "The excursion is the same when you go looking for your sorrow as when you go looking for your joy."
>
> —Eudora Welty

CHAPTER

CLARE CRAIG

October 22nd

I've been spending a lot of time at the hospital with Michael, doing what I can, which seems damn little at this point. The boys are here, too, as much as possible, although it's difficult for them to see their father like this. I'm proud of them. It isn't easy to watch your parent die and they're handling this with an inner strength I didn't know they possessed.

Mick and Alex both decided to take the first semester off from college; they didn't want to leave their father, knowing that Michael's time is very short now.

Because of the drugs, Michael's out of it most days,

but every now and then, the fog clears and he's aware of who's with him and what's happening.

This evening was one of those times. He's so weak now. The fight is gone and with it the will to live. I always thought that when death came, it would be as "a thief in the night," stealing away what is most precious. I thought death would be resisted to the final moment, the final gasp. It's not true. Michael has accepted his death.

In those few moments of clarity, Michael told me he doesn't fear it anymore. After everything he's endured, the pain of liver cancer, the treatment, followed by the riptide of hope and despair—after all that, dealing with death seems almost easy.

We laughed about that. Until tonight I could never imagine laughing about death. But it was either laugh or cry, and I knew Michael needed the laughter more than my tears. Then he did the most unexpected thing.

He reached for my hand and without a word of explanation whispered that he was sorry.

He didn't need to elaborate. I knew what he was saying. He was sorry for the affair, sorry for the divorce, sorry for the grief he'd heaped upon me.

I remember when he first told me he was moving out. The shock of his falling in love with Miranda had left me speechless. I was stunned and bewildered long before I felt the pain of his betrayal. Perhaps that should have told me something. I remember that, as he was packing, he claimed I didn't need him and Miranda did. At the time that incensed me. Of all the ridiculous things to say! If he wanted a clinging, insecure little girlfriend instead of a grown-up wife, then he was welcome to her.

Only now do I truly understand what he meant. It wasn't that I didn't need him, because I did in all the ways that mattered. It was that I didn't let him know it. I didn't let him know I enjoyed his company and valued his opinion. I'd slipped into the habit of making all the important decisions when it came to our family. I was the one who handled the finances, dealt with our sons, the house and just about everything else. Without knowing what I'd done, I stripped Michael of his pride.

I'm not justifying the affair, but I'm admitting I played a role in what led up to it. It's easy to excuse Miranda. She was young, vulnerable and grieving her father's death. Because of that, she confused dependence with love and latched onto Michael.

As Michael coped with the cancer, he seemed to need forgiveness. He's talked to the boys, talked it all out with them, but not me. Not until tonight.

I forgave him, and then I asked him to forgive me. He held my hand, nodded briefly and turned his head away, but not before I saw the tears. I would have said more, but I was crying, too.

Death is approaching. I can feel it now, sense it. Everything inside me is screaming that it's too soon and Michael is far too young to die. But if he can welcome death, surrender to it, can I do less?

Who would have thought the end would come like this? I've hated Michael, and I've loved him. Now as death grows closer, I've discovered that my love is stronger than my hate

* * *

"Mom." Alex gently tapped her shoulder and Clare started, unaware she'd fallen asleep.

As she'd sat vigil at Michael's bedside, she'd drifted off. Her sons stood on the other side of the raised bed, looking at her, their eyes filled with dread and pain.

"Dad's breathing has slowed," Mick told her.

Clare chewed on her lower lip. This was exactly what they'd been told would happen. Michael was in the final stages of the disease and had, several days earlier, quietly slipped into a coma.

Her pulse racing, Clare glanced at the heart monitor and watched the irregular beat of his heart. She reached for Michael's hand, holding it firmly between her own as his body released its life.

"No..." Alex sobbed, his agony nearly undoing Clare's forced calm.

Then there was nothing. A beat. One solitary beat, followed by a flat line. A nurse stepped into the room and stood with them, noting the time of death on a chart.

This was it? The end? Somehow Clare had expected there to be more as Michael Craig moved serenely from life to death. Then the reality of it suddenly overwhelmed her and with it came a flood of pain, the current so strong it threatened to pull her under, to consume her. Alex broke down and crumpled into the chair, his shoulders racked with sobs. Mick stood tall and silent. Clare wanted to reach out to both her children, but was lost in her own agony.

"We will always love you." She choked out the words and leaned down to kiss Michael's forehead. Kiss him goodbye.

"It's over," Mick announced as though this was the end when in some ways it was only the beginning.

Clare nodded and walked around to the other side of the bed. Her two sons hugged her, the three of them forming a tight circle. The same circle they'd formed the afternoon Michael had moved out of the family home. Only this time Michael was gone forever.

The funeral took place two days later, and the service was crowded with people from the business community, family and friends. The *Willow Grove Independent* ran a full-column obituary and the dealership closed for the day. Clare hosted the wake at her house.

Liz, Karen and Julia were all there, helping with the setup, seeing to the guests and lending Clare their love and support. She would never have asked them to help, but was grateful her dearest friends could be with her.

It was evening before the last of the relatives and business associates had left. Mick and Alex were in the living room talking with Karen and Julia when Clare sat down in the kitchen.

"It's about time you took a rest," Liz said, joining her. "How are you holding up?"

Rather than answer, Clare simply nodded.

"It hurts, doesn't it?"

"More than I ever thought it could," Clare whispered. "We were divorced. I assumed I'd done my grieving.... I didn't have a clue."

"I don't think anyone really does."

Clare looked away. She wasn't a woman who easily shed tears, but after a day in which she'd held back all the pain, she could no longer restrain her emotion. "I accepted a long time ago that Michael was dying," she said. "I was prepared—as prepared as anyone can be. Yet when he died, I felt as though someone had shot me in the gut."

Liz nodded, and they sat across from each other, their hands wrapped around coffee mugs.

"I remember when the police officer came to tell me Steve was gone. I heard the words, saw his mouth move and understood what he was saying, but I couldn't take it in. I just couldn't absorb it."

They were quiet for several moments, and Clare suspected her friend was dealing with the impact of her own memories.

"I'll say one thing for Michael. He was full of surprises right to the end," she murmured after a while.

"How do you mean?" Liz asked.

"Our attorney told me Michael altered his will during the last month of his life. He left the dealership to me." She almost smiled. As part of the divorce settlement, Michael had been required to buy out her half of the enterprise. And now...he'd given it back.

"He didn't leave it to the boys?"

"No," Clare said, still amazed. "He didn't give Fred any explanation, but I know what he was thinking. Mick and Alex have no interest in selling cars. Their talents and desires lie in other areas. Being stuck with Craig Chevrolet would be nothing but a burden. It's just not a career either of them wants."

"They could always sell it," Liz suggested.

Clare knew that was exactly what *wouldn't* have happened. Michael feared the boys would keep it out of a sense of obligation and misplaced loyalty. Despite their feelings, they would've held onto it in an effort to honor their father's memory.

"You love the car business."

Clare nodded. "Yes, and I'll make a success of it."

"You already have," Liz reminded her.

All Clare had done was pick up the pieces. Yes, she'd worked long hours, but she'd thrived on the challenge, just as Michael had known she would.

"How are Mick and Alex holding up?"

Clare wasn't sure how to answer. Like her, they'd thought they were prepared for Michael's death, but it had shaken them more than they'd expected.

"They're dealing with it, but they'll need time." As would Clare. She would go on, struggle forward and find her way through this grief, the same as her children.

"How about another cup of coffee?" Liz asked. "I made a fresh pot. Seems a shame to let it go to waste."

Although she'd had enough coffee, Clare felt the need for company. She didn't feel a need to talk, she realized; she just wanted someone to sit with her. Suddenly the thought of being alone seemed terrifying.

Liz poured their coffee and sat down at the table.

Clare tried to speak and couldn't. Then Liz, who seemed to read the agony in her heart, reached across the table and touched her arm. Clare tried to hold back the tears, but it was too hard. She hurt too much.

"Go ahead," Liz said softly. "You don't have to be strong anymore. Let it go."

Clare broke into sobs and felt the comforting arms of her friend around her.

"May the hinges of friendship never grow rusty."
—Unknown

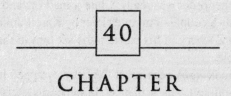

CHAPTER

THURSDAY MORNING BREAKFAST CLUB

It was barely November, and already Christmas decorations were up. Clare pulled into the strip mall where Mocha Moments was located, noting that Liz Kenyon's Seville was parked out front. Knowing her friend, Clare suspected Liz had ordered her croissant and coffee, and had their window table secured.

The air was cool and damp this morning, with a breeze coming in from the Pacific, but Clare didn't mind. The Santa Ana winds had dried out the valley these past few months, and the moisture was a refreshing change.

Clare entered the coffee shop, waving to Liz, and read over the menu, although she always ordered the same thing. When the group had first started meeting, her double-shot espresso, bitter and strong, had matched her mood.

"Espresso and currant scone, right?" the young man behind the counter said, obviously proud of his memory.

"Normally yes, but I'm in the mood for something different this morning."

The teenager's face showed surprise.

"I'll have a pecan roll and coffee," she told him, deciding quickly. It was time for a change.

"Coming right up," he said, bouncing back with a cheerful smile.

When her order was ready, Clare joined Liz and was followed only a couple of minutes later by Karen. Julia arrived last, with Zachary in his carrier; she set him in the middle of the table.

They took turns peeking at the baby, wrapped in his exquisite hand-knit, yellow blanket. In some ways, this precious little boy belonged to the entire Thursday morning group. Like the other women, Clare had invested a great deal of emotion in Zachary. The infant's successful struggle for life brought balance to the loss she had so recently suffered. She was thrilled to see that he was thriving.

"It's almost time for us to come up with another word for the year," Liz said once they'd all sat down with their orders. "For next year, I mean."

"Already?" Clare protested. "You're as bad as these mall people putting up Christmas decorations before Thanksgiving."

"What are we supposed to do with the word from this year?" Karen asked.

"What was your word?" With so much on her mind, Clare had forgotten.

"Acceptance," Karen told her.

"Did you learn anything from it?" This came from Liz.

Karen took a sip of her peppermint-flavored latte and mulled over the question. "Yes, I think I have. A year ago, I was constantly arguing with my mother over which direction I should take. I was so sure I knew what was right for me. *She* thought I should be a teacher. Go figure." Karen made a mocking face. "Then there was Victoria." She paused, apparently thinking it all out. "When I chose *acceptance,* I wanted my mother to accept me for who I am. I wanted her to appreciate me."

"She apparently knows you better than you know yourself."

Karen nodded. "I never realized how much I'd enjoy a classroom, but I'm loving every minute of it. My mother has her annoying little habits, but then we all do. She only wants what's best for me and for Victoria."

Clare exchanged a look with Liz. This was Karen speaking? Wow, what a difference in less than a year!

"Over the last few months, I've learned that I needed to accept myself first. I wanted Mom to be proud of me, the way she was of my sister. At the same time, I resisted that feeling and tried to be as different from Victoria as possible."

"I don't know what Victoria would have done without you," Liz said.

Karen dismissed the praise and seemed almost embarrassed by it. "She's my sister."

"Get back to your word," Julia urged. "I want to know what you learned."

"What I learned," Karen repeated slowly. "Okay. I thought I wanted to act, to work in theater and film, and I do, but I don't need to look for my self-worth in a credit scrolling down some screen. I've discovered something better."

"Teaching high-school drama classes," Julia supplied.

"No," Karen teased, "regular meals."

They all laughed.

"Being on stage is great fun, but sharing my love of the stage with others is even more compelling."

"That's great." Clare was genuinely pleased for her.

"What's the latest on your sister?" Liz asked.

"Ah, yes," Karen said, frowning. "As you already know, Roger's serving a six-month jail term. Victoria's seeing a counselor and with the help of my parents and Roger's, she's back in her own home. She loves her job selling commercial real estate, and seems to have a real knack for it. Mom and I are both confident that she's going to be just fine."

"What about Bryce?" Julia asked.

"He's in a day care facility three days a week and my mother takes him on Monday and Fridays."

"Sounds like an excellent solution," Liz said.

"Is Victoria going to file for divorce?" Clare wanted to know.

"I don't think she's decided yet," Karen said. "She'd prefer not to go the divorce route, but she might not have any option. Naturally, the twit is saying all the right things—he would, with his job on the line—but Victoria needs proof that he's changed first. They'll continue living apart while Roger proves himself."

"I'd hate to see a repeat of the abuse."

"Victoria's being very careful. She's taking it nice and slow, and not making any major decisions until she's had time to work everything through with her counselor."

"Good for her," Liz said.

Karen heaved a sigh. "There's something else about *acceptance*. Glen and I are seriously discussing marriage."

"He proposed?" Julia cried excitedly.

"Well...yes."

"And you've accepted," Clare finished for her. Making the connection.

Karen's face beamed with happiness and she nodded. "He's perfect for me. It's amazing how well we balance each other. Oh guys, I'm so in love."

"That's the way it's supposed to be," Liz said. "When's the wedding?"

"May," Karen informed them. "I already have my new word. *Bride.*"

Clare exchanged smiles with Liz. It wouldn't surprise her if next year Liz announced that she was marrying Dr. Jamison.

"What was your word again, Liz?" Clare asked,

"Time," Liz reminded them. "Last January I hit a real low point in my life."

Clare remembered how lost Liz had been without her family around her.

"It seemed as if all the good years had somehow slipped through my fingers. I felt as though time was disappearing and taking with it everything I'd wanted to accomplish and never would." She frowned. "I suppose I was afraid of living the rest of my life alone. It was bad enough when I lost Steve, but then without the children around me, the loneliness seemed so much worse."

Clare would soon face that herself when both Mick and Alex left for college. The thought of coming home to an empty house every night filled her with dread, and yet the boys were so seldom there that in practical terms it woudn't make much difference.

"Do you still feel lonely?" Julia asked.

"No." Liz's look was thoughtful. *"Time* is still a good word for me, but not for the reasons I assumed. This is *my time.* In the last twelve months, I've learned to relax and enjoy every single minute."

"You forgot to mention that it's also your time to fall in love."

Liz smiled. "Falling in love," she echoed. "I feel like I'm in high school again. Silly, isn't it?"

"No," Julia insisted with a wistful sigh of her own. "I think it's wonderful."

"And so unexpected," Liz added. "I always said I didn't need a man in my life and I don't."

"But it's certainly a bonus," Karen piped up.

"I think what stands out the most for me," Liz said with a glimmer of amusement, "is that it takes a hell of a man to replace no man."

"What?" Karen asked, frowning. "I don't get it."

"I do," Clare said.

"A hell of a man to replace no man," Karen repeated thoughtfully, then slowly nodded. "I understand now. You discovered that you liked your life, and Dr. Jamison sort of complements the...the *serenity* you found all on your own."

"I couldn't have said it better myself," Liz agreed.

"Well, I've discovered I like my life, too," Karen said, happiness shining in her eyes. "Who would've believed I'd marry a man my mother approved of? Certainly not me, and Mom's wild about Glen. She thinks he's the best thing that ever happened to me. Which he is."

"What about you, Clare?" Liz asked. "What was your word for the year?"

Talk about ironies. *"Faithful,"* she reminded her friends. "I chose it in anger on New Year's Day. At the time, I was trapped in bitterness. I remember thinking *I* was the one who'd always been faithful—to Michael, to our family and to myself."

"You *were* faithful—right to the very end." Julia's voice was so quiet, the others had to strain to hear.

"Yes," Clare replied, "but not in the way I'd anticipated."

"I can't tell you how much I admire what you did for Michael," Liz told her.

Clare looked away, embarrassed by the praise. A year ago she would've laughed in the face of anyone who dared to suggest she'd bring Michael back into the family home. Yet she had. She'd nursed him, loved him and together with her sons, she'd buried him.

"I did learn a valuable lesson this year," Clare said, struggling to keep the emotion out of her voice.

"What was that?" Liz asked.

She wasn't sure she could adequately put her thoughts into words. "I hated Michael for what he'd done to me and the boys. I mean, I *really* hated him. I didn't dare let any of you know how intense my anger with him was for fear you'd think I should be locked away."

Her friends silently studied her and Clare had the feeling that her confession hadn't come as any big shock. They knew and had always known.

"And I loved him," she said. "Deeply and totally. Despite everything. In the end I forgave him—and I forgave myself. In ways I thought were impossible, I *was* faithful—to both of us. To what we'd been and…and to the people we really were." Flustered, she waved her hand and looked away. "I'm not expressing myself very well."

"Yes, you are," Liz countered, reaching for her hand and briefly squeezing it. "You're making perfect sense."

Clare laughed, the sound deep and throaty, and the noise startled Zachary awake. Julia deftly dealt with her son, bringing him into her arms.

"I had an epiphany of my own this last year. My word was *gratitude* but it should have been *surprise!*"

They all laughed again, garnering interest from the people who sat around them.

"I remember the day you told us you were pregnant," Karen said, grinning down at Zachary who looked back at her with big beautiful blue eyes.

"A baby at this time of my life. Oh, pleasssse, say it isn't so."

The laughter rang out again.

"Our family's working as a team now," Julia said. "I'm amazed at Adam and Zoe and how unselfish they've become for Zack. What an incredible blessing he's been."

He gurgled as though to add his own comment.

"The last few months have been hectic," she continued. "It isn't easy having a newborn in the house, especially a preemie who needs a lot of extra care. Starting over with another child is a challenge, I'll grant you that—but I wouldn't change a thing."

"You said you had an epiphany?"

"Basically that's it," Julia said. "I realized that I *can* have it all. The big beautiful home, the husband and family, plus the career. Just not at the same time. I will return to my shop, but not until it's right for Zack."

"That is so wise," Karen said, as though in awe.

"You'd be surprised how smart we all are," Clare said, "you included." She wanted Karen to realize her contribution to the group.

So here they were, the four of them, each at a different place in her life. They could laugh together and cry together and often did, sometimes both at once. To everything there is a season, and these were the seasons of their lives.

Four women, all friends, who met every Thursday morning at eight.

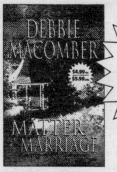
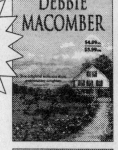

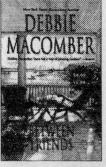

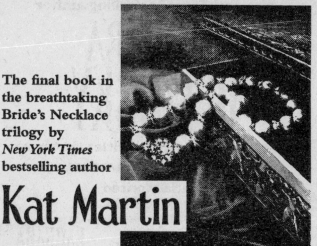

The final book in the breathtaking Bride's Necklace trilogy by *New York Times* bestselling author

Kat Martin

Trying to win back the trust of his jilted love, Rafael, Duke of Sheffield, presents her with a stunning necklace rumored to hold great power. As much as Dani wants to believe it can right the wrongs of the past, she fears there is one truth it cannot conceal, a truth that could cost her this second chance with Rafe, the only man she has ever loved....

The Handmaiden's Necklace

"Kat Martin is one of the best authors around! She has an incredible gift for writing."
—*Literary Times*

Available the first week of January 2006 wherever paperbacks are sold!

www.MIRABooks.com

MKM2207

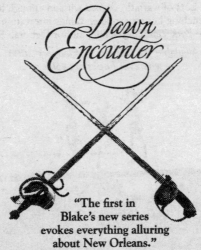

LUANNE JONES

"No better than a pack of heathens." That's what their grandmother called Charma Deane, Bess and Minnie, three cousins growing up in rural Orla, Arkansas. To them, nothing could be better than being a heathen girl. But when Charma Deane is betrayed several times by her cousin Bess, she leaves Orla.

Now, years after leaving the "Aunt Farm" behind, Charma Deane's back to make peace with the past and repair the strained ties with Bess, and they remind each other of their old vow: live without limits, love without question, laugh without apologies and make sure that whoever dies first won't be sent to heaven looking like hell.

Heathen Girls

"Reading Luanne Jones is like an afternoon with a best friend. Lots of warmth, wicked wit and enough heart-wrenching honesty to keep things interesting."
—*New York Times* bestselling author Deborah Smith

Available the first week of January 2006
wherever books are sold!

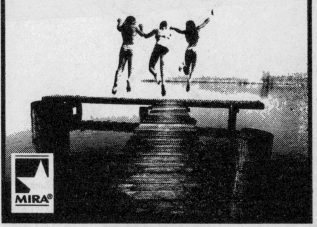

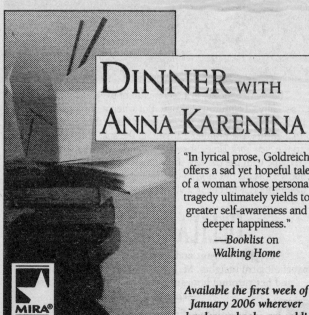

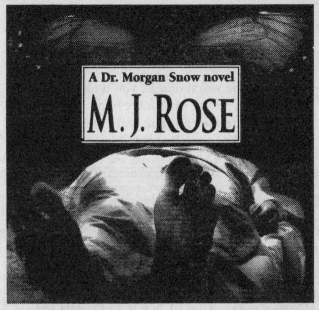